W9-AAA-779

THE HUMAN NERVOUS SYSTEM
Basic Principles of Neurobiology

THE HUMAN NERVOUS SYSTEM
BASIC PRINCIPLES OF NEUROBIOLOGY
THIRD EDITION

Text by **Charles R. Noback, Ph.D.**
Department of Anatomy
College of Physicians and Surgeons
Columbia University

Illustrated by **Robert J. Demarest**
Director of Medical Illustration
College of Physicians and Surgeons
Columbia University

McGRAW-HILL BOOK COMPANY
New York St. Louis San Francisco Auckland Bogotá Hamburg
Johannesburg London Madrid Mexico Montreal New Delhi
Panama Paris São Paulo Singapore Sydney Tokyo Toronto

NOTICE

Medicine is an ever-changing science. As new research and clinical experience broaden our knowledge, changes in treatment and drug therapy are required. The editors and the publisher of this work have made every effort to ensure that the drug dosage schedules herein are accurate and in accord with the standards accepted at the time of publication. Readers are advised, however, to check the product information sheet included in the package of each drug they plan to administer to be certain that changes have not been made in the recommended dose or in the contraindications for administration. This recommendation is of particular importance in regard to new or infrequently used drugs.

THE HUMAN NERVOUS SYSTEM
Basic Principles of Neurobiology

Copyright © 1981, 1975, 1967 by McGraw-Hill, Inc. All rights reserved. Printed in the United States of America. No part of this publication may be reproduced, stored in a retrieval system, or transmitted, in any form or by any means, electronic, mechanical, photocopying, recording, or otherwise, without the prior written permission of the publisher.

1234567890   VHVH   89876543210

This book was set in Aster by Progressive Typographers.
The editors were Richard W. Mixter and John J. Fitzpatrick;
the designer was Charles A. Carson;
the production supervisor was Robert A. Pirrung.
Von Hoffmann Press, Inc., was printer and binder.

Library of Congress Cataloging in Publication Data

Noback, Charles Robert, date
    The human nervous system.

    Includes bibliographies and index.
    1. Neurobiology. I. Demarest, Robert J.
II. Title. [DNLM: 1. Nervous system—Physiology.
2. Nervous system—Anatomy and histology.   WL101 N744h]
QP361.N58   1981   612'.8   80-10285
ISBN 0-07-046851-6

WL
101
N 744h
1981

To Eleanor and Alice

3 0001 00003 7772

64790

CONTENTS

PREFACE

The third edition is the culmination of the efforts of a neuroanatomist and a medical illustrator to incorporate many of the recent advances in basic neuroanatomy and neurobiology into the format of the first two editions. Special attention has been directed to the organization of a concise account with illustrations of the subject matter. Thus the information contained in the current sustained, explosive expansion of the neurobiologic literature cannot be presented comprehensively. New drawings illustrate many recent findings and modern concepts. An atlas of Weigert-stained sections of the human brain in several planes has been added. For the photographs of the brain and the transverse sections of the brainstem, we are indebted to Dr. Howard A. Matzke of the University of Kansas Medical Center and Dr. Joyce E. Shriver of the Mount Sinai School of Medicine. For the CAT scan of the brain we thank Dr. Sadek K. Hilal of the Neurological Institute of New York.

Only a sampling of the articles of the thousands of investigators whose research has contributed important information and concepts to neurobiology is included in the bibliographies accompanying each chapter. The cited literature has been selected to comprise handbooks, monographs, reviews, and general sources in addition to some original research contributions. Many of the references contain informative articles on topics discussed in other chapters in addition to the one in which each is listed. Many of the books noted in Chapter 1 contain comprehensive bibliographies. Valuable sources with articles on recent advances in a broad spectrum of subjects are *The Neurosciences—Study Programs* (1967, 1970, 1974, and 1978), *Neurosciences Research Program Bulletin* (1966 to date), *Annual Reviews of Neurosciences* (1978 to date), and *Trends in Neurosciences* (1978 to date).

For their valuable suggestions, we wish to thank Drs. Norman L. Strominger, James P. Kelly, Judith-Ann Silverman, Gary Pickard, Dominick P. Purpura, and F. Hermann Rudenberg and Mr. Donald Wong.

For their patience and constructive efforts toward the realization of this book, we are appreciative of the editorial staff and others of the McGraw-Hill Book Company, especially Mr. John Fitzpatrick.

Charles R. Noback
Robert J. Demarest

ON TERMINOLOGY

The long axis through the brain and spinal cord is called the *neuraxis*. It takes the form of a T, the vertical axis being a line passing through the entire spinal cord and brainstem (medulla, pons, and midbrain) and the horizontal axis being a line extending from the frontal pole to the occipital pole of the cerebrum (see Chap. 1, Fig. 1-19). In essence, the cerebral axis is oriented at a right angle to the long axis of the brainstem–spinal cord axis. The bend in the axis occurs at the junction of the midbrain and the diencephalon (Chap. 1).

The term *rostral* ("toward the beak") means in the direction of the cerebrum. *Caudal* means in the direction of the coccygeal region. These terms are used in relation to the neuraxis, not the body. In this usage, the cerebrum is rostral to the brainstem and the frontal pole of the cerebrum is rostral to the diencephalon.

Coronal sections are those cut at right angles to the neuraxis; thus a coronal section of the cerebrum is at right angles to a coronal section of the brainstem or spinal cord. *Horizontal sections* are those cut parallel to the neuraxis. Horizontal sections through the cerebrum are cut from the frontal pole to the occipital pole, parallel to a plane passing through both eyes. Horizontal sections through the brainstem and spinal cord are cut rostrocaudally parallel to the front and back of the neuraxis. A *sagittal section* is cut in a vertical plane along the midline; it divides the central nervous system into two symmetric right and left halves. Midsagittal is sometimes used for sagittal. Parasagittal sections, then, are also in the vertical plane but lateral to the sagittal section.

Within the central nervous system, a group or column of cell bodies and dendrites of neurons is variously known as a *nucleus, ganglion, lamina, body, cortex*, or *center*. *Afferent* (or *-petal*, as in centripetal) refers to bringing to or into a structure such as a nucleus; afferent is often used for sensory but not necessarily conscious sensations. *Efferent* (or *-fugal*, as in centrifugal) refers to going away from a structure such as a nucleus; efferent is often used for motor.

Bundles of nerve fibers in the central nervous system which are characterized by anatomic or functional criteria are called by such terms as *tract, fasciculus, brachium, peduncle, column, lemniscus, commissure, ansa*, or *capsule*. A *commissure* is a bundle of fibers crossing the midline at right angle to the neuraxis, often interconnecting similar structures on each side. A *decussation* refers to fibers crossing the midline either at right angles or obliquely. *Contralateral* refers to the opposite side; it is used primarily to indicate, for example, that pain is lost or paralysis occurs on the side opposite to that of the lesion. *Ipsilateral* refers to the same side; it is used primarily to indicate, for example, that pain is lost or paralysis occurs on the same side as that of the lesion.

A *modality* refers to the quality of a stimulus and the resulting forms of sensation (e.g., touch, pain, sounds, vision). Some pathways (tracts, nuclei, or areas of cortex) are *somatotopically* (*topographically*) organized; specific portions of these structures are associated with restricted regions of the body. For example, (1) fibers conveying position sense from the hand are in definite locations within the posterior columns (ascending sensory pathway), and (2) certain areas of the motor cortex regulate movements of the thumb. Some structures of the visual pathways are topographically related to specific regions within the retina (retinotopic organization), and similarly some structures of the auditory pathways are organized functionally with respect to different frequencies or tones (tonotopic organization).

CHAPTER ONE

THE BRAIN: GROSS ANATOMY, BLOOD SUPPLY, AND MENINGES

The average adult brain weighs about 1400 g (3 lb), or approximately 2 percent of the total body weight. This semisolid, pinkish gray organ is invested by a succession of three membranes called *meninges* and is protected by an outer rigid capsule, the bony skull. The meninges are, from the brain outward, the *pia mater, arachnoid,* and *dura mater* (see Figs. 1-37 and 1-38). The brain floats in a fluid; this *cerebrospinal fluid* (*CSF*) supports the soft delicate brain and acts as a shock absorber against external blows to the head. The CSF is located within the subarachnoid space (between the pia mater and the arachnoid) and within the ventricular cavities deep in the brain (see Figs. 1-17 and 1-18). The major arteries and veins which supply the brain are associated with the meninges.

The brain has a gelatinous consistency because its soft nervous tissues are held together and supported by only a meager connective tissue matrix. Because of the paucity of connective tissue, brain tissue cannot be sutured. As a result, neurosurgeons generally use an aspirator instead of a scalpel to excise pieces of damaged brain tissue, and an electric cautery or inert silver clips instead of surgical sutures to control bleeding.

Neurosurgery may be performed under local anesthesia, in part, because the brain is insensitive when directly stimulated; it has no sensory receptors. In contrast, the meninges and the blood vessels, which are innervated by sensory nerves are sensitive to "pain" stimuli.

MAJOR SUBDIVISIONS OF THE BRAIN

The brain, or *encephalon,* is conventionally divided into five major divisions: telencephalon or endbrain, diencephalon or inter- (twixt-) brain, mesencephalon or midbrain, metencephalon or afterbrain, and myelencephalon or medulla oblongata (see Fig. 1-1). The *telencephalon* and the *diencephalon* form the *prosencephalon,* or forebrain. The *metencephalon* and *myelencephalon* form the *rhombencephalon,* or hindbrain (see Fig. 1-1). The *metencephalon* comprises the pons and cerebellum.

The *cerebrum* includes the telencephalon, diencephalon, and upper midbrain. The *cerebrum* is partially divided into halves—the cerebral hemispheres—by the deep vertical *longitudinal fissure* (see Fig. 1-5). The *cerebral hemispheres* include such telencephalic structures as the cerebral cortex, white matter deep to the cortex (see Figs. 1-1, 1-24, and 16-7), the corpus striatum, and the corpus callosum (see Figs. 1-6 and 1-20). A cerebral hemisphere is less than half the cerebrum, for it does not include the diencephalon and the midbrain. The *ventricular system* is a continuum of cavities within the brain filled with cerebrospinal fluid. It is subdivided as follows: the lateral ventricles are the cavities of the cerebral hemispheres, the third ventricle is the cavity of the diencephalon, the cerebral aqueduct (iter or aqueduct of Sylvius) is the cavity of the mesencephalon, and the fourth ventricle is the cavity of the rhombencephalon

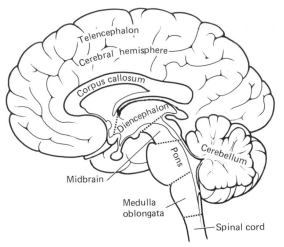

FIGURE 1-1 The major subdivisions of the central nervous system as viewed in sagittal section.

(see Figs. 1-17 and 1-18). The *cerebellum* is the expanded dorsal portion of the metencephalon (see Figs. 1-1, 1-2, and 1-6).

The *brainstem* is a collective term for the diencephalon, mesencephalon, and rhombencephalon exclusive of the cerebellum (see Figs. 1-1 and 1-2). (The diencephalon is sometimes not included with the brainstem.) The brainstem is the part of the brain which remains after the cerebral hemispheres and the cerebellum are removed. The brainstem is subdivided by its topographic relation to the tentorium (see Figs. 1-6 and 1-37) into the *supratentorial* and *infratentorial divisions*. The diencephalon is the supratentorial division, and the midbrain, pons, and medulla oblongata form the infratentorial division (see Figs. 1-6 and 1-11). All the cranial nerves except the olfactory and optic nerves, emerge from the infratentorial brainstem (see Figs. 1-11 and 1-13). The pons and the medulla are also called the *bulb*. Often, the infratentorial division is called the brainstem.

TOPOGRAPHY OF THE OUTER SURFACE OF THE BRAIN AND OF THE MEDIAL SURFACE OF THE MIDSAGITTALLY SECTIONED BRAIN

Each *cerebral hemisphere* is conventionally divided into six lobes: frontal, parietal, occipital, temporal, central (insula or island of Reil), and

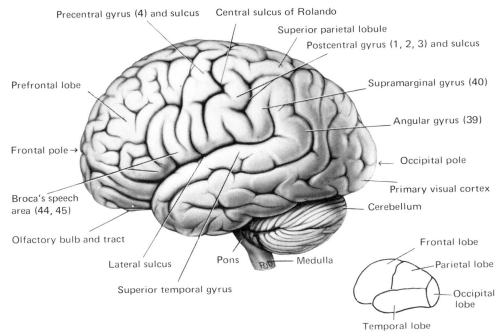

FIGURE 1-2 Lateral surface of the brain. Numbers refer to Brodmann's areas (refer to Figs. 1-3, 16-3, and 16-7).

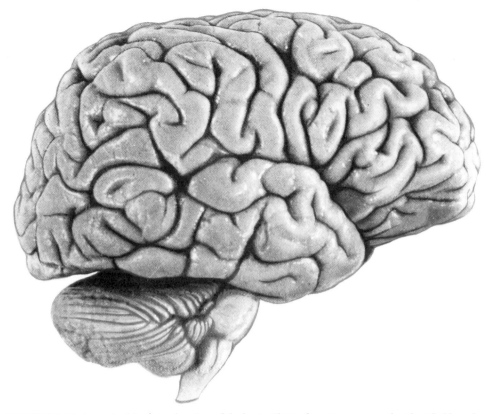

FIGURE 1-3 Photograph of the lateral surface of the brain. The surface structures can be identified by referring to Figs. 1-2, 16-1, and 16-3. (*Courtesy of Dr. Howard A. Matzke, University of Kansas Medical Center.*)

limbic (see Figs. 1-2, 1-4, and 1-8). The cerebral cortex, or the gray matter on the surface of the cerebrum, is marked by slitlike incisures called *sulci* (fissures). The raised ridges are called *gyri* (convolutions). The patterns formed by the sulci and gyri are variable, with no two brains having precisely identical patterns; not even the two hemispheres of one brain have the same pattern. Gyri and sulci are a manifestation of the great size and complexity of the cerebral cortex, whose surface area, including that exposed to the sulcal depressions, totals over 2 ft² (2200 cm²). A cerebral cortex with gyri and sulci is called a *gyrencephalic cortex.* Two-thirds of the cortical surface is obscured from view because it faces the sulcal spaces.

This division into lobes is largely arbitrary and is used for descriptive purposes. The convolutional patterns of the cerebral cortex in mammals with relatively large brains are related to the greater increase during evolution in the vol-

ume of the gray matter (*cortex*) as compared to the lesser increase in volume of the underlying white matter. A *cortex* is a mantle of gray matter (nerve cell bodies, dendritic trees, terminals of axons, and glial cells, described in Chap. 2) on the outer surface of the brain—hence cerebral cortex of the cerebrum, cerebellar cortex of the cerebellum, and cortex of the superior and inferior colliculi of the midbrain (see Figs. 1-15 and 1-24; see also Fig. 9-3).

Lateral aspect of the cerebral hemisphere (see Figs. 1-2 to 1-4)

Several major sulci are boundaries which divide the cerebral cortex into lobes. In turn, the lobes are subdivided by secondary and tertiary sulci into gyri. The "end" of each of three lobes is called a pole, viz., *frontal pole, temporal pole,* and *occipital pole* (see Fig. 1-2; see also Fig. 16-3).

The boundaries of the frontal, parietal, temporal, and occipital lobes on the lateral surface of the cerebral hemispheres are the *lateral sulcus (lateral fissure of Sylvius)*, *central sulcus of Rolando*, and the *parietooccipital line* (see Fig. 1-2; see also Fig. 16-3).

The *lateral sulcus* comprises the short stem and the posterior, horizontal, and posterior rami (see Figs. 16-1 and 16-3). The *stem of the lateral sulcus* is located between the orbital surface of the frontal lobe and the anterior temporal lobe and reaches the basal surface of the cerebrum. The stem continues as the long posterior ramus between the parietal and temporal lobes and terminates after curling upward into the parietal lobe. The horizontal and ascending rami extend forward and upward, respectively, for a short distance into the frontal lobe (see Fig. 16-3). Deep in the lateral sulcus is the *central lobe (insula, island of Reil)*; it is hidden in a surface view (see Fig. 1-4).

The central sulcus extends from the medial surface with a forward slope to just short of the lateral sulcus (Figs. 1-2 and 1-4; see also Fig. 16-3). The *frontal lobe* is located rostral to the central sulcus (Fig. 1-2). The *parietal lobe* lies between the central sulcus and the parietooccipital line. The *occipital lobe* is located posterior to the parietooccipital line and sulcus. The *parietooccipital line*, a line of convenience on the lateral surface, extends from the preoccipital incisure (notch) to the transverse occipital sulcus (see Fig. 16-3). It parallels the parietooccipital sulcus, a prominent landmark on the medial surface (see Fig. 1-8; see also Fig. 16-4).

The *temporal lobe* lies below the lateral sulcus and rostral to the parietooccipital line (see Fig. 16-3). The boundaries separating the parietal, occipital, and temporal lobes on the lateral surface of the hemisphere are not precise or meaningful.

The large frontal lobe is indented by three major sulci: the *precentral sulcus* and the *su-*

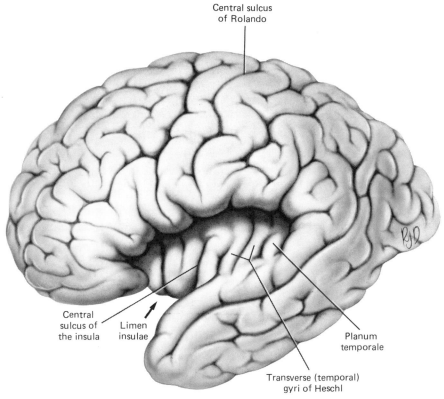

FIGURE 1-4 Lateral view of the cerebrum with opercula bordering the lateral sulcus separated to expose the insula (central lobe), transverse gyri of Heschl, and planum temporale (see Chap. 16).

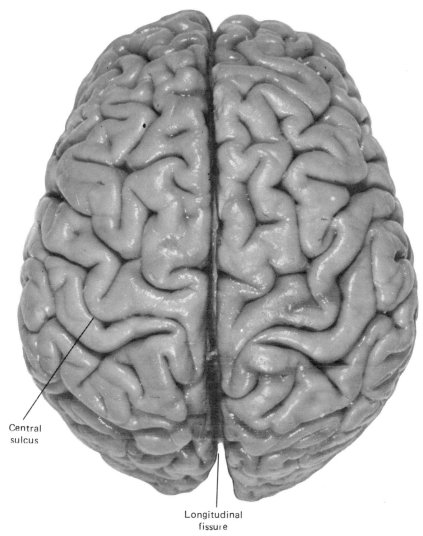

Central
sulcus

Longitudinal
fissure

FIGURE 1-5 Photograph of the dorsal view of the cerebrum. The surface structures can be identified by referring to Fig. 16-6. (*Courtesy of Dr. Howard A. Matzke, University of Kansas Medical Center.*)

perior and *inferior frontal sulci* (see Fig. 1-2; see
also Figs. 16-1 and 16-3). These sulci divide the
frontal lobe into the *precentral gyrus* (known as
the *motor cortex*) and the *superior, middle*, and *inferior frontal gyri*. These gyri extend onto the medial aspect of the hemisphere. The ascending
and horizontal rami of the lateral sulcus subdivide the inferior frontal gyrus into the *pars oper-
cularis, pars triangularis*, and *pars orbitalis* (see
Fig. 16-3). The opercular and triangular parts
are called *Broca's speech area* (Chap. 16 and Fig.

16-7, areas 44 and 45). The portion of the frontal
lobe located rostral to the precentral sulcus is
called the *prefrontal cortex* (prefrontal lobe or *hyperfrontal cortex* (see Figs. 1-2 and 16-3).

The parietal lobe has two major sulci—the
postcentral sulcus and the *intraparietal* (or *interparietal*) *sulcus* (Fig. 1-2; see also Figs. 16-1 and
16-3). These divide the lobe into the postcentral
gyrus and two lobules, called the *superior and inferior parietal lobules*. The inferior parietal lobule
is further subdivided into a *supramarginal gyrus*

and an *angular gyrus.*

The occipital lobe is divided by secondary occipital sulci into several unnamed gyri. A small sulcus in front of the occipital pole, called the *lunate sulcus,* is often present (see Fig. 16-3).

The taut extension of the inner dura mater, called the *tentorium* (tent), is located between the occipital lobe (which it helps to support) and the cerebellum (see Figs. 1-6, 1-38, and 1-39). The portions of the frontal, parietal, and temporal lobes that override the depths of the *central sulcus* are called *opercula*—hence frontal, parietal, and temporal opercula. When the opercula are raised (see Fig. 1-4), the central lobe is viewed as a pyramidal lobe with its apex directed toward the anterior perforated substance (see Figs. 15-4 and 16-6). The region of the apex is called the *limen insulae* (gyrus ambiens) (see Fig. 1-4; see also Fig. 15-4). The insula is surrounded, except at the limen, by the circular sulcus. The cortical convolutions of the insulae form three short gyri anteriorly and a long posterior gyrus separated by the central insular

sulcus (see Fig. 1-4). The insular cortex is continuous with that of the opercula.

The temporal lobe has two sulci which form boundaries of three gyri. These include the *superior and inferior sulci* and the *superior, middle, and inferior gyri* (see Figs. 1-2 and 16-1; see also Fig. 16-3). Near the posterior end of the superior temporal gyrus, on its superior surface and within the banks of the lateral sulcus, are the superior transverse temporal gyri (anterior and posterior) (see Fig. 1-4). They extend obliquely forward from the circular sulcus of the insula. The anterior gyrus—also known as the *transverse gyrus of Heschl*—and the adjacent portion of the superior temporal gyrus are the primary cortical centers for hearing (see Chap. 10 and Fig. 16-7, area 41).

Medial aspect of the cerebral hemisphere

The medial aspect of the cerebral hemisphere can be subdivided into the limbic lobe and por-

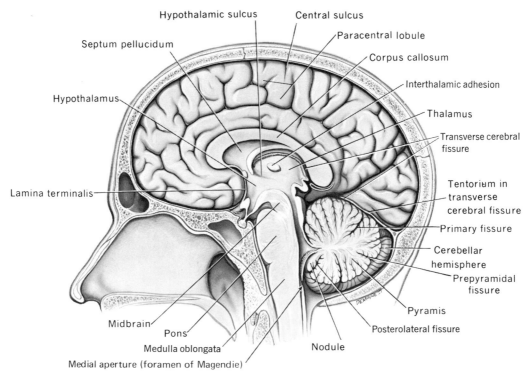

FIGURE 1-6 Median sagittal section of the brain and part of the head.

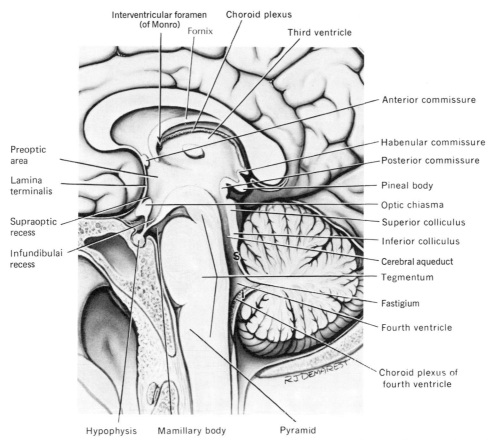

Interventricular foramen
(of Monro)   Choroid plexus

Fornix   Third ventricle

Anterior commissure

Habenular commissure

Posterior commissure

Preoptic area

Pineal body

Lamina terminalis

Optic chiasma

Superior colliculus

Supraoptic recess

Inferior colliculus

Cerebral aqueduct

Infundibulai recess

Tegmentum

Fastigium

Fourth ventricle

Choroid plexus of fourth ventricle

RJ DEMAREST

Hypophysis   Mamillary body   Pyramid

FIGURE 1-7 Median sagittal section of the brainstem. The brainstem consists of a (1) *roof* [choroid plexus of the third ventricle, superior and inferior colliculi, cerebellum, superior (S) and inferior (I) medullary velum and choroid plexus of fourth ventricle], (2) *central canal* (cerebral aqueduct and third and fourth ventricle), (3) *tegmentum*, and (4) *basilar portion* (internal capsule, crus cerebri, pons, and pyramid) (refer to Fig. 8-3).

tions of the frontal, parietal, and occipital lobes (see Figs. 1-8 and 1-10). The *limbic lobe* is the ring of cortex and associated structures surrounding the central core of the cerebrum. It comprises the hippocampus, dentate gyrus, parahippocampal gyrus, uncus, isthmus, fasciolar gyrus, cingulate gyrus, supracallosal gyrus, subcallosal gyrus, and parolfactory cortex or area (see Figs. 1-8 and 1-10; see also Figs. 15-2 and 16-4).

The curved line formed by the cingulate sulcus, anterior half of the collateral sulcus, and the rhinal sulcus forms the border between the limbic lobe and the cortices of the frontal, parietal, and temporal lobes (see Fig. 16-4). The *paracentral lobule* is continuous with the precentral and postcentral gyri of the lateral surface (see Figs. 1-6 and 1-8; see also Fig. 16-4). It is partially divided by the continuation of the central sulcus. Thus, the superior frontal gyrus and paracentral gyrus rostral to central sulcus are included in the frontal lobe, while the paracentral gyrus behind the central sulcus and the precuneus belong to the parietal lobe (see Figs. 1-2, 1-8, and 1-9). The *occipital lobe* on the medial aspect comprises the wedge-shaped *cuneus*, located between the *parietooccipital sulcus* and the *calcarine sulcus*, and the lingual and occipitotemporal gyri behind the plane of the *preoccipital notch* (see Figs. 1-8 and 1-9; see also Fig. 16-4). The cortex on both banks of the calcarine sulcus are the locale of the primary visual cortex (see

Fig. 12-13, Chap. 12). The lingual gyrus (located between the collateral and calcarine sulci) is continuous with the parahippocampal gyrus (see Fig. 16-6). Between the inferior temporal gyrus and the more medially placed collateral and rhinal sulci is the *occipitotemporal (fusiform) gyrus* (see Figs. 1-10, and 16-6).

The limbic lobe

The limbic lobe—literally meaning bordering lobe—is composed of gyri and associated structures on the medial aspect of the cerebral hemispheres roughly surrounding the diencephalon and corpus callosum (see Figs. 1-8 to 1-10; see also Figs. 15-2, 15-3, and 16-4). In turn, the temporal, occipital, parietal, and frontal lobes encircle the limbic lobe on its outer rim.

In the temporal lobe there are three structures of the limbic lobe located parallel to the collateral and rhinal sulci (see Fig. 16-4). They are, in order from lateral to medial, the parahippocampal gyrus, the dentate gyrus, and the hippocampus (see Fig. 1-10; see also Fig. 15-3). The hippocampal sulcus is between the parahippocampal and dentate gyri (see Fig. 1-10; see also

Fig. 15-3). The latter has a corrugated appearance, which is the basis for the name dentate gyrus. The *hippocampus* forms the floor of the inferior horn of the lateral ventricle (see Fig. 1-31). The rostral portion of the hippocampus has several shallow grooves and elevations having a pawlike appearance, the so-called *pes hippocampus* (Fig. 1-10). The hippocampus is also known as the Ammon's horn (*cornua ammonis*, abbreviated CA; see Fig. 15-5), or ram's horn.

The cortical band of parahippocampal gyrus located adjacent and parallel to the hippocampal sulcus is called the *subiculum* (see Fig. 1-10; see also Fig. 15-3). The subiculum is a transitional cortex between the neocortex of the parahippocampal gyrus and the archicortex of the hippocampus (Chap. 15). The rostral parahippocampal gyrus and an adjacent portion of the uncus is called the *entorhinal area* (see Fig. 1-10, area 28; see also Figs. 15-3 and 16-8). The general region medial to the rhinal sulcus comprising primarily the uncus and entorhinal area is called the *piriform area* (lobe)—named for its pear shape in mammals with a well-developed olfactory sense (Fig. 1-10; see also Chap. 15 and Fig. 15-4). The *limen insulae* (threshold of the in-

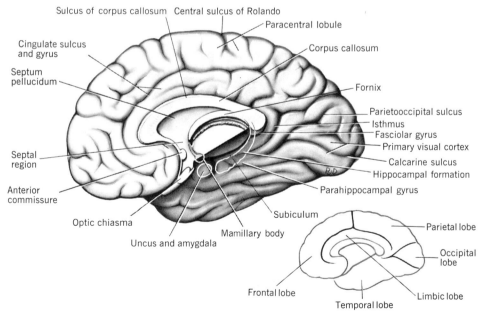

FIGURE 1-8 Median surface of the cerebral hemispheres. The amygdaloid body and the hippocampus are outlined by white lines. The subcortical amygdaloid body is located within the uncus. The hippocampal formation is located in the floor of the temporal horn of the lateral ventricle (see Figs. 1-11 and 16-4).

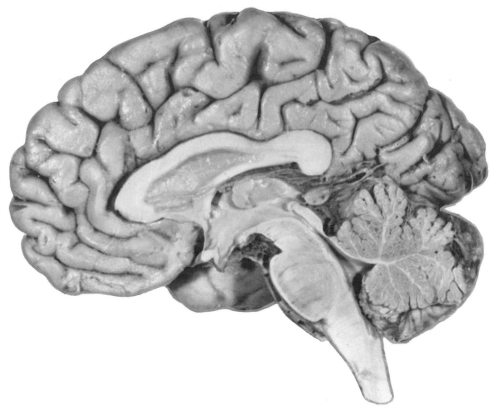

FIGURE 1-9 Photograph of midsagittal view of the brain. Structures can be identified by referring to Figs. 1-6, 1-7, 15-2, 16-2, and 16-4. (*Courtesy of Dr. Howard A. Matzke, University of Kansas Medical Center.*)

sula) is the apex of the insula located adjacent to the piriform area and deep in the lateral sulcus (see Fig. 1-4).

Several sequences of structures parallel the curvature of the lateral ventricles to form four arcs of the limbic lobe, further described in Chap. 15: (1) The uncus, parahippocampal gyrus, isthmus, and cingulate gyrus form an arc (see Fig. 1-10), often called the *gyrus fornicatus.* (2) Another sequence comprises the hippocampus, dentate gyrus, fasciolar gyrus, supracallosal gyrus, and subcallosal gyrus (see Figs. 1-10 and 1-11). The isthmus and fasciolar gyri are located behind the splenium of the corpus callosum. The thin supracallosal gyrus comprises a lamina of gray matter, called the *indusium griseum,* and two pairs of nerve fiber bundles called the *medial* and *lateral longitudinal striae* (see Fig. 1-10). The supracallosal and subcallosal gyri are called the *hippocampal rudiment* because they are thin extensions of the hippocampal gray matter located adjacent to the corpus callosum. (3) From the region of the hippocampus there extends an arc band of fibers called the *fornix* (see Figs. 1-8 and 1-10). It continues to the region on the anterior wall of the interventricular foramen of Monro, where it divides into a small precommissural and a large postcommissural bundle on either side of the anterior commissure (see Fig. 1-10; see also Fig. 15-3). The postcommissural fornix recurves before terminating in the mamillary body of the hypothalamus (see Fig. 1-10). In the region of the hippocampus, the fornix commences as the *alveus* and the *fimbria of the hippocampus;* it continues as the *body of the fornix* and then as the *column of the fornix* (see Figs. 1-10 and 1-31; see also Fig. 15-3). The alveus is a thin mantle of white matter on the ventricular surface of the hippocampus. The converging columns interconnect by means of the thin sheet called the *hippocampal (fornical) commissure,* which is located just beneath the corpus callo-

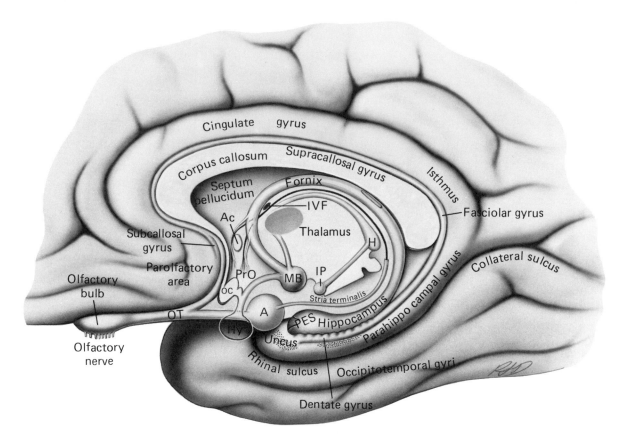

FIGURE 1-10 Configuration of the basic structures associated with the limbic lobe (refer to Figs. 1-8, 15-2, and 15-3). Note the arcs formed by sequences of limbic structures: (1) uncus, parahippocampal gyrus, isthmus, and cingulate gyrus; (2) hippocampus, dentate gyrus, fasciolar gyrus, supracallosal gyrus, and subcallosal gyrus; (3) hippocampus, fornix, and mamillary body; and (4) amygdala (A), stria terminalis, and preoptic area of hypothalamus. The two stippled areas represent the entorhinal area (area 28 of Brodmann, Fig. 16-7) in the uncus and the subiculum in the parahippocampal gyrus. The amygdala (A) is actually located deep to the uncus. A, amygdala; AC, anterior commissure; H, habenula; Hy, hypothalamus; IP, interpeduncular nucleus; IVF, interventricular foramen of Monro; MB, mamillary body; OC, optic chiasma; OT, olfactory tract; PES, pes hippocampus; P$_r$O preoptic area of hypothalamus.

sum (see Fig. 15-3). The two columns and the commissure form the *lyra* or *psalterium* (the harplike instrument). From the *amygdaloid body*, the gray mass within the uncus (see Figs. 1-8 and 1-9), a small bundle called the *stria terminalis* (stria semicircularis) parallels the fornix along the medial margin of the caudate nucleus and then passes along the caudal wall of the interventricular foramen. The stria then divides into precommissural and postcommissural bundles before terminating in the preoptic hypothalamus (see Fig. 1-10).

The region in the vicinity of the lamina terminalis is a phylogenetically old area which var-

ious authorities have given different names. The following is a reasonable account which can be readily modified. The region is incorporated into the limbic system. Rostral to the lamina terminalis is the *parolfactory* area (precommissural septum in front of anterior commissure) with its anterior and posterior parolfactory gyri and sulci (see Fig. 16-4). The *anterior olfactory sulcus* is roughly at the boundary between the neocortex of the frontal lobe and the paleocortex of the parolfactory and subcallosal gyri. The *subcallosal gyrus* and the *anterior parolfactory gyrus* combined have been called the *subcallosal area*. The subcallosal gyrus continues as the prehippocampal rudiment into the *anterior parolfactory gyrus* (also called *parateminal body, area, or gyrus*). (Figs. 1-10, 15-3, and 16-4). This hippocampal rudiment is the extension of the *indusium griseum* (supracallosal gyrus) in the region rostral to the lamina terminalis. This rudiment and the parateminal body form the subcallosal gyrus (see Fig. 16-4). The parateminal body is continuous with the *diagnonal band of Broca*, which leads into the cortex of the uncus (see Fig. 15-4). The diagonal band is located in the caudal anterior perforated space parallel to and in front of the optic tract (see Fig. 15-4). The olfactory tubercle is a hillock in the rostral anterior perforated space (see Fig. 15-4).

The *septal region (area)* comprises those neural tissues just anterior and posterior to the lamina terminalis and the anterior commissure (see Figs. 1-8 and 15-3); it includes the parolfactory and subcallosal gyrus (called the *precommissural septum*) and the region surrounding and above the medial aspects of the anterior commissure (called the *postcommissural septum*). The *septum pellucidum* is the thin narrow plate composed of glial cells and a few fibers of the fornix (see Fig. 1-6; see also Fig. 16-4); although technically a part of the postcommissural septum, it is generally considered to be a separate entity referred to as the *supracommissural septum*. The important septal nuclei are located in the postcommissural septum just dorsal to and in front of the anterior commissure, and they extend into the anterior parolfactory gyrus of the precommissural septum. The septal nuclei are divided into medial and lateral nuclei (Chap. 15).

Telencephalic structures visible from midsagittal aspect

The *corpus callosum* is a bundle of nerve fibers that traverses the midplane (commissure), interconnecting the neocortex of one hemisphere with that of the other hemisphere (see Figs. 1-6 and 1-9). The corpus callosum is divided into the *rostrum, genu, body,* and *splenium* (see Figs. 15-2 and 16-4). The genu and the U-shaped bundles of callosal fibers radiating to the frontal lobe form the forceps minor. The splenium and the callosal fibers radiating to the occipital lobe form the forceps major. The genu blends into the rostrum, which is continuous with the lamina terminalis.

Some callosal fibers, called the tapetum (see Fig. 1-29), radiate laterally and inferiorly to form a thin sheet on the outer border of the inferior and posterior horns of the lateral ventricle. The *anterior commissure* is a bundle of the limbic lobe cortex and of part of the temporal lobe neocortex (see Figs. 1-7, 1-8, and 1-10).

The lamina terminalis is a thin plate of neural tissue that forms the anterior boundary of the third ventricle (see Figs. 1-6 and 1-10). The median telencephalon includes the anterior commissure, the lamina terminalis, and the neural tissue in front of a line from the interventricular foramen (of Monro) to the optic chiasma called the preoptic area (see Fig. 1-10). (The interventricular foramen is for the passage of cerebrospinal fluid from the lateral ventricle of a cerebral hemisphere to the third ventricle seen in Figs. 1-18, 1-31, and 1-37.)

The fornix (seen only in part) is a bundle of fibers forming an arc from the hippocampus (archicortex) to the mamillary body of the diencephalon (see Figs. 1-7, 1-10, and 1-31).

The septum pellucidum consists of paired thin plates in the midplane extending from the corpus callosum to the fornix (see Fig. 1-8). The midline slit between the two septa of the septum pellucidum is the self contained cavum septum pellucidum; it is not connected to the ventricular system or to a subarachnoid space.

The *transverse cerebral fissure* separates the thalamus, midbrain, and cerebellum, located below, from the cerebral hemispheres (see Fig. 1-6).

The *tentorium* is primarily located between the cerebellum and the occipital lobes (see Fig. 1-6 and "Meninges," further on in this chapter).

The *velum interpositum* is the fold of pia mater occupying the transverse cerebral fissure between the diencephalon and corpus callosum (caudal to the interventricular foramen; see Fig. 1-37 and "Meninges").

Basal view of the cerebral hemisphere

The *frontal lobe* is demarcated by the olfactory sulcus, which extends parallel to the medial border (see Figs. 1-11 and 1-12), and an irregular group called the *orbital gyri and sulci* (see Fig. 16-5). The *gyrus rectus* is located medial to the olfactory sulcus, in which are located the olfactory

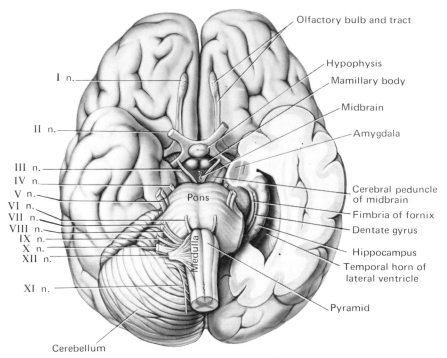

Olfactory bulb and tract

Hypophysis

Mamillary body

Midbrain

Amygdala

I n.

II n.

III n.
IV n.
V n.
VI n.
VII n.
VIII n.
IX n.
X n.
XII n.

XI n.

Pons

Medulla

Cerebellum

Cerebral peduncle
of midbrain

Fimbria of fornix

Dentate gyrus

Hippocampus

Temporal horn of
lateral ventricle

Pyramid

FIGURE 1-11 Basal surface of the brain. A horizontal section has been made through the right temporal and occipital lobes, exposing the hippocampus, dentate gyrus, fornix, and temporal horn of the lateral ventricle; n., cranial nerve (refer to Figs. 1-12 and 16-6).

bulb and tract (Fig. 16-6); the orbital gyri are located among the orbital sulci.

The rhinal sulcus and the collateral sulcus may be discontinuous or continuous. The *rhinal sulcus* and the *collateral sulcus* form the boundary between the parahippocampal gyrus and the occipitotemporal (fusiform) gyrus (see Figs. 1-10 to 1-12). The latter gyri may be further divided into a medial and lateral occipitotemporal gyrus by an occipitotemporal sulcus (see Figs. 16-4 and 16-6). The medial bulge in the most anterior portion of the parahippocampal gyrus is the *uncus*, which is located near the incisura (notch) of the tentorium. The midbrain "passes" through the notch (see Figs. 1-37 and 1-38; see also Fig. 16-4).

Functional subdivisions of the neocortex

The general functional significance of various portions of the cerebral neocortex is schematically outlined in Chap. 16. The frontal lobe is subdivided into (1) the precentral gyrus (including part of the paracentral lobule) (see Fig. 1-8;

see also Fig. 16-4), (2) the cortical area in front of the precentral gyrus, and (3) the prefrontal "lobe," or cortex (see Fig. 1-2).

The precentral gyrus has a motor function and hence is called the *motor cortex* (see Fig. 1-2, area 4). If it is stimulated electrically, precise movements can be elicited in the conscious patient. For example patients respond to cortical stimulation by moving their fingers because they say they had to move them.

The area in front of the precentral gyrus, also associated with motor activities, is called the *premotor area* (Fig. 16-12, area 6). The portion of the premotor area in the vicinity of the ascending ramus (the inferior frontal gyrus) of the lateral sulcus, known as *Broca's speech area* (see Fig. 1-2, area 44), has a role in the motor aspects of vocalization.

The *prefrontal lobe* (cortex) has a role in such subtle expressions as anxiety, placidity, drive, and concern with social attitudes. The prefrontal lobe is structurally and functionally integrated with the anterior temporal lobe. Intractable visceral pain may be alleviated by bilateral prefrontal lobotomy (disconnection of the prefrontal cortex by surgical transection of its nerve fibers).

The parietal, occipital, and temporal lobes may be functionally subdivided into primary receptive and association areas. The postcentral gyrus and the posterior portion of the paracentral lobule are known as the primary receptive area for the general senses, including touch, pressure, and others. The *transverse gyri of Heschl*, located in the upper part of the temporal lobe in the depth of the lateral cerebral sulcus, constitute the primary receptive area for audition (see Fig. 1-4). The cortex on either side of the calcarine fissure (including portions of the cuneus and lingual gyrus) is known as the primary receptive area for vision. The remaining parts of the neocortex in these lobes are called the association areas. These association areas are essential to such general sensations as the recognition and comprehension of weight, shape, texture, and form, and to the elaboration of the sensations of vision and audition (e.g., recognition of the written and spoken word). No solid evidence exists relating specific regions of the cortex with learning or creative ability. The temporal lobe is associated with memory. The limbic lobe is integrated into systems involved with behavior and emotional expressions.

The cerebral cortex has been subdivided

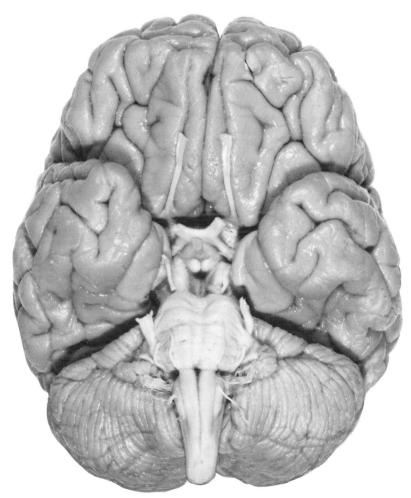

FIGURE 1-12 Photograph of basal view of brain. Structures can be identified by referring to Figs. 1-11, 7-1, and 16-5. (*Courtesy of Dr. Howard A. Matzke, University of Kansas Medical Center.*)

into areas by the use of microscopic anatomic criteria (cytoarchitecture). The numbered areas proposed by Brodmann are often used (see Figs. 16-7 and 16-8): precentral gyrus or motor cortex as area 4; premotor cortex as areas 6 and 8; precentral gyrus or general sensory cortex as areas 1, 2, and 3; the primary receptive area for vision as area 17; and the primary receptive area for audition as comprising areas 41 and 42.

MEDIAL ASPECT OF THE DIENCEPHALON, MESENCEPHALON, METENCEPHALON, AND MYELENCEPHALON

Diencephalon

The *diencephalon* is surrounded laterally and dorsally by the cerebral hemispheres. Its anterior aspect is exposed (see Fig. 1-1). It is continuous caudally with the midbrain. In the median view (see Figs. 1-1, 1-6, and 1-7; see also Fig. 11-1), the perimeter of the diencephalon (midsagittal view) includes, in order, the choroid plexus of the third ventricle, habenular commissure, pineal body, posterior commissure (roof), a hypothetic line from the posterior commissure to the mamillary bodies (caudal margin), mamillary bodies, tuber cinereum, hypophysis (pituitary gland), and optic chiasma (floor), and the line from the optic chiasma to the interventricular foramen (anterior margin). The midsagittal plane of the diencephalon is occupied by the slit-like third ventricle, which is the central canal of the diencephalon. Note that the choroid plexus of the third ventricle is continuous through each interventricular foramen with the choroid plexus of each lateral ventricle of the cerebral hemispheres (see Figs. 1-17, 1-18, and 1-21). Each choroid plexus is composed of extensions of the pia mater and its vascular network which are covered by the cuboidal epithelial cells of the ependyma lining the ventricular cavity.

Three of the four subdivisions of the diencephalon are visible in a midsagittal view of the brain: epithalamus (adjacent to the choroid plexus), thalamus (dorsal thalamus), and hypothalamus. The subthalamus is not visible in this view.

The *epithalamus* is the narrow band on the roof of the diencephalon, including the stria medullaris thalami (which parallels the entire attachment of the choroid plexus), habenula, habenular commissure, pineal body, and posterior commissure; the first three are associated with the limbic system (see Figs. 1-7 and 1-10; see also Chap. 15, especially Fig. 15-3). The function of the pineal body is discussed in Chap. 11. The posterior commissure is associated with reflexes of the optic system (Chap. 12).

The *thalamus*, the largest subdivision of the diencephalon, is located above the hypothalamic sulcus. The thalamus is the major integrative station that is intercalated between many subcortical structures and the cerebral cortex. For example, all sensory impulses except those of olfaction are relayed to the thalamus before reaching the cerebral cortex. The *interthalamic adhesion* (*massa intermedia*) is merely a site of secondary fusion (soft commissure) of the dorsal thalamus across the midline in about 70 percent of brains (see Fig. 1-6). The *hypothalamus* is located below the hypothalamic sulcus and includes the floor structures. Through the optic chiasma pass the fibers from the eyes to the brain. The hypothalamus contains the highest integrative centers of the autonomic nervous system (Chaps. 6 and 11); it is involved in such functional activities as the regulation of body temperature, emotional expressions, and endocrine gland activities. The *hypophysis*, or pituitary gland, is the master endocrine gland.

The *subthalamus*, which flanks the hypothalamus laterally and hence is not visible, is a significant subcortical station in the motor activities of voluntary muscles (see Fig. 1-27; see also Figs. 13-2 and 14-1).

Mesencephalon, metencephalon, and myelencephalon

These segments of the brainstem have similar basic features; each has a roof, a central canal (ventricular system), a tegmental portion, and a basilar portion (see Fig. 1-7). The *tegmentum* of the brainstem comprises some structures functionally integrated into somatic and visceral reflex activities, into ascending systems associated with conscious and unconscious afferent pathways, and into descending systems associated with autonomic and somatic motor activities.

The *basilar portion of the brainstem* (crus cerebri, basilar portion of pons, and pyramid of medulla; see Fig. 1-7) consists of descending pathways originating in the cerebral cortex, including the corticospinal, corticobulbar, and corticopontine-pontocerebellar pathways (see Chaps. 5, 8, and 9).

Mesencephalon (midbrain) (see Figs. 1-1 and 1-7)   The roof consists of the *lamina quadrigemina* (*tectum*), which includes a pair of *superior colliculi* (*optic system*) and a pair of *inferior colliculi* (*auditory system*). The superior colliculus is associated with optic systems, visual guidance, and tracking activities related to eye and head movements. The inferior colliculus is involved with auditory and acousticomotor activities. Caudal to the inferior colliculus is the exit for the fourth cranial nerve (trochlear nerve). Rostral to the superior colliculus is a small region called the pretectum. The *posterior commissure*, located at the junction between the midbrain (pretectum) and the diencephalon, is composed of fibers interconnecting several tectal nuclei (Fig. 1-7). A small *intercollicular commissure*, located at the level of the inferior colliculi, interconnects the nuclei of the inferior colliculus. The central canal is the *cerebral aqueduct* (*iter*, aqueduct of Sylvius), which extends from the third ventricle to the fourth ventricle (see Figs. 1-17 and 1-18). The midbrain tegmentum is prominent. The basilar portion comprises paired crura cerebri (crus cerebri, singular). The tegmentum and crura form the cerebral peduncles. Between the two peduncles is the interpeduncular fossa; the rootlets of the oculomotor (third) cranial nerve emerge from the base of the midbrain into the *interpeduncular fossa* (see Fig. 1-13). The *substantia nigra* is located between the tegmentum and the crura cerebri. The *cerebral peduncle* is composed of the midbrain tegmentum, substantia nigra, and crus cerebri (Figs. 1-7 and 8-12); in brief, the cerebral peduncle is half of the midbrain, excluding the tectum.

Metencephalon (pons)   The roof is basically the cerebellum, the superior and inferior medullary veli, and part of the choroid plexus of the fourth ventricle. The canal is the rostral half of the fourth ventricle. The tegmentum is continuous with that of the midbrain and the medulla. The basilar portion is the *pons proper*.

Myelencephalon (medulla oblongata)   The roof consists of the rest of the choroid plexus of the fourth ventricle (see Fig. 1-1). The apex of the roof of the fourth ventricle extending into the cerebellum is called the *fastigium* (see Fig. 1-7). The canal is the caudal half of the fourth ventricle and its caudal continuation is the central canal of the medulla and spinal cord. The tegmentum comprises the bulk of the medulla. The pyramids form the basilar portion.

The boundaries between any two divisions of the brainstem are not defined precisely (see Figs. 1-1, 1-7, 1-13, and 1-14). The boundary between the diencephalon and the mesencephalon is a plane passing through the posterior commissure and the caudal aspect of the mamillary bodies; that between the mesencephalon and the metencephalon is a plane passing caudal to the fourth cranial nerve and the rostral border of the pons; that between the metencephalon and the myelencephalon is a plane passing through the eighth cranial nerve and the caudal border of the pons; and that between the myelencephalon and the spinal cord is roughly a transverse plane in the region between the caudal end of the twelfth cranial nerve and the first cervical nerve in the vicinity of the foramen magnum.

BASAL ASPECT OF THE BRAIN

The telencephalic structures, visible in a basal view, are portions of the frontal, temporal, and the occipital lobes (see Figs. 1-11 to 1-13; see also Figs. 7-1, 15-4, and 16-6). Significant landmarks are the *rhinal sulcus* and the *collateral sulcus* (sulci delineating the limbic lobe from the neocortex (see Fig. 15-3). Elements of the olfactory pathways include the olfactory nerve (first cranial nerve), olfactory bulb, olfactory tract, and the three olfactory striae (lateral, medial, and intermediate). In the region of the olfactory trigone lateral to the optic tract is the *anterior perforated substance;* it is indented and stippled by small arterial branches of the middle cerebral artery.

The diencephalic structures include the

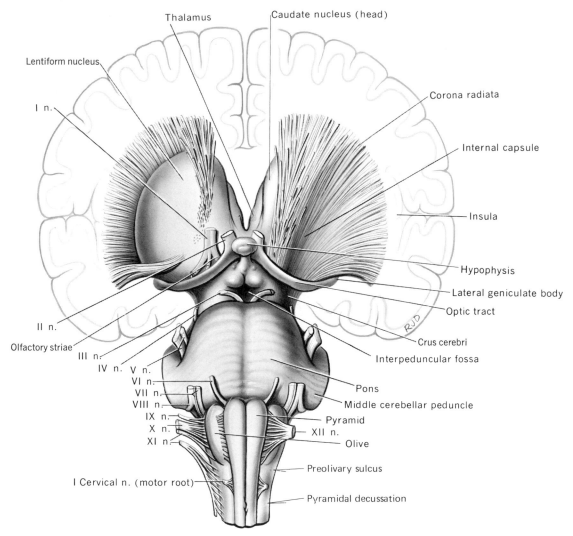

Thalamus

Caudate nucleus (head)

Lentiform nucleus

Corona radiata

I n.

Internal capsule

Insula

Hypophysis

Lateral geniculate body

Optic tract

II n.

Crus cerebri

Olfactory striae

Interpeduncular fossa

III n.

IV n. V n.

VI n.

VII n.

VIII n.

Pons

Middle cerebellar peduncle

IX n.

Pyramid

X n.

XII n.

XI n.

Olive

Preolivary sulcus

I Cervical n. (motor root)

Pyramidal decussation

FIGURE 1-13 Basal surface of the brainstem and roots of cranial nerves.

optic nerve (second cranial nerve) and optic tract of the visual system; and the hypophysis (pituitary gland and infundibulum), tuber cinereum, and mamillary bodies of the hypothalamus. Two areas on the base of the brain—the *anterior perforated substance* and *posterior perforated substance*—are perforated by numerous small blood vessels (see Fig. 1-12; see also Figs. 7-1 and 15-4). The former is located behind the olfactory trigone adjacent to and in front of the optic tract, and the latter is in the floor of the *in-terpeduncular fossa* of the midbrain (see Fig. 1-13).

The *mesencephalic structures* include the crura cerebri of the cerebral peduncle, the third cranial nerve (oculomotor nerve) emerging in the interpeduncular fossa, and the fourth (trochlear) cranial nerve (see Figs. 1-13 and 1-14).

The *metencephalic structures* include the pons proper, cerebellum, and fifth (trigeminal) cranial nerve. This nerve emerges on the lateral aspect of the pons. Note the sensory ganglion, sensory root, and motor root of the trigeminal nerve (see Fig. 1-13; see also Figs. 7-1 and 7-6).

The *myelencephalic (medullary) structures* include the pyramids, olives, and roots of seven cranial nerves (see Fig. 1-13). The pyramids are formed by the fibers of the motor pyramidal tract that crosses the midline at the pyramidal decussation in the lower medulla. The *olive* is a protuberance formed by the inferior olivary nucleus (Chap. 8). The sixth (abducent), seventh (facial), and eighth (vestibulocochlear) cranial nerves emerge at the pontomedullary junction. The ninth (glossopharyngeal) and tenth (vagus) nerves emerge as a series of rootlets from the posterolateral (postolivary) sulcus on the posterior margin of the olive. The eleventh (spinal accessory) cranial nerve emerges in the form of rootlets from the medulla (posterolateral) and from the spinal cord (between the dorsal and ventral roots of the first six cervical spinal nerves). The twelfth (hypoglossal) cranial nerve emerges from the preolivary sulcus on the anterior margin of the olive.

Note that the third, sixth, and twelfth cranial nerves emerge from the anterior aspect of the brainstem in a longitudinal line just lateral to the midsagittal plane; the fifth, seventh, ninth, tenth, and eleventh cranial nerves emerge from the lateral aspect of the brainstem (Figs. 1-11 through 1-14; see also Fig. 7-1). All cranial nerves (except the first and second) emerge from the infratentorial brain stem.

LATERAL ASPECT OF THE BRAINSTEM

Of the subdivisions of the diencephalon, only the dorsal thalamus and subthalamus extend to the lateral surface of the diencephalon adjacent to the internal capsule (see Fig. 1-27). The epithalamus and hypothalamus are not visible from this view because they are medial structures

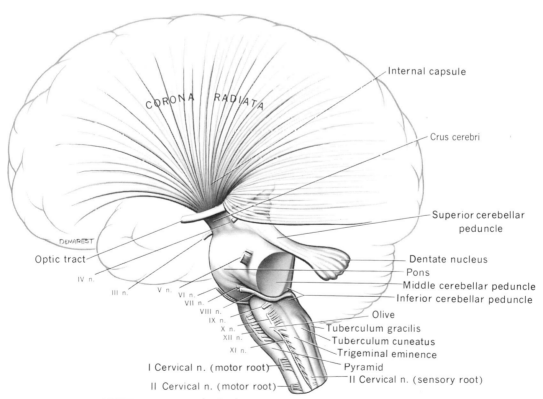

FIGURE 1-14 Lateral surface of the brainstem and roots of cranial nerves.

bordering the third ventricle. The thalamus is the only diencephalic subdivision which extends throughout the width of the diencephalon from the internal capsule to the third ventricle.

Note the *pulvinar*, a posterior extension of the thalamus proper. The optic nerve, optic chiasma, optic tract, and lateral geniculate body are structures of the visual pathways (see Figs. 1-14 and 1-15). The *lateral geniculate body* is a thalamic nucleus located below the pulvinar. Each *internal capsule*, which flanks the diencephalon laterally, is continuous with the crus cerebri of the midbrain and the *corona radiata* of the white matter of the cerebral hemisphere (see further

on in this chapter, "The Brain as a Three-Dimensional Structure: Solid Geometry of the Brain").

The mesencephalic structures viewed (see Figs. 1-14 and 1-15) include the superior and inferior colliculi (or the corpora quadrigemina) and the fourth cranial nerve (all roof structures), tegmentum, and crus cerebri of the basilar portion (see "Solid Geometry of the Brain," further on). The brachium of the superior colliculus, which extends from the lateral geniculate body of the thalamus to the superior colliculus, consists of fibers of the optic pathways (see Fig. 1-15). The brachium of the inferior colliculus, which extends from the inferior colliculus to the

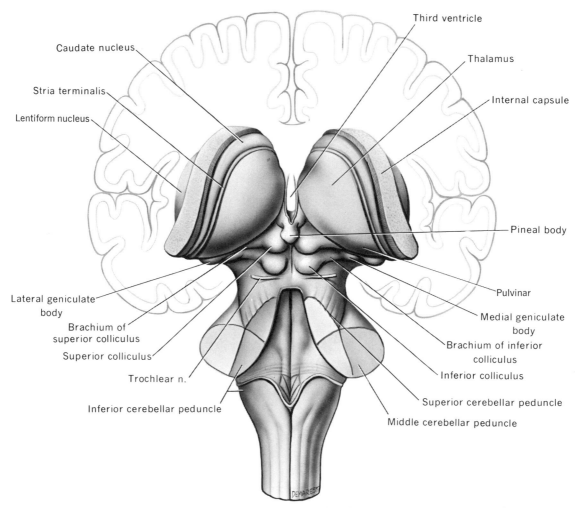

FIGURE 1-15 Dorsal surface of the brainstem.

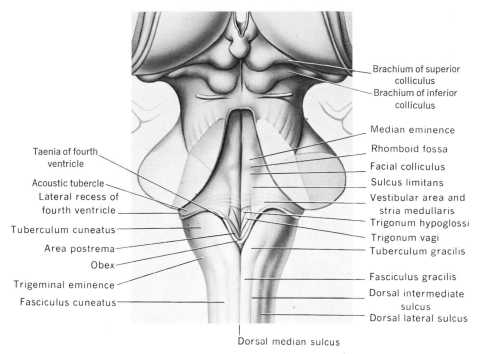

Brachium of superior colliculus
Brachium of inferior colliculus
Median eminence
Rhomboid fossa
Facial colliculus
Sulcus limitans
Vestibular area and stria medullaris
Trigonum hypoglossi
Trigonum vagi
Tuberculum gracilis
Fasciculus gracilis
Dorsal intermediate sulcus
Dorsal lateral sulcus

Taenia of fourth ventricle
Acoustic tubercle
Lateral recess of fourth ventricle
Tuberculum cuneatus
Area postrema
Obex
Trigeminal eminence
Fasciculus cuneatus

Dorsal median sulcus

FIGURE 1-16 Dorsal surface of the lower brainstem.

medial geniculate body of the thalamus, consists of fibers of the auditory pathways (see Fig. 1-15). The fourth cranial nerve is the only cranial nerve that emerges from the posterior aspect of the brainstem.

The metencephalic structures viewed include the cerebellum, pons, three brachia of the cerebellum, and fifth cranial nerve. The *superior cerebellar peduncle* (brachium conjunctivum) consists of fibers that project mainly from the cerebellum to the upper brainstem. The *middle cerebellar peduncle* (brachium pontis) of fibers that project from the pons proper to the cerebellum. The *inferior cerebellar peduncle* (restiform body) consists of a bundle that extends from the lower brainstem to the cerebellum.

The myelencephalic structures viewed include the choroid plexus, tuberculum gracilis, tuberculum cuneatus, eminentia trigemini, olive, and pyramids. The *tuberculum gracilis* and *tuberculum cuneatus* are hillocks produced by nuclei associated with ascending sensory pathways from the spinal cord (see Fig. 1-14). The *eminentia trigemini* (tuberculum cinereum) is a ridge produced by the spinal (descending) nu-

cleus and tract of the fifth cranial nerve (Chap. 8).

POSTERIOR ASPECT OF THE BRAINSTEM

The diencephalic structures viewed include the epithalamus, which is flanked laterally by the thalamus proper. The mesencephalic structures viewed include the superior and inferior coliculi and their brachia, the fourth cranial nerve, and the lateral surfaces of the tegmentum and the crura cerebri (see Figs. 1-15 and 1-16).

The metencephalic and myelencephalic structures viewed include the three cerebellar peduncles and some landmarks on the floor of the fourth ventricle. The floor is marked by a groove, the sulcus limitans (see Figs. 1-15 and 1-16). Medial to this groove are located the trigonum vagi and trigonum hypoglossi, and lateral to it is the area vestibularis. The *trigonum hypoglossi* is a short ridge formed by the underlying hypoglossal nucleus; the *trigonum vagi* is formed by the underlying motor (parasympathetic) nucleus of the vagus nerve (Chap. 8). The *area vestibularis* is the region of the vestibular nuclei. The *facial (or abducent) colliculus* is a hillock formed by the genu (Chap. 8) of the facial nerve and the nucleus of the abducent nerve.

On the dorsal surface of the inferior medulla are the tuberculum gracilis and tuberculum cuneatus. Note the diamond-shaped fourth ventricle (rhomboid fossa). The lateral recesses of the ventricle extend laterally at the level of the upper medulla. The eminence formed by the dorsal cochlear nucleus lateral to the vestibular area is the *acoustic tubercle* (see Fig. 1-16). The *taenia of the fourth ventricle* is the line of attachment of the tela choroidea to the medulla (see Fig. 1-16). The *obex* is a fold of tissue overhanging the site at the apex where the fourth ventricle funnels into the central canal of the medulla; it is used as a landmark by neurosurgeons.

CEREBELLUM

The *cerebellum* is a fissured and lobated structure which is a modulator and coordinator of motor activities (Chap. 9). The cerebellar surface is marked by numerous fissures separating long narrow folds called *folia* (see Figs. 9-1 and 9-3). Only one-sixth of the cerebellar cortex is exposed to the surface; five-sixths faces the fissural clefts.

The contours of the lobes, lobules, and fissures of the cerebellum have been colorfully named and subdivided. Most of them have no special functional significance. Three schemas for grossly subdividing the cerebellum are helpful (see Fig. 9-1).

1. The centrally placed median subdivision is the wormlike *vermis*, which is flanked laterally by the expansive cerebellar hemispheres.
2. The cerebellum consists of an anterior lobe, a middle (posterior) lobe, and a flocculonodular lobe. Each of these lobes includes portions of the vermis and the hemispheres. The *anterior lobe* is the rostral segment of the cerebellum, delineated from the posterior lobe by the primary fissure (fissura prima). The *middle lobe* consists of the rest of the cerebellum except for the small flocculonodular lobe located on the underside of the cerebellum near the brainstem. The *flocculonodular lobe* (vestibulocerebellum) consists of a small median lobule, called the *nodule of the vermis*, and of the laterally extended lobule, called the *flocculus*, of each hemisphere (see Fig. 1-6). The fissure delineating the middle lobe from the flocculonodular lobe is the posterolateral fissure; its medial extension was called the prenodular fissure.
3. A phylogenetically based schema subdivides the cerebellum into archicerebellum, paleocerebellum, and neocerebellum. The *archicerebellum* is the *flocculonodular lobe*. It is phylogenetically the oldest lobe of the cerebellum and is functionally associated with the vestibular system. The *paleocerebellum* roughly consists of the vermis less the nodule. This lobe, too, is old phylogenetically; it is associated generally with fibers from the spinal cord and lower brainstem. The *neocerebellum* includes the cerebellar hemispheres less the flocculi. These lobes are new phylogenetically, and they are functionally associated largely with the upper brainstem and cerebrum, including the cerebral cortex.

The precise boundaries of these various divisions of the cerebellum are not defined similarly by all authorities. The surface of the cerebellum is covered by the cerebellar cortex. The *tonsil* is a lobule located on the medial inferior aspect of the cerebellum (see Fig. 9-1). On the inferior surface of the cerebellum between the tonsils is a medial subarachnoid space called the *vallecula*. Deep to the cortex is a mass of nerve fibers forming the white matter (corpus medullare) of the cerebellum. Within this white matter are the four pairs of deep cerebellar nuclei, from medial to lateral: the nuclei fastigii, globosus, emboliformis, and dentatus (Chap. 9). The cerebellum is connected with the brainstem by the three cerebellar peduncles (brachia or pillars) previously noted.

A thin lamina—the superior medullary velum—extends rostrally from the cerebellum to the midbrain tectum; another lamina—the inferior medullary velum—extends caudally from the cerebellum to the choroid plexus of the fourth ventricle (see Fig. 1-7). These veli roof the fourth ventricle.

VENTRICULAR SYSTEM

The ventricular system (see Figs. 1-17 and 1-18) is the series of cavities within the brain lined by the ependyma and filled with cerebrospinal fluid. Each cerebral hemisphere contains a *lateral ventricle*, each of which is connected through one of the paired interventricular foramina (of Monro) with the third ventricle of the diencephalon. The *third ventricle* is continuous with the tubelike cerebral aqueduct of the midbrain, and the latter with the large *fourth ventricle* of the pons and medulla. The *central canal* of the spinal cord joins the fourth ventricle slightly rostral to the junction of medulla and spinal cord.

The lateral ventricle is subdivided into four parts: the anterior horn, located rostral to the interventricular foramen, is in the frontal lobe; the body, located posterior to the interventricular foramen is in the parietal lobe; the inferior or temporal horn is in the temporal lobe; and the occipital horn is in the occipital lobe. The *atrium*, or *trigone*, of the lateral ventricle is located at the junction of the temporal horn, the occipital horn, and the body of the ventricle.

The pia mater, which is in direct apposition with the ependymal lining of the ventricles, is known as the *tela choroidea*. The vascular cores of the choroid plexuses are located within the tela choroidea.

Each ventricle contains a *choroid plexus*, a rich network of blood vessels of the pia mater which are in contact with the ependymal lining of a ventricle (see Figs. 1-7, 1-17, 1-18, and 1-29). These plexuses have a role in the elaboration of the cerebrospinal fluid. The choroid plexus of each lateral ventricle is located in the body and temporal horn; it is continuous through an interventricular foramen with the choroid plexus of the third ventricle. The choroid plexus of the fourth ventricle is a T-shaped structure located in the roof of the medulla. In this roof are three foramina through which the cerebrospinal fluid escapes from the fourth ventricle into the subarachnoid space. One of these three apertures is located at one of the ends of the T (Fig. 1-18). The two lateral openings are the lateral apertures (Luschka); the probable midline opening is the medial aperture (Magendie). Some choroid plexus extends through the lateral aperture into the subarachnoid space.

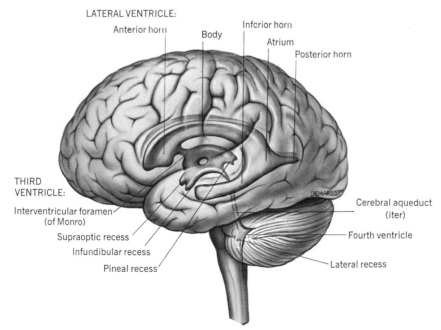

FIGURE 1-17 Lateral view of the ventricles of the brain.

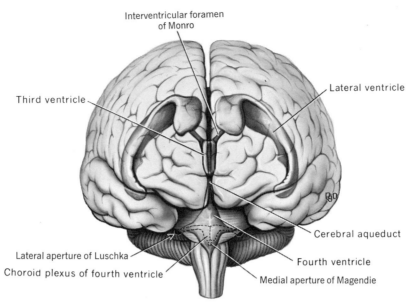

Interventricular foramen
of Monro

Lateral ventricle

Third ventricle

Cerebral aqueduct

Lateral aperture of Luschka

Fourth ventricle

Choroid plexus of fourth ventricle

Medial aperture of Magendie

FIGURE 1-18 Frontal view of the ventricles of the brain.

THE BRAIN AS A THREE-DIMENSIONAL STRUCTURE: SOLID GEOMETRY OF THE BRAIN

Axes of the brain (Fig. 1-19)

The brain may be visualized as a geometric figure with two main axes: vertical and horizontal (see Fig. 1-19). Description of the relation of the major structures of the brain to these axes is the purpose of the following schema, which outlines some pertinent aspects of the topographic anatomy of the brain. The vertical axis is the line which extends caudally from the region of the pre- and postcentral gyri through the brainstem and spinal cord. The horizontal axis extends from the frontal pole toward the occipital pole of the cerebrum; this axis bifurcates in the region deep to the angular gyrus into (1) an extension which reaches the occipital pole and (2) a recurved arc which is directed toward the temporal pole. The latter is illustrated by the broken line in Fig. 1-19.

A major pathway which parallels the vertical axis is the corticospinal (pyramidal) tract. This motor pathway originates mainly from the pre- and postcentral gyri and descends successively through portions of the corona radiata,

internal capsule, crus of the midbrain, pons, pyramid of the medulla, and spinal cord (see Figs. 1-14 and 1-23; see also Fig. 5-25).

The visual pathway from the eyes to the primary visual cortex in the vicinity of the calcarine sulcus (see Fig. 12-13) is oriented parallel to the horizontal axis from the frontal pole to the occipital pole. The long axis of the diencephalon [from the interventricular foramen (of Monro) to the pineal body] is roughly parallel to this axis (Fig. 1-7). The lateral ventricle of the cerebral hemisphere parallels the horizontal axis and its arc into the temporal lobe (Figs. 1-17 and 1-23). The sequence of frontal lobe, parietal lobe, and temporal lobe also follows this curve. Other structures oriented to this curve are outlined below as arc structures. The arc shape of the cerebral hemispheres and the arc structures are formed during early ontogeny. The cerebral hemispheres develop from the region in the vicinity of the interventricular foramen. From this region cells migrate rostrally to develop into the frontal lobe and caudally along the horizontal axis to the occipital pole and to the temporal pole.

The junctional region between the midbrain and diencephalon forms an angle between the infratentorial brainstem, which is oriented

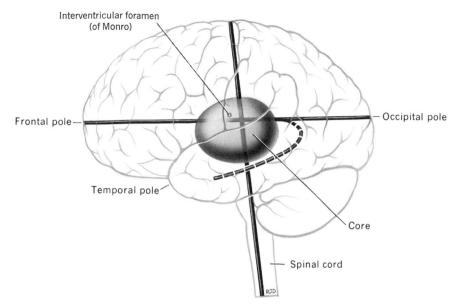

Interventricular foramen
(of Monro)

Frontal pole

Temporal pole

Occipital pole

Core

Spinal cord

RJD

FIGURE 1-19 Geometry of the brain. Vertical axis is parallel to the long axis of the brainstem and spinal cord. Horizontal axis is parallel to the long axis of cerebrum from frontal pole to occipital pole. For explanation of broken line, see text.

parallel to the vertical axis, and the diencephalon, which is oriented parallel to the horizontal axis. This is illustrated in Fig. 1-7; note that the long axis of the third ventricle and its choroid plexus is oriented approximately at a right angle to the long axis of the cerebral aqueduct and fourth ventricle and to the sequence of superior colliculus, inferior colliculus, cerebellum, and choroid plexus of the fourth ventricle.

Core structures and arc structures

Anatomically the cerebrum may be subdivided into a group of central or core structures and a group of arc structures. The diencephalon and the lentiform nucleus are considered to be core structures located centrally in the cerebrum. Each cerebral hemisphere forms an arc, which flanks the core structures.

Knowledge of the anatomic relation of the core structures to one another is useful in identifying them in sections of the brain. In the following sequence, the core structures are listed in order, from the most medially located third ventricle to the most laterally located cortex of the central lobe (insula). The sequence is third ventricle, thalamus of the diencephalon, internal capsule, lentiform nucleus (globus pallidus and putamen), external capsule, claustrum, extreme capsule, and cortex of central lobe (see Figs. 1-13, 1-15, and 1-31).

The *arc structures of the cerebral hemispheres* are illustrated in Figs. 1-17, 1-20, and 1-21. These include (1) the lateral ventricle, (2) the choroid plexus of the lateral ventricle, (3) the caudate nucleus, (4) the sequence of hippocampus, fimbria, body, and column of the fornix and mamillary body, (5) the sequence of amygdaloid body, stria terminalis, and hypothalamus (see Figs. 1-10 and 15-3), and (6) the corpus callosum (Fig. 1-6). Many of these structures form boundaries of the lateral ventricles. Because these structures curve and extend into the temporal lobe, each arc structure may be viewed twice in some sections through the cerebrum (see Figs. 1-22, 1-27, 1-28, and 1-31).

Note that the anterior horn and body of the lateral ventricle and its associated arc structures are located in a sagittal plane which is medial to the internal capsule (see Figs. 1-13, 1-15, 1-23, 1-27, and 1-28).

The cerebrum peripheral to the core structures just noted includes the white matter deep to the cortex (subcortical white matter) and the

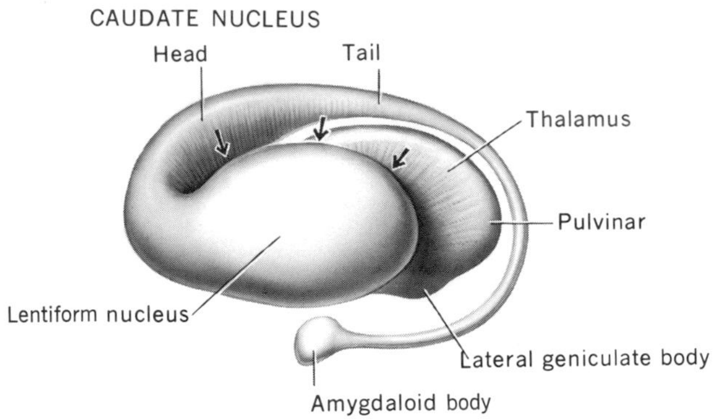

CAUDATE NUCLEUS

Head   Tail

Thalamus

Pulvinar

Lentiform nucleus

Lateral geniculate body

Amygdaloid body

FIGURE 1-20 Geometry of the brain. The thalamus and lentiform nucleus are included in the core structures. The caudate nucleus and the amygdaloid body (amygdala) are included in the arc structures (see text and Fig. 1-21). Arrows indicate the location of the cleft where the internal capsule is located. The lentiform nucleus and the caudate nucleus comprise the *corpus striatum.*

cerebral cortex. Three general categories of fibers are present in this white matter: (1) the *projection fibers*, which project from (and to) the cortex to (and from) deep cerebral structures, brainstem, and spinal cord (most of them passing through the internal capsule); (2) the major *commissural fibers*, which originate in the cortex or a subcortical nucleus of one cerebral hemisphere and terminate in the cortex of the contralateral hemisphere [these are the *corpus callosum, anterior commissure, fornical (hippocampal) commissure, posterior commissure,* and *habenular commissure*]; and (3) the *association fibers*,

which arise in the cortex of one hemisphere and terminate in the cortex of the same hemisphere (Figs. 1-10, 15-3, and 16-10; Chap. 16).

The *corpus callosum* is the largest commissure in the brain; it interconnects most of the neocortical areas of one hemisphere with those of the other hemisphere (refer to Chap. 16). The corpus callosum comprises several portions called the rostrum, genu, body, and splenium (see Figs. 15-2 and 16-4).

The *anterior commissure* consists of two portions. The smaller anterior portion interconnects olfactory structures of the two sides. The larger

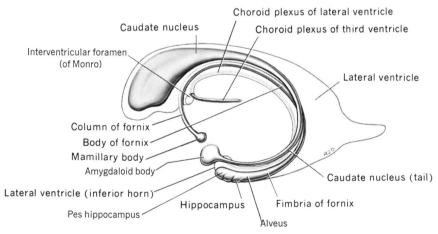

Caudate nucleus

Choroid plexus of lateral ventricle

Choroid plexus of third ventricle

Interventricular foramen (of Monro)

Lateral ventricle

Column of fornix

Body of fornix

Mamillary body

Amygdaloid body

Lateral ventricle (inferior horn)

Pes hippocampus

Hippocampus

Fimbria of fornix

Alveus

Caudate nucleus (tail)

FIGURE 1-21 Geometry of the brain. The horizontal axis is modified into an arc by the curved extension into the temporal lobe. Structures of the cerebral hemisphere which parallel this arc (arc structures) include the lateral ventricle, fornix-hippocampus complex, stria terminalis (not illustrated), amygdaloid body, caudate nucleus, and choroid plexus of lateral ventricle.

posterior portion interconnects the neocortex of the anterior aspects of the temporal lobe (neocortical areas not interconnected by the corpus callosum). In a midsagittal section of the brain the anterior commissure is seen to be located just behind the upper part of the lamina terminalis and in a plane rostral to the interventricular foramen and the column of the fornix (see Fig. 1-7). As viewed from above, the anterior commissure has the form of an arc with a slight posterior curve extending laterally. It extends laterally along the inferior aspect of the globus pallidus and putamen to the inferior border of the claustrum.

The *fornical (hippocampal) commissure* consists of some fibers interconnecting the hippocampus of both sides (see Fig. 15-3). They pass from the hippocampus successively through the fimbria and crus of the fornix (at the site where the crura are close to the corpus callosum), cross the midline as the fornical commissure, and

continue through the crus and fimbria to the opposite hippocampus (archicortex).

The *habenular commissure* interconnects the paired habenular nuclei; it is located in the upper leaflet of the pineal stalk (see Figs. 1-7 and 1-10).

The *posterior commissure* is located in the lower leaflet of the pineal stalk at the junctional zone between the midbrain and diencephalon; it interconnects structures of the roof of the midbrain (see Figs. 1-7 and 1-10).

CEREBRUM AS VIEWED IN CORONAL SECTIONS AND HORIZONTAL SECTIONS

The topographic relations of the major cerebral structures can be understood by examining the selected series of coronal sections and horizontal sections of the cerebrum (see Figs. 1-22 and 1-24 through 1-31). The analysis of these sections, ac-

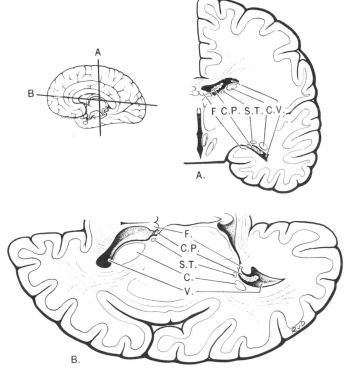

FIGURE 1-22 Sections illustrating that the arc structures may be visualized twice in a section through the cerebrum (see Fig. 1-21). *A.* Coronal section (see Figs. 1-27 through 1-29 for other details). *B.* Horizontal section (see Fig. 1-31 for other details). F., fornix; C.P., choroid plexus; S.T., stria terminalis; C., caudate nucleus; V., lateral ventricle.

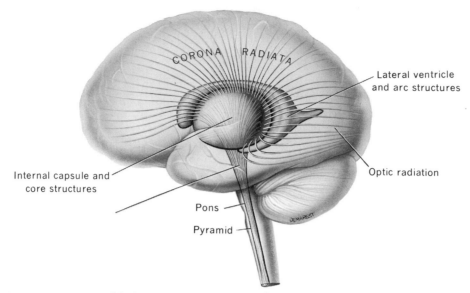

CORONA RADIATA

Lateral ventricle
and arc structures

Optic radiation

Internal capsule and
core structures

Pons

Pyramid

FIGURE 1-23 Geometry of the brain. The internal capsule passes through the central core and fans out to the cerebral cortex as the corona radiata.

companied by reference to the following five topics, should prove helpful.

Boundaries of lateral ventricle as viewed in coronal sections

The *anterior horn* has a triangular outline, with the superior border formed by the corpus callosum, the medial wall by the septum pellucidum, and the posterolateral floor by the head of the caudate nucleus (see Fig. 1-25).

The *body* of this ventricle has a transverse slitlike outline, with the superior border formed by the corpus callosum, the medial wall by the narrow septum pellucidum and body of the fornix, the ventral floor by the superior aspect of the thalamus, the stria and vena terminalis, and the tail of the caudate nucleus (see Fig. 1-28). The choroid plexus, which is attached medially to the fornix and the tissue over the thalamus, extends into the cavity of the ventricle (see Fig. 13-2).

The *temporal horn* has a commalike outline, with the superior border formed by the tail of the caudate nucleus, stria terminalis, and white matter, and the floor and medial border formed by the fimbria of the fornix, the hippocampal formation, and white matter (see Fig. 1-27). The

choroid plexus extends into the ventricle from the medial aspect. The amygdaloid body forms a bulge into the rostral tip of the inferior horn.

The *posterior horn* is bordered laterally by the corpus callosum, called the *tapetum* in this region, and the white matter (see Fig. 1-30).

Basal ganglia and corpus striatum

The term *basal ganglia* refers to several masses of subcortical gray matter deep in the cerebral hemispheres. These basal ganglia (telencephalic nuclei) are in the main functionally integrated into motor activities (Chap. 14).

The basal ganglia include the caudate nucleus, the subthalamic nucleus, the lentiform (lenticular) nucleus, and, according to some authorities, the amygdaloid body (amygdaloid complex, corpus amygdaloideum, amygdala), and the claustrum. The substantia nigra is now considered to be a basal ganglion. The *caudate nucleus* consists of a head (floor of the anterior horn of the lateral ventricle) and a tail (see Figs. 1-21 and 1-28). The tail is long and attenuated (commencing at the level of the interventricular foramen), forming a boundary of the body and the temporal horn of the lateral ventricle (see Fig. 1-21). The *lentiform* nucleus is subdivided

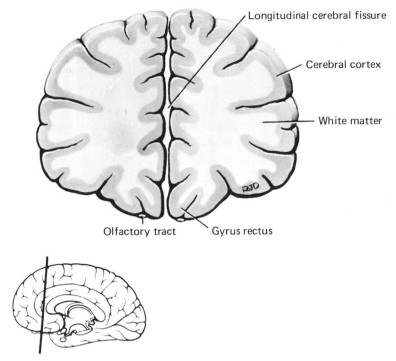

FIGURE 1-24 Coronal section through cerebrum. Level in frontal lobe rostral to corpus callosum.

into a medial nucleus, called the *globus pallidus* (pallidum), and a lateral nucleus called the *putamen* (see Fig. 1-26).

The *amygdaloid body* is located deep in the uncus rostral to the temporal horn, where it is seemingly fused with the tip of the tail of the caudate nucleus (see Figs. 1-8, 1-11, 1-20, and 1-21).

The claustrum is a thin plate of gray matter located between the cortex of the central lobule (insula) and the putamen (see Fig. 1-26).

The *lentiform (lenticular) nucleus* and the *caudate nucleus* are collectively called the *corpus striatum* (see Figs. 1-20 and 1-21 and 1-25 through 1-28). The globus pallidus is referred to as the *paleostriatum*, the amygdaloid body as the *archistriatum*, and the caudate nucleus and the putamen as the *neostriatum* or *striatum*.

Internal capsule (Figs. 1-31, 13-7, 13-8, 16-14)

The internal capsule, so named because it is internal (or medial) to the lentiform nucleus, is di-

vided into an anterior limb, a genu, a posterior limb, a retrolentiform (postlentiform) part, and a sublentiform part (see Figs. 1-13, 1-14, and 1-31; see also Figs. 13-7 and 16-14). The *anterior limb* (caudato-lenticular limb) is located between the head of the caudate nucleus and the lentiform nucleus (Figs. 1-21 and 16-9). The *genu* (knee) is located between the anterior and the posterior limbs—medial to the lentiform nucleus, posterior to the head of the caudate nucleus, and anterior to the thalamus (see Fig. 1-31; see also Fig. 16-14). The *posterior limb* (thalamolenticular limb) is located between the lentiform nucleus, located laterally, and the thalamus and tail of the caudate nucleus, located medially (see Figs. 1-27 and 1-31). The *postlentiform (retrolenticular) part* is lateral to the thalamus and posterior to the lentiform nucleus (see Fig. 1-31; see also Fig. 16-9). The *sublentiform part* is the portion below the lentiform nucleus. The locations of the fiber tracts that pass through the internal capsule are outlined in Chap. 16 (see Fig. 16-14).

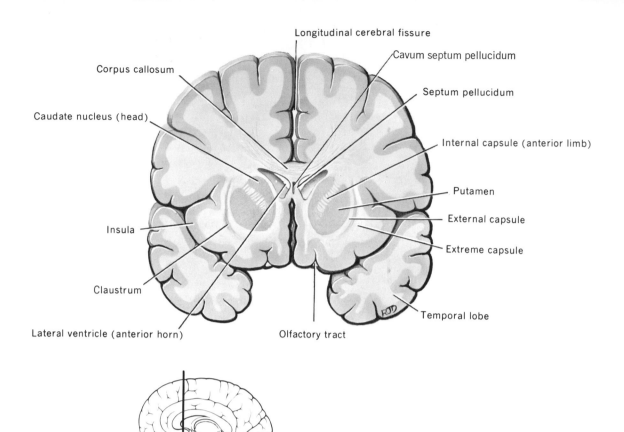

FIGURE 1-25 Coronal section through cerebrum. Level of anterior horn of lateral ventricle and anterior limb of internal capsule.

THE BLOOD SUPPLY

A rich blood supply is required to sustain the ever-active brain. The blood flow is not absolutely uniform, but it is invariably ample. Irreversible damage to the brain results when it is deprived of its circulation for more than a few minutes. Paradoxically the blood circulation provides such a slight margin of physiologic safety that consciousness is lost if the supply is cut off for about 5 s.

The brain requires about one-fifth of the blood pumped by the heart (one-third of the output of the left side of the heart), for the brain consumes approximately 20 percent of the oxygen utilized by the body (as much as 50 percent in the young infant). It takes about 7 s for a drop of blood to flow through the brain from the internal carotid artery to the internal jugular vein. Roughly 800 mL of blood flows through the brain each minute, with 75 mL being present in the brain at any given moment. Approximately 50 mL of blood flows through 100 g of brain each minute. This copious blood flow is necessary because the brain possesses little metabolic reserve and derives its energy almost exclusively from sugar glucose. The brain utilizes about 400 kcal a day, or about one-fifth of a 2000-kcal diet. Because the normal brain is never at rest, the availability of oxygen and glucose must be maintained by a constant blood flow, for the demand is the same whether one is resting, sleeping, thinking, or daydreaming.

The blood flow to the brain is largely regu-

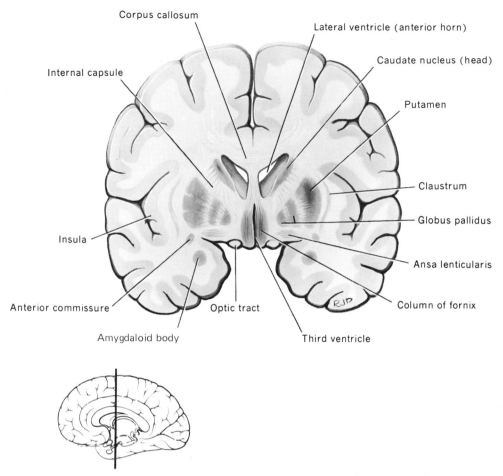

Corpus callosum

Lateral ventricle (anterior horn)

Internal capsule

Caudate nucleus (head)

Putamen

Claustrum

Globus pallidus

Insula

Ansa lenticularis

Anterior commissure

Optic tract

Column of fornix

Amygdaloid body

Third ventricle

FIGURE 1-26 Coronal section through cerebrum. Level of genu of internal capsule.

lated by the effect of metabolic products in the bloodstream on the vascular (arteriolar) tone of the cerebral blood vessels. For example, carbon dioxide is not only the prime physiologic driver of respiration; it is, in addition, a potent relaxant and dilator of the arterioles of the brain. In humans, the role of the autonomic nervous system proper in cerebral vasodilatation is said to be superimposed on those caused by chemical factors. The delicate adjustments of the blood flow of CO_2 and other metabolites are the main means by which the brain ensures that its blood flow is adequate and sufficient with respect to the normal blood pressure (see "Blood Flow in Cortex," Chap. 16). The vascularity and blood flow vary in different regions of the brain. The gray matter, with its higher metabolic activity,

has a richer blood supply than the white matter. The central nervous system has no lymphatic vessels.

The organism has several lines of defense so that the brain can obtain its required oxygen:

1. *Pressure receptors in the carotid sinus* and *chemoreceptors in the carotid body* at the bifurcation of the common carotid artery are integrated into reflexes through the respiratory and cardiovascular centers in the medulla; these function to maintain a constant blood flow to the brain. Pressure (baro-) receptors are also located in the aortic arch.
2. Autoregulatory control of the blood flow to the brain is achieved through the response of the smooth muscles within the cerebral ves-

sels to the blood pressure exerted by these vessels. When the pressure drops, the smooth muscles relax, the vessels dilate, and resistance to blood flow decreases. When the pressure increases, the smooth muscles contract, the vessels constrict, and the resistance to blood flow increases. When the intracranial pressure increases (rise in cerebrospinal fluid pressure), the vessels respond by dilating.

3. Metabolic control of blood flow to the brain is most important. Cerebral vessels dilate when the blood levels of CO_2 are high and of O_2 are low. They constrict when the levels of CO_2 are low and of O_2 are high.

4. When the blood flow through the brain is reduced, the brain compensates by extracting more O_2 from the available O_2 in the blood than otherwise.

5. A severe pressure drop evokes the *cerebral ischemic reflex*. Neurons in the medulla respond by stimulating the sympathetic nervous system outflow to the heart, which, in turn, increases the blood flow from the heart to the brain.

Arterial supply of the brain

The arterial blood supply to the brain is basically derived from two pairs of trunk arteries, located at the base of the brain: the *vertebral arteries (vertebral arterial system)* and the *internal corotid arteries (carotid arterial system)* (see Figs. 1-32 and 1-33). The vertebral arteries enter the cranial cavity through the foramen magnum and become located on the anterolateral aspect of the medulla. The blood flowing through the ver-

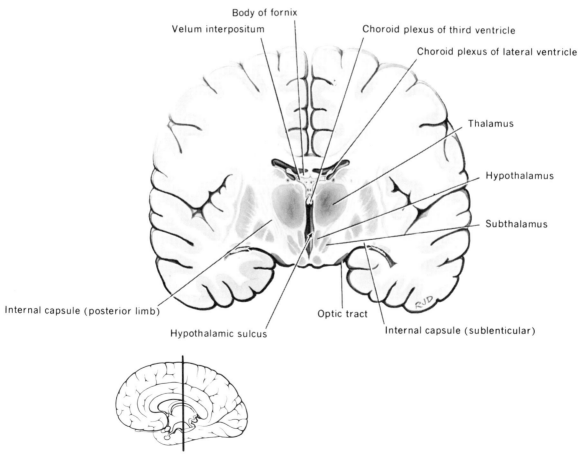

FIGURE 1-27 Coronal section through cerebrum. Level of body of lateral ventricle and posterior limb of internal capsule (see Fig. 1-22).

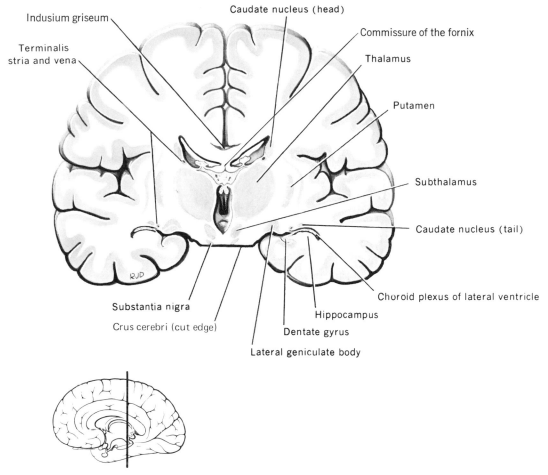

Indusium griseum

Terminalis stria and vena

Caudate nucleus (head)

Commissure of the fornix

Thalamus

Putamen

Subthalamus

Caudate nucleus (tail)

Choroid plexus of lateral ventricle

Substantia nigra

Crus cerebri (cut edge)

Hippocampus

Dentate gyrus

Lateral geniculate body

RJD

FIGURE 1-28 Coronal section through cerebrum. Level of occipital aspect of posterior limb of internal capsule (see Fig. 1-22).

tebral arterial system supplies the medulla, pons, midbrain, caudal portion of the diencephalon, cerebellum, medial and inferior regions of the temporal and occipital lobes, and small variable portions of the lateral regions of the temporal, parietal, and occipital lobes. The internal carotid arteries enter the base of the cranial cavity and become located just lateral to the hypophysis of the hypothalamus. The blood flowing through the carotid arterial system will supply most of the cerebrum (including most of the diencephalon) except for that supplied by the vertebral arterial system (see Figs. 1-32 and 1-33).

The vertebral arteries unite at the ponto-medullary junction to form the basilar artery, which continues to the midbrain level, where it bifurcates into the two posterior cerebral arteries. The intracranial portion of each *vertebral artery* gives rise to the *anterior spinal artery*, the *posterior spinal artery*, the *posterior inferior cerebellar artery*, and a small meningeal branch. The branches of the basilar artery include the *labyrinthine (internal auditory) arteries*, the *anterior inferior cerebellar arteries*, small pontine branches, and the *superior cerebellar arteries*. The *labyrinthine artery* passes through the facial canal to vascularize the inner ear.

Each posterior cerebral artery gives off a number of blood vessels to the midbrain, diencephalon, and cerebrum (temporal, occipital, and parietooccipital branches) and a *posterior*

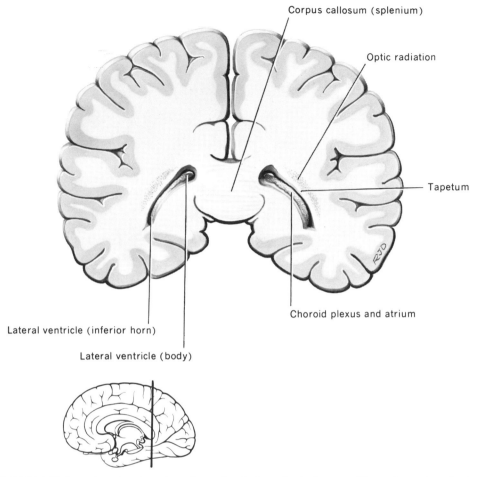

Corpus callosum (splenium)

Optic radiation

Tapetum

Choroid plexus and atrium

Lateral ventricle (inferior horn)

Lateral ventricle (body)

FIGURE 1-29 Coronal section through cerebrum. Level of retrolenticular part of internal capsule and splenium of corpus callosum (see Fig. 1-22).

choroidal artery. The branches of the vertebral, basilar, and posterior cerebral arteries supply the medulla, pons, and midbrain in patterns which may be conceptually summarized as follows: the *paramedian branches* are distributed to a medial zone on either side of the midsagittal plane, the *short circumferential branches* to an anterolateral zone, and the *long circumferential branches* to a posterolateral zone and to the cerebellum (see Fig. 8-23). The superior cerebellar, anterior inferior cerebellar, and posterior inferior cerebellar arteries may be considered to be long circumferential arteries.

Two small vessels from the vertebral arteries join to form the anterior spinal artery. It supplies the median zone, in which are located the pyramids, medial lemniscus, medial longitudinal fasciculus, hypoglossal nucleus and nerve, caudal portions of the dorsal motor nucleus of the vagus nerve, and solitary nucleus (see Fig. 8-23). Each *posterior spinal artery* supplies the posterior region of the lower medulla, in which are located the nuclei and fasciculi gracilis and cuneatus. Each *posterior inferior cerebellar artery* supplies the lateral zone dorsal to the inferior olive in which are located the spinothalamic tract, spinal trigeminal nucleus and tract, nucleus ambiguus, dorsal motor nucleus of the vagus nerve, and roots of cranial nerves XI, IX, and X (see Fig. 8-23). Each *vertebral artery* has

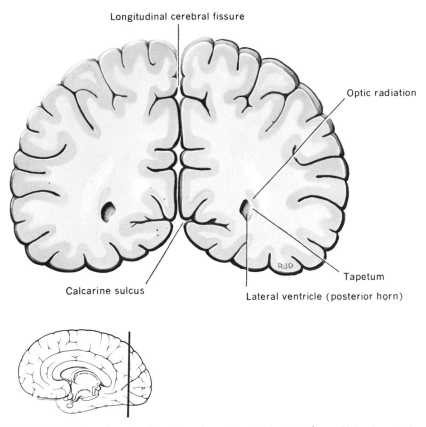

Longitudinal cerebral fissure

Optic radiation

Tapetum

Lateral ventricle (posterior horn)

Calcarine sulcus

FIGURE 1-30 Coronal section through cerebrum. Level of posterior horn of lateral ventricle.

branches which supply portions of the antero-lateral zone of the medulla; in this zone are located portions of the pyramid, hypoglossal nucleus, inferior olive, reticular formation, solitary nucleus, and dorsal motor nucleus of the vagus nerve (see Fig. 8-23).

The *paramedian branches of the basilar artery* supply the medial pons (excluding most of the tegmentum), in which are located the cortico-spinal, corticobulbar, and corticopontine tracts, and the pontine nuclei (see Fig. 8-23). The *short* and *long circumferential arteries* supply the anterolateral, lateral, and posterior regions of the pons, respectively; the anterior inferior cerebellar and superior cerebellar arteries also supply vessels (see Fig. 8-23). Structures located in this region include the medial lemniscus, medial longitudinal fasciculus, spinothalamic and posterior spinocerebellar tracts, middle and superior cerebellar peduncles, reticular formation,

and some cranial nerve nuclei. The *labyrinthine arteries* join cranial nerves VII and VIII and are distributed to the internal ear.

The cerebellum is supplied by the posterior inferior cerebellar, anterior inferior cerebellar, and superior cerebellar arteries.

The vascular network within the midbrain is organized with the basic brainstem pattern of paramedian, short circumferential, and long circumferential branches. The blood vessels include the *posterior cerebral, posterior communicating,* and *superior cerebellar arteries.*

In its proximal position, the *posterior cerebral artery* has branches which, after penetrating through the posterior perforating substance, supply the upper midbrain and posterior thalamus. The *posterior choroidal artery* is a branch to the central part of the choroid plexus of the lateral ventricle and choroid plexus of the third ventricle. Its distal branches supply the cortex

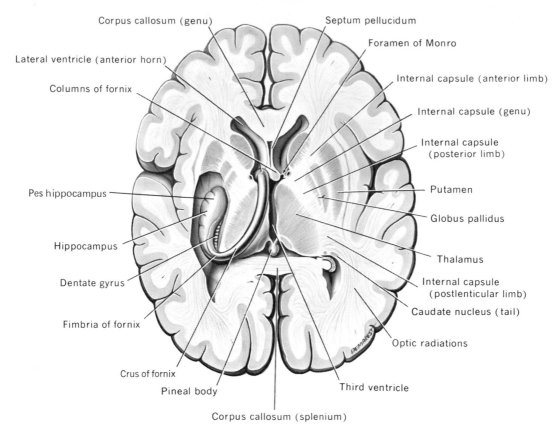

Corpus callosum (genu)
Septum pellucidum
Foramen of Monro
Lateral ventricle (anterior horn)
Internal capsule (anterior limb)
Columns of fornix
Internal capsule (genu)
Internal capsule (posterior limb)
Pes hippocampus
Putamen
Globus pallidus
Hippocampus
Thalamus
Dentate gyrus
Internal capsule (postlenticular limb)
Caudate nucleus (tail)
Fimbria of fornix
Optic radiations
Crus of fornix
Pineal body
Third ventricle
Corpus callosum (splenium)

FIGURE 1-31 Horizontal section through cerebrum. On the left side, note that the hippocampus, dentate gyrus, inferior horn of the lateral ventricle, and the fimbria of the fornix are below the plane of the section, and the crus of the fornix is above the plane of the section. The pes hippocampus is the rostral hippocampus (see Fig. 1-21).

and white matter on the medial aspect and small portions on the lateral aspect of the occipital and temporal lobes (see Figs. 1-32 and 1-33).

Each *internal carotid artery* (see Fig. 1-32) ascends to the base of the skull, passes through the carotid canal, and then curves as a sigmoid-shaped vessel (curving upward, backward, and upward) close to the medial wall of the cavernous sinus and enters the middle cranial fossa. After passing through the sinus, it bifurcates in the region of the anterior perforating substance into the anterior and middle cerebral arteries. The sigmoid contour of the artery within the sinus—known as the *carotid siphon*—probably accounts for the resilience of the artery.

After emerging from the cavernous sinus, the internal carotid artery gives off the hypophysial, ophthalmic, posterior communicating,

and anterior choroidal arteries. Just beyond this, lateral to the optic chiasma, it bifurcates into the anterior cerebral artery and the large middle cerebral artery. The latter is considered to be the continuation of the internal carotid artery. An important branch of the internal carotid artery is the *ophthalmic artery* (Fig. 1-32), which supplies the eyes and orbits. Its most important branch is the *central retinal artery* (Fig. 1-32), which pierces the optic nerve about half-way along its intraorbital course. This central artery runs with its companion vein in the center of the nerve to the retina (a central nervous system structure), where this "end artery" arborizes to supply the neuroretina (Chap. 12 and Fig. 1-32). Some other branches of the ophthalmic artery are components of the *ophthalmic anastomoses* with branches of the external carotid artery. The

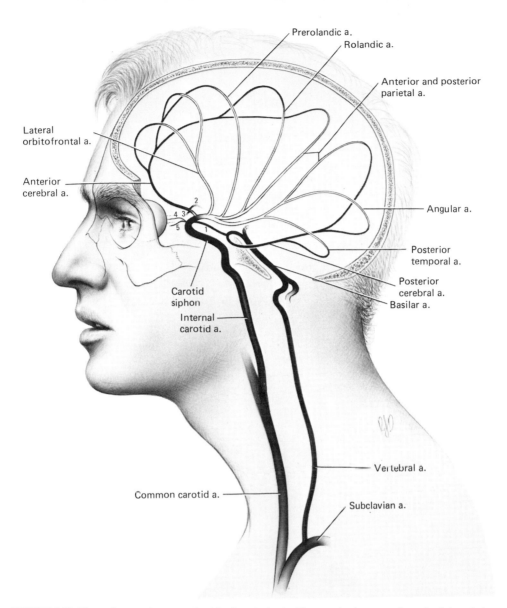

FIGURE 1-32 The major arteries conveying blood to the brain. The vertebral artery, a branch of the subclavian artery, ascends through the foramina of the upper six cervical vertebrae. At the base of the skull the artery winds around the lateral mass of the atlas, passes through the foramen magnum, pierces the dura mater and arachnoid, enters and continues forward within the subarachnoid space to join the opposite vertebral artery to form the basilar artery. The internal carotid artery, a terminal branch of the common carotid artery, ascends to the base of the skull, traverses the carotid canal and cavernous sinus, and enters the middle cranial fossa. Note the ophthalmic artery (5), a branch of the internal carotid artery, and one of its branches, the central retinal artery (4). The middle cerebral artery ramifies through its frontal, parietal, and temporal branches over the lateral surface of the cerebral hemisphere. Its branches include the orbitofrontal, prerolandic, rolandic, anterior parietal, posterior parietal, angular, and posterior temporal arteries. The anterior cerebral artery is mainly found on the medial aspect of the hemisphere. The numbered arteries in the illustration comprise (1) the posterior communicating artery, (2) the anterior communicating artery, (3) the recurrent artery of Heubner —an artery that penetrates the anterior perforated substance, (4) the central retinal artery, and (5) the ophthalmic artery. A., artery. (*Adapted from R. D. Adams and M. Victor, Principles of Neurology, McGraw-Hill Book Company, New York, 1977.*)

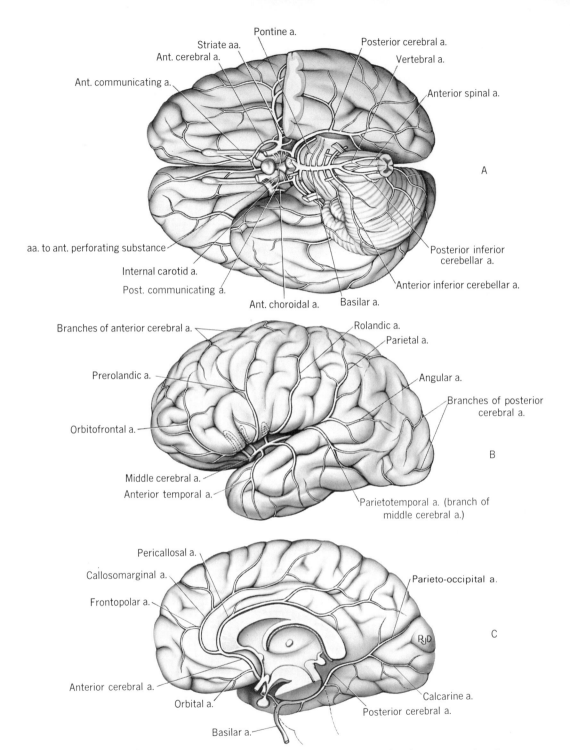

FIGURE 1-33 Distribution of the arteries on the surface of the brain. *A*. Basal surface. *B*. Lateral surface. *C*. Medial surface. * Superior cerebellar artery.

anterior choroidal artery supplies the choroidal plexus of the lateral ventricle and a number of cerebral structures along its course (including the optic tract, cerebral peduncle, lateral geniculate body, and posterior limb and retrolenticular portion of the internal capsule).

A ring of blood vessels is present on the base of the brain which is known as the *cerebral arterial circle (of Willis)* and which includes part of the posterior cerebral arteries, posterior communicating branches between the posterior cerebral arteries and the internal carotid artery, part of the internal carotid arteries, anterior cerebral arteries (but not the middle cerebral artery), and a short anterior communicating branch between the two anterior cerebral arteries. The "classic" cerebral arterial circle is bilaterally symmetric with well-developed communicating branches in only about 20 percent of individuals. The right vertebral artery is often hypoplastic. Absence of a portion of the circle is not uncommon. Generally the circle is unsymmetric; a communicating branch may be narrow or absent. The cerebral arterial circle does not act as a circle for blood flow, but it may act as a safety valve when differential pressures are present in these arteries. Numerous small arteries (striate, ganglionic, and thalamic) from the circle and the proximal portions of its branches penetrate into the base of the brain, supplying the diencephalon, internal capsule, basal ganglia, and surrounding deep structures.

The *anterior cerebral artery* gives off (1) the medial (recurrent) striate artery, which supplies portions of many structures including the head of the caudate nucleus, internal capsule, putamen, globus pallidus, and septal nuclei; and (2) the orbital branches, frontal branches, pericallosal artery, and callosomarginal artery to portions of the frontal and parietal lobes (see Fig. 1-33).

The *middle cerebral artery* runs laterally on a transverse course along the base of the cerebrum and depths of the lateral sulcus before dividing into branches which supply the insular lobe and large regions of the frontal, parietal, temporal, and occipital lobes on the surface of the cerebrum (see Figs. 1-33 and 1-34). The *lenticulostriate (striate) arteries* of the transverse course supply large segments of the globus pallidus, putamen, caudate nucleus, thalamus, and internal capsule. Occlusion or rupture of the striate arteries of the middle cerebral artery may interrupt the motor pathways of the internal capsule, and this may result in the paralysis associated with the classic stroke.

The large arteries and their branches on the surface of the brain are known as *superficial* or *conducting arteries*. The branches of these arteries that penetrate into the substance of the brain are small vessels known as *penetrating* or *nutrient arteries*. These vessels branch roughly at right angles from the superficial arteries and continue through the brain as graceful curves resembling the silhouette of an elm tree. The nutrient arteries branch into extensive capillary networks, which anastomose with each other. The gray matter, with its high metabolic rate, is more vascular than the white matter. One cubic centimeter of gray matter may have more than 1000 mm of capillaries.

Anastomotic connections are extensive in the brain. The anastomoses among the large branches of the superficial arteries are usually physiologically effective, so that occlusion of a vessel need not result in any impairment of the blood supply to the neural tissues. Rich anastomoses exist among the capillary beds of adjacent nutrient arteries and between the deep and superficial circulation. In all probability, true end arteries are not present in the human brain. However, occlusion of the large nutrient vessels often results in neural damage, because the anastomotic connections are not sufficient to allow enough blood to reach the deprived region rapidly enough to meet the high metabolic requirements of the region.

In general, the occlusion of an artery results in a brain lesion which is usually less extensive than the region supplied by that artery. This occurs because the peripheral regions normally supplied by the occluded artery are adequately supplied by collateral circulation from bordering arteries.

The *ophthalmic artery* may serve as an anastomotic channel between the internal carotid circulation to the brain and the external carotid circulation to the face and scalp. This so-called *ophthalmic anastomosis* can help to furnish blood from the external carotid circulation of the facial region to the brain via the sequence of ophthalmic artery, anterior cerebral artery, and cerebral arterial circle in the course of obstructive diseases of the internal carotid artery system. An entire hemisphere can be adequately supplied through the ophthalmic anastomosis following the gradual occlusion of an internal carotid artery.

Considerably more blood to the brain flows through the internal carotid system than through the vertebral arterial system. Although the arterial trees formed by these two systems are basically similar in the brains of most individuals, many variations of these basic patterns exist. In fact, variation may be the rule. For example, a posterior cerebral artery may be a branch of the middle cerebral artery in one in five brains; in this situation the cerebral arterial circle is incomplete. The anterior cerebral arteries of both sides may be supplied with blood from only one internal carotid artery; in this case, the anterior communicating artery continues as the contralateral anterior cerebral artery.

Venous drainage of the brain

The venous drainage of the brainstem and cerebellum roughly parallels the arterial supply. On the other hand, the venous trees in the cerebrum do not usually parallel the arterial trees. In general the venous trees have short, stocky branches that come off at right angles, resembling the silhouette of an oak tree. Venous anastomoses of the deep veins and the superficial veins are *extensive* and *effective*. The veins of the brain drain into superficial venous plexuses and the dural sinuses (see Fig. 1-34). The dural (venous) sinuses are valveless channels located between two layers of the dura mater, the outer meningeal layers. Most of the venous blood of the brain ultimately drains to the base of the skull and into the internal jugular veins of the neck.

The cerebral veins are classified as a *superficial (external surface) cerebral group* and a *deep cerebral group*. Rich anastomoses between the two groups occur through the vascular networks within the brain substance (see Fig. 1-35). The blood from the cortex on the upper lateral and medial aspects of the cerebrum drains to the *superior sagittal (dural) sinus*, which drains blood to the occipital region (*confluence of the sinuses*) and then to the *right transverse* and *sigmoid si-*

nuses into the *right internal jugular vein* (see Fig. 1-34). Blood from the other regions of the cerebral cortex drains into the other dural sinuses in the vicinity of the veins and finally into the internal jugular veins. The deep cerebral veins drain toward the regions of the interventricular foramina to form the two internal cerebral veins located within the velum interpositum just above the choroid plexus of the third ventricle. These vessels join in the vicinity of the pineal body to form the *great cerebral vein of Galen* (see Fig. 1-34). Blood then flows in order through the straight dural sinus, confluence of sinuses, left lateral sinus, and sigmoid sinuses to the *left internal jugular vein*. Blood from the superficial veins tends to drain through the right jugular vein, and blood from the deep cerebral veins tends to drain through the left jugular vein in the neck.

Some venous sinuses are located in the basal region of the cranial cavity. The spongelike *cavernous sinuses* are a bilateral network of venous channels on either side of the sphenoid body next to the sella turcica. *Intercavernous sinuses* surrounding the hypophysis and the *basilar venous plexus* behind the sella turcica interconnect the two cavernous sinuses across the midline (see Figs. 1-33 and 1-34). A number of venous channels communicate with the cavernous sinuses. Although the blood may flow in either direction in these venous channels, there is a general pattern of drainage. The *ophthalmic vein* from the orbit, the *sphenoparietal sinus* (connected with the meningeal veins), and the middle cerebral vein drain into the cavernous sinus. Each *superior petrosal sinus* and *inferior petrosal sinus* drains posteriorly from the cavernous sinus to the transverse sinus and bulb of the internal jugular vein, respectively. Anastomotic connections via *emissary veins* are made with the *pterygoid* and *pharyngeal venous plexuses* in the facial portion of the head.

Several important structures are associated with the cavernous sinuses. The *internal carotid artery*, its accompanying sympathetic plexus and the abducent nerve pass through the cavernous sinus; the oculomotor, trochlear, ophthalmic, and maxillary nerves course within the lateral wall of the cavernous sinus in which they are embedded.

Some of the dural sinuses connect with the

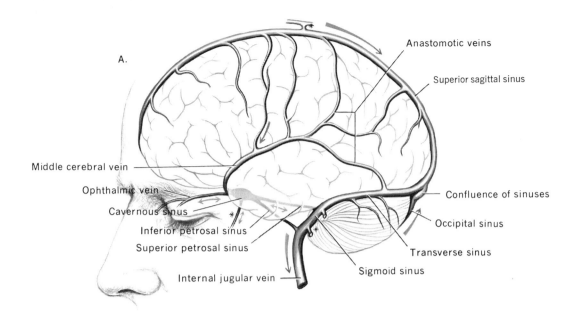

A.

Anastomotic veins

Superior sagittal sinus

Middle cerebral vein

Ophthalmic vein

Cavernous sinus

Inferior petrosal sinus

Superior petrosal sinus

Internal jugular vein

Confluence of sinuses

Occipital sinus

Transverse sinus

Sigmoid sinus

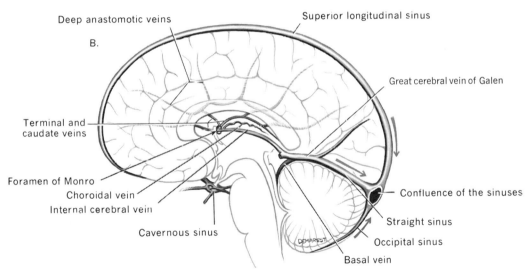

Deep anastomotic veins

B.

Superior longitudinal sinus

Great cerebral vein of Galen

Terminal and
caudate veins

Foramen of Monro

Choroidal vein

Internal cerebral vein

Cavernous sinus

Confluence of the sinuses

Straight sinus

Occipital sinus

Basal vein

FIGURE 1-34 Venous drainage from the brain. *A.* Lateral view of the brain. *B.* Medial view of the brain.
* Emissary veins.

veins superficial to the skull by emissary veins (see Fig. 1-35). These veins act as pressure valves when intracranial pressure is raised, and also as pathways for the spread of infection into the brain case. (Infection in the nose may spread via an emissary vein high in the nose into the menin-

ges and may result in meningitis. This spread may be dangerous, even life-threatening.)

The blood may flow in either direction through the *emissary veins*, depending upon the differential venous pressure within the cranial cavity as compared to that outside the skull.

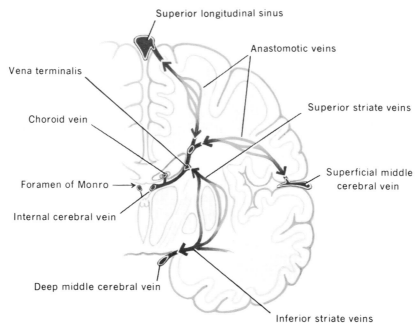

FIGURE 1-35 Coronal section of the monkey brain. Note the anastomoses between deep veins and superficial veins.

Some emissary veins are (1) a frontal vein interconnecting the superior sagittal sinus with the veins in the nasal cavity, (2) parietal veins interconnecting the superior sagittal sinus with the occipital veins of the scalp, (3) the mastoid veins interconnecting the sigmoid sinus with the postauricular and occipital veins of the scalp, (4) condylar and hypoglossal veins interconnecting the sigmoid sinus with the suboccipital plexus of veins, and (5) veins interconnecting the cavernous sinus with the ophthalmic vein and pharyngeal veins.

MENINGES AND CEREBROSPINAL FLUID

Meninges

The *meninges* are the three layers of noneural (connective tissue) membrane that surround and protect the soft brain and spinal cord (see Figs. 1-36 and 1-37). Each of these layers—pia mater, arachnoid, and dura mater—is a separate continuous sheet. The pia mater and arachnoid are collectively called the *leptomeninges*, and the dura mater is called the *pachymeninx*.

The *pia mater* is intimately attached to the brain and the spinal cord, following every sulcus and fissure. It is a vascular layer of delicate connective tissue through which pass the blood vessels that nourish the neural tissues. Astrocytes of the central nervous system have processes that terminate as end feet in the pia mater to form the pia-glial membrane (Chap. 2; see also Figs. 2-16 and 2-17). This membrane apparently prevents the entrance of harmful materials into the central nervous system.

The *arachnoid* (from the Greek *arachnes,* "spider") is a thin, delicate layer, so named because of the numerous fine trabeculae that extend from it to the pia mater. The arachnoid layer does not follow each indentation of the central nervous system, but rather skips from crest to crest. The subarachnoid space between the pia mater and the arachnoid contains the cerebrospinal fluid and the major blood vessels.

The *velum interpositum* is a triangular fold of pia mater interposed between the corpus callosum and fornix above and the roof of the third ventricle and thalamus below (see Fig. 1-37). The subarachnoid space between these two laminae is filled with cerebrospinal fluid and blood ves-

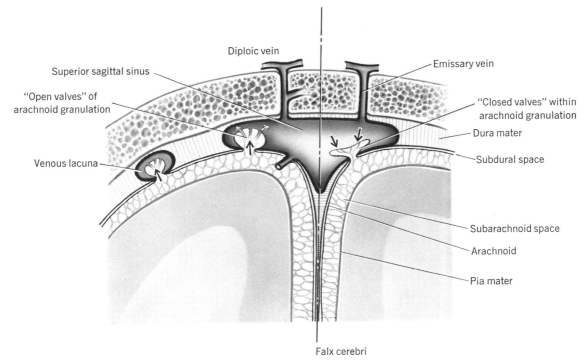

Diploic vein

Superior sagittal sinus

"Open valves" of arachnoid granulation

Venous lacuna

Emissary vein

"Closed valves" within arachnoid granulation

Dura mater

Subdural space

Subarachnoid space

Arachnoid

Pia mater

Falx cerebri

FIGURE 1-36 Coronal section through superior sagittal sinus and associated structures. The arachnoid granulation (left of the vertical line) expands and its "valves" open when the cerebrospinal fluid in the subarachnoid space exceeds venous pressure in the sinus. The arachnoid granulation (right of the vertical line) collapses and its "valves" close when the venous pressure in the sinus exceeds the pressure of the cerebrospinal fluid within the subarachnoid space. The dura mater represents the combined inner and outer dura mater.

sels; it is continuous posteriorly with the superior cistern. This side forms the base of the triangle. The apex of the triangle is located rostrally at the two interventricular foramina, while the two sides of the triangle extend laterally into each lateral ventricle. The pial vascular bed of the apex and two sides combines with the ependyma of the lateral ventricles and interventricular foramina to form the choroid plexuses of the lateral ventricle and interventricular foramina. After passing through these foramina, the choroid plexus continues as a single midline structure extending from the apex to the middle of the base of the triangle. This is the choroid plexus of the third ventricle, formed by the union of the vascular plexus of the pia with the ependyma in the roof of the third ventricle of the diencephalon.

Several large spaces, called *cisterns*, are located in the subarachnoid space. Cisterns are located in regions where indentations are present on the surface of the brain; at these sites the pia hugs the surface of the brain closely and a large subarachnoid space is formed because the arachnoid skips from promontory to promontory.

Three cisterns are located on the anterior aspect of the brainstem and hypothalamus: the *pontine cistern*, located at the medullary-pontine junction; the *interpeduncular cistern*, in the interpeduncular fossa of the midbrain; and the chiasmatic cistern, in the region of the optic chiasm (see Fig. 1-37). Two cisterns are located on the posterior aspect of the brainstem. *The cerebellomedullary (magna) cistern* is located between the choroid plexus of the medulla and the cerebellum. The *superior cistern* of the great cerebral vein is found posterior to the midbrain tectum. The *cistern of the lateral cerebral fossa* is located in the region of the lateral cerebral sulcus. In front of the optic chiasma is the prechiasmic cistern.

The *spinal cistern* is located in the lumbar

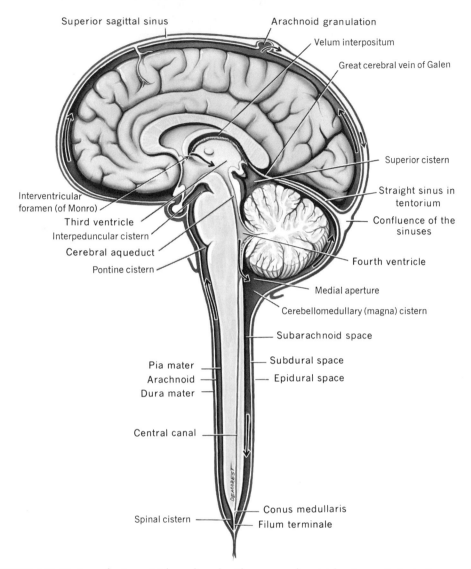

Superior sagittal sinus

Arachnoid granulation

Velum interpositum

Great cerebral vein of Galen

Superior cistern

Straight sinus in tentorium

Confluence of the sinuses

Fourth ventricle

Interventricular foramen (of Monro)

Third ventricle

Interpeduncular cistern

Cerebral aqueduct

Pontine cistern

Medial aperture

Cerebellomedullary (magna) cistern

Subarachnoid space

Subdural space

Epidural space

Pia mater

Arachnoid

Dura mater

Central canal

Conus medullaris

Spinal cistern

Filum terminale

DEARMEST

FIGURE 1-37 Meninges, brain ventricles, subarachnoid spaces, and ventricles. Arrows indicate the normal direction of flow of the cerebrospinal fluid.

and upper sacral regions caudal to the spinal cord (second lumbar to sacral vertebral levels). This cistern is formed because the spinal cord and its pia mater terminate at the second lumbar level (except for the filamentous *filum terminale*—a hairlike extension of the pia mater to the sacral region), and the arachnoid layer continues as a membrane sac to the sacral levels. The spinal cistern contains the cauda equina

(roots of the lower spinal nerves) and the cerebrospinal fluid (CSF). The CSF can be aspirated from the spinal cistern by a lumbar puncture (tap). Many blood vessels are present in the subarachnoid space.

The tough nonstretchable *dura mater* consists of two layers in the head—the outer and inner dura mater. The dura, skull, and vertebral column act as an inelastic case enclosing the brain, spinal cord, cerebrospinal fluid, and blood vessels. The outer dura mater is actually the membrane of the skull bones (periosteum). The inner surface of the bony vertebral canal is the periosteum of the vertebrae.

The inner dura mater is reflected from the skull's surface to form the falx cerebri, tentorium cerebelli, and diaphragma sellae (Fig. 1-38).

The sickle-shaped *falx cerebri* is a midline partition located in the longitudinal fissure between the cerebral hemispheres. This falx extends from the rostrally located crista galli of the ethmoid bone posteriorly to the internal occipital protuberance and the tentorium cerebelli. Its free border roughly follows the corpus callosum.

The *tentorium* is a partition located within the transverse fissure between the occipital lobe of the cerebrum and the cerebellum (see Figs. 1-37 and 1-38). The tentorium is attached to the upper edges of the petrous bone and to the ridges along the occipital bones. Within the attachments to the petrous bones are the superior petrosal dural sinuses, and within the attachments to the occipital bones are the transverse dural sinuses. The tentorium resembles a tent, with its medial ridge drawn upward and taut by its attachment to the falx cerebri. Within this attachment is the straight dural sinus. The inner free border of the tentorium is called the *tentorial incisure;* this incisure rings a space which is occupied by the midbrain near its junction with the diencephalon.

The *diaphragma sellae* forms the roof of the pituitary fossa (sella turcica); it is a dural reflection with a perforation through which passes the infundibular stalk of the hypophysis.

The relatively rigid dura mater divides the cranial cavity into three major compartments— the tentorium separates the supratentorial spaces from the infratentorial space, and the falx cerebri divides the supratentorial space into right and left halves. These compartments act to restrict movement of the brain from side to side and from fore to aft. Should the pressure in any of these three compartments differ from that in the others, brain tissue may shift or herniate from a region of high pressure to one of lower pressure. A most critical shift is the so-called tentorial herniation, in which the uncus of the temporal lobe is forced through the tentorial

notch. The result can be life-threatening when the push of the midbrain against the tentorium damages tissues and obstructs blood circulation. Another serious herniation is the *cerebellar–foramen magnum herniation* (or *pressure cone*), in which the downward-displaced portion of the cerebellum through the foramen magnum can compress the medulla.

The *subdural space* is the potential thin space located between the inner dura mater and the arachnoid. The film of fluid in the subdural space is *not* cerebrospinal fluid. Recent evidence indicates that the subdural space is actually between two thin layers of the dura adjacent to the arachnoid. The *epidural space* surrounding the spinal cord is the space between the dura mater and the periosteum of the vertebral column, occupied by blood vessels and fat (see Fig. 1-37). There is no epidural space in the head because the inner dura and outer dura are fused, except where they form the walls of the dural venous sinuses, which drain the venous blood from the brain. The dura mater is continuous over the cranial and spinal nerves as a dural sleeve that is actually continuous with the epineurium of the peripheral nerves (Chap. 2). The epidural space in the sacral region of the vertebral column is utilized clinically as a site for the injection of anesthetics to block sensory input from the periphery (as in painless childbirth).

In head injuries, bleeding may occur into the subarachnoid space (*subarachnoid hemorrhage*), into the subdural space (*subdural hemorrhage*), between the outer dura and the skull (*extradural* or *epidural hemorrhage*), or into the brain substance itself. The common cause of a subarachnoid hemorrhage is arterial bleeding following the rupture of an aneurysm, which is a congenital weakness of a main branch of the internal carotid or vertebral arteries. Such bleeding into the leptomeningeal space can be confirmed by obtaining blood-stained cerebrospinal fluid from the lumbar cistern (lumbar puncture). *Subdural hemorrhage* is usually caused by a tearing of the bridging veins crossing from the cerebral cortex to the superior sagittal sinus. An abrupt fore-and-aft movement of the brain relative to the dura may occur following a blow which does not fracture the skull. Extradural hemorrhages result from torn meningeal vessels, which result from a fracture of the skull. Bleeding within the substance of the brain itself is frequently caused by hypertension. This can be rapidly fatal because of the destruction of brain tissue.

Innervation of the dura mater

The dura mater and the cerebral vessels are supplied with a rich innervation by branches of the trigeminal, vagal, and spinal nerves, and by sympathetic nerves (see Fig. 1-38). The sensory and autonomic fibers to the meninges pass via the blood vessels of the carotid and vertebral plexuses. The sympathetic fibers accompany the middle meningeal arteries which supply the skull and dura mater but not the blood vessels to the brain. The ethmoidal nerves of the ophthalmic nerve innervate the anterior cranial fossa and rostral part of the falx cerebri. Recurrent tentorial branches of the ophthalmic nerve course close to the tentorial incisure and then spread out to supply the tentorium cerebelli and the posterior part of the falx cerebri. Branches of the maxillary and mandibular nerves supply the innervation to the middle cranial fossa. A recurrent meningeal branch of the vagus nerve supplies some of the innervation to the posterior cranial fossa. The posterior cranial fossa is primarily innervated by ascending branches of the first three cervical spinal nerves. Recurrent branches of the spinal nerves innervate the dura mater surrounding the spinal cord. The large blood vessels of the brain also have a rich sensory innervation. Irritation of these sensory nerves from the distention or constriction of these arteries is the source of many common *headaches*. The ophthalmic branch of the trigeminal nerve is reported to be the one most frequently involved. The brain is actually insensitive to pain; it has no sensory receptors. The cerebral blood vessels have receptor sites for many neurotransmitters (Chap. 3). The *locus coeruleus* (Chap. 8) partially influences the tone of some cerebral blood vessels.

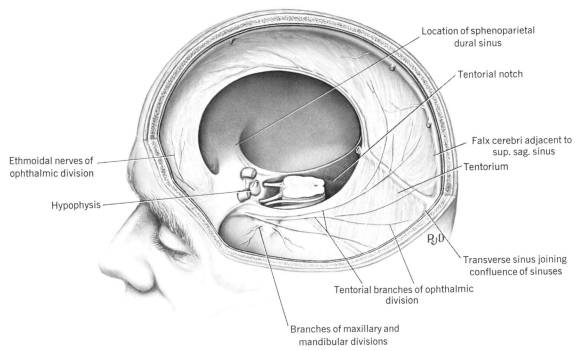

FIGURE 1-38 Innervation of the dura mater and the cranial fossae. Branches of the ophthalmic division of the trigeminal nerve innervate the anterior cranial fossa, falx cerebri, and tentorium. Branches of the maxillary and mandibular divisions innervate the middle cranial fossa. The first three cervical nerves and a few branches of the vagus nerve innervate the posterior cranial fossa.

Cerebrospinal fluid

The *cerebrospinal fluid* (CSF) is a crystal-clear, colorless, almost protein-free solution which looks like water and is found in the ventricular system and the subarachnoid space. The brain and spinal cord are shock-mounted against injury, for they literally float in this medium (like a log submerged in water); the 1400-g brain has a net weight of about 50 to 100 g while suspended in the cerebrospinal fluid. The specific gravities of the brain and CSF are 1.040 and 1.007, respectively. The soft, nonrigid brain, which is 80 percent water, is able to stand the stresses incurred during movements of the head because of the buoyancy of this fluid jacket and the protection of the meninges, and the rigid bony skull. In addition, the CSF prevents the brain from tugging on the meninges, nerve roots, and blood vessels, which are innervated by sensory nerves. Should some fluid be removed, as in certain diagnostic procedures, the patient suffers from intense pain and excruciating headaches with every shift of the brain resulting from a movement of the head. These painful symptoms last until the CSF is naturally replaced.

The pressure of the fluid is lower than that of the blood. In individuals lying on their side the pressure varies from about 60 to 180 mmH$_2$O (not mmHg) throughout the subarachnoid space. In seated individuals the pressure may reach 400 mmH$_2$O in the lumbar cistern, may be zero in the cisterna magna, and is below atmospheric pressure in the ventricles of the brain. Fluctuations in the pressure of this fluid are directly related to and synchronous with changes associated with the heartbeat and the respiratory cycle. High abdominal and thoracic pressures that result during the lifting of a heavy object can raise the pressure in the subarachnoid space to such a level that the venous drainage of blood from the spinal cord is impeded. These shifts in pressure occur because the rigid skull box (dura and bone) does not yield and therefore any addition to or subtraction from inside the cranial box results in a change in the internal pressure.

The volume of CSF in the average adult is estimated to be about 135 mL (75 to 150 mL), of which roughly 80 mL is in the ventricles and 55 mL is in the subarachnoid space. Daily production is roughly estimated at about 300 mL.

In all probability most of the fluid is produced at the choroid plexuses and a significant amount by the brain. The latter diffuses through the ependyma and pia mater (Chap. 2).

The CSF consists of water; a small amount of protein; gases in solution (oxygen and carbon dioxide); sodium, potassium, calcium, magnesium, and chloride ions; glucose; a few white blood cells (mostly lymphocytes and some monocytes); and many other organic constituents. Because the CSF is essentially isotonic to blood plasma, with minimal amounts of protein and cells, it has been characterized as a cell-free, protein-free ultrafiltrate of blood. This is not an accurate description, because the composition of nascent CSF from the choroid plexus, where it is primarily formed, differs significantly from an ultrafiltrate of blood.

Although some CSF is probably the product of extrachoroidal tissues (the brain itself), most CSF is elaborated at the choroid plexus of the lateral, third, and fourth ventricles. The choroid plexus is large; its surface area ranges from 150 to 300 cm^2. Its structural organization is illustrated in Fig. 2-16 and outlined in Chap. 2, under "Blood-Brain Barrier." The *choroid plexus* is a functionally complex structure specialized to secrete, to dialyze, and to absorb; some of these roles are performed by active transport operating bidirectionally. The epithelial layer of the choroid plexus is a key structure for the transcellular transport of solvents and solutes from the choroidal vessels to the ventricular CSF. Some substances are known to "flow" in the opposite direction from the CSF to the choroidal blood vessels.

Following its formation by the choroid plexuses, the composition of the CSF becomes modified during its passage through the ventricular system and subarachnoid space. The active transport and diffusion of the molecular and ionic constituents take place in both directions —between the blood plasma and the CSF, and between the CSF and the brain tissues. The capillaries and associated tissues of the choroid plexuses and pia mater are the sites for the exchange between the blood vascular system and the CSF. The pia-ependymal membrane lining the ventricular system and the pia-glial membrane lining the subarachnoid space are the sites for the exchange between the brain tissues and the CSF. In general, those substances with high lipid solubility (such as CO_2, volatile anesthetics, and barbiturates) shift from the blood stream to the brain to the CSF. Hydrophilic substances of limited solubility (such as electrolytes, sugars, and amino acids) shift from the bloodstream to the CSF to the brain.

The cycle of formation, flow, and disposal of CSF follows the pressure gradient from the arterial stream, where the pressure is highest, to the ventricles and subarachnoid space, where the pressure is less, to the venous blood of the dural sinuses, where the pressure is least. The classical concept of the "faucet" system, although not necessarily correct in detail, has utility. The CSF formed at the choroid plexus (which acts as a faucet) of each ventricle enters the ventricles and flows from the lateral ventricles through the interventricular foramina into the third ventricle, through the aqueduct, and into the fourth ventricle. The CSF passes through the lateral and medial apertures in the roof of the fourth ventricle into the cisterna cerebellomedullaris and slowly circulates rostrally through the subarachnoid space to the region of the superior sagittal sinus at the top of the skull, where the CSF percolates through the channels of the arachnoid granulations to join the venous blood of the superior sagittal sinus (see Figs. 1-36 and 1-37). A minor route of CSF absorption appears to be the lymphatics associated with the dural sleeves of the cranial nerves and the roots of the spinal nerves.

The *arachnoid granulations* are extensive tufts of piarachnoid which, along with the thinned-out inner dura, project into the superior sagittal sinus and some of its outpockets, called *lateral lacunae* (see Fig. 1-36). A *granulation* (Pacchionian body) comprises a number of arachnoid villi, each of which is composed of loose connective tissue permeated by a meshwork of channels 10 to 20 μm in diameter. This meshwork has a valvelike role; it permits the one-way bulk flow of CSF from the subarachnoid space into the venous blood of the superior sagittal sinus, and it prevents the regurgitation of blood from the sinus into the subarachnoid space (see Figs. 1-36 and 1-37). When the CSF pressure exceeds the venous pressure, the "valves" open and CSF flows to the dural sinus. When the venous pressure is elevated (as in coughing or lifting a heavy object), the arachnoid villi are compressed and the channel meshwork becomes occluded (the "valve" closes). The unidirectional flow is, in a sense, regulated by the pressure of the CSF.

The ventricular system and the subarachnoid space can be visualized on an x-ray plate by withdrawing some CSF and replacing it with air. The air may be introduced by passing a needle (1) through a small hole drilled in the skull and then through the brain into a lateral ventricle; or (2) between two lower lumbar vertebrae (*spinal tap*) into the *spinal cistern* (caudal to the spinal cord). The air in the lumbar region can ascend and outline the subarachnoid space of the spinal and cranial cavities (by *pneumoencephalography*); it can also pass through the medial and lateral apertures (foramina of Magendie and Luschka) to outline the ventricular system (*ventriculogram*).

By adjusting the position of the head to manipulate the air into particular locations, desired x-ray films can be made. Many topographic details are revealed. In the subarachnoid space, the following are examples of some structures visualized: proximal portions of cranial nerves V through X, internal auditory meatus, all cisterns, valleculae, subarachnoid space of velum interpositum, and the pineal gland. The following ventricular structures can be outlined: medial aperture, lateral recess and choroid plexus of fourth ventricle, fastigium, aqueduct in the midbrain, supraoptic recess, infundibular recess, lamina terminalis, anterior commissure of the third ventricle, interventricular foramen, and many structures in the walls of the lateral ventricles.

The secretion of CSF is an active process requiring energy. It can be continuous even in the face of an adverse pressure gradient as in hydrocephaly, in which its outflow is obstructed. In hydrocephaly the ventricles are dilated by an abnormal amount of CSF. The increased pressure may result in cranial enlargement in the fetus and infant because the sutures in the cranium have not yet closed. Irreparable damage can occur because the cerebrum is compressed between the cranium and the enlarging ventricles. Hydrocephalus is usually caused by an obstruction at the cerebral aqueduct or, less commonly by blockage of the foramina of the choroid plexus of the fourth ventricle.

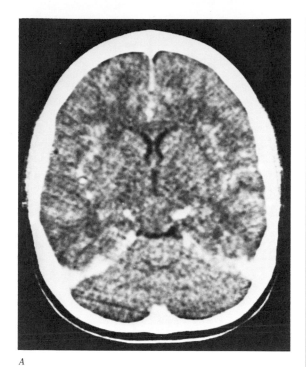

A

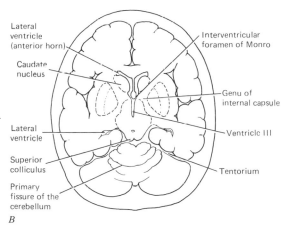

Lateral
ventricle
(anterior horn)

Caudate
nucleus

Lateral
ventricle

Superior
colliculus

Primary
fissure of the
cerebellum

B

Interventricular
foramen of Monro

Genu of
internal capsule

Ventricle III

Tentorium

FIGURE 1-39 *A.* Computerized axial tomography (CAT) scan of the brain. *B.* Diagram illustrating some major structures in *A* (refer to Figs. 1-31 and A-35). (*Courtesy of Dr. Sadek K. Hilal, Department of Radiology, Neurological Institute, Columbia-Presbyterian Medical Center, New York.*)

Computerized axial tomography (*CAT scan*) is a radiological procedure which combines rapid scanning of an anatomic area, such as the head, by a narrow, pencil-thin x-ray beam connected with a photon detector and a computer. The instrumentation translates the differences in tissue density detected along the beam path into a permanent numerical or pictorial display (see Fig. 1-39). The procedure permits visualization of such structures as ventricles, subarachnoid space, cisterna, sulci, hemorrhages, and gray and white matter as well as certain landmarks like the pineal body and choroid plexus.

BIBLIOGRAPHY

Anson, B.: *Morris' Human Anatomy*, McGraw-Hill Book Company, New York, 1966.

Barr, M. L.: *The Human Nervous System*, Harper & Row, Publishers, Incorporated, New York, 1979.

Carpenter, M. B.: *Human Neuroanatomy*, Williams and Wilkins Company, Baltimore, 1976.

Crosby, E. C., T. Humphrey, and E. Lauer: *Correlative Anatomy of the Nervous System*, The Macmillan Company New York, 1962.

Cserr, H. F.: Physiology of the choroid plexus. Physiol Rev, 51:273–311, 1971.

Curtis, B. A., S. Jacobson, and E. M. Marcus: *An Introduction to the Neurosciences*, W. B. Saunders Company, Philadelphia, 1972.

Davson, H.: *Physiology of the Cerebrospinal Fluid*, Little, Brown and Company, Boston, 1967.

DeArmond, S. J., M. M. Fusce, and M. M. Dewey: *Structure of the Human Brain. A Photographic Atlas.* Oxford University Press, New York, 1976.

Ford, D. H., and J. P. Schadé: *Atlas of the Human Brain*, Elsevier Publishing Company, Amsterdam, 1966.

Kuhlenbeck, H.: *Central Nervous System of Vertebrates*, vols. 1–5, Karger, Basel, 1967–1977.

Matzke, H. A., and F. M. Foltz: *Synopsis of Neuroanatomy*, Oxford University Press, New York and London, 1979.

Mettler, G. A.: *Neuroanatomy*, The C. V. Mosby Company, St. Louis, 1948.

Miller, R. A., and E. Burack: *Atlas of the Central Nervous System in Man*, The Williams and Wilkins Company, Baltimore, 1977.

Minckler, J. (ed.): *Introduction to Neuroscience*, The C. V. Mosby Company, St. Louis, 1972.

Netter, F. H.: *Nervous System*, Ciba Pharmaceutical Products, Summit, N.J., 1958.

Noback, C. R., and R. J. Demarest: *The Nervous System: Introduction and Review*, McGraw-Hill Book Company, New York, 1977.

Peele, T. L.: *The Neuroanatomic Basis for Clinical Neurology*, McGraw-Hill Book Company, New York, 1977.

Roberts, M., and J. Hanaway: *Atlas of the Human Brain in Section*, Lea and Febiger, Philadelphia, 1970.

Sidman, R. L., and M. Sidman: *Neuroanatomy: A Programmed Text*, Little, Brown and Company, Boston, 1965.

Singer, M., and P. I. Yakovlev: *The Human Brain in Sagittal Section*, Charles C Thomas, Publisher, Springfield, Ill., 1954.

Sobotta, J.: *Atlas of Descriptive Human Anatomy*, Hafner Publishing Company, New York, 1954.

Stephans, R. B., and D. L. Stilwell: *Arteries and Veins of the Human Brain*, Charles C Thomas, Publisher, Springfield, Ill., 1969.

Villiger, E., E. Ludwig, and A. T. Rasmussen: *Atlas of Cross Section Anatomy of the Brain*, McGraw-Hill Book Company, New York, 1951.

Warwick, R., and P. L. Williams (eds.): "Neurology," in *Gray's Anatomy* 35th ed, W. B. Saunders Company, Philadelphia, 1973, chap. 7, pp. 745–1109.

Willis, W. D., and R. G. Grossman: *Medical Neurobiology*, The C. V. Mosby Company, St. Louis, 1977.

CHAPTER TWO

BASIC MICROSCOPIC ANATOMY

THE STRUCTURAL ELEMENTS

The nervous system is composed of three basic elements: (1) nerve cells, called *neurons* (see Fig. 2-1), (2) interstitial cells, including neuroglia cells, neurolemma cells, and satellite cells, and (3) connective tissue elements, including fibroblast cells and their fibrous products (collagenous fibers and reticular fibers), microglia, blood vessels, and extracellular fluids.

The *neuron* is the keystone; it is the *morphologic* unit, the *functional* unit, and the *ontogenetic* unit of the nervous system. Morphologically, each neuron is in contact (synapse) through its processes with other neurons, so that each neuron is an interconnecting segment in the network of the entire nervous system. Functionally, each neuron is an integrator, conductor, and transmitter of coded information. Ontogenetically, all neurons develop from one primordial cell type, the matrix cell.

The *interstitial cells* are in intimate contact with the neurons and their processes. Actually, the entire surface of each neuron, with a few exceptions (synapses and nerve endings), is enveloped and insulated from other tissues by the interstitial cells. These cells are interposed between each neuron and the immediate blood capillaries and adjacent neurons. The interstitial cells of the central nervous system are the two glial cell types (astroglia and oligodendroglia); those of the peripheral nervous system are the neurolemma cells (Schwann cells) of the peripheral ganglia.

The *connective tissue elements* are similar to the connective tissue proper present in other regions of the body. They have several ancillary roles in the functional economy of the nervous system. The fibroblasts and their collagenous and reticular fiber products are the supporting and structural binding elements of the nervous system. For example, the meninges surrounding the central nervous system and the capsule of some of the peripheral sense organs are connective tissues. Blood vessels transport and exchange gases, nutrients, and numerous metabolic products. The microglia of the central nervous system and the histiocytes of the peripheral nervous system are the scavenger cells, capable of ingesting particulate matter.

The neurons and interstitial cells are embryologically derived from ectoderm; the connective tissue elements are of mesodermal origin. The central nervous system develops from a pseudostratified epithelium, called the ventricular zone (Chap. 4). This "epithelial" origin is expressed later by similarities between the central nervous system and structures composed of epithelium (e.g., epidermis). Both consist of closely packed cells with a minimal amount of extracellular space intercalated among their cellular elements. No connective tissue cells and fibers are located in these spaces. In addition, the cells of both are joined by cell-to-cell junctions.

NEURON

The diversity of form and size of neurons is probably greater than for any other cell type in the body (see Figs. 2-1 and 2-2). However diverse, all neurons have common qualities designed to express the three fundamental properties of nerve cells, viz., the specialized capacity to react

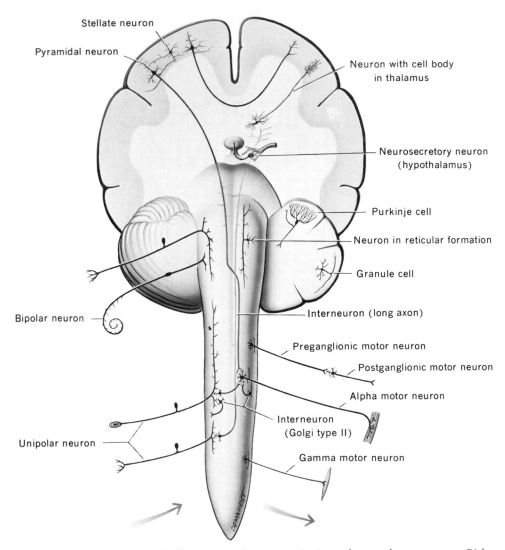

FIGURE 2-1 Typical neurons. Left, afferent (sensory) neurons projecting to the central nervous system. Right, efferent (motor neurons) and hypothalamic neurosecretory neurons (Chap. 11) projecting from the cental nervous system.

to stimuli, to transmit the resulting excitation rapidly to other portions of the cell, and to influence other neurons, muscle cells, and glandular cells.

The typical neuron consists of a *cell body* (*soma*, and *nerve cell*) and thin, threadlike processes—one axon and several dendrites (Figs. 2-3 and 2-4). *Soma* is often used in its combining form, "somatic"; e.g., an axosomatic synapse is a synapse between an axon and a cell body.

Perikaryon refers to the cytoplasm around the nucleus. The cell body (nucleus and perikaryon), the portion of the neuron essential to the life of the neuron, is usually just beyond the range of visibility of the unaided eye. In man, cell bodies vary in size from 4 to 135 μm in diameter; the cell size is roughly correlated with the length of the axonal process. A neuron with a cell body of less than 25 μm in diameter generally has a short unmyelinated axon, while one with a cell

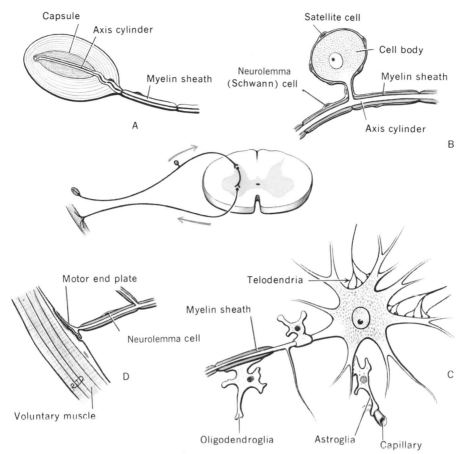

FIGURE 2-2 Structures associated with a three-neuron spinal reflex include the sensory neuron, interneuron, and alpha motor neuron. *A.* Pacinian corpuscle contains an unmyelinated axis cylinder with the corpuscle. *B.* The cell body and its processes of the unipolar spinal neuron within a spinal ganglion are associated with the neurolemma (Schwann) cells and the satellite cells. *C.* Alpha motor neuron (multipolar neuron) within the anterior horn. Note (1) the telodendritic endings of the interneuron synapsing with the dendrites (axodendritic synapses) and with the cell body (axosomatic synapses) of the motor neuron, (2) astrocyte with a process extending to a blood capillary and another process to the neuron, and (3) oligodendroglia with process extending to myelin sheath of axon within spinal cord. *D.* Motor end plate is a neuromuscular synapse between the nerve terminal and a voluntary muscle.

body of over 25 μm in diameter has a myelinated axon. The axonal and dendritic processes are from 0.1 to 3 μm thick (many are below the resolution of the light microscope) and range from a fraction of an inch to several feet in length. The fine processes can attain a sizable bulk. In a large neuron, the total volume of the processes may be from 100 to over 1000 times that of the cell body. The entire neuron—cell body and processes—is surrounded by the *plasma membrane.* The axon and its plasma membrane are often called the *axis cylinder* and *axolemma,* respectively.

Some idea of the relative proportions of various parts of a neuron can be gained from this well-known comparison. If the cell body of a motor neuron of the spinal cord were enlarged to the size of a baseball, the axon would be about 1 mile long; the dendrites and their branches would arborize throughout a large amphitheater. The smallest neurons in the mammalian nervous system are in the hypothalamus.

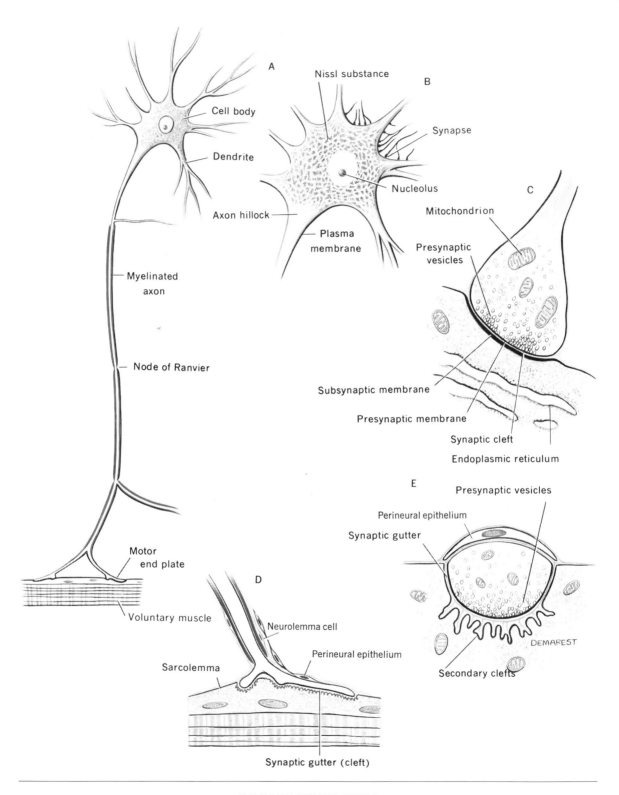

A

Nissl substance

Cell body

Dendrite

B

Synapse

Nucleolus

Axon hillock

Plasma membrane

C

Mitochondrion

Presynaptic vesicles

Subsynaptic membrane

Presynaptic membrane

Synaptic cleft

Endoplasmic reticulum

Myelinated axon

Node of Ranvier

E

Presynaptic vesicles

Perineural epithelium

Synaptic gutter

Secondary clefts

DEMAREST

Motor end plate

Voluntary muscle

D

Neurolemma cell

Perineural epithelium

Sarcolemma

Synaptic gutter (cleft)

THE HUMAN NERVOUS SYSTEM

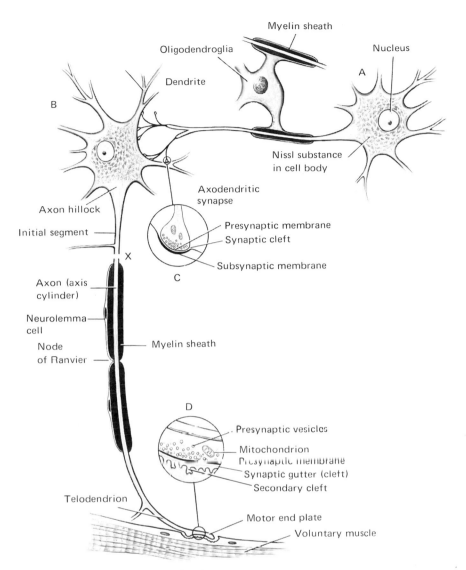

FIGURE 2-4 *A*. A neuron located within the central nervous system. *B*. A lower motor neuron located in both the central and peripheral nervous systems. *C*. Axosomatic synapse. *D*. The synapse with a voluntary muscle cell forms a motor end plate. The hiatus in the nerve at X represents the border between the central nervous system above and the peripheral nervous system below.

FIGURE 2-3 A motor neuron (lower motor neuron, alpha motor neuron) of the anterior horn of the spinal cord. *A*. The neuron includes a cell body and its processes (dendrites and axons). Note the axon collateral process branching at a node of Ranvier. *B*. Axons terminate as telodendria; each telodendritic terminal has a bulbous ending, forming either an axosomatic or an axodendritic synapse. *C*. The synapse as reconstructed from electron micrographs. Note similarities between synapse and motor end plate in *E*. *D*. Motor end plate as visualized with the light microscope. The sarcolemma (plasma membrane of muscle cell) is the postsynaptic membrane of the motor end plate. *E*. Section through motor end plate as based on electron micrographs. Portion of terminal ending fits into synaptic gutter of muscle fiber. Neurolemma (Schwann) cells cover portion of axon not in the gutter. The secondary clefts (junctional folds) are modifications of the sarcolemma.

Plasma membrane (cell membrane)

The *plasma membrane* is the continuous outer layer of the cell body and its processes. Estimates indicate that about 10 percent of the surface area of a large neuron is located on the cell body and the remaining 90 percent on the dendrites and axon. The plasma membrane is a highly organized and dynamic structure of about 5 nm in thickness, consisting of two layers of lipid molecules containing some associated proteins (see Fig. 2-5). The lipids are oriented with their hydrophilic ends directed toward the water on the inside and the outside of the cell, and with their hydrophobic ends directed away from the water and toward the interior of the membrane. The lipid regions of the plasma membrane are essentially similar in all types of cells. The differences among membranes of different cells between different portions of the membrane of a given cell resides primarily in the arrangement of the various specific proteins that are associated with the membrane. These proteins are related to various functions expressed by the membranes. The proteins embedded in the lipid bilayer are called *integral* or *intrinsic proteins* and those attached to the integral proteins are called *peripheral proteins* (see Fig. 2-5). The integral proteins may extend throughout and beyond the bilipid layer or may be present in only one lipid lamina (see Fig. 2-5). Because the membrane lipid is fluid, an integral protein may move by diffusion within the membrane. Integral proteins have specialized roles; among these are acting as transmembrane channels (ionophores) and as a coupled sodium-potassium pump (see Fig. 2-5 and Chap. 3 for more details). On the external side of the plasma membrane is a layer of carbohydrates, which are linked either with integral proteins (glycoprotein; see Fig. 2-5) or with a lipid (glycolipids). This external coat is often called a glycocalyx.

Cell body

Within the cell body are located the nucleus and a number of cytoplasmic structures, including neuroplasm, mitochondria, Nissl substance,

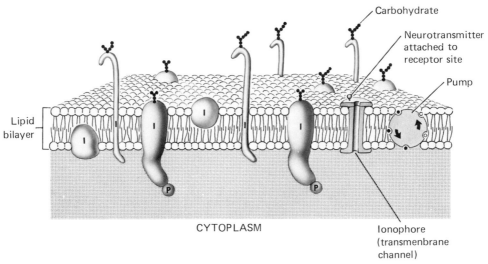

FIGURE 2-5 Plasma membrane of a neuron. Several types of integral proteins (I) are embedded in the bilipid layer of the 5-nm-thick plasma membrane. The carbohydrate chains of the glycoproteins are located on the outer membrane surface. The differential distribution of specific proteins is a basis for regional differences in the functional activities expressed by the membrane (see text). The carbohydrate chains of the glycolipids are not illustrated.

On the right of the figure integral proteins are schematized as (1) a transmembrane channel (ionophore) with about a 0.5-nm-wide pore and (2) a coupled sodium-potassium pump (Chap. 3). An ionophore acts as a selective channel for the preferential passage of an ion such as sodium or potassium (Chap. 3). The disk on the outer margin of the ionophore represents the receptor site (receptor protein) acting as a binding subunit for a neurotransmitter, which is represented as an irregular object above the receptor site (Chap. 3). The pump is specialized to transport sodium ions (open circles) out of the neuron in exchange for pumping potassium ions (solid circles) into the neuron (Chap. 3). Peripheral proteins (P) are attached to the integral proteins.

Golgi apparatus, lysosomes, lipofuscin granules, microtubules, neurofilaments, and, at times, cilia (see Figs. 2-3, 2-4, and 2-6).

The nucleus is spherical and proportional to the neuron it occupies. Its clear vesicular appearance with widely dispersed fine chromatin material is indicative of active transcriptional activity. The *chromatin* is composed of deoxyribonucleic acid (DNA), the chemical carrier of hereditary characteristics. Neurons normally have a diploid number of chromosomes. Certain neurons, previously thought to be tetraploid, are now known to be diploid cells.

The large nucleus is characteristically located in the center of the cell body. Exceptions to this rule include the neurons of the dorsal nucleus of Clarke, cells of the sympathetic ganglia, and injured neurons; in these cells the nuclei are in an eccentric location.

The prominent *nucleolus* is composed largely of ribonucleic acid (RNA) and associated proteins, the chemical substances involved with the synthesis of proteins. Some neurons may have up to three nucleoli. Adjacent to the nucleolus are one or more small DNA-containing bodies, called the *nucleolar satellite, female sex chromatin, paranucleolar body,* or *Barr body*— named after the neuroanatomist who first described it. This Barr body, present in the female but seldom seen in the male, represents sex chromatin. By noting the presence or absence of this satellite in various cells of the body, medical geneticists can determine the genetic sex in the intersexual state and in patients with certain sex-linked congenital diseases (Fig. 2-6).

The *nuclear envelope* is the boundary structure between the nucleus and the cytoplasm; *nuclear pores,* with a fine diaphragm spanning each "opening," are located in the nuclear envelope. These pores may act as channels of communication between the nucleus and the cytoplasm.

The *neuroplasm* is the microscopic structureless cytoplasm in which are located the Nissl substance, mitochondria, and other inclusions. In the axon the neuroplasm is called axoplasm. In the neuroplasm are found the potassium ions and other chemical entities so critical to impulse transmission and to the metabolism of the cell.

The *mitochondria* are present in large numbers and are located randomly throughout the cell body in the vicinity of nodes of Ranvier and nerve terminals and varicosities. Their structure and metabolic role are basically the same as in other metabolically active cells. Energy is stored in the form of energy-rich adenosine triphosphate (ATP); hence, mitochondria are associated with those organelles which utilize the ATP as an energy source for their metabolic activities. In this respect mitochondria are the powerhouses of all cells, including neurons, because they are the main suppliers of energy. The membrane contains *monoamine oxidase (MAO)*, which is important in the degradation of catecholamines (Chap. 6).

The *Nissl substance* (chromophilic or chromidial substance) comprises the intensely basophilic aggregates located in the cell bodies and dendrites of all neurons. It is absent in the axon and in that portion of the cell body, called the axon hillock, near the site of emergence of the axon (see Figs. 2-3, 2-4, and 2-6). As viewed under the light microscope, the Nissl substance ranges in appearance from small rhomboid blocks (Nissl bodies) in large neurons to dustlike particles in the cell bodies in smaller neurons. Electron micrographs indicate that the Nissl bodies are nodal points in the *endoplasmic reticulum (ER)*, which permeates the cell body and dendrites. Each Nissl body comprises (1) broad sheets of *granular ER* (so-called *rough ER*, with ribosomes attached on the outer surface of the cisternae) piled one upon the other in a regular pattern, (2) free ribosomes, and (3) ribosomes in clusters or rosettes of five or six granules surrounding a central granule (*polyribosomes*) located in the neuroplasm between the ER cisternae. Ribosomes are RNA-rich granules. The granular ER is continuous with the agranular ER (so-called smooth ER, without ribosomes).

In general, the Nissl aggregates are larger near the nucleus and smaller near the periphery of the cell and the dendrites. The Nissl substance is the principal protein-synthesizing organelle; it manufactures in 1 to 3 days an amount of protein equal to the protein content in the cell at any one time. Much of it is transported down the axon by axoplasmic flow or transport. Among the cells of the body, large neurons rank among those with the highest concentrations of protein-synthesizing RNA. Neurons are actually glandular cells synthesizing proteins, including "trophic substances" and enzymes essential to

64790

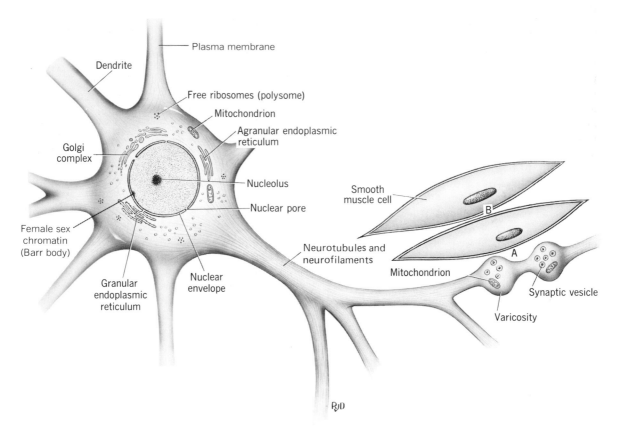

FIGURE 2-6 Some of the cytoplasmic organelles and associated structures of a postganglionic neuron of the autonomic nervous system. The junction between the varicosity and smooth muscle cell (A) is a typical synapse. The junction between two smooth muscle cells (B) is an electrical synapse (gap junction, nexus). The small circles in cell body represent lysosomes.

the formation of neurotransmitters (Chap. 6). Nerve cells require large amounts of protein to maintain their integrity and to perform their functional activities.

When a neuron is injured (e.g., the axon is cut), the Nissl substance seems to disappear in a process known as *chromatolysis*. Actually the total amount of RNA within the cell body is the same. Its concentration decreases because the cell imbibes water and may triple its volume. Within a few days, the RNA responds by synthesizing protein to reconstitute the neuron (see "Degeneration" and "Regeneration" at the end of this chapter). After the neuron is reformed, the cell body and the Nissl substance return to their original form.

The *Golgi apparatus* is a prominent organelle in all neurons which is located near the nucleus and in the proximal portions of the den-

drites but is absent in the axon. At any locale, it consists of stacks of five to seven broadflattened cisternae without granules, oriented roughly parallel to the nuclear envelope. The cisternae are interconnected by agranular ER, which in turn is continuous with granular ER. Some of the protein manufactured by the Nissl bodies is transported via the channels within the cisternae of the rough ER and smooth ER to the cisternae of the Golgi apparatus, where the protein product is concentrated and packaged. However, much of the protein synthesized by the neuron is not conveyed to the Golgi apparatus. In an injured neuron the Golgi apparatus undergoes a dissolution; by the time the neuron recovers, the Golgi apparatus is reconstructed.

Numerous *lysosomes* are present in all neurons. These spherical or oval bodies (0.3 to 0.5 μm in diameter) are membrane-bound multivescicular bodies containing hydrolytic enzymes. The lysosomal system is an intracellular digestive system designed to ensure the removal of injured organelles, insoluble cytoplasmic residues and other "waste products." Its enzymes can break down proteins, RNA, and DNA. As long as the lysosomes are intact, access of their enzymes to the cytoplasmic substrates is prevented. At the death of a neuron, these lysosomes, acting as "suicide bags," release enzymes that can autolyze the cell.

Pigmented inclusions are present in some neurons. *Lipofuscin* pigment is first found ontogenetically in some neurons of young adults and continues to accumulate throughout life. Because the yellow-to-brown granules accumulate during aging, they are considered to be "wear-and-tear" pigments; they may be either the products of the degradation of neuronal cytoplasm by lysosomal activity, or a form of lysosome. These pigments are probably not injurious to the neuron; they are readily found in the aging but viable motor neurons of the spinal cord and cells of the inferior olivary nucleus. Almost all neurons of senile animals contain lipofuscin pigment in varying amounts. *Melanin* is present in certain cells as a dark brown pigment. These include certain neurons of the olfactory bulb, pars compacta of the substantia nigra, locus ceruleus, dorsal motor nucleus of the vagus nerve, spinal ganglia, and sympathetic ganglia. These cells begin to accumulate such pigment at about the fourth or fifth year of life. *Iron-containing granules* are found in nerve cells of the pars reticularis of the substantia nigra and the globus pallidus. Cells containing melanin pigment show very little lipofuscin pigment.

Neurotubules (*microtubules*) and *neurofilaments* (*microfilaments*) are filamentous protein structures found in the dendrites, cell bodies, and axons of all neurons. They are oriented parallel to the long axis of each cell process.

Neurotubules are unbranched tubules 25 nm in diameter with a 15-nm-diameter core. They are not present in the spine or in axon terminals. Neurotubules may have a role in maintaining the characteristic shape of a neuron by acting as a cytoskeleton. They are also presumed to be important in intracellular transport—especially with the rapid phase of plasmic flow; (this is discussed later in this chapter). The activity at the interface between the tubules and the cytoplasm is thought to facilitate the direction and speed of the movement of large molecules and such organelles as mitochondria. The movements may be either *orthograde* (away from the cell body) or *retrograde* (toward the cell body).

Plasmic flow is drastically altered by colchicine and vinblastine, presumably because these drugs, which bind with tubulin, inactivate the neurotubules. Another suggested role for these tubules is in the elongation in the length of nerve processes during development.

Neurofilaments are spiral protein threads about 10 nm in diameter, with a central core of 3 nm. They differ chemically from neurotubules. The neurofilaments do contain actin or actinlike substance and do demonstrate contractility. Their precise function has not been established. Several roles have been suggested: (1) as cytoskeletal elements, (2) involvement with the micromovements of the tips of developing and regenerating nerve fibers, and (3) importance in changing the shape of the embryonic neuron by reducing one dimension of the cell. For example, during the to-and-fro nuclear movement of the matrix cell and its subsequent maturation the neurotubules may be involved with the elongation of the cell and the neurofilaments with the narrowing (purse-string effect) of certain dimensions (Chap. 4).

Cilia are often found in the ependymal cells and in the neurons from many regions of the central nervous system. They are probably vestigial and functionless remnants associated with the epithelial origin of neurons.

Dendrites and axons

Neurons have two types of processes, viz., *dendrites* (*dendrons*) and *axons*. An axon is often called a *nerve fiber*. The typical neuron has two or more branching dendrites extending out from the cell body and only one axon (*axis cylinder, neuraxon*). In these neurons, the cell body and its dendrites form the receptor, or dendritic, zone of the neuron, and the axon is the conducting zone. The receptor zone receives and processes input which evokes a graded, decremental (not all-or-none) response (Chap. 3). The conducting zone conveys influences from the receptor zone via nondecremental (all-or-none) action potentials

(Chap. 3). Some specialized neurons lack an axon; each *anaxonic neuron* consists of a cell body and dendrites. Such neurons are the bipolar amacrine and horizontal neurons of the retina and the granule cells of the olfactory bulb.

The primary sensory neurons conveying information from the sensory receptors in the body to the central nervous system are organized in a different manner (see Chap. 3, Figs. 3-9 and 3-10).

Dendrites are actually "drawn-out" protoplasmic extensions of the cell body; they have the same structural and functional features as the cell body. In a sense, dendrites are the structural expression by which the neuron attains a large surface area for the receptor zone (see Chap. 3). In most neurons, the total dendritic length exceeds the total axonic length. In contrast, the axon is a process of the neuron.

Dendrites The dendrites are relatively short branched extensions which rarely extend more than 700 μm from the perikaryon. From thick bases of from 5 to 10 μm in diameter, the dendritic trunks taper and then divide. The trunks and their branches divide several times. Two daughter branches diverge at an acute angle, with the fork of the angle located on the side distal to the cell body. Small excrescences of various sizes and shapes—called *dendritic spines*, *thorns*, or *gemmules*—are present on many dendrites. They are synaptic structures. There are no spines at the bases of large trunks or on cell bodies. Some spines consist of a threadlike segment with a bulbous ending; these "musical note" spines are the most common. Other spines are thick, stubby segments with bulbous endings of various sizes (see Fig. 2-11). Dendritic spines may be labile structures; they can disappear following deafferentiation or sensory deprivation or even with increasing age.

Many pyramidal neurons of the cerebral cortex have about 4000 spines per cell (see Fig. 16-13). In such a neuron, the surface area of the spines accounts for about 40 percent of the total surface area of dendrites and cell body. In effect, the spines and the dendrites serve the role of increasing the area of the receptor zone of the neuron, which is usually greater than that of the axon. Most neurons are mutipolar because many dendrites emerge and spread out from their cell bodies. Dendrites have the same organelles as the cell body. They are rarely myelinated. Like the cell body, dendrites contain some rough ER and free ribosomes.

The spatial volume occupied by all the dendrites of a neuron is known as the dendritic field of that neuron. The field may be symmetric (spherical or ovoid) as in many stellate cells or eccentric and flattened in two dimensions as in a cerebellar Purkinje cell (see Fig. 2-7).

Neurons have been classified into three groups, on the basis of the patterns of their dendritic fields (Ramón-Moliner and Nauta): generalized or isodendritic neurons; specialized or allodendritic neurons; and highly specialized or idiodendritic neurons (see Fig. 2-7).

1. *Isodendritic neurons* are characterized by long straight dendrites which spread out either from the cell body in all directions or along a given plane. The dendrites show a medium degree of branching, with daughter branches longer than trunk branches. Only a moderate number of spines are present. These cells are the basic neuron of the reticular core of the brainstem (Chap. 8).
2. *Allondendritic neurons* have a heterogeneous configuration of various types; they have a few main dendritic trunks which branch. Examples of these neurons include the pyramidal cells of the cerebral cortex and neurons of many of the processing (relay) nuclei within the brainstem (see Fig. 16-9).
3. *Idiodendritic neurons* have dendrites which branch to form arbors. These specialized neurons include mitral neurons of the olfactory bulb, Purkinje cells of the cerebellum, and bipolar cells of the retina and auditory nerve (see Fig. 2-7).

Axons (Figs. 2-3 and 2-4) The axon of a typical multipolar neuron arises from a cone-shaped region of the cell body, called the *axon hillock*, attains a small diameter within 0.1 mm from the hillock to form the *initial segment*, and then usually enlarges slightly to the diameter that is, in general, maintained throughout most of the length of the axon. Some axons arise from a dendrite; the axon hillock of a stem dendrite is located in the basal portion. The diameter may be reduced in size in the terminal branches of the axon.

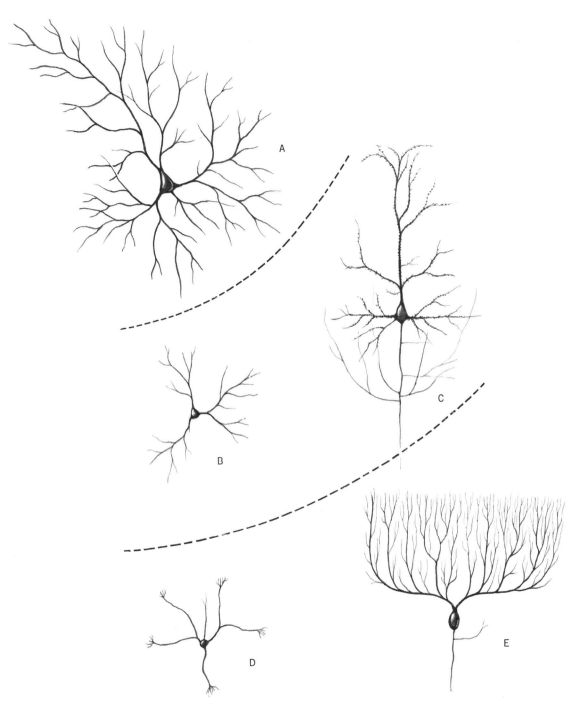

FIGURE 2-7 Dendritic patterns. *A.* Generalized or isodendritic neuron. *B.* Allodendritic neuron of the medulla. *C.* Allodendritic neuron–pyramidal cell of cerebral cortex. *D.* Idiodendritic neuron–tufted neuron of a sensory nucleus. *E.* Idiodendritic neuron–Purkinje cell of the cerebellum.

The axon is usually ensheathed by a segmented, discontinuous layer called the myelin sheath, which is interrupted at regular intervals by the nodes of Ranvier (described further on under "Peripheral Nerves"). Along its course, side or collateral branches may emerge from the axon at nodes of Ranvier. Distally, each axon branches profusely and in an irregular manner into terminal arborizations. The terminal sprays of individual axonal branches are often referred to as *telodendria* (singular *telodendron*, Fig. 2-6D). The initial, or proximal, branches of the telodendria are *preterminal* (*nonsynaptic*) *segments*, and the distal branches are *terminal* (*synaptic*) *segments*. The final tip of each branch is called *the terminal*. A large axon terminal that covers a large surface of a postsynaptic cell is called a *calyx* (Chap. 8) or a *basket* ("Basket Cells," Chap. 9).

In large neurons the axon hillock is deficient in Nissl substance, but in small neurons the ribosomal content is essentially the same as in the cytoplasm of the cell body. A diagnostic feature of the axon hillock is the funnel arrangement of many fascicles of neurotubules and microtubules which extend into and are oriented parallel to the long axis of the initial segment. In some cells the axon may arise from a dendrite. The unmyelinated initial segment (axon neck) is the nodal site, or trigger zone, associated with the initiation of the nerve impulse (action potential). Ribosomes are usually absent from this axon neck as well as the entire axon. The *initial segment* is characterized by several features: (1) it is the narrowest portion of region; (2) it is free of an oligodendroglial sheath; (3) it contains numerous neurotubules linked by cross bridges; (4) an electron-dense undercoat is adjacent to the plasma membrane; and (5) it is physiologically a locale of low-threshold excitability (Chap. 3).

In myelinated fibers the myelin sheath commences just distal to the initial segment. The axoplasm of an axon contains longitudinally oriented neurofilaments, microtubules, and agranular endoplasmic reticulum. The myelin sheath may extend along the preterminal segments but not necessarily along the terminal segments. Internodal distances are shorter in the telodendria than on the axon. The terminal segment has beaded dilatations (varicosities), or bulbous knobs, along its course before it termi-

nates in an enlargement. The presynaptic terminals of an axon have the form of bulblike expansions called *synaptic boutons, bouton terminaux, end feet,* or *neuropodia* (see Fig. 2-8). Some axons have small expansions along their course called *bouton en passage, synaptic knobs,* and *bouton de passant*. Each bouton is the presynaptic element of a synapse. *Boutons en passant* may be located at the node of Ranvier of a myelinated presynaptic segment. In the extensive axonal network of each postganglionic sympathetic fiber, the varicosities have diameters of 1 μm, the axon between varicosities is 0.1 μm in diameter, and the distance between two varicosities may average about 3 μm. Mitochondria are present especially in the vicinity of each node of Ranvier and in the boutons en passant and terminal bouton of the synaptic segments. Some neurons may have as many as 25,000 varicosities (see Fig. 2-6).

Collateral and axonal branches emerge from a node of Ranvier at approximately right angles to the axon. A *recurrent collateral branch* may bifurcate at the first node of Ranvier, recurve, and arborize in the vicinity of the cell body before synapsing with neurons other than the parent neuron. These recurrent branches are often called *sustaining collaterals* because with these branches the cell body of the neuron remains viable, even when the main axonal branch is severed.

Neurons with long axons (up to 3 ft in length) are known as Golgi type I cells, and those small neurons with short axons are known as Golgi type II cells. Unmyelinated axons in the central nervous system lack any form of cellular ensheathment.

Neuropil

Within the gray matter of the nervous system are complex, highly organized entanglements of dendritic, axonal, and glial processes which act as the structural substrate where neural processing of organized physiologic activity takes place. This ordered meshwork of processes is called the *neuropil*. The high concentration of synaptic junctions among the plethora of neuronal processes is associated with the many sophisticated, subtle nuances processed through the functional interactions within this fiber matrix.

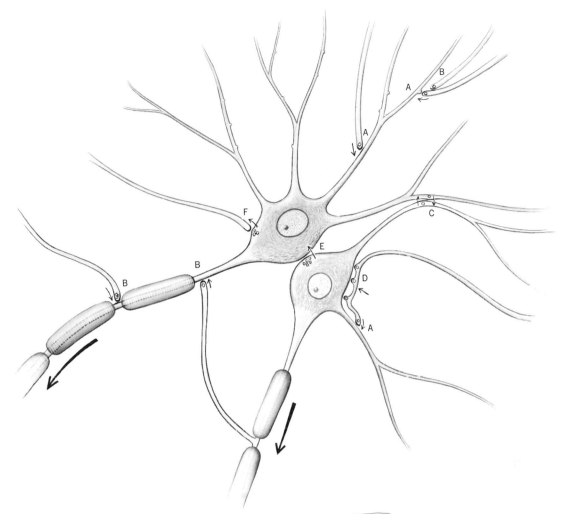

FIGURE 2-8 Several types of synapses: A, axodendritic synapses; B, axoaxonic synapse; C, reciprocal dendro-dendritic synapses (refer to Fig. 2-9); D, *en passant* axosomatic synapses; E, somatosomatic synapse; F, soma-toaxonic synapse.

PLASMIC (AXOPLASMIC, DENDROPLASMIC) TRANSPORT AND FLOW

A neuron is an actively secreting cell which has all the biosynthetic organization and high RNA content needed for the manufacture of enzymes, neurosecretions, and neurotransmitters. The products of the cell body are distributed to the axon terminals via unidirectional (orthograde, anterograde) flow of axoplasm (bulk flow) and transport (not bulk flow). This process of *axoplasmic flow and transport* occurs at two general rates: (1) a *slow rate* of 1 to 10 mm per day, and (2) *fast rates* of about 100 to 2800 mm per day. The slow rate may be accounted for by "peristaltic-like waves" of the axon by which the axoplasm is "massaged forward" like a slug toward the nerve endings. Evidence indicates that fast rates are associated with transport along the neurotubules and neurofilaments. The neurotubules are involved in plasmic transport. This is indicated by the observation that this flow is inhibited by such drugs as colchicine. These chemicals cause the selective breakdown of neurotubules.

Many neurotubules are present in postganglionic sympathetic motor neurons, in which dense core vesicles are transported down the axon at the rate of 100 to 200 mm per day; and also in hypothalamic neurons, in which the transport of secretion granules occurs at rates of 2800 mm per day.

Somatofugal axoplasmic flow from cell body through axon may serve several functions: (1) maintenance of neural integrity, (2) distribution of neurosecretory granules, (3) transport of enzymes and chemicals involved with the formation of neurotransmitters, and (4) distribution of substances associated with trophic activity.

Plasmic flow is actually bidirectional, with some substances being transported (1) from the cell body somatofugally through the axons and dendrites or (2) from the terminals back to the cell body. Thus, flow can be both orthograde and retrograde. Some transport may be saltatory; mitochondria can be observed to move in short jumps.

Basically, the varieties of plasmic transport are expressions of the unity of each neuron and are the means for the maintenance of neuronal integrity. The mechanisms serve to distribute chemicals, enzymes, fluids, and trophic substances to their proper destinations so that the neuron can perform its functional roles. The retrograde fast transport may be, in part, the way information of the state of the distant portions of the processes is conveyed to the cell body. This feedback can affect the cell body so it can modulate its activity to make the critical adjustments in regulating the metabolic state of the neuron—as just stated, an expression of the unity of the neuron.

Synapse

Synapses (*synaptic junctions*) are regions of specialized contact between neurons, between neurons and effector organs, or between two muscle fibers. According to one estimate, the human brain may have as many as 10^{14} synapses. They are one means by which cell-to-cell communication takes place. Many varieties of synapse are recognized (see Figs. 2-8 through 2-11).

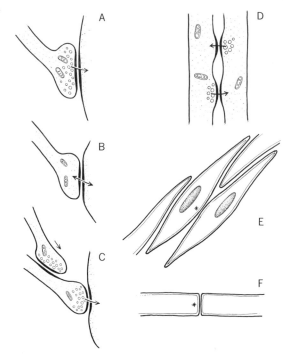

FIGURE 2-9 Several types of synapses. *A.* An asymmetric chemical synapse in which transmission occurs across a 200-Å-wide synaptic cleft in one direction (arrow). *B.* A symmetric electrical synapse in which transmission occurs across a 20-Å-wide cleft (gap junction) in either direction (arrow). *C.* Serial chemical synapses ("nests" or "glomeruli") in which transmission occurs serially across 200-Å-wide synaptic clefts in one direction. *D.* Reciprocal dendrodendritic asymmetric chemical synapses across 200-Å synapses (arrows). *E.* Symmetric electrical synapse (*) with a 20-Å-wide cleft (gap junction) between two smooth-muscle cells. *F.* Symmetric electrical synapse (*) with a 20-Å-wide cleft (gap junction) between two cardiac muscle cells.

Synapse may utilize chemicals or electrical currents as vehicles for communication. In a *chemical synapse* (junction), a chemical neurotransmitter is released by the presynaptic neuron and this substance is capable of evoking a response in the postsynaptic cell. In this type of synapse the presynaptic cell is always a neuron; the postsynaptic cell may be a neuron, a muscle cell, or a glandular cell. In an *electrical synapse* (junction), two cells are electrically coupled so that an electronic spread of nerve impulses directly crosses the synapse from the presynaptic cell to the postsynaptic cell. In this type of synapse, the presynaptic cell to postsynaptic cell linkage may be a neuron to neuron synapse, a

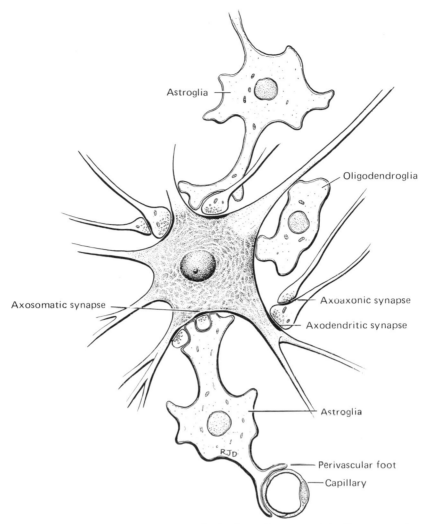

FIGURE 2-10 Relation of a neuron, astrocyte, oligodendroglia, and nerve terminals. The axosomatic synapse, axodendritic synapse, and axoaxonic synapse in the central nervous system have thickened subsynaptic membranes. Astrocytes are glial cells with thin processes extending to the walls of the capillaries as perivascular feet, and others to neurons. The perineuronal oligodendroglia are glial cells with thick, stubby processes.

cardiac muscle cell to cardiac muscle cell synapse (*intercalated disk*), or a smooth muscle cell to smooth muscle cell synapse (*nexus*).

The axon of a neuron may terminate in only a few synapses or in up to 200,000 synapses (Purkinje cells of cerebellum). On the other hand, the dendrites and cell body of a single neuron may receive synaptic contacts from many neurons—from several hundred to as many as 200,000 separate axon contacts. In some neurons, as much as 40 percent of the surface of the cell body is covered with synapses. An average neuron is said to make from 1000 to 10,000 synaptic contacts with other neurons and may receive synaptic input from about 1000 other neurons.

On the basis of the linkage of a neuron with some other cell, there are three types of synapse: (1) an interneuronal synapse, between two neurons; (2) a neuromuscular junction, between a neuron and a muscle cell; and (3) a neuroglandular junction between a neuron and a glandular cell.

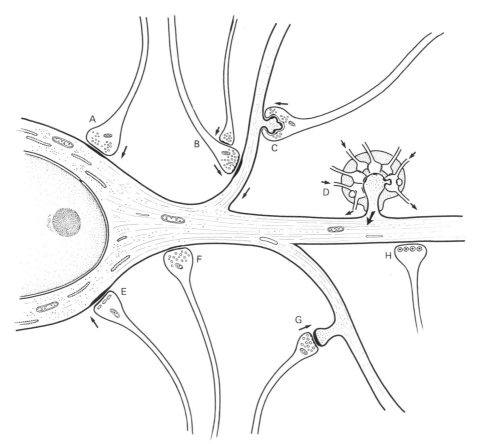

FIGURE 2-11 Types of synapses associated with various regions of a neuron. *A*. Axosomatic synapse. *B*. Series of two synapses consisting of an axoaxonic synapse and an axodendritic synapse. This "serial synapse" is associated with presynaptic inhibition (Chap. 3). *C*. Complex axodendritic synapse between an axon terminal and a dendritic spine. Several postsynaptic thickenings are present on the spine. *D*. Synaptic glomerulus composed of multiple groups of synaptic contacts placed about a centrally located dendritic expansion. A glial capsule surrounds the entire structure. Both excitatory and inhibitory synapses are present in this glomerular processing complex. *E*. Type II symmetric axosomatic synapse. The symmetric synapse (both presynaptic and postsynaptic membranes are equally thin and electron-dense) is associated with flattened synaptic vesicles. The type II synapse is said to be usually inhibitory (Chap. 3). *F*. Type I asymmetric axodendritic synapse. The asymmetric synapse (postsynaptic membrane is thicker and more electron-dense than the presynaptic membrane) is associated with round, clear synaptic vesicles. The type I synapse is said to be usually excitatory (Chap. 3). *G*. Type I axodendritic (axospinous) synapse between an axon terminal and a dendritic spine. *H*. Axodendritic synapse with electron-dense care vesicles (dense core of vesicle within a clear surround).

Chemical synapses (Figs. 2-3 and 2-8) *Chemical synapses* are the classic synapses. They comprise three components: a *presynaptic element*, a *postsynaptic element*, and a *synaptic cleft* of about 200- to 300-Å width between the two elements. In the central nervous system the presynaptic element of an axon is either a bouton en passant or a bouton terminal. Within the boutons are microvesicles, called *synaptic vesicles*, which contain putative neurotransmitter chemicals. These vesicles are clustered close to the presynaptic membrane and lie between some electron-dense membrane projections which form a grid internal to the presynaptic membrane. The synaptic vesicles are ordered among the channels of the grid and make contact with the presynaptic membrane. The contents of the vesicle are extruded by exocytosis into the synaptic cleft while the wall of the vesicle is incorporated into the presynaptic membrane for recycling (see Fig.

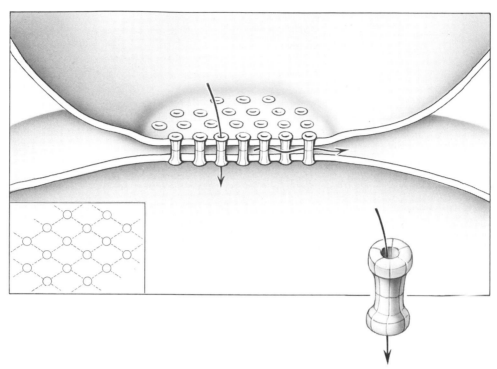

FIGURE 2-12 Gap (electronic) junction associated with electrotonic synapse. This junction consists of a 2-nm-wide continuous extracellular space and a 1-nm hydrophilic pore through a connexon bridging two adjacent cells. The pore within each connexon (enlarged in lower right) bridges between the cytoplasm of the two cells. The connexons form a hexangonal lattice (lower left). The gap junction is essentially a pair of differentiated plasma membrane sites specialized for intercellular communication. *Connexons* are specialized intrinsic membrane proteins (Chap. 3).

3-5). Mitochondria are present within each bouton.

The postsynaptic element is either the dendritic spine or the smooth segment of a dendrite, a cell body, or an axon. The plasma membrane of the bouton is the *presynaptic membrane*, and that of the postsynaptic cell at the synapse is the *subsynaptic membrane*. This subsynaptic membrane is that region of the postsynaptic membrane that is juxtaposed against the presynaptic membrane at the synapse. In general usage, the subsynaptic membrane is referred to as the postsynaptic membrane. No concentration of synaptic vesicles is present in the postsynaptic cytoplasm near the subsynaptic membrane.

The synaptic cleft may contain fine filaments derived from the outer glycoprotein coats of the two membranes. These pre- and postsynaptic membranes contain integral proteins that presumably differ from the proteins in the rest of the plasma membrane. The subsynaptic portion of the postsynaptic membrane contains the specialized receptor proteins at the receptor sites and transmembrane channels (see Fig. 2-5 and Chap. 3).

In some dendritic spines, there is a specialized postsynaptic structure called the spine apparatus; it comprises several flattened sacs separated by dense material. On the basis of their sizes and shapes in electron micrographs, several types of synaptic vesicles are recognized. Among these are (1) *spherical (or agranular) vesicles*, of about 400 to 600 Å in diameter, with clear centers; (2) *dense-core (or granular) vesicles*, of from 500 to 800 Å in diameter, with a dense granule of about 280 Å in diameter; (3) *flat vesicles*, of from 200 to 400 Å; and (4) *large dense-core vesicles* up to 2000 Å in diameter. Some spherical vesicles and flattened vesicles are associated with the neurotransmitter acetylcholine; such associations are called "cholinergic synapses." The dense-core vesicles are associated with such biogenic amine neurotransmitters as norepinephrine or serotonin; these are called "adrenergic synapses." The small dense-core vesicles are found in the peripheral postganglionic sympathetic neurons, and the large dense-core vesicles may be associated with adrenergic endings in the central nervous system. The spherical agranular vesicles are usually associated with excitatory synapses. The flattened vesicles are usually associated with inhibitory synapses. The large dense-core vesicles are found in certain neurons of the hypothalamus which elaborate the hormones oxytocin and vasopressin (Chap. 11). The motor end plate "synapse" is described below in this chapter, and the synapse associated with postganglionic autonomic fibers is discussed in Chap. 6, The Autonomic Nervous System.

Electric (electronic) synapse (Figs. 2-6, 2-9, and 2-12) An *electric synapse* is composed of three components: a presynaptic element, a postsynaptic element, and a narrow gap of 20 Å between the two elements. Because these plasma membranes are so closely apposed, they form a *gap junction* (electronic junctions). The two cells are *"electrically coupled"*; the ionic flow from the presynaptic cell readily spreads to the postsynaptic cell. In mammals, electrical synapses are known to be present in a few places—in the lateral vestibular nucleus, the mesencephalic nucleus of the fifth nerve, and the bipolar cell–ganglion cell junction in the primate retina. The junction (nexus) between two smooth muscle cells and that between two cardiac muscle cells (intercalated disks) are gap junctions which function as electrical synapses.

The *gap junction* is structurally organized so that there are (1) channels with cytoplasmic continuity between two adjoining cells and (2) other channels permitting the passage of extracellular fluid through the gap between the cells. There are no channels connecting the extracellular gap with the cytoplasm of the cells. The channels between the cells are in the form of hexangular "pipes" of protein subunits called *connexons*; each "pipe" extends as a continuous tubule through the plasma membranes of neurons and the 2-nm extracellular gap (see Fig. 2-12). Each connexon has a 1-nm diameter intercellular channel through which ions and small molecules may pass from one cell to another. By this pas-

sage the electrical activity set up in the presynaptic cell can readily spread to the postsynaptic cell without any synaptic delay (Chap. 3). Thus, the two cells are "electrically coupled" by these low-resistance gap junctions. Although infrequent in the mammalian central nervous system, electrical synapses are found in the lateral vestibular nucleus, the mesencephalic nucleus of the fifth nerve, and the bipolar cell–ganglion cell junction on the primate retina. The junction between two smooth muscle cells (*nexus*) and that between two cardiac muscle cells (*intercalated disks*) are gap junctions which function as electrical synapses.

Interneuronal synapse (Figs. 2-8 through 2-11) These synapses are named on the basis of the parts of the neuron associated with the presynaptic and postsynaptic elements. Three of these synapses are numerous: (1) the *axosomatic synapse*, between an axon and a cell body; (2) the *axodendritic synapse*, between an axon and a dendrite; and (3) the *axoaxonic synapse*, between an axon and an axon. Other, less numerous synapses include (4) the *dendrodendritic synapse*, between a dendrite and a dendrite; (5) the *somatosomatic synapse*, between one cell body and another; (6) the *somatoaxonic synapse*, between a cell body and an axon; and (7) *somatodendritic synapse*, between a cell body and a dendrite.

These junctional complexes are identified as chemical synapses because two closely apposed parallel plasma membranes of the two structures are separated by a synaptic cleft, and synaptic vesicles are concentrated near the plasma membrane of the presynaptic element. Dendrodendritic synapses have been noted in the posterior horn of the spinal cord, lateral geniculate body, ventral posterior and ventral lateral thalamic nuclei, superior colliculus, retina (amacrine cells), and olfactory bulb. Reciprocal dendrodendritic synapses (see Figs. 2-8 and 2-9) are present in the olfactory bulb, retina, lateral geniculate body, and ventral lateral thalamic nucleus. Their possible functional roles are discussed under "The Olfactory System," in Chap. 15.

Two morphologic types of synapses have been described in the pyramidal cells of the cerebral cortex. The *type I synapse* is present in the axodendritic synapses on the spines of the pyramidal cells (see Fig. 2-11). The *type II synapse* is formed at the axodendritic synapses of the dendritic trunk and mainly at the axosomatic synapses on the pyramidal cells (see Fig. 2-11). The type I synapse is characterized by thick, dense, and extensive subsynaptic membranes separated by a synaptic cleft 300 Å wide. The type II synapse is characterized by thin, dense patches on the presynaptic and subsynaptic membranes separated by a 200-Å synaptic cleft. In these pyramidal cells, the spines always have type I synapses; cell bodies always have type II synapses; and the dendritic membranes between spines have both type I and type II synapses. Intermediate types of synapses between type I and type II are present in the central nervous system. The type I synapse is called an asymmetric synapse because of the thin presynaptic and thick postsynaptic membranes. The type II synapse is called a symmetric synapse because both membranes are relatively thin (see Fig. 2-11).

A specific synapse need not be a permanent structure; it may be replaced by a new synapse. The degree to which this occurs normally is not known. For example, synapses are lost and new synapses are formed at the junctions between the sensory neurons and the neuroepithelial cells in the taste buds; neuroepithelial taste cells are replaced every few days, necessitating the formation of new synapses to maintain a functional end organ (Chap. 8).

Forms of neurons

Neurons assume a vast array of forms (see Fig. 2-1). The cell bodies have a variety of shapes, with ovoid, pyramidal, stellate, spherical, bulbous, or irregular contours. The axons and dendrites exhibit an apparently endless number of arborization patterns. Some common types will be described.

The *bipolar neuron* is a nerve cell with just two processes. Bipolar cells are found in the retina of the eye and in the cochlear, vestibular, and olfactory nerves. In each of these examples the dendrite commences peripherally as a terminal arborization and the axon usually extends centrally (see Fig. 3-10D).

The *unipolar neuron* (or *pseudounipolar neuron*) is a nerve cell with one short process that divides into two long processes (see Fig. 3-10C).

Basically this is a modified bipolar cell in which the axon and the dendrite are in common for a short distance from the cell body; hence the term "pseudounipolar neuron." The cell body of this neuron type is located in the spinal ganglia of the spinal nerves or in some sensory ganglia of the cranial nerves (Chap. 7). The nominal "dendrite" in this neuron is the long process that extends to the sensory endings. Because nerve impulses are conducted via this process to the cell body, the process warrants the term "dendrite." The length, the relatively constant diameter, and the all-or-none conducting property (Chap. 3) of this long process account for its being called an axon. In brief, the distal process of a unipolar cell may be called either an axon or a dendrite. The other branch that terminates in the central nervous system is an axon (see Fig. 5-13).

Neurons are often classified as *Golgi type I* and *Golgi type II* neurons. The Golgi type I has a long axon which extends well beyond the region of the parent cell body and dendritic field. The axon terminates in another part of the nervous system or in the peripheral organs; for example, the pseudounipolar cells of dorsal root ganglion and pyramidal cortical cells projecting to the brainstem or spinal cord. The Golgi type II neuron has a short axon which arborizes and terminates on other neurons in the vicinity of the parent cell body and dendritic field. These Golgi type II cells are also known as *interneurons, intercalated neurons, internuncial neurons,* and *local circuit neurons.* Some local circuit neurons have axons which may terminate outside the territory of its dendritic arborization (see "Renshaw Cells" and "Gelatinosa Cells" in Chap. 5). Many Golgi type I and II neurons are called multipolar because the cell body appears multipolar, since numerous dendrites extend out in all directions from the soma.

The *Purkinje cell* is a neuron located in the cortex of the cerebellum (Fig. 2-7). It has a dendrite with an extensive arborization in one plane, resembling the branches of a vine on a trellis. Its axon has a recurrent collateral branch. A Purkinje cell may have several hundred thousand synaptic endings on its dendritic tree.

The *pyramidal cell* of the cerebral cortex is a neuron named from the shape of its cell body (Fig. 2-7). Each cell has a number of dendrites.

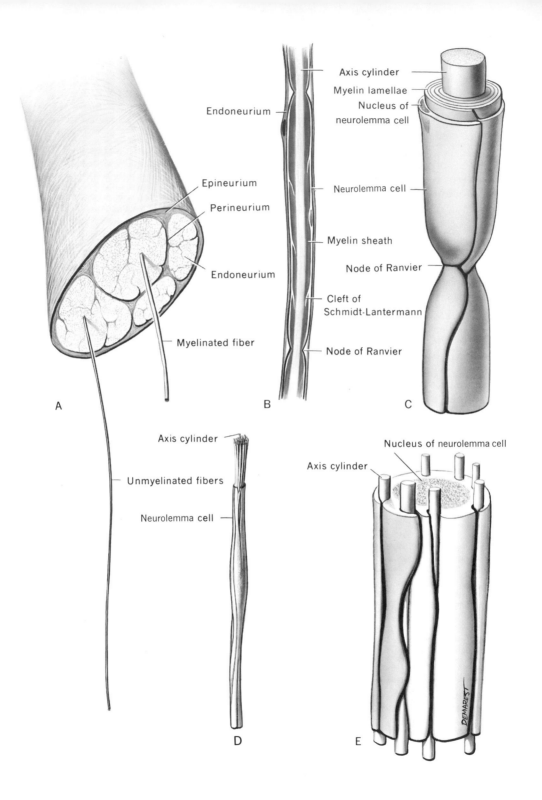

Endoneurium

Epineurium

Perineurium

Endoneurium

Myelinated fiber

A

Axis cylinder

Myelin lamellae

Nucleus of
neurolemma cell

Neurolemma cell

Myelin sheath

Node of Ranvier

Cleft of
Schmidt-Lantermann

Node of Ranvier

B

C

Axis cylinder

Unmyelinated fibers

Neurolemma cell

D

Nucleus of neurolemma cell

Axis cylinder

E

The one apical dendrite extends from the apex of the pyramid to arborize in several branches; many collateral branches extend from one *apical dendritic* process. The other branched dendrites that extend from the cell body are called *"basilar dendrites"* (Chap. 16). The axons of some pyramidal cells may exceed 3 ft in length. Axon collateral branches are present.

PERIPHERAL NERVOUS SYSTEM

The peripheral nerves are the cranial and spinal nerves, including their branches. The peripheral ganglia are the collections of cell bodies associated with the peripheral nerves. A *peripheral nerve* also comprises the three basic tissue elements, as noted at the beginning of the chapter (see Fig. 2-13): (1) axons (neuron); (2) neurolemma (Schwann) cells and the myelin sheaths (interstitial elements); and (3) the endoneurium, perineurium, and epineurium (connective tissue elements). A *peripheral ganglion* also comprises the three basic elements: (1) cell bodies, proximal portions of axons and dendrites (of the neuron); (2) the inner satellite cells (interstitial elements); and (3) the outer satellite cells (connective tissue elements).

Peripheral nerves

A *peripheral nerve* with its numerous nerve fibers is comparable to a telephone cable (see Fig. 2-13). The axons are analogous to the wires, and the neurolemma cells and the endoneurium to the insulation encapsulating each wire. Groups of the insulated nerve fibers are bound into fascicles by the perineurium. Groups of fascicles are in turn encapsulated by the epineurium. Each of these layers is continuous with a counterpart in most peripheral ganglia.

The *nerve fiber* includes an axon (axis cylinder), its neurolemma sheath, and its endoneural connective tissue sheath. The neurolemma sheath may elaborate myelin, a fatty layer surrounding an axis cylinder. A nerve fiber with a myelin sheath is called a myelinated or medullated nerve fiber, and that with little or no myelin is called an unmyelinated or nonmyelinated nerve fiber (see Fig. 2-13). Nearly all nerve fibers over 2 μm in diameter are myelinated, and those under 2 μm are unmyelinated.

The *myelin sheath* is a segmented, discontinuous layer, interrupted at regular intervals by the *nodes of Ranvier* (see Fig. 2-13). The distance from one node to the next is an internode, whose length is roughly proportional to the diameter of the axon. The longer the internodal distance, the thicker is the diameter of the myelin sheath. The length of the internodes varies from 50 to 1500 μm. The diameters and lengths of internodes of the various fibers are directly related to the speed of conduction of the nerve impulse (Chap. 3). Each internode is formed by and surrounded by one neurolemma (Schwann) cell. Between the neurolemma cell proper and the axis cylinder is the myelin sheath, which consists of fine concentric layers. These myelin sheath lamellae are submicroscopic structures consisting of protein and lipid layers that are the repeating units of the myelin sheath (see Fig. 2-13*C*). Each layer is actually derived from the cell membrane of the neurolemma cell. The spiral wrapping ("jelly roll") of these cell membranes encapsulates the axon (see Fig. 2-13*C*). In effect, the myelin sheath is a helical arrangement of successive double cell membranes of the neurolemma cell from a few to 100 spirals per internode; the fused lamellae remain after the neurolemma cell cytoplasm is squeezed out, and the membranes fuse. The *clefts of Schmidt-Lantermann* are present in living nerves (see Fig. 2-13*B*). These clefts are small pockets of cytoplasm formed by local separations of the myelin lamellae. The axon is almost naked at each node of Ranvier, for the myelin sheath is absent at each node. Only the fingerlike processes of the adjacent neurolemma cells interdigitate over the

FIGURE 2-13 Peripheral nerve as visualized under light microscope and under electron microscope magnifications. *A.* A myelinated nerve fiber and several unmyelinated nerve fibers extending out of the peripheral nerve trunk. *B.* Myelinated nerve fiber as visualized with light microscope. *C.* Myelinated nerve fiber as reconstructed from electron micrographs. The helically laminated myelin sheath (jelly roll) is continuous with the cell membrane of the neurolemma cell. *D.* Several unmyelinated nerve fibers as viewed with the light microscope. One neurolemma cell ensheaths several nerve fibers. *E.* Several unmyelinated nerve fibers ensheathed by one neurolemma cell, as reconstructed from electron micrographs.

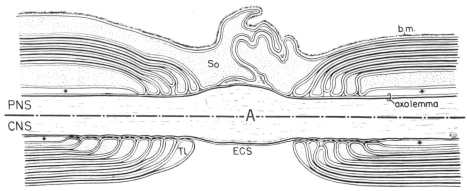

FIGURE 2-14 Regions of the nodes of Ranvier in the peripheral nervous system (PNS) compared with those in the central nervous system (CNS). In the PNS, the neurolemma cell has an outer collar (So) of cytoplasm which loosely interdigitates in the nodal region with the outer collar of the adjacent neurolemma cell. In the CNS, the axis cylinder (A) in the nodal region is exposed directly to the extracellular space (ECS). In both the PNS and CNS the compact-layered myelin surrounding the axis cylinder forms terminal loops (T.L.), which are in close apposition to the axolemma; this apposition may form a "seal," preventing ready movement of materials between the periaxonal space (*) and the nodal region. The neurolemma cell is covered by a basement lamina (b.m.). (*Courtesy of Dr. R. P. Bunge and the American Physiological Society.*)

nodal area in the peripheral nervous system (see Fig. 2-14); the nodes are naked in the central nervous system (see Fig. 2-14).

Four features of the nodes are important: (1) nerve fibers branch at a node; (2) concentrations of mitochondria in the axis cylinder at these sites suggest local high metabolic activity; (3) the close proximity of extracellular fluids to the axon at each node is critical to saltatory conduction (Chap. 3); and (4) the possible isolation of the periaxonal space of the internode from the node of Ranvier by the close appostion of the terminal loops of the myelin sheath to the axolemma (see Fig. 2-14) may be critical to saltatory conduction.

Whereas a myelinated fiber is ensheathed by its private layer of neurolemma cells, a group of *unmyelinated fibers* share a common neurolemma cell (see Fig. 2-15). As many as 20 or more unmyelinated fibers may share one neurolemma cell. These fibers are separated from one another, for each is embedded in a private sleeve of the surface of the neurolemma cell's plasma membrane. The fibers are not within the cytoplasm of the neurolemma cell, for the cell membrane of the neurolemma cell is intact everywhere. In effect, a theoretical myelin sheath is represented by the cell membrane of the neurolemma cell. The axons comprising the olfactory nerve present an unusual arrangement. Up to

several dozens of axons are organized into a fascicle surrounded by one neurolemma cell; the axons in each fascicle are essentially in direct contact with each other (axons are separated by spaces 100 Å wide). The olfactory nerve comprises many fascicles (Chap. 15).

The *peripheral nerves and ganglia* of both the somatic and autonomic nervous system consist of myelinated and unmyelinated fibers bound together by several layers composed of connective tissue elements and by a layer of epithelium (see Fig. 2-13). The *endoneurium* (*sheath of Henle*) surrounds each neurolemma cell as a private sheath; it comprises the basal lamina associated with the neurolemma cell, some scattered mesenchymal cells, fibroblasts, histiocytes, and a few delicate connective tissue fibers. The *perineurium* surrounds nerve fibers grouped into fascicles; it comprises an *outer lamina of connective tissue* and an *inner lamina of epithelium*. The inner lamina is a thin, continuous, multilayered sheet of squamous epithelial cells—called the *perineural epithelium*. It extends centrally along the dorsal and ventral roots, where it is continuous with the piarachnoid layers, and peripherally to form the capsules of the sensory receptors (e.g., Pacinian and Meissner's corpuscles and neuromuscular spindles) and motor end plates (see Fig. 2-3). The perineural epithelium is thought to provide a barrier to the passage of

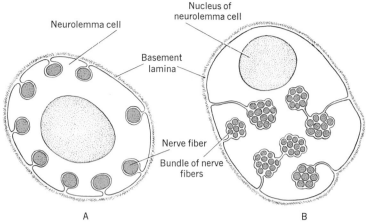

FIGURE 2-15 Unmyelinated fibers of peripheral nervous system. *A.* Nine myelinated fibers enclosed in individual troughs of a neurolemma cell. *B.* Clusters of groups of fine fibers enclosed in troughs of a neurolemma cell as in the olfactory nerve. (*After Dr. R. P. Bunge.*)

many substances from the connective tissue of the epineurium and perineurium to the nerve fibers. The *epineurium* binds together large numbers of fascicles into the named peripheral nerves of gross anatomy. The connective tissue lamina of the perineurium of these layers are continuous with the dura mater. The connective tissue serves several useful purposes: a supportive role, a nutritive role by providing a network of blood vessels, and a role in the conductile activity of the nerve fiber through the electrolytes in the interstitial fluids.

Peripheral ganglia

The *ganglia* of the peripheral nervous system are the structures consisting of the cell bodies and their adjacent cell processes. Two types of ganglia are present: (1) the sensory (afferent) ganglia of the cranial nerves and the spinal ganglia of the spinal nerves, and (2) the motor ganglia of the autonomic nervous system.

The *sensory ganglia*, located close to the central nervous system, are usually aggregations of unipolar cells (Chap. 5). No synapses are found in these ganglia. One process of these unipolar cells extends distally through a peripheral nerve to a sensory ending; the other process projects into the central nervous system (see Fig. 2-2).

The *autonomic motor ganglia*, located at a distance from the central nervous system, are aggregations of multipolar (postganglionic) neurons of the autonomic nervous system (Chap. 6). The dendrites and cell bodies of these multipolar neurons, which are located wholly within a ganglion, make synaptic connections with the axons of preganglionic neurons (Chap. 6).

Each cell body of each ganglion is encapsulated by a single layer of inner satellite (capsular) cells which is continuous with the neurolemma cell layer of a peripheral nerve fiber. No myelin sheath is associated with the cell bodies, except in two cases: The cell bodies of the vestibular and spiral ganglia of the eighth cranial nerve are myelinated. Surrounding the layer of the inner satellite cells is the layer of outer satellite cells, which is continuous with the endoneurium surrounding the peripheral nerve fiber. The connective tissue binding the ganglia is continuous with the perineurium and epineurium of the peripheral nerve. These layers are often absent or scant in the small ganglia (parasympathetic ganglia) in smooth muscle.

THE CENTRAL NERVOUS SYSTEM

The central nervous sytem is composed of the same three basic elements as the peripheral nervous system: neurons, neuroglia (astroglia, oligodendroglia, and radial glia) of the interstitial elements, and microglia and blood vessels of the connective tissue elements.

Neuroglia and other elements
(Figs. 2-10 and 2-16)

The neuroglial (glial) cells outnumber the neurons and comprise about half the total volume and weight of the brain and spinal cord. Literally the neurons are in a sea of glial cells (Figs. 2-10, 2-16, 2-17, and 2-18). Depending upon the region glial cells outnumber neurons by 10 to 100 times.

The neuroglia cells—"nerve-glue"—are metabolically supportive cells of the nervous system, assisting the neurons to perform their roles. Glial cells do not form synapses or generate action potentials. They do form and sustain the myelin sheaths. In ways not fully defined, the glial cells have significant roles in regulating the ionic concentration within the extracellular space so critical to the electrophysiologic activity of neurons. In addition, they may act as intermediary stations for conveying nutrients, gases, and waste products between the neurons and the vascular system and cerebrospinal fluid. Most tumors originating within the central nervous system arise from neuroglial elements. In brief, the glial cells provide the structural and metabolic support for the extensive and delicate network of the neurons.

Neuroglia—"nerve glue"—are classified into the following types: (1) oligodendrocytes, (2) astrocytes, (3) microglia, (4) radial glia, and (5) peripheral glia. The glial cells were initially named by their appearance in silver-stained sections viewed with a light microscope. Glial cells called tanacytes extend from the cavity of the third ventricle to the pia surface in the hypothalamus (see Chap. 11). Special glial cells are Muller's cells of the retina (see Chap. 12) and Bergmann cells of the cerebellar cortex (see Chap. 9).

Oligodendrocytes (oligodendroglia) Three general types of oligodendrocytes are recognized: perineuronal (satellite) oligodendrocytes, adjacent to the cell bodies of neurons; interfascicular oligodendrocytes, associated with the myelin sheaths; and perivascular oligodendrocytes, in the vicinity of blood vessels.

The perineuronal (satellite) oligodendrocytes are found in gray matter, whereas the interfascicular oligodendrocytes are located between nerve fibers of the white matter and with groups of myelinated fibers located in the gray matter (see Figs. 2-10 and 2-14). An oligodendrocyte can be distinguished from an astrocyte by several criteria. It has a smaller, rounder, denser nucleus; only a few delicate processes extend from its cell body. Within their denser cytoplasm are many microtubules, mitochondria, and ribosomes but no filaments nor glycogen. Except for the form of their processes, these types of oligodendrocytes are morphologically similar.

Oligodendrocytes are presumed to perform two roles: forming and maintaining the myelin in the central nervous system; and sustaining neurons by supplying nutrition and possibly some unknown factors. A symbiotic association between these cells and neurons is an intriguing possibility.

The perineuronal oligodendrocytes that encapsulate the cell bodies are equivalent to the satellite cells of the spinal ganglia and autonomic peripheral ganglia. The interfascicular oligodendroglia surrounding the nerve fibers are the equivalent of the neurolemma (Schwann) cells of the peripheral nerves. All these cells are derived from ectoderm.

The myelin sheaths of the axons in the central nervous system are the products of layers of the plasma membranes of oligodendrocytes. Each oligodendroglial cell forms and maintains more than 50 internodal segments of many axons (see Fig. 2-16). Extending from each of these glial cells are several cytoplasmic tongues surrounded by the plasma membrane; each tongue extends to an axon, where it spreads out as a flat, thin sheath and a myelin membrane spiral. This is the myelinated internode. In brief, myelin sheaths of the central nervous system and peripheral nervous system are similar; both are compacted layers of plasma membranes. The nodes of Ranvier in the central nervous system are exposed directly to the extracellular space; the node is not ensheathed by the plasma membrane of the glial cell. The tongue probably serves as the route through which material from the cell body passes to sustain the myelin sheath. Unmyelinated fibers of the central nervous system lack any form of cellular ensheathment.

Astrocytes (astroglia) Two types of astrocytes include protoplasmic astrocytes, located primarily in the gray matter of the brain and spinal

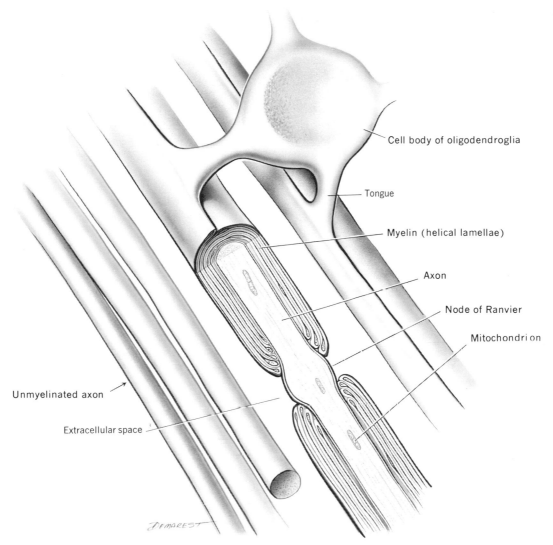

Cell body of oligodendroglia

Tongue

Myelin (helical lamellae)

Axon

Node of Ranvier

Mitochondrion

Unmyelinated axon

Extracellular space

FIGURE 2-16 Relation of oligodendroglia to the axons of the central nervous system, as reconstructed from electron micrographs. The three unmyelinated axons on the left are naked. The two myelinated axons on the right share one oligodendroglial cell. The myelin sheaths of each of the myelinated fibers are continuous through the protoplasmic tongue with the glial cell body. This glial tongue spreads out as a ridge, which extends throughout the entire length of an internode. The loop of the cell membrane at the ridge makes the site where the glial cell membrane is doubled (myelin unit of two plasma cell membranes) and is continuous as the laminated myelin sheath. (*Adapted from Bunge, Bunge, and Ris.*)

cord, and *fibrous astrocytes,* found chiefly in the white matter. As compared to an oligodendrocyte, an astrocyte has a larger, irregular ovoid nucleus, which is less compact; many cytoplasmic processes extend from its cell body. Cytoplasmic filaments and glycogen are characteristic.

The processes of the glial cells may extend to the blood capillaries to form *vascular feet, end feet,* or "sucker feet"; the *pia-glial membrane* (*external limiting gliosal membrane, glia limitans*) adjacent to the subarachnoid space (see Fig. 2-17); and the nonsynaptic surface of a neuron (see Fig. 2-18). In some regions of the brain, gap

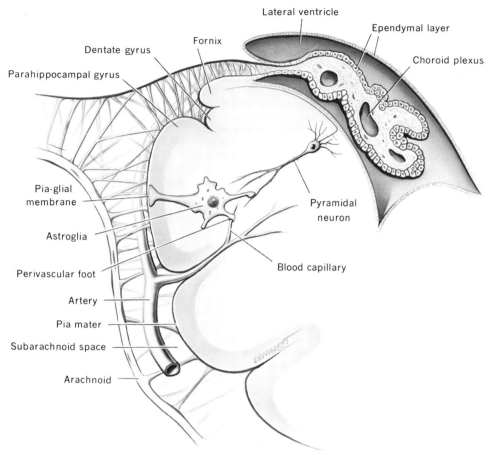

FIGURE 2-17 Relations of the leptomeninges, subarachnoid, choroid plexus, ventricle, astroglia, and neurons of the central nervous system. The subarachnoid space is located between the arachnoid and pia mater. The choroid plexus is composed of an ependymal layer and a highly vascularized connective tissue core. Subarachnoid blood vessels and subarachnoid space are continuous with the core of the choroid plexus. The astrocyte has several processes: one extends to a blood capillary and terminates as a perivascular foot; another process extends to and contacts the pyramidal neuron; and another extends to the pia mater.

junctions interconnect two glial cells (refer to "Blood-Brain Barrier," further on).

The *ependymal* cells lining the ventricular system and choroid plexuses, tanacytes of the hypothalamus (Chap. 11), pituicytes of the neurohypophysis (Chap. 11) and Muller's cells of the retina (Chap. 12 and Fig. 12-8) are considered to be forms of astrocytes.

Microglia The *microglia* are phagocytic cells which are related to the macrophages of the connective tissues. The microglia are found throughout the central nervous system; under proper stresses, as in an injury, they function to phagocytize, transform, and remove disintegration products of the neurons. They act as scavengers.

Radial glia The radial glial cell consists of a cell body usually located close to the ventricular surface of the developing central nervous system (see Figs. 4-4 and 4-6). It has an elongated radial fiber which extends distally and terminates as conical end feet at either the pial surface or on the wall of a blood vessel. The Bergmann cells of the cerebellum cortex are a form of radial glia. The fibers of these radial glial cells have a significant role in providing guidance for migrating neurons in the central nervous system. These cells are considered by some to be specialized astrocytes.

Peripheral glia   The peripheral glial cells are the inner satellite cells of the peripheral ganglia and the neurolemma (Schwann) cells of the peripheral nervous system. In a sense, the neurolemma cells are the oligodendrocytes of the peripheral nervous system.

Several recognized functions of the glial cells include:

1. *Formation of the myelin sheath.* The lamellated myelin sheath around the axons is formed by the neurolemma cells of the peripheral nervous system and the interfascicular oligodendrocytes of the central nervous system.
2. *Removal of debris of severely diseased or injured cells.* As previously noted, microglia are the phagocytes of the central nervous system.
3. *Repair following damage from injury.* The fibrous astrocytes are considered to be the scarring cells of the nervous system which repair the gaps caused by destruction of neural tissues from a variety of insults. Connective tissue may also contribute to the central nervous system scarring, which is called sclerosis.
4. *Guides during embryonal and fetal development.* As previously noted, the glial fibers of the radial glia act as guides for the migration of neurons and the growth of their processes.
5. *Structural support.* Strong doubts are now cast on the old concept that glial cells have a role in the mechanical support of neural tissues.
6. *Putative roles.* Some evidence suggests that there is macromolecular communication between glia and neurons. This may occur (*a*) by the actual transfer of macromolecules from one cell to another or (*b*) by action of macromolecules of glia on the surface constituents of neurons. Communication may occur via gap junctions between glial cells (see Fig. 2-12), between glial cells and neurons, and between neurons and neurons. These gap junctions suggest that neurons and glia may be energy-coupled and metabolically coupled

units (Hyden). Glial cells may have putative roles in the development and maintenance of the nervous system, in the signaling activity of neurons and in trophic activities (Chap. 6).

Other considerations   The freshly cut brain has areas that are grayish in appearance (gray matter) and others that are whitish (white matter). Gray matter is composed mainly of cell bodies of neurons and dendrites; white matter is made up largely of myelinated and unmyelinated axons. Glial cells and blood vessels are located in both white matter and gray matter.

The numerous blood vessels are accompanied, once they enter within the substance of the central nervous system, by a minimal amount of perivascular connective tissue. The pia mater, arachnoid, and dura mater, which envelop the central nervous system, are formed of connective tissue elements.

Blood-brain barrier (brain barriers)

The concept of the *blood-brain barrier* (*hematoencephalic barrier*) was originally based on observations that many chemical substances which readily pass out of the bloodstream into the interstitial fluid and parenchyma of many organs do not do so in the brain and spinal cord. Thus barrier sites of graded permeability are said to exist between the vascular system and the brain. The concept has since been modified to include the various anatomic features and physiologic and biochemical systems which operate to subdivide the central nervous system and associated structures into a number of compartments; hence, the existence of *brain barriers* which demarcate these compartments. Among these are (1) the *blood-brain barrier* between the vascular and the brain compartments, (2) the *blood-cerebrospinal fluid* (*CSF*) *barrier* between the vascular and the CSF compartments, and (3) the *brain-CSF barrier* between the brain and CSF compartments. Furthermore, the central nervous system has been divided into a *neuronal compartment*, a *neuroglial compartment*, and an *intercellular* (*extracellular*) *fluid compartment* (see Fig. 2-18). Some authorities think of the "barrier" as comprising both the structural entities and the physiologic processes that slow down rather than

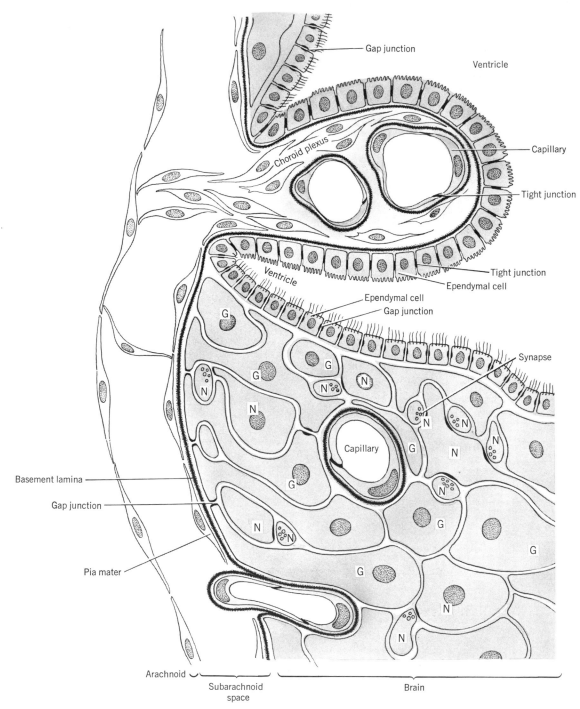

FIGURE 2-18 Some ultrastructural features in the brain, choroid plexus, piaarachnoid layer, and ventricle. The continuous extracellular space of the central nervous system is located among the glial cells (G) and neurons or their processes (N). Many of these features are basic to modern concepts of the blood-brain barrier. See the text for details. (*After Brightman and Reese.*)

stop the movement of certain substances from one compartment into another compartment. The movement of these substances takes place by diffusion and/or active transport.

Recent studies on the ultrastructure of the brain, meninges, and choroid plexus (see Fig. 2-18) illustrate some of the morphologic features associated with the brain-barrier concepts. As the blood vessels penetrate into the brain and spinal cord, they lose their muscular coats and the accompanying perivascular space; the capillaries are now invested by a continuous basement lamina and are ensheathed by end feet of astrocytes (see Fig. 2-17).

The capillaries of the brain (parenchymal vessels) and choroid plexuses and those entering the brain through the pia-glial membrane (leptomeningeal vessels) are surrounded by a perivascular basement lamina (membrane) composed of a mucopolysaccharide matrix. The endothelial cells of these capillaries are joined throughout by tight junctions (in a tight junction, there is an actual fusion between the outer protein leaflets of the plasma membranes of the adjoining cells). This intercellular seal implies that no intercellular space is available for the passage of substances between the blood and extracellular space. The basement lamina is not an effective barrier because it acts as a porous sieve. The so-called blood-brain barrier has as its main structural basis the occluding tight junctions between the nonfenestrated capillary endothelial cells. These nonfenestrated capillaries function with a markedly reduced pinocytotic activity. In effect, the transcapillary exchange is essentially through the endothelial cells with the major barrier being the plasma membranes of the endothelial cells. Much of the transport is probably energy-dependent, as expressed by the presence of numerous endothelial mitochondria. Apparently there is relatively free communication of CSF in the subarachnoid space and central canal system with that of the extracellular spaces and channels between the astrocytes of the central nervous system (see Fig. 2-17). These fluids act as large ionic buffer pools serving to maintain the constancy of the environment of the nervous system. Homeostasis of the neuronal environment is considered to be the functional role of the blood-brain barrier.

The choroid plexus is characterized by having *fenestrated capillaries;* the endothelial cells have fenestrations, or pores, closed by diaphragms thinner than the plasma membrane. Fenestrated capillaries are located in structures noted for fluid transport. The capillaries in the brain are not fenestrated. The *basement lamina* is also found adjacent to the epithelial cells of the choroid plexus and continuous with the pia-glial membrane, where it is intercalated between the pial cells and the glial cells.

The *choroid plexus* consists of two layers: (1) The fenestrated capillaries are located within a connective tissue stromal layer. Its interface with the subarachnoid space is formed by a thin layer of flattened connective tissue cells joined together by gap junctions. (2) The single layer of cuboidal epithelium has a continuous basement lamina on its basal side. These cells are joined to adjacent cells by tight junctions. These junctions act to restrict intercellular movement of material. Microvilli are present on the free border of the cells facing the ventricles. The fenestrated capillaries, adequate stromal space, and active transport systems within the cuboidal epithelial cells are geared to enhance the passage of materials from the vascular system to the CSF of the ventricles (and vice versa). The belts of tight junctions between the endothelial cells and cuboidal choroidal cells form limiting sheets which are barriers to the intercellular movement of proteins. Passage across the epithelial cells may take place by selective active transport and by pinocytosis. In the latter, the cell "drinks" a small quantity of fluid, forms a vesicle, transports it across the cell, and discharges the vesicle into the ventricle (or vice versa).

The brain and spinal cord contain an extracellular space located among nonfenestrated capillaries, glial cells, and neurons. They are surrounded by a pia-glial membrane and other meninges. The extracellular space probably occupies about 15 percent of the brain volume (depending upon the method used to obtain data, other estimates range from about 5 to 25 percent). These extracellular spaces are open and act as channels for the rapid diffusion of ions (e.g., Na^+ and K^+) and certain small molecules among the cells or to the CSF in the ventricles or subarachnoid space (see Fig. 2-16). These substances in these extracellular spaces have an outlet to the CSF of the ventricular cavities; this is the intercellular space among the discontinuous gap junctions between adjacent ependymal cells lining the ventricles. Another outlet to the CSF of the subarachnoid space is through the intercellular spaces and basement lamina at the pia-glial membrane. The flattened pial cells, like the ependymal cells, are also joined together by discontinuous gap junctions (see Fig. 2-18).

The capillaries of the central nervous system consist of a continuous endothelial lining surrounded by a continuous basement lamina. Physiologic evidence indicates that the basement lamina is not a barrier to diffusion. About 85 to 99 percent of the perivascular surface is covered with the end feet of astrocytes. These end feet are linked to one another by discontinuous gap junctions (unobstructed intercellular clefts are present between some portions of the end feet). Transport across the capillaries occurs by diffusion or by pinocytosis. All neurons and glial cells are no farther than 25 to 50 μm away from a blood capillary, but many are considerably farther away from the CSF. Evidence indicates that the exchange of materials is considerably more rapid between the CSF and the brain than between the capillaries and the brain.

The astrocytes have a significant location. They form a special compartment or pool (1) between the capillaries and the neurons, (2) between the capillaries and the pia-glial membrane, and (3) between the neurons and the pia-glial membrane. Discontinuous gap junctions join two astrocytes (1) at their end feet adjacent to a capillary, (2) at the glial processes of the pia-glial membrane, and (3) between their cell bodies or processes. Glial cells are similar to neurons in that they have high resting potentials, a high concentration of potassium ions, and a low concentration of sodium ions. In contrast to neurons, glial cells do not generate propagated impulses. Some substances probably pass from the astroglial compartment to the other compartments and the extracellular space.

The primary role of the brain barriers is to provide the control systems which regulate and maintain the optimal stable chemical environment for the neurons of the central nervous system. Homeostatic mechanisms utilize the molecular transport systems and various physical constraints (e.g., gap junctions) to regulate the ion fluxes between the blood plasma, extracellular space within the brain, and the CSF. The exquisite control of the chemical environment of the central nervous system is essential to minimize the effects of any potential variations, because neurons are most sensitive to their chemical milieu.

Recent studies suggest that certain substances are discharged into the CSF and transported within the ventricle to other sites. Hormones of the posterior lobe of the hypophysis, hypothalamic hormones, and melatonin of the pineal body may be discharged into the CSF and transported to other sites by intracerebral transport.

In summary, the CSF performs several functional roles: (1) its buoyancy protects the brain; (2) it is a link in the control of the chemical environment of the central nervous sytem; (3) it acts as a medium for the exchange of nutrients and waste products with the central nervous system; and (4) it may serve as a channel for intracerebral transport. In general, it seems that neuroglia function primarily as regulating systems rather than as indispensable adjuncts to the neuronal elements.

Meninges (functional morphology)

The *meninges* consist of a thick *dura mater*, two thin layers of *arachnoid* and the *pia mater* and their two spaces—"*subdural*" and *subarachnoid spaces*. The pia mater comprises a network of squamous cells with long processes and some bundles of collagenous fiber. Its outer layer is continuous. Most blood vessels are in the subarachnoid space near the glial border of the brain. The arachnoid consists of two layers of flattened cells—an outer barrier lamina and an inner lamina (Nabeshisma et al.). The closely packed cells of the outer layer are connected to form a continuous system of cells attached by tight junctions; this suggests the cell layers of this lamina are the structural basis for the "*meningeal barrier*" to the passage of large molecules from the dura to the subarachnoid space. The inner lamina of more loosely packed cells bonding the subarachnoid space is tied together by gap junctions.

The dura mater consists of elongated cells with finely branched processes (probably fibroblasts) and many crisscrossing bundles of collagenous fibers. An inner layer of flattened dural cells form the dural border layer which is snugly apposed to the arachnoid barrier layer. The separation of the dural border layer from the bulk of the dura mater forms the "subdural space." Thus, the subdural space is formed by a cleavage within the dura mater; it is not located between the dura and the arachnoid, which do not readily separate (Nabeshima et al.).

NERVE ENDINGS OF THE PERIPHERAL NERVES

The pseudounipolar ganglion cells are the receptor neurons and their peripheral terminals are specialized sensory receptors. The nerve endings in the peripheral tissues may be characterized by functional and structural criteria. The afferent, or sensory, endings are those nerve terminals that are involved in the transduction of various forms of environmental energy into neural activity.

The efferent, or motor, endings are those nerve terminals that stimulate muscles or glands (a form of synapse between a nerve fiber and an effector). One sensory neuron, its branches, and its sensory endings constitute a unit known as a *sensory unit*. One motor neuron, its branches, and the muscles innervated by its endings constitute a unit known as a *motor unit*.

Structurally the nerve endings may be classified as *free (nonencapsulated) nerve endings* and *encapsulated nerve endings*. The free nerve endings are the endings of the axis cylinders without any apparent structural modification of the adjacent tissues. The encapsulated endings are the endings of axis cylinders which are surrounded by organized connective tissue capsules. All nerve endings are naked in the sense that they are devoid of a neurolemmal (Schwann) sheath.

AFFERENT (SENSORY) ENDINGS

Morphologically there are three types of nerve endings: (1) *free nerve endings*, (2) *expanded tip endings*, and (3) *encapsulated endings* (see Fig. 2-19).

Free nerve endings

The *free nerve endings* are the branched terminations of myelinated and unmyelinated fibers that finally lose their neurolemma (Schwann) sheaths and terminate as naked axis cylinders. These simple endings are found in the epithelium of the skin, cornea of the eye, mucous membranes, intermuscular connective tissues, and pulp of the tooth. The unmyelinated nerves to the viscera (heart, intestinal tract) ramify and terminate in the same way (details of the junctional endings are controversial). Cold, warmth, touch, and pain are probably the subjective effects that follow the stimulation of these endings. Axons that terminate as a plexus around the hair follicle act as sensitive tactile receptors when a hair is moved. A parent myelinated fiber may divide into numerous unmyelinated terminal branches innervating over a hundred hair follicles. In turn, a hair follicle may receive terminals from several parent fibers. Depending upon the specific hair follicle, hair endings may respond optimally to slow hair movement, to fast hair movement, or to movement mainly in one direction (*movement detectors*).

Those endings known as interoceptors are free nerve endings in the wall of viscus, as in the stomach (where they may give rise to discomfort and pains of distention, hunger sensations, and cramps of contraction), the bronchi of the lungs (where they monitor the tension in the lungs during respiration), and the aorta, other large arteries, and the right atrium of the heart (where they are sensitive to changes in blood pressure).

Expanded tip endings

The *expanded tip endings* are found primarily in the skin. They include (1) *Merkel's corpuscle*, which is a touch-pressure receptor, and (2) a *"cold"* receptor. When in the vicinity of the epithelial specializations of several Merkel's corpuscles, the myelinated sensory nerve branches into several unmyelinated branches that lose their Schwann cells before penetrating into the basal lamina of the epidermis. Each terminal forms a flattened disk or plate which contacts and is partially enclosed by a specialized epithelial cell called a Merkel's cell. The cell contains dense core vesicles located close to the nerve disk. These cells may release a transmitter that

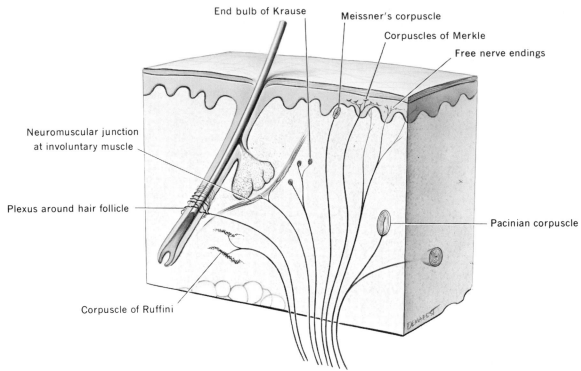

Labels on figure:
End bulb of Krause
Meissner's corpuscle
Corpuscles of Merkle
Free nerve endings
Neuromuscular junction at involuntary muscle
Plexus around hair follicle
Pacinian corpuscle
Corpuscle of Ruffini

FIGURE 2-19 Nerve endings in the skin. Free nerve endings subserve pain; Meissner's corpuscles, Merkel's corpuscles, and plexus around hair follicle subserve the tactile sense; Pacinian corpuscles subserve pressure and vibratory sense; corpuscles of Ruffini act as movement detectors. Free nerve endings form the motor innervation of involuntary (smooth) muscle.

depolarizes the nerve terminal. Many desmosomes extend from this cell to the adjacent epithelial cells.

A simpler form of an expanded nerve terminal receptor–epithelial cell nerve ending is said to respond to cold stimuli. No specific specialized receptors responding to warmth have been documented.

Encapsulated endings

There are three main types of *encapsulated nerve endings* in the skin and connective tissues: Pacinian, Meissner's, and Ruffini corpuscles. They are characterized by the presence of lamellated connective-tissue sheaths surrounding the nerve terminal. Each is supplied by one myelinated nerve fiber derived from a nerve which divided into branches innervating the similar endings. Other named encapsulated endings (such as endings of Krause or Golgi-Mazzoni) are said to be variants of these three endings. The encapsulated endings

associated with muscles are the neuromuscular spindles and those associated with tendons are the Golgi tendon organs.

Pacinian corpuscles are the largest encapsulated receptors (from 1 to 4 by 2 mm), large enough to be seen by the naked eye (see Fig. 2-19; see also Fig. 3-11). They resemble miniature onions in being formed by as many as 30 or more concentric lamella enclosing a cylindric central core in which is found an unmyelinated nerve fiber. The nerve fiber enters one pole of the capsule, has one or two internodes, and becomes unmyelinated. The ending is exquisitely sensitive to mechanical displacement and responds to vibratory stimuli (tuning fork) up to about 400 per second. The nerve can respond without the capsule to mechanical stimuli applied directly to the nerve. The capsule has the role of a mechanical filter—its elastic components ensure that the ending responds both when stimuli are applied and when they are removed.

Meissner's corpuscle (tactile) are ovoid

bodies located in the dermal papillae of glabrous skin (see Fig. 2-19). These are most numerous on the tips of the fingers and toes, where from 20 to 30 corpuscles may be concentrated in a square millimeter. Although several nerve fibers may enter each capsule, it is probable that all fibers may be branches of the same axon. These unmyelinated fibers spiral among the inner lamellar cells. Numerous tonofibrils extend from the outer cells of the capsule to the overlying epidermal cells. Meissner's corpuscles respond optimally to low frequencies of about 30 to 40 per second—this is known as *flutter sense*. These sensitive receptors adapt rapidly.

Ruffini corpuscles are elongated, fusiform structures 1 to 2 mm long. These thinly lamellated corpuscles are located in skin, subcutaneous tissues, and joint capsules. The myelinated fibers enter the ending and break up into unmyelinated branches which twist among the collagenous fibers of the capsule. These collagenous fibers pass outside the capsule and join the collagenous bundles of the skin and joint capsule. The Ruffini corpuscles are slowly adapting mechanoreceptors which are activated by the mechanical displacement of the surrounding connective tissue, presumably through the displacement induced by the collagenous fibers. In the joints, some of these endings discharge following movement in one direction while other endings respond when the joint is held in a fixed position.

Neuromuscular spindles are encapsulated, elongated, fusiform receptors found in all voluntary muscles of humans (Fig. 2-20). They average about 1.5 mm in length and 0.5 mm in width. Each spindle is an association of specialized striated muscle cells, afferent and efferent nerve endings, and a fluid-filled space. To perform its functional role, not only is each spindle mounted within a voluntary muscle, but its long axis is oriented *in parallel* to the muscle fibers of the voluntary muscle. The capsule of the spindle is continuous at its two tapered ends with the connective tissue surrounding the normal muscle fibers. Within this structural orientation to the voluntary muscle, the spindle will stretch when the muscle relaxes (lengthens). It will shorten when the voluntary muscle contracts (see Fig. 2-20). On this basis it performs its role as a stretch receptor monitoring tension (Chap. 5).

Two afferent nerve endings innervate the muscle fibers of each spindle. The *primary sensory ending* (*annulospiral ending*) terminates as a spiral wrap around the *central region* (*bag region, equatorial region*) of a nuclear bag fiber and as a side branch to a nuclear chain fiber. The *secondary sensory ending* (*flower-spray ending*) terminates on the polar segment of a nuclear chain fiber and nuclear bag fiber. Each spindle has one and only one primary nerve fiber innervating the central region of all intrafusal fibers, and from none to five secondary nerve fibers. The secondary fibers may terminate in the form of spirals, as a spray of fine branches, or as both (see Fig. 2-20).

Motor nerves, called *gamma efferent fibers* (*fusimotor neurons*, γ motor neurons) innervate each intrafusal muscle fiber in the polar regions (not in or near the bag region). From 1 to 25 gamma efferent fibers innervate a spindle. One gamma efferent fiber may branch and innervate several spindles within the same muscle. These gamma efferent fibers terminate as plate endings or as diffuse multiterminal endings. The plate endings are similar to the motor plate endings on the voluntary muscles. The multiterminal endings—also called *trail endings* or *en grappe* endings—have a number of varicose-like enlargements making the nerve-muscle synaptic junctions. Several motor endings may be located on each intrafusal fiber.

The miniature striated muscle cells of the spindle are called *intrafusal fibers,* and those of the voluntary muscles are called *extrafusal fibers.* From 2 to 20 (average 6) long intrafusal fibers are located within the enveloping connective tissue capsule of each spindle. The intrafusal muscles extend toward the poles of the spindle capsule and then beyond to blend with the endomyseal or perimyseal connective tissue of the muscle. Occasionally, a nuclear bag muscle fiber may be continuous from one spindle to another more distant spindle. Such a tandem muscle fiber is incorporated into the normal organization of both spindles with a bag region in each spindle.

Two types of intrafusal fibers are recognized: nuclear bag fibers and nuclear chain fibers. The *nuclear bag muscle fibers* extend the entire length of the neuromuscular spindle. In the thickened equatorial region of each intrafusal fiber is the noncontractile *nuclear bag,* so

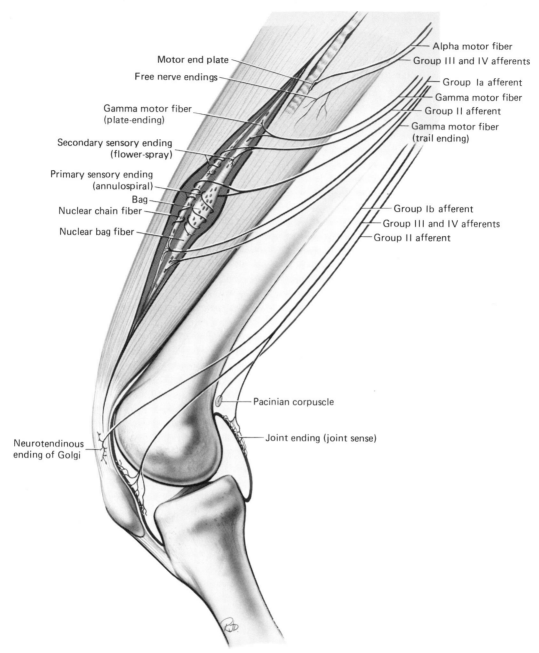

Labels (top, left to right):

Motor end plate

Free nerve endings

Gamma motor fiber
(plate-ending)

Secondary sensory ending
(flower-spray)

Primary sensory ending
(annulospiral)

Bag

Nuclear chain fiber

Nuclear bag fiber

Alpha motor fiber

Group III and IV afferents

Group Ia afferent

Gamma motor fiber

Group II afferent

Gamma motor fiber
(trail ending)

Group Ib afferent

Group III and IV afferents

Group II afferent

Pacinian corpuscle

Joint ending (joint sense)

Neurotendinous
ending of Golgi

FIGURE 2-20 Nerve endings in voluntary muscles, tendons, and joints. The neuromuscular spindle, which is disproportionately enlarged, is illustrated, with only two intrafusal muscle fibers—one nuclear bag fiber and one nuclear chain fiber. The nerve endings associated with the neuromuscular spindle include the primary sensory (annulospiral) endings, the secondary sensory (flower spray) endings, and motor end plates.

called because of its large concentration of cell nuclei. This bag is separated from the spindle capsule by a tissue fluid–filled space transversed by nerve fibers. The two ends of the nuclear bag are continuous with the polar segments of the intrafusal muscle fibers; the polar segments are striated and contractile. When active, the pull from the intrafusal fibers is on the bag. The *nuclear chain muscle fibers* do not extend the length of the spindle; they are shorter and thinner than nuclear bag fibers. The thin equatorial region of each fiber is the noncontractile region, with muscle nuclei arranged in a single-file chain. This region is continuous with the polar segments.

The *primary sensory ending* is the terminal of a group Ia fiber on the bag region while the *secondary sensory ending*, which terminates on the chain fiber predominately, is the terminal of a group II fiber. Functionally, the primary endings and their group Ia fibers respond most actively during the dynamic phase of muscle stretch (exhibit *dynamic sensitivity*, Chap. 5). The secondary endings and their group II fibers respond more actively to the maintained stretch of a muscle (exhibit *static sensitivity*, Chap. 5). The "motor plate type" endings terminate mainly on the nuclear bag fibers, whereas the *diffuse trail endings* make *en passant synapses* mainly on the nuclear chain fibers. Functionally, the activity of the efferent fibers stimulates the intrafusal fibers to contract and thereby effectively stretch the section of the fiber innervated by the sensory endings. This results in the increased sensitivity of these endings so they discharge more readily at increased stretch (Chap. 5). The nuclear chain fibers contract more rapidly and in a twitchlike fashion, whereas the nuclear bag fibers contract less rapidly and in a tonic fashion.

The number of spindles per gram of muscle is high in those small muscles subserving fine delicate movements, such as the intrinsic muscles of the hand, the eye muscles, and muscles at base of skull and neck. The latter muscles are involved in regulating the delicate postural adjustments of the head upon the vertebral column.

The *Golgi tendon organ* (*GTO, neurotendinous endings of Golgi*) is a 1-mm-long capsulated ending in a tendon located at the junction of a muscle and tendon or within a muscle sheath (see Fig. 2-21). Each GTO is innervated by one myelinated group Ib afferent fiber which upon entering the capsule becomes unmyelinated, and whose branches terminate in small sprays among the twisting, dividing, and regrouping intracapsular bundles of collagenous fibers. These collagenous fibers enter and leave the end of the capsule through tight-fitting collar seals to join the collagenous bundles of the tendon, which are, in turn, attached to extrafusal muscle fibers. It is postulated that the increased tensile forces on the collagen bundles following the muscle contraction tighten the braided collagen bundles and thereby squeeze and activate the nerve terminals (Schoultz and Swett).

The GTOs are mechanoreceptors monitoring the forces exerted during passive muscle stretch or active muscle contraction (Chap. 3). These endings are tension recorders (biological force transducers) active during both contraction and stretching of the muscles. Because the GTOs are located in the tendon, they are said to be *in series* with the muscle fibers. The strain of the collagenous fibers appears to be the effective stimulus for initiating activity in the nerve endings of the Golgi tendon organ.

EFFERENT (MOTOR) ENDINGS (Fig. 2-3)

The *motor end plates* are the specialized efferent endings which terminate on the voluntary (striated) muscles. Each branch terminates as one motor end plate. Practically all muscle fibers are innervated by just one motor end plate. This ending is actually a synapse between a nerve fiber and a muscle fiber. The myelin sheath ends just before the axon reaches the muscle fiber. Distal to the myelin sheath are neurolemma cells (called *teloglia*), which are associated with the axonal branches. The nerve fiber terminates as a flattened plate in a depression, called a *trough, synaptic gutter*, or *primary synaptic cleft*, which indents the surface of the muscle fiber. The primary synaptic cleft is about 200 to 500 Å wide. Within the synaptic cleft is an amorphous material which is continuous with the basement lamina of the muscle cell on the outer surface of the sarcolemma. The axon tip just proximal to the presynaptic mem-

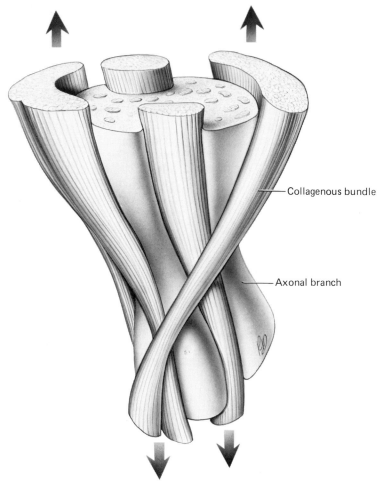

Collagenous bundle

Axonal branch

FIGURE 2-21 Golgi Tendon Organ (GTO). This receptor consists of the branches of a nerve fiber intertwined among braided collagen bundles. Increase in tensile forces (arrows) straightens and tightens the bundles with the resultant pinching of the nerve fibers of this mechanoreceptor. Each GTO is surrounded by a thin capsule. (*Adapted from Schoultz and Swett.*)

brane contains many mitochondria and synaptic vesicles. These agranular vesicles, of 400 to 500 Å in diameter, contain acetylcholine.

The postsynaptic membrane (postjunctional membrane) on the muscle fiber is thickened, and its surface area is increased by secondary foldings (*secondary clefts, "subneural apparatus,"* or *junction folds*). Close to the secondary foldings in the muscle fiber are many nuclei and mitochondria. The muscle portion of the end plate is called the *sole plate*. A motor unit to the muscle of the eye, with its delicate and dexterous movements, includes three to six muscle fibers. A

motor unit to the gastrocnemius muscle, with its massive and cruder movements, may include over 2000 muscle fibers (motor units of leg muscles average 250 fibers). Muscles innervated by one motor unit are intermingled among the muscle fibers innervated by other motor units. Muscles innervated by relatively more motor units are capable of exerting fine gradations of tension.

The motor endings of the autonomic nervous system terminate as free nerve endings, often in the form of beads and varicosities. These are the endings that innervate muscles (smooth involuntary muscle), glands, and cardiac muscle.

DEGENERATION, REGENERATION, AND SPROUTING

An injured neuron reacts to insult, whether it is a transection, a crush, a toxic substance, or a deprivation of blood supply. The entire neuron responds, for the trauma acts as a potent stimulus, through a series of events, which are basically directed to the preservation of the neuron.

Degeneration

Some of the changes which occur following the simple transection of an axon will be outlined. The reactions, known as the axon reaction, following a transection may be divided into changes in (1) the cell body (chromatolysis), (2) the nerve fiber on the side of the cell body proximal to the trauma (primary degeneration), and (3) the nerve fiber distal to the trauma (secondary, or Wallerian, degeneration).

The cell body imbibes water, triples in volume, and becomes turgid. The Nissl bodies undergo "dissolution" or chromatolysis. The cell swelling precedes the *chromatolysis*. The nucleus may be displaced to the side of the cell body; it assumes an excentric location. The Golgi apparatus is disrupted and dispersed. The poor staining of the cell body exhibiting chromatolysis is a result of the disassociation of the ribosomes from the rough endoplasmic reticulum. Chromatolysis is greater the closer to the cell body the axon is severed. If severance is too close with loss of sustaining collaterals, the neuron dies. In some situations, the sustaining collaterals, if preserved, are sufficient to offset any overt retrograde neuronal changes.

Following the axotomy, there is an increase in ribonucleic acid synthesis in the nucleus, in ribonucleic acid content in the nucleolus, and in the rate of passage in newly synthesized ribonucleic acids from the nucleus to the cytoplasm. The increase in the cytoplasmic ribonucleic acid is followed by an increase in the protein and enzyme content of the cell body. Many of these newly synthesized substances are conveyed by axoplasmic transport and flow down the axon. These are manifestations of metabolic activities

which can ultimately lead to the regeneration of the severed process. The chromatolysis is indicative of the enhanced protein synthesis in the cell body. The nerve fiber proximal to the cut usually shows only a few degenerative changes, including the breakdown of the myelin sheath and the axis cylinders in several internodes bordering the injury.

The nerve distal to the cut undergoes several anterograde changes (see Fig. 2-22). One of the initial reactions, occurring during the first day following trauma, is swelling of the axonal terminals and synaptic vesicles. The axis cylinders and terminal arborizations swell and, after the first week, fragment and disintegrate. The myelin sheath breaks up after a few days into elongated segments and during the next few weeks into smaller spherical and oval fragments. Macrophages phagocytize these breakdown products and remove them from the nerve. Some myelin-sheath fragmentation products may persist for many months after the initial trauma. The disintegration of the myelin sheath suggests that there may be a close trophic relation between the Schwann cells and oligodendroglia—the myelin-forming cells and the axis cylinder.

Transneuronal degeneration

An injured or degenerating neuron may produce conditions resulting in changes in postsynaptic and presynaptic neurons. In the case of the postsynaptic neuron, such *transneuronal or transynaptic effects* are known as *anterograde or orthograde transynaptic changes:* they may be expressed by the degeneration of the neuron or cell or by a hyperresponse of the postsynaptic neuron or muscle, known as *degeneration hypersensitivity* (Chap. 6). The effect on the presynaptic neuron, if degeneration should occur, is known as *retrograde transneuronal degeneration.* Both types of transneuronal degeneration have been observed in certain neuronal sequences in the central nervous system such as some neurons of the visual and auditory systems. Two explanations for this phenomenon have been proposed: (1) The deprivation of critical physiological neuronal influences produces physiological changes that result in degeneration of a neuron; (2) the alteration or removal of certain trophic substances evokes degenerative changes.

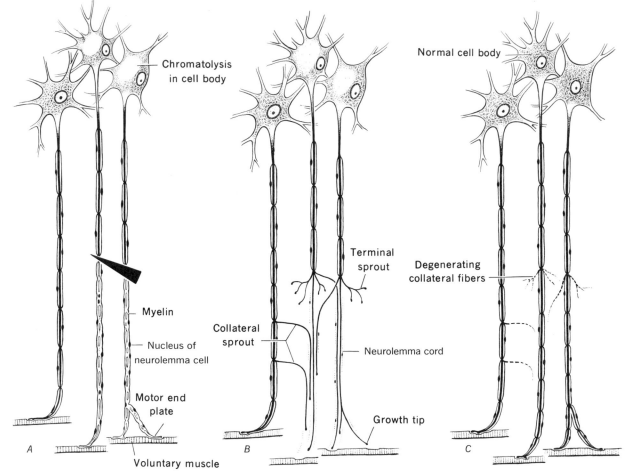

FIGURE 2-22 Degeneration and regeneration of peripheral somatic motor nerve fibers. *A.* Several days after transection (at the wedge). Note the chromatolysis and eccentric nuclei, increase in number of neurolemma cells, and fragmentation of myelin sheaths. *B.* Several weeks later the neurolemma cord receives regenerating axis cylinders from the transected fibers and collateral branches from the adjacent normal fiber. *C.* Several months later collateral branches of axis cylinders that failed to innervate motor end plates degenerate. The regenerated portions of the fibers contain more internodes than before; hence they conduct nerve impulses more slowly.

Regeneration

It is not possible to segregate degenerative processes from regenerative processes, for, in a real sense, all the activities of the neural tissue are primarily directed to reconstitution of the nerve. Regeneration is essentially a process of reorganization and growth (see Fig. 2-22).

Regeneration of nerve fibers can occur when a fully functional cell body is preserved, when there is minimal obstruction at the site of trauma, when the capacity for the generation of nerve sprouts is expressed, and when there is an adequate supply of substances essential for axonal growth.

Depending upon the severity of the trauma, degeneration in the stump proximal to the trauma may occur back for a distance of a few internodes to about 3 cm. The severed end of the axis cylinder is sealed by new plasma membrane within 12 h. Leakage of axonal cytoplasm is negligible and inconsequential.

The neurolemma cells in the segment near the trauma and those throughout the entire distal segment undergo mitotic activity and increase to more than 10 times the original population.

The proliferating neurolemma cells form continuous cords or "tubes" of cells that maintain the orderly longitudinal pattern of the nerve. These cells also migrate into the gap between the distal and proximal stumps and may form a bridge between the two stumps. The cell body synthesizes proteins and other metabolites that flow distally into the injured nerve process. The severed axon tip or terminal forms a new cell membrane, and within a few days several axonal branches or sprouts extend from each original nerve process. Each nerve fiber commences to regenerate by sending out many fine sprouts with tips called *growth cones* or *filopodia*. These advancing tips, growing at a rate of about 3 to 4 mm per day, extend out; several tips find a substrate (fibrous lattice or neurolemma cell) and continue to lengthen with a tip that also develops many fine sprouts. Many sprouts retract.

When conditions are favorable, many of these growing tips will enter the distal stump. Each of these regenerating processes will contact a neurolemma cord band. This cord will act as a guide, for the regenerating axon continues to grow along the cord to a nerve ending at the optimal rate of 3 or 4 mm per day. Many processes will enter the distal stump and follow the neurolemmal cords to the nerve endings. If the gap between the two stumps is too long, the regenerating axons may not be able to bridge it. Hence, approximating the cut ends is desirable. Later the neurolemma cells surround the regenerating nerve fibers. Some regenerating fibers become myelinated within 10 days. In time the axon diameters and the myelin sheaths thicken. Each regenerated nerve fiber tends to have an internodal length, a diameter, and a conduction velocity of about 80 percent of those of the original fiber.

The functional effectiveness of peripheral nerve regeneration is related to some other factors. Each regenerating axon of the proximal stump may divide many times, to form as many as 50 branches. Each neurolemmal cord in the distal stump may act as a guiding scaffold for many regenerating axons. If regeneration is successful, there may be more nerve fibers in the distal stump than in the proximal stump several months later. Neurolemmal cords can remain for months awaiting regeneration. If regeneration is unsuccessful, the cords are reduced in size by the enveloping connective tissues.

By a year later, many of these fibers will have degenerated. The survivors are those axons that terminate in the proper nerve endings and form functional endings. In effect, the numerous regenerating branches from one axon are a means by which the parent axon increases the possibilities of reaching a proper nerve ending. The capacity of each neurolemma cord to guide many axons is the means of increasing the possibility of the nerve ending's being innervated by a proper nerve fiber. Motor fibers will eventually degenerate if they are located in a neurolemma cord that terminates in a sensory ending.

Physiological changes are also a consequence of axotomy. The normal action potentials of the axon (with continuity with the cell body) are replaced by graded potentials (Chap. 3). Some segments of the dendrites may produce action potentials. A reduction in the density of the synaptic population on the cell body and dendrites is said to occur. Normal physiological expressions do not return to the regenerated axon for many months or years (see end of chapter). The readjustments of the reflex arcs utilizing the central nervous system require further adaptations to obtain functional recovery.

Collateral sprouting

Collateral branches from an axon may sprout from an intact undamaged nerve and enter into an adjacent denervated neurolemma cord (see Fig. 2-22). This is known as *collateral nerve sprouting* or *preterminal axonal sprouting*. This collateral sprouting may occur at any node of Ranvier along the axon in the vicinity of the degenerating fibers.

According to one concept, the nearby degenerating nerve fibers exert a stimulus to which the normal nearby fibers respond by forming collateral sprouts that are, in turn, attracted to the axonless neurolemma cord. This stimulus is presumed to be elicited by chemical substances released by the degenerating nerve fibers, interstitial cells, or denervated structures.

According to another concept, the primary

stimulus for activating nerve fibers to sprout collateral branches is provided by tissues of the target organ which is being innervated. In a sense these substances activate each nerve to express its inherent potentiality to generate more collateral branches. In this view, the expression of the potentiality to sprout is inhibited by chemical substances "secreted" by adjacent nerve fibers. Each normal nerve fiber releases such substances, which tend to inhibit adjacent nerve fibers from sprouting. Experimental evidence indicates that these chemical substances are transported from the cell body with the help of the microtubules by fast axoplasmatic flow.

These concepts provide the theoretical bases of understanding why axons utilize their potential to form new collateral branches and to reinnervate the denervated peripheral nerve endings. They offer an explanation for the fact that many muscle fibers denervated in poliomyelitis, for example, may be reinnervated by a branch of an adjacent normal fiber, so that the initial paralytic symptoms are ameliorated. The anesthetic area in the skin following a nerve injury may gradually shrink as a result of collateral sprouting.

Transected nerve fibers in the adult mammalian central nervous sytem attempt to regenerate. Some axons form *sprouts* and growing tips. Many are apparently incapable of mobilizing the metabolic responses which sustain extensive axonal regeneration. The most widely accepted explanation for the failure of fibers to regenerate for any distance is that the regenerating axon tip is unable to penetrate through the glial scar formed at the site of injury.

Thus collateral nerve sprouting occurs in both the peripheral and the central nervous systems. Functional synaptic connections may occur after collateral regeneration in both systems.

Functional considerations of nerve regeneration

Return of function after regeneration of severed nerves may be excellent. Sensory, motor, and autonomic functional activity may closely resemble that of the original state. However, functional recovery may be poor, especially if the injury is very traumatic and the cut nerve stumps are not properly approximated.

Cross unions of the proximal part of one nerve with the distal segment of another nerve (*crossed-nerve anastomoses*) are followed by successful regeneration of the nerve fibers; e.g., anastomosis of the proximal portion of the hypoglossal nerve (to the tongue) to the distal portion of the facial nerve (responsible for facial expression). The muscles of facial expression, when reinnervated, will regain their lost muscle tonus and can then be contracted voluntarily. However, the integrated complex functional activity will be modified. The movement of facial muscles can occur only when the patient attempts to move the tongue. The mammalian nervous system is limited in its ability to readapt the function of its disarranged nerves.

Functional recovery following the regeneration of the nerves may take a year or so in some situations in humans. For example, this amount of time is required for the return of sensations and motor control of the hand subsequent to a severe trauma of the ulnar nerve in the arm. In the interim, skillful use of physical therapy is required to maintain the musculature in proper condition for eventual rehabilitation.

BIBLIOGRAPHY

Bloom, W., and D. W. Fawcett: *A Textbook of Histology*, W. B. Saunders Company, Philadelphia, 1975.

Bennett, M. V. L., and D. A. Goodenough (eds.): *Gap Junctions, Electronic Coupling and Intercellular Communication*, Neurosciences Research Program Bulletin, The M.I.T. Press, Cambridge, Massachusetts, 1978.

Bourne, G. H. (ed.): *The Structure and Function of Nerve Tissue* (6 vols.), Academic Press, Inc., New York, 1968, 1969, 1972.

Brightman, M. W., and T. S. Reese: Junctions between intimately opposed cell membranes in the vertebrate brain. J Cell Biol, 40:648–677, 1969.

Brightman, M. W., and T. S. Reese: "Membrane Specializations of Ependyman Cells and Astrocytes," in D. B. Tower (ed.), *The Nervous System, vol. I: The Basic Neurosciences*, R. O. Brady (vol. ed.), Raven Press, New York, 1975, pp. 267–277.

Bunge, M. B., R. P. Bunge, and H. Riss: Ultrastructural study of remyelination in an experimental lesion in adult cat spinal cord. J Biophys Biochem Cytol, 10:67–94, 1961.

Bunge, R. P.: Glial cells and the central myelin sheath. Physiol Rev, 48:197–251, 1968.

Clemente, C. D.: Regeneration in the central nervous system. Int Rev Neurobiol, 6:257–301, 1964.

Copenhaver, W. M., D. E. Kelly, and R. L. Wood: *Bailey's Textbook of Histology*, The Williams and Wilkins Company, Baltimore, 1978.

Gray, E. G., and R. W. Guillery: Synaptic morphology in the normal and degenerating nervous system. Int Rev Cytol, 19:111–182, 1966.

Guth, L.: Regeneration in the mammalian peripheral nervous system. Physiol Rev, 36:441–478, 1956.

Hubbard, J. I. (ed.): *The Peripheral Nervous System*, Plenum Press, New York, 1974.

Jones, E. C., and W. M. Cowan: "Nervous Tissue," in L. Weiss and R. O. Greep (eds.), *Histology*, McGraw-Hill Book Company, 1977, Chap. 8, pp. 283–372.

Minckler, J. (ed.): *Pathology of the Nervous System*, vol. 1, McGraw-Hill Book Company, New York, 1968.

Nabeshima, S., T. S. Reese, D. M. Landis, and M. W. Brightman: Junctions in the meninges and marginal glia. J Comp Neurol, 164:127–170, 1975.

Peters, A., S. L. Paley, and H. DeF. Webster: *The Fine Structure of the Nervous System. The Neurons and Supporting Cells*. W. B. Saunders, Philadelphia, 1976.

Ramon-Moliner, E., and W. J. H. Nauta: The isodendritic core of the brain stem. J Comp Neurol, 126:311–336, 1966.

Schoultz, T. W., and J. E. Sweet: The fine structure of the Golgi tendon organ. J Neurocytol, 1:1–28, 1972.

Winkelmann, R. K.: *Nerve Endings in Normal and Pathological Skin: Contributions to the Anatomy of Sensations*, Charles C Thomas, Publisher, Springfield, III., 1960.

CHAPTER THREE

BASIC NEUROPHYSIOLOGY

The ability to react to a stimulus is a fundamental property of all living organisms. Glands secrete, muscles contract, cilia sweep, and certain cells ingest foreign organisms. Two systems are specialized to enable the organism to coordinate and to mobilize its resources in responding to the internal and external environments. These are the nervous system and the endocrine system. In fact, the two systems are interrelated and integrated (Chap. 11). The *endocrine system* is a coordinator, utilizing *chemical messengers (humoral agents or hormones)* that are transmitted through the bloodstream from their source in an endocrine gland to their site of action in a target organ. The reactivity of this system is slow. The *nervous system* is a rapid coordinator utilizing *chemical messengers (neurotransmitter agents)* for interneuronal communication via synaptic junctions (synapses); an agent is secreted by a nerve cell into a narrow synaptic cleft where it acts to influence another nerve cell, a muscle cell, or a glandular cell. Another adaptation for intercellular communication is the gap (electronic) junction, in which direct ultramicroscopic continuities between some neurons and certain muscle cells (in smooth and cardiac muscles) are present (Chap. 2).

PHYSIOLOGIC SIGNAL OF A NEURON

Each neuron generates several types of signals in performing its functional role. They consist of a baseline potential, called the *resting potential*, and some specialized signals, including *integrated potential*, *action potential*, and *graded postsynaptic and receptor potentials*. Electric impulses are the universal language of the known nervous system.

Resting potential

The baseline signal is the *resting membrane potential*, which is the background level of activity from which the other signals take off. In general, this potential is present along the entire plasma membrane of the neuron, unless other signals are superimposed on it. Mammalian neurons are polarized with a resting potential of about -60 to -80 mV, with the inside of the neuron being negative in relation to the extracellular fluid (see Fig. 3-1).

Integrated potential

Integrated potential is generated at a specialized segment of a neuron called the *trigger zone*, which is usually located at the initial segment of an axon or at the first node of Ranvier in a sensory receptor (see Figs. 2-4, 3-2, and 3-10). The integrated potential may trigger the generation of an action potential (nerve impulse).

Action potential

Neurons convey signal information over long distances via an *all-or-none action potential* (*nerve impulse, spike*). An action potential is a depolarizing signal of up to $+30$ to $+40$ mV (see Figs. 3-2 and 3-7) in which the polarity is the reverse of that in the resting potential (inside, the neuron is positive in relation to the extracellular fluid). This signal is conveyed via unmyelinated and myelinated fibers for distances ranging from a few millimeters to several meters or more.

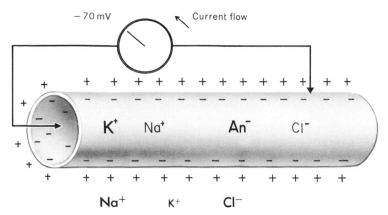

FIGURE 3-1 Resting (steady) potential. The intracellular neuroplasm potential of the normal nerve fiber "at rest" is negative to the extracellular potential. Sodium (Na^+) and chloride (Cl^-) ions are in high concentration in the extracellular fluid, and the potassium (K^+) ions and protein (An^-) are in high concentrations in the neuroplasm. The potential across the plasma membrane is about -70 to -90 mV.

Such long-distance transmission is called a *propagated (action) potential*.

Graded postsynaptic and receptor potentials

The initial response of a neuron to stimulation is generally via a *graded potential* that spreads passively for short distances up to about 1 mm before fading out. Hence, graded potentials are *nonpropagating potentials*. Several graded potentials are named for some structural or functional feature. Graded potentials generated in a sensory receptor are called *receptor* or *generator potentials*. Because these potentials occur mainly, but not exclusively on dendrites and cell bodies and are associated with the transduction of neural activity at synapses, they are sometimes called *postsynaptic dendritic, transducer,* or *input potentials*. These potentials are perturbations from the basic resting potentials. They may influence the trigger zone.

Resting potential

All cells have a transmembrane potential with neurons which express it in a specialized form. The "resting" neuron is a charged cell surrounded by an excitable plasma membrane. The *resting potential* is the result of the difference in the electric (bioelectric) potentials between an extracellular fluid outside the neuron and the intracellular fluid (neuroplasm) inside the neuron.

The plasma membrane of the neuron acts as a selectively permeable boundary (5 to 10 nm thick) capable of maintaining a differential distribution of ions in the fluids on either side of it. Sodium (Na^+) and chloride (Cl^-) ions are in higher concentration in the interstitial fluid (which is similar to sea water); potassium (K^+) and protein (organic) ions are in higher concentration in the intracellular fluid (see Fig. 3-1). Because ions tend to diffuse away from regions of high concentration, sodium ions tend to diffuse across the plasma membrane into the neuron, and potassium ions tend to diffuse out of the neuron into the interstitial fluid. However, this diffusion gradient is modified by the plasma membrane of the resting axon; the resting membrane has a higher selective permeability for potassium ions than for sodium ions. As a result, potassium ions tend to leak out of the axon rapidly. The potassium leakage continues until an equilibrium is attained when the inside of the axon reaches an electrically negative potential relative to the interstitial fluid. This equilibrium is the resting potential measured in millivolts (thousandths of a volt). As a result, the interstitial fluid has a positive charge in relation to the net negative charge of the intracellular fluid.

The ions diffuse across the plasma membrane through *aqueous channels (pores)* that are composed of integral proteins. There are separate sodium channels and potassium channels (Figs. 2-5, 3-1, 3-6, and 3-7). Actually, they occupy only a small fraction of the plasma mem-

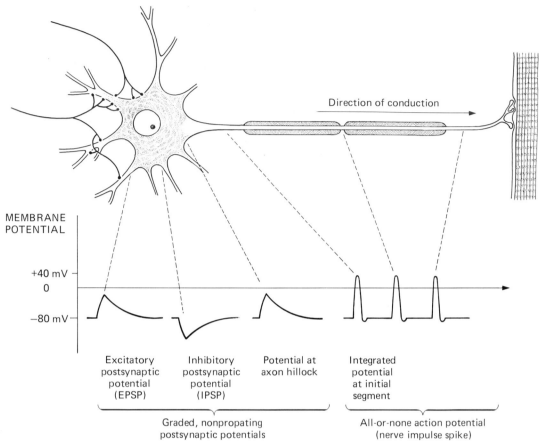

MEMBRANE
POTENTIAL

+40 mV
0
−80 mV

Direction of conduction

| Excitatory postsynaptic potential (EPSP) | Inhibitory postsynaptic potential (IPSP) | Potential at axon hillock | Integrated potential at initial segment |

Graded, nonpropating
postsynaptic potentials

All-or-none action potential
(nerve impulse spike)

FIGURE 3-2 Schema demonstrating the types of electric potential changes which are recorded across the plasma membrane at various sites of a motor neuron. On the surface of the dendrites and cell body are excitatory and inhibitory synapses, which, when stimulated, produce local, graded, nonpropagating potentials. These are exhibited as an excitatory or depolarizing postsynaptic potential (EPSP) and an inhibitory or hyperpolarizing postsynaptic potential (IPSP). These local potentials are summed at the axon hillock and, if adequate, may trigger an integrated potential at the initial segment and an all-or-none action potential, which is conducted along the axon to the motor end plate. (*Adapted from Gray's Anatomy, W. B. Saunders, Philadelphia, 1973.*)

brane. The concept of separate Na$^+$ and K$^+$ channels is based in part on the action of certain drugs. Tetrodotoxin (TTX), a poison found in the puffer fish, selectively blocks Na$^+$ conductance but not K$^+$ conductance. On the other hand, tetraethylammonium (TEA) selectively blocks K$^+$ conductance but not Na$^+$ conductance. TTX acts on the outer surface of the membrane and TEA on the inner surface—indicating that the plasma membrane is asymmetric.

The *resting membrane potential* across the plasma membrane of the resting neuron is about 0.1 V (from 70 to 100 mV). The potential differ-

ence of this biologic battery across a membrane that is one-millionth of a centimeter thick is actually high, for it is equivalent to a field of 100 kV across a membrane 1 cm thick.

While the resting potential is maintained, the permeability (conductance) pattern for potassium and chloride ions is high while that for anions and sodium ions is low. *Conductance* is a measure of the ease with which a current flows. The differential concentrations of sodium ions and potassium ions are maintained by the metabolic activity of the neuron by which the sodium is pumped out of the cell and the potassium into the cell by the metabolically fueled sodium-potassium transport system. The energy for the pump is derived from the hydrolysis of adenosine triphosphate (ATP). This transport system is also called the *sodium pump*. The exchange process involving the transport of sodium ions out of the cell and of potassium ions into the cell is called the *coupled sodium-potassium pump* (Fig. 2-5).

In short, the interstitial fluid has high concentrations of sodium ions (10 times as high as that on the outside) and chloride ions (14 times as high as that on the outside) than in the intracellular fluid of the neuron, which has high concentrations of potassium ions (30 times as high inside in some neurons) and large organic protein ions. The inorganic ions (Na^+, K^+, and Cl^-) can pass across the cell membrane with relative ease but are prevented from doing so by metabolic activity. The potassium ions are held in the neuron by the strong electrostatic attraction of the organic ions which are too large to leak across the plasma membrane.

The transmembrane potential of the "resting neuron" is the result of the ionic concentration differences across the selectively permeable plasma membrane. This membrane acts as a *capacitor* (a structure which stores charges) and has *capacitance*—the property of the cell membrane to store electrical charges and to keep them separate. This combined ability of the plasma membrane to have capacitance and to permit diffusion of ions is, in part, related to mosaic organization of large regions of bilipid layers interspersed with aqueous protein channels (pores) (see Fig. 2-5). The bilipid regions lack permeability channels and are effective electrical insulators with high capacitance per unit area (high resistance). The aqueous protein channels permit the passage of ions between the two conducting media—extracellular and intracellular fluids—while the electrical charges can be stored on the two sides of the membrane. The capacitor is thus a resistance insulator (the lipid bilayer) which separates two conducting layers (extracellular and intracellular fluids) (see Fig. 2-5).

Simply described, the degree of *resistance* to the passage of ions across the plasma membrane is probably related to the bilipid layer (with its high resistance) and to the number of ionic chan-

nels (composed of integral proteins) open to a particular ion (Na^+, K^+, Cl^-, and Ca^+). When resistance is high, the number of closed channels is high and the conductance is low (conductance is a reciprocal of resistance). The greater the number of open channels (pores) the greater the conductance. Thus the plasma membrane may be conceived as a mosaic of capacitance and resistance regions (lipid bilayer) and scattered sites of Na^+ and K^+ channels (integral proteins).

INTEGRATED POTENTIAL AND ACTION POTENTIAL

An *action potential* is normally initiated by the excitatory activity of the dendritic or generator potentials activating the trigger zone of the neuron, namely by an *integrated potential*. An action potential in the axon follows (see Figs. 3-3, 3-6, and 3-7). In essence the integrated potential produces a *depolarization* of the plasma membrane by a rapid increase in the sodium conductance that results in an inward sodium ion (Na^+) current. In depolarization there is the thrust to decrease the membrane polarization, thereby making the region inside of the membrane more positive with respect to the tissue fluid outside the cell membrane (see Fig. 3-2). The inward sodium current causes a further depolarization and even more inward current. This so-called *regenerative process* produces the action potential with a reversal in the polarity from that in the resting potential (−80 mV) to that in the action potential (+30 to 40 mV) (see Fig. 3-2). It is significant that the sodium and the potassium channels in the plasma membrane sustaining action potentials are *voltage-sensitive* (*voltage-dependent conductance channels*). This means that the membrane voltage of the ongoing action potential operates to open sodium and potassium channels in the resting plasma membrane. In essence, the action potential impulses are propagated along the axonal plasma membrane (unmyelinated fibers) by the longitudinal spread of the current without decrement (regenerative process). As each site of the membrane generates a spike, it depolarizes and excites adjacent nonactive sites to increase their conduction and give rise to a new regenerative action potential. The sequence of permeability changes during the im-

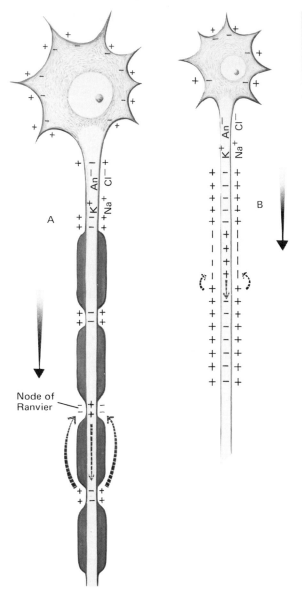

A

Node of
Ranvier

B

pulse may be summarized as follows: The *integrative potential* and resulting action potential open up sodium in the channels, resulting in an inward current; this is followed by further depolarization with the opening of more channels until most or all are open. As the action potential approaches the Na^+ equilibrium potential, the Na^+ channels begin to close (conductance decrease). This depolarization at each point along the membrane results, with a slight delay, in the opening of the potassium channels (increase in K^+ conductance). The potassium current tends to repolarize the plasma membrane and the return of the resting potential. At any one site the sequence of the opening followed by the closure of both the Na^+ and K^+ channels takes place within milliseconds.

Note that the current flows from a region of positive potential to a region of negative potential (see Figs. 3-3 and 3-4); current is a *consequence* of the differences in potentials; it does not *create* the differences in potentials. Current is the movement of positive charges. Once the spike has passed, the closed channels are immediately ready to open again. The nerve fiber gains sodium and loses potassium during the passage of the action potential. Later the small amount of sodium which entered the cell is metabolically pumped out (see Fig. 2-5). If the stimulus does not lower the membrane potential to the critical level, then the resultant *local response* fades and dies (*cable property*) within a few millimeters of the stimulus site. The normal resting potential returns immediately. The local response of a nerve propagates with decrement. Gland cells and muscle cells are similar in this respect. The resting potential in muscle cells is about -70 to -90 mV, with the minus sign signifying intracellular negativity with respect to the extracellular potential.

In the central nervous system the astroglial cells act as a "potassium sink"; this is important because these cells have the capacity to take up excess potassium from the extracellular fluid which may accumulate after prolonged neuronal activity.

During the interval prior to the critical point, sodium ion permeability (inrush) is dominant, while during the interval following the critical point, potassium permeability (outrush) is dominant. Once this critical threshold is

FIGURE 3-3 *A.* A neuron with a myelinated axon. *B.* A neuron with an unmyelinated axon. Note the charges on the cell membrane and the location of certain ions in each neuron "at rest" and at active sites (one on each neuron) during conduction of an all-or-none action potential. The minus ($-$) sign within the neuron signifies negativity with respect to the extracellular fluid outside the neuron. The solid arrows outside the neurons indicate the direction in which the nerve impulses are propagated. The interrupted arrows indicate the direction of flow of the current. Sodium, Na^+; potassium, K^+; chloride, Cl^-; and protein anions, An^-. By definition, current is the direction in which the positive charge flows.

reached, the depolarization continues until the intracellular fluid adjacent to the cell membrane is negative to the interstitial fluid. A reversal in the polarity occurs from that of the resting potential (-80 mV) to that of the action potential ($+40$ mV). Thus an action potential is triggered when the depolarization reaches a critical point. At the excited locus, the flow of current is inward into the neuron; at the adjacent nonexcited membrane, the flow of current is outward into the interstitial fluid point. The action potential is a sequence of point-to-point flow down the axon with each point acting as a site of sodium inrush into the axon, followed by potassium outrush. This is an electrical signal of the action potential which travels along the cell membrane as a chain reaction and regenerates itself from point to point along the axon (continuous conduction) without loss of amplitude and at a constant speed for that axon (see Fig. 3-2). The nerve fiber gains sodium and loses potassium during the passage of the action potential. Later the small amount of sodium which entered the cell is metabolically pumped out.

The amounts of potassium, sodium, and chloride involved in maintaining the potentials are insignificant as compared with the amount of the ionic stores. Even when the sodium pump (or coupled sodium-potassium pump) is not working, an axon can be stimulated to produce over 100,000 action potentials before its ionic stores are exhausted. Hence such systems as the sodium pump have plenty of time to redistribute and replenish the ionic stores. In its effect, the pump is electrically neutral, because the pumping of sodium ions out of the neuron is accompanied by an inflow of an equal amount of potassium ions. In an axon the local response is a depolarization that precedes the action potential. It is significant that the nerve impulse is not an electric current like one that passes through an electrical wire but is rather a sequence of ionic exchanges in which the electrical charges are indicative of an action potential. Actually, nerve fibers are very poor conductors of electricity. Within a millisecond or so after the action potential has passed by, the cell membrane is restored to its resting potential, in which state the extracellular fluid is positive to the intracellular fluid. This smooth progressive movement of the action potential is the method of conduction in unmyelinated nerves.

Saltatory conduction The propagation of the action potentials by continuous spread along the axon applies to unmyelinated fibers. This spread is relatively slow. Nature has evolved two strategies to increase the speed of conduction. The first is to increase the cross-sectional size of the axon; this method has been utilized in the giant axon of the squid. The second is to add myelin around a nerve fiber. By this strategy the conduction velocity is greater in the myelinated than in the unmyelinated axons of the same cross-sectioned size. The latter means is utilized by vertebrates.

The action potential in a myelinated nerve is propagated by *discontinuous spread, or saltatory (hop or jump) conduction* (Figs. 3-3 and 3-4), in which the nerve impulse hops along the nerve fiber from node of Ranvier to node of Ranvier. The current apparently spreads electronically from active to inactive node. This, along with increasing fiber diameter, is nature's way of obtaining higher speeds of conduction; the greater the distance between nodes of Ranvier in a nerve fiber, the faster its speed of conduction. The mye-

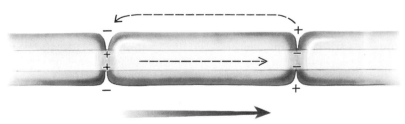

FIGURE 3-4 Saltatory conduction. The conduction of the nerve impulse in a myelinated nerve fiber probably occurs as a local circuit "leaps" from one node of Ranvier to the next node of Ranvier. Arrow below figure indicates direction in which nerve impulse is propagated.

lin sheath acts as an insulator with considerable electric resistance, which constrains ionic flow.

The *node of Ranvier* is the site where ionic interchange between the interstitial fluid and the intracellular fluid readily occurs. This discontinuous ionic movement at the node is efficient from the energy point of view. The nodes are sites of high capacitance and low electrical resistance. No inward current passes through the myelin, and the underlying plasma membrane is not excited as the spike passes by. The extraneuronal path for local current propagation is outside the myelin sheath—not deep to it.

The local bioelectrical circuits generated at the node where the impulse is passing can reach out for a considerable distance in advance of the action potential. Eddy currents are produced by the movements of potassium and sodium cations from two or three resting nodes of Ranvier ahead. Each node is a site of self-regeneration. In saltatory conduction, the nerve impulse hops because only small patches of plasma membrane of nerve at the nodes can be depolarized to propagate the impulse. The nodes with low thresholds are linked together by myelinated internodes (segmented insulating jackets) that act as passive conductors. Saltatory conduction may be enhanced by the restraint of extracellular fluid within the periaxonal space of the internode (see Fig. 2-12).

The distance from node to node (internodal distance) varies from 200 to over 1000 μm. The ratio of the internodal distance to the diameter of the nerve fiber is approximately 100:1. The more a fiber is myelinated, the longer is its internodal distance, and the faster it conducts an action potential. The myelin improves the signaling efficiency of the nerve fiber.

"Baby" action potentials

Dendrites generally have plasma membranes which do not conduct action potentials. However, long branching dendrites of some neurons do conduct small action potentials, called "baby" action potentials. These neurons comprise Punkinje cells of the cerebellar cortex (Chap. 9), pyramidal cells of the hippocampus (Chap. 15), motor neurons of the oculomotor nerves, and spinal motor neurons (Chap. 5). These dendrites generate baby action potentials

which act to propagate potentials to the cell body and initial segment of each neuron.

Refractory periods

Each point on the nerve fiber is not reexcitable for a millisecond after the peak of the action potential has passed it, no matter how intense the stimulus. This millisecond interval is known as the *absolute refractory (hyperpolarized) period*.

The hyperpolarized period results because the potassium conductance is slow in cutting off and takes a few milliseconds to return to resting levels. This period ends when the number of sodium ions is great enough to generate outward current sufficient to overcome the outward current generated by the "slowly" closing potassium channels. This period implies that a nerve fiber cannot transmit more than 1000 impulses per second (some nerve fibers are thought to have an absolute refractory period of a fraction of a millisecond to a few tenths of a second and hence may transmit up to 2000 impulses per second). Thus, for example, a fiber of the auditory nerve cannot transmit a sound of 10,000 cycles per second in the form of 10,000 impulses per second.

Other periods, called *relative refractory periods*, have higher or lower than normal excitability thresholds. This is related to the readjustments made by the conductance channels.

Transmitter release

Communication between nerve cells and between nerve cells and effectors (muscle and glandular cells) is generally by chemicals (neurotransmitters). When the action potential invades the axon's presynaptic terminal, the depolarization increases the permeability of the Ca^{2+} channels in the presynaptic membrane. The calcium conductance is voltage dependent. Calcium ions move inward and trigger the synaptic vesicles to release their neurotransmitter contents into the synaptic cleft. The calcium aids in the binding (fusing) of the synaptic vesicles to specific release sites on the presynaptic membrane. Na^+ and K^+ ions are not required for the actual release. In less than 100 μs the acetylcholine released from the vesicle diffuses across the synaptic cleft and binds with the acetylcholine receptor proteins on the postsynaptic membrane.

Neurotransmitters are released as biological quanta rather than as a continuous stream from the vesicles. Apparently all transmitters are stored in vesicles in a precursor form. After the vesicles fuse with the presynaptic membrane, the neurotransmitters are discharged as the vesicle opens up into the synaptic cleft by exocytosis (Fig. 3-5). Quantal release is the rule. A quantum appears to be the number of transmitter molecules per vesicle and is the smallest quantity of units released.

It has been calculated that, at the motor end plate synapse, a quantum contains slightly less than 10,000 molecules of acetylcholine. This quantum activates approximately 2000 ionic channels (channel proteins) in the postsynaptic membrane; these channels remain open for about 1 ms and then shut down. During the brief period that a channel is open about 20,000 Na^+ ions and about the same number of K^+ ions pass through the 0.4- to 0.6-nm pore of the channel. This produces an ionic flow that results in a change in the voltage difference on the two sides of the plasma membrane so that it approaches zero (see Fig. 3-2). The acetylcholine, released by the nerve impulse, produces a postsynaptic potential (voltage change) that lasts for about 5 ms. The resulting activity in the postsynaptic membrane (graded potential; see Fig. 3-2) is chemically dependent (channel chemically gated by acetylcholine); it is not voltage-dependent (channel not voltage-gated).

A large number of peptides, called *neuropeptides*, are involved in some way with neural activity. These peptides, found throughout the vertebrate nervous system, are presumed to have essential roles either as neurotransmitters, neurohormones, or neuromodulators. As yet, their precise roles have not been elucidated. A *neurohormone* is a chemical released by a nerve cell that acts like a neurotransmitter but does not require direct contact between nerve cell releasing the agent and the target cells (endocrine system). A *neuromodulator* is a chemical agent that alters the responsiveness of a nerve cell to a neurotransmitter but does not itself carry the nerve signals.

Neurotransmitters capable of evoking EPSPs include acetylcholine and norepinephrine. All EPSPs are summational (see page 101). The first impulse arriving at the synapse produces an EPSP. If a second impulse arrives at the synapse before the first EPSP has decayed, it positively adds (summates) to whatever remains of the first. In turn a third EPSP adds to what remains of the other two. The addition of successive EPSPs at the same synapse is called *temporal summation*. The addition of EPSPs at different synapses on the same neuron is called *spatial summation*. If the summation of EPSPs can reach the critical level at a nodal point such as the initial segment, an action potential is generated (see Figs. 3-2 and 3-7).

The postsynaptic membrane of the dendrites and cell body is presumed to have different properties from the presynaptic membrane of the axon. These differences are significant in the integrative activity of the neuron. The action potential of an axon is a traveling potential, is not graded (i.e., has an all-or-none response), and exhibits refractoriness immediately following a stimulation. In contrast, the postsynaptic potential is a standing potential (i.e., it does not travel), is graded, and lacks refractoriness immediately following a stimulation. These properties are most significant, for they mean that a second postsynaptic potential can be added to the first potential (temporally, summated subliminal stimuli). The graded responses provide a greater flexibility and plasticity of reaction to the neuron and to the nervous system than the rigidity of the stereotyped all-or-none pulse.

Decremental conduction and the receptor membrane

The *all-or-none nerve impulse* (*digital spike or pulse*) is characteristic of the axon, which is specialized for conducting long distances. The remainder of the neuron, cell body, and dendrites of a typical neuron may not respond in an all-or-none manner but propagates a response with decrement. Unlike the response of the axon, the local response is not necessarily followed by an action potential. Stimulation of receptor sites on the cell body and dendrites of a motor neuron evokes a *graded response* (*local response*) which spreads with decrement (cable property) and fades out in a short distance. The graded response generated at one synapse does not generally reach the initial segment of the axon because, except for the few synapses near an initial segment, most synapses are too far from the initial segment. The initial segment on the axon is the critical site at which an action potential is initiated and generated in the axon. If the decremental spreading activity of the neuron reaches the initial segment, an action potential may result. The dendrites and the cell body are adapted not for long-distance transmission but rather for integrating synaptic activity.

The terminal segment of a sensory nerve ending may also exhibit decremental conduction without all-or-none activity. The terminal segments, or telodendria, are the unmyelinated portions of the nerve process. Stimulation of the terminal segment results in decremental conduction. Should the activity reach the node of Ranvier (initial segment) in the myelinated portion, an all-or-none action potential is generated in the nerve fiber and is conducted to the central nervous system. The critical site for the initiation of the action potential in many nerve fibers is the first node of Ranvier. The portion of the neuron exhibiting decremental conduction may be called the *receptor membrane* (see Fig. 3-10), because it is influenced by synaptic activity of other neurons (dendrites and cell body) and environmental stimuli (terminal segment of peripheral nerve ending). The precise location of the "initial segment" in an unmyelinated nerve is not known.

PHYSIOLOGY OF THE CHEMICAL SYNAPSE

Of prime significance in the integrative activities of the nervous system is the synapse. Although each nerve fiber may transmit an impulse in either direction within the neuron (toward or away from the cell body), conduction in a sequence of neurons is transmitted in only one direction (unidirectional conduction). In effect, the synapse is rectifying in that it allows the current to flow in one direction only. This one-way transmission occurs because the chemical transmitter, released only by the presynaptic neuron, triggers the postsynaptic neuron to respond in some manner. The synapse acts as a one-way valve, permitting the action potential of an axon to exert its influence across the synaptic cleft on a dendrite (axodendritic synapse) or on a cell body (axosomatic synapse). *Unidirectional conduction* across the synapse from the presynaptic neuron to the postsynaptic neuron results in the functional or dynamic polarity of any sequence of neurons.

With the arrival of the action potential, neurotransmitters (transmitters) are released from each bouton in packets or quanta (number of molecules contained in one presynaptic vesicle), rather than in a continuous stream (see Fig. 3-5). Each packet is a *biologic "quantum"* in the sense that it is the minimal unit of release. These quanta are released from the synaptic vesicles within the bouton into the synaptic cleft by exocytosis (Chap. 2). The *putative transmitters* include acetylcholine, norepinephrine, dopamine, 5-hydroxytryptamine (serotonin), aminobutyric acid (GABA), glycine, and others.

According to *Dale's principle*, each neuron elaborates and releases the same transmitter at all its synaptic terminals. This does not imply that the effects of this neurotransmitter are the same on all postsynaptic cells innervated by each neuron, because the effects are largely determined by the postsynaptic cell ("Graded Postsynaptic and Receptor Potentials" further on.) The Dale principle does not apply to all neurons. The existence of two neurotransmitters in the same neuron has been demonstrated in some neurons.

Transmission of neurotransmitters across the chemical synapse usually requires from 0.3 to 1.0 ms (synaptic delay or synaptic latency). Synaptic delays of several milliseconds may occur in the autonomic ganglia. The synapse has a lower safety factor than the axon, for, unlike the axon, which is essentially not fatigable, the synapse is fatigable. During anoxia resulting from an insufficient blood supply or from general anesthesia, synaptic transmission succumbs much sooner than does axonal conduction. This coincides with the fact that the synaptic physiology is altered by many pharmaceutical agents.

Receptor potential

Sensory nerve endings are stimulated by some form of energy. Such endings usually respond with an excitatory *receptor (generator) potential*. Some receptors that respond to stimulation by evoking inhibitory activity (see "Rods and

Cones" in Chap. 12). The excitatory receptor potential is generated by the inflow of Na^+ and outflow of K^+ through their respective channels on the nerve ending (see Fig. 3-11). This receptor potential, actually an EPSP, when active spreads passively for 1 or 2 mm along the plasma membrane. If the potential reaches a low-threshold site, such as a node of Ranvier, an action potential can be generated (Fig. 3-11 and page 101).

ROLE OF INHIBITION

Although excitation is an active form of expression, inhibition has a major role in the refinement of that expression. In fact, the nervous system is largely an inhibitory system. Excitation sets the tone while inhibition does the sculpturing. For example, in learning the skill of writing, inhibition is critical. Actually a child can make most motions but is unable to control them efficiently. In the learning process the inhibition of the nonessential motions is a critical key to the essential focal act. In many neural afflictions the impairment of inhibitory influences explains the state. The loss of inhibition is crucial in epilepsy and the abnormal movement diseases (Chap. 14). We are, in a way, restrained by inhibition, like Gulliver when he was tied down. Processing is largely inhibitory.

Electric (electronic) synapse

In the *electric synapse*, the currents generated by the action potential in the presynaptic nerve spread directly into the postsynaptic neuron through the low-resistance, high-conductance channels of the connexons of the gap junction (see Chap. 2, Figs. 2-9 and 2-12). Transmission at these synapses can be bidirectional. However, only a small amount of transmission actually occurs in either direction; in such cases the backward transmission usually has no effect. Although these high-speed electrotonic junctions are infrequent in the mammalian, including the human, central nervous system, they are found between some neurons of the olfactory bulb, sensory neocortex, cerebellar cortex, inferior olivary nucleus, lateral vestibular nucleus, and the mesencephalic nucleus of the trigeminal nerve.

Electronic coupling in other tissues is common—most epithelial cells, cardiac muscle, and smooth muscle—and in the embryo. Electric synapses are called *intercalated disks* in cardiac muscle and *nexuses* in smooth muscles. In embryonic tissues such coupling is most frequent; it may be the significant way by which messages are communicated for the regulation of induction, differentiation, and development. This electronic coupling in the embryo disappears at critical times during development.

Postsynaptic and presynaptic inhibition

Inhibition may be expressed upon a neuron as either postsynaptic or presynaptic. *Postsynaptic inhibition* operates through axosomatic or axodendritic synapses on the receptive segment of a neuron (see Figs. 3-2, 3-6, and 3-7). In this type of inhibition the presynaptic neuron hyperpolarizes the receptive segment and decreases the likelihood that the postsynaptic cell will fire. On the other hand, presynaptic inhibition operates through axoaxonic synapses at the nerve terminal just proximal to an excitatory (axosomatic or axodendritic) synapse (see Figs. 2-8B and 2-10). In *presynaptic inhibition* the presynaptic (inhibitory) axon slowly depolarizes the presynaptic terminals of the excitatory neuron. The action of the axon is ultimately to reduce the transmitter output of the excitatory neuron. The action potential of excitatory neuron then stimulates a reduced release of transmitter—probably because the terminal membrane of the excitatory neuron is somewhat inactivated (presumably due to slight inactivation of Ca^{2+} conductance at the terminal). In effect, the action of the presynaptic inhibitory synapse is to excite through a neurochemical transmitter the excitatory synapse which now becomes less effective in releasing neurotransmitters for a brief period. Presynaptic activity is a means by which selective control can be exerted on restricted locales of a neuron.

Recycling of vesicles

The neurotransmitter in the synaptic cleft has a number of possible fates. It can (1) accomplish its designated role as activating a receptor site on the postsynaptic membrane, (2) diffuse away into the interstitial fluid, or (3) be inactivated by

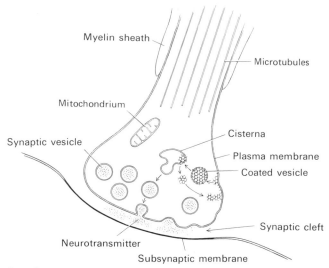

Myelin sheath

Microtubules

Mitochondrium

Synaptic vesicle

Cisterna

Plasma membrane

Coated vesicle

Synaptic cleft

Neurotransmitter

Subsynaptic membrane

FIGURE 3-5 Recycling of synaptic vesicles. Neurotransmitters are synthesized in a neuron, stored and packaged in vesicles, and released by exocytosis. The transmitters and vesicles are recycled (Fig. 6-5). Following exocytosis, the vesicle membrane fuses with the plasma membrane. New vesicle membranes are reformed by pinocytosis (endocytosis) and form the plasma membrane and its intermediary structures called cisternae. The coat of the newly formed vesicle is also recycled. (*After Heuser and Reese.*)

enzymes (Chap. 6) as, for example, acetylcholine by the enzyme cholinesterase. The neurotransmitter or one of its breakdown products can be taken up by the axon terminal and recycled (see Fig. 3-5).

The release of neurotransmitter at each synapse is a rapid and constantly ongoing activity. The amount of transmitter and vesicle membrane involved is large, especially with respect to the size of a nerve terminal. Although the raw materials do contribute to the formation of new vesicles, means have evolved to conserve and to reutilize the vesicle membrane and the neurotransmitter by recycling. Information on the recycling of some neurotransmitters (acetylcholine and norepinephrine) and their breakdown products are illustrated in Fig. 6-5. The vesicle membrane is apparently similar both structurally and functionally to a plasma membrane. According to one concept (see Fig. 3-5), the vesicle membrane fuses with the plasma membrane and, following release of the transmitter by exocytosis, is incorporated into the presynaptic membrane. The former vesicle membrane is then reincorporated by endocytosis into cisternae within the cytoplasm of the nerve terminal (see Fig. 3-5). New vesicles are generated from the cisternae.

Graded postsynaptic and receptor potentials

Postsynaptic potentials Receptor sites are present in the postsynaptic membranes of neurons, muscle fibers, and gland cells. Receptor sites are membrane-bound molecules that specifically recognize and bind a neurotransmitter, hormone, or drug. These sites are composed of specialized receptor proteins. In a neuron, these receptor proteins are present on the dendrites and cell body but essentially absent from any axon except at the initial segment or in the sensory endings. After crossing the synaptic cleft, the neurotransmitter interacts with receptor molecules and, in turn, this leads to a conductance change in the postsynaptic membrane (see Fig. 2-5).

Receptor sites (see Fig. 2-5) have several important features: (1) they are protein in nature; (2) they are located in the plasma membrane with the binding subunit, containing the binding site for the transmitter, facing outward so that the transmitter can reach the binding subunit; (3) they contain another subunit which can form a channel for the passage of ions through the plasma membrane (called an *ionophore*). The transmitter stimulates the binding subunit that, in turn, triggers the channel subunit to open and widen the ionophore channel. The transmitter is the key that fits into the binding subunit, which is the lock. Several different kinds of receptor sites may be present on a postsynaptic membrane, with each receptive to a different transmitter. The receptor site specifies (1) the kind of neurotransmitter that can elicit an action and (2) the nature of the response (excitatory or inhibitory). To state the matter otherwise, "only the receptor knows." For example, the transmitter norepinephrine acts to excite (depolarize) pacemaker cells in the heart and smooth muscle cells of the vas deferens, whereas it inhibits (hyperpolarizes) the smooth muscle of the gut and the secretory cells of the sublingual gland. Acetylcholine excites the contraction of voluntary muscles while it acts, through inhibition, to lower the heart rate.

The response of the postsynaptic membrane is either to evoke *excitatory graded potentials* called *excitatory postsynaptic potentials* (*EPSPs*) or *inhibitory graded potentials* called *inhibitory postsynaptic potentials* (*IPSPs*) (Figs. 3-2, 3-6, 3-7).

An *EPSP* is the result of a simultaneous increase in Na^+ and K^+ ion conductance with both Na^+ and K^+ channels open. This potential is not all-or-none (not regenerative). Rather, it is a graded decremental potential that lasts from a few to tens of milliseconds and extends for only a short distance along the postsynaptic membrane. Postsynaptic potentials are *not* voltage-dependent. As a corollary, the postsynaptic membrane is not responsive to electric stimulation like the plasma membrane of an axon. If the wave of depolarization reaches the integrative site of the neuron (spike-generating membrane, initial segment, first node of Ranvier) at threshold, then an action potential is initiated. The EPSP is generated by an inward flow of Na^+ and an outward flow of K^+.

An *IPSP* is the result of increase in the conductance of Cl^- ions and/or K^+ ions. When the inhibitory synapse is activated, the resultant inward flow of Cl^- through the chloride channels tends to make the interior of the cell adjacent to the plasma membrane more negative (see Figs. 3-6 and 3-7). This hyperpolarization drives graded postsynaptic potential away from threshold and thereby tends to prevent the integrative site from reaching the threshold essential for evoking an action potential. Inhibition raises the dendritic and somal potential from about the normal resting level of -60 to -80 mV or even higher.

Inhibitory gabanergic neurons—those releasing the neurotransmitter GABA—include all cerebellar inhibitory neurons (Chap. 9), many local circuit neurons such as Renshaw cells in the spinal cord (Chap. 5) and such Golgi type I cells as the Purkinje cells of the cerebellum.

Neuromuscular synapse

Voluntary muscle The *motor end plate* is a synapse between a nerve and a voluntary muscle fiber; it is called a *neuromuscular synapse or junction*. When the action potential of the motor nerve reaches this junction, a large amount of acetylcholine is released into the synaptic cleft. This triggers the postjunctional membrane (postsynaptic membrane, end plate of the muscle fiber) to generate a muscle action potential, which is conducted along the plasma membrane. This action potential sets off a series of reactions resulting in the contraction of the muscle fiber (see Fig. 3-8). The action potential of the alpha motor neuron always evokes an *obligatory response* (viz., the muscle fiber contracts) because more than enough neurotransmitter is always liberated to get a muscle action potential and a contraction.

The sequence of events within a lower motor neuron, motor end plate, and voluntary muscle illustrates some basic phenomena of activities of the nervous system. The motor end plate is actually a neuromuscular synapse between a nerve and a muscle. Acetylcholine is synthesized within the lower motor neuron (or any cholinergic neuron) by the combination of choline and acetyl coenzyme A (acetyl CoA). The reaction is catalyzed by choline acetyltransferase (choline acetylase). Choline is primarily transported into the neuron, whereas acetyl CoA is a product of mitochondrial oxidative activity of the neuron. The choline acetyltransferase originates in the cell body and, either by active transport or axoplasmic flow, flows down to the nerve terminals, where it is present within the cytoplasm and not in the synaptic vesicles (see Fig. 6-5).

After being synthesized, the acetylcholine is bound to a protein and stored in the storage

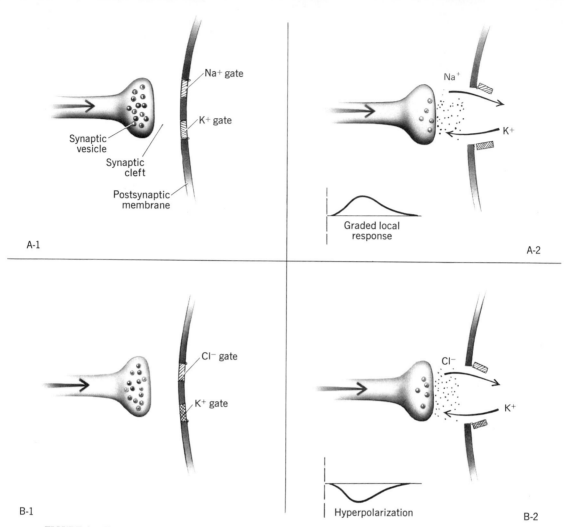

FIGURE 3-6 Excitatory synapses (*A*) and inhibitory synapses (*B*). *A-1* and *B-1.* Synapses prior to release of neurotransmitter. *A-2.* Excitatory postsynaptic response following release of neurotransmitter with Na⁺ ion inrush through Na gate and K⁺ ion outrush through K gate. *B-2.* Inhibitory postsynaptic response following release of neurotransmitter with Cl⁻ ion inrush through Cl⁻ gate and K⁺ ion outrush through K⁺ gate.

granules (synaptic vesicles) of about 400-Å diameter. These spherical vesicles with clear centers contain acetylcholine plus a protein called *vesiculin* and ATP.

Vesicles may possibly be formed, in part, from neurotubules. Some acetylcholine is continuously liberated from the synaptic vesicles into cytoplasm, from which it crosses the presynaptic membrane into the synaptic cleft (gutter). Each quantum consists of about 10,000 acetylcholine ions. This small amount of acetylcholine stimulates the postjunctional membrane

(end plate) of the muscle fiber to produce random generator potentials (nonpropagated depolarization), which are called *miniature end plate potentials* (*MEPPs*). Each MEPP is graded, shows rapid decrement, and lasts only a few milliseconds; an MEPP does not result in muscle contraction. The acetylcholine is released into the synaptic cleft in quanta. Each quantum produces one MEPP. These small transient MEPP are a normal feature of the "resting" postsynaptic membrane. At least 40 to 50 quanta of acetylcholine are required to initiate the synaptic ac-

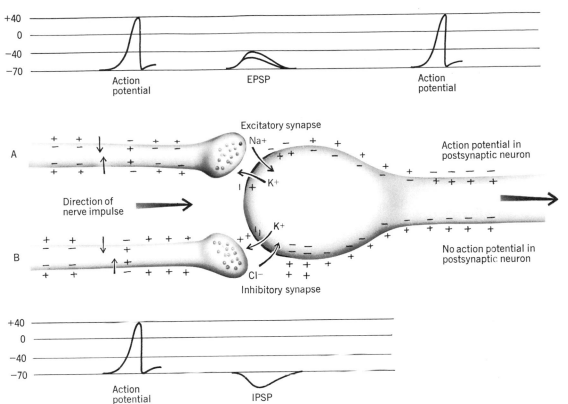

FIGURE 3-7 Sequences in (*A*) excitatory and (*B*) inhibitory transmission from presynaptic neurons (left) across synapses to postsynaptic neuron (right). *A.* The action potential conducted along the presynaptic axon to an excitatory synapse produces an EPSP, which, in turn, can contribute to the generation of an action potential in the postsynaptic neuron. *B.* The action potential conducted along the presynaptic axon to an inhibitory synapse produces an IPSP, which, in turn, suppresses the generation of an action potential in the postsynaptic neuron.

tivity which results in the contraction of a muscle fiber. Each nerve impulse activates the release of from 100 to 250 quanta of acetylcholine within a millisecond; this liberated amount is known as *quantal content.* Thus there is a substantial safety margin in neuromuscular transmission; hence an obligatory response.

As in other synapses, the inward flow of extraneuronal *calcium ions* across the presynaptic membrane in response to depolarization is prerequisite to the release of acetylcholine from the vesicles into the cleft. In the absence of calcium ions there is no release of acetylcholine following depolarization of the nerve terminals. *Magnesium* ions, acting as antagonists to the calcium ions, inhibit the release of acetylcholine. *Botulinus toxin*, a potent poison, blocks the release of acetylcholine from the nerve terminals, whereas

the venom of the black widow spider stimulates the rapid release of acetylcholine, causing depletion of the transmitter.

The events linking the excitation of the muscle plasma membrane (sarcolemma) to the contraction and relaxation of the muscle fibers are known as *excitation-contraction coupling* (*EC coupling*) or *electrochemomechanical coupling.* The EC coupling can be divided into (1) depolarization of plasma membrane, (2) release of Ca^{2+} and activation of contraction of the myofibrils, and (3) relaxation of myofibrils (Fig. 3-8).

Depolarization of the plasma membranes The muscle fiber is stimulated by the nerve action potentials which trigger, as in a typical chemical synapse, the release of many quanta of acetylcholine into the synaptic cleft of the motor end plate. The quanta content is sufficient to depolarize the postsynaptic plasma membrane (sarcolemma) to produce a normal end plate potential. The resulting wave of depolarization is conveyed along the sarcolemma and along the *tranverse tubules* (*T tubules*) of the muscle cell. The plasma membrane lining each T tubule is a continuation of the sarcolemma extending into the center of the fiber. The cavity of the T tubule contains "extracellular fluid" which is in communication with the extracellular fluid surrounding the muscle fiber. T tubules are located at each Z line of a muscle fiber. In effect, the surface area of a muscle fiber is increased manifold by the T tubules because the surface area of the tubules is five to seven times that of the outer surface of the muscle cell. These T tubules are the morphologic means by which the wave of depolarization is rapidly conveyed from the muscle surface to the interior of the fiber to initiate contraction and ensure the synchronous contraction of the fiber as a unit.

Calcium release and the activation of contraction The wave of depolarization stimulates the release of Ca^{2+} out of the sarcoplasmic reticulum (SR) into the space surrounding the myofilaments. The SR is a continuous system of membrane-limited tubular network—a specialized form of endoplasmic reticulum (see Fig. 3-8), with a segment adjacent to a T tubule (terminal cisterna) and longitudinal extensions oriented parallel to the plane of the contractile myofibrils (see Fig. 3-8). Each T tubule is flanked by two terminal cisternae to form the so-called triads of the voluntary muscle. Calcium ions are stored within the sarcoplasmic reticulum. The action potential of a T tubule stimulates Ca^{2+} ion release from the SR into the region of the thick-thin myofilament overlap. This translocation of the Ca^{2+} ions activates the contractile mechanism of the myofilaments. The conversion of adenosine triphosphate (ATP) to adenosine diphosphate (ADP) releases the energy required for this contraction.

Relaxation After the action potential is gone, the uptake of Ca^{2+} occurs; a calcium pump shifts the Ca^{2+} out of the myofilament space by active transport into the longitudinal part of the SR. The reduction in the calcium ion concentration

in the vicinity of the myofibrils prevents further contraction and thereby brings about relaxation of the muscle fibers. Finally, the Ca^{2+} ions shift back into their storage sites in the terminal cisternae.

Involuntary (smooth) muscles Smooth muscles are spindle-shaped cells which are in such close apposition with one another as to form gap junctions (nexus, Figs. 2-6B and 2-9E). These electrical junctions permit the spread of excitatory waves (contractions) from one muscle cell to another throughout the entire muscle mass. Smooth muscles can be stimulated to contract by postganglionic autonomic neurons (see "Enteric Nervous System," Chap. 6), by certain hormones, and by local changes within the muscle itself. Local contraction may be initiated in response to stretching of the muscle fibers. These muscles are capable of slow, sustained contractions; they are efficient because their contraction can be sustained with a minimal expenditure of energy. Smooth muscles maintain an "intrinsic tone" which is the basal tension upon which the other contractions are added.

The basic principles of excitation-contraction coupling and contraction by the sliding-filament principle expressed by voluntary muscles apply to smooth muscles. Although prominent filament bundles are present in smooth muscle cells, the actin and myosin filaments are not organized in parallel arrays. Excitation at the nerve-muscle junctions produces a membrane depolarization, which is followed by the release (contraction) and uptake (relaxation) of calcium ions so critical to muscle contraction and relaxation. The differences between the voluntary and involuntary muscle contractions—such as force, speed, and holding economy—are probably caused by the less regular arrangement of the myofilaments and the lesser number of contractile linkages in the involuntary muscle filaments.

On the basis of functional criteria, the smooth muscles have been classified as either *unitary muscles* or *multiunit muscles*. Unitary muscles are so called because contraction waves spread throughout the muscle mass as if the muscles were a single unit. These muscles are characterized by spontaneous activity, apparently initiated in pacemakers within the

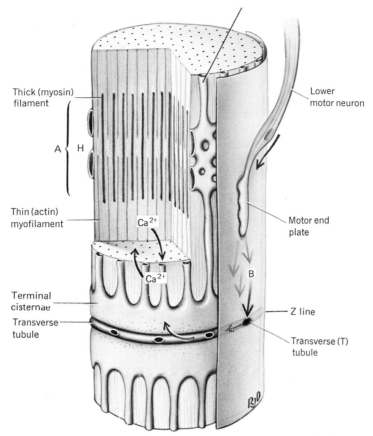

Thick (myosin) filament

A { H

Thin (actin) myofilament

Ca²⁺

Ca²⁺

Terminal cisternae

Transverse tubule

Lower motor neuron

Motor end plate

B

Z line

Transverse (T) tubule

FIGURE 3-8 Neuromuscular linkage. Sequence of events from the action potential of a motor nerve (A), to motor end plate, to action potential of muscle cell membrane (B), to T tubule and to sarcoplasmic cisternae. The release and uptake of calcium ions are involved with excitation-contraction (EC) coupling.

muscle, and by contractile responses to rapid stretch. Neural influences do not initiate contraction in these muscles, but rather, act to coordinate and regulate their contractile activity. Unitary musculature is found in the gastrointestinal tract, ureter, and uterus. *Multiunit muscles* are so called because each muscle mass, which is dependent upon its innervation for activation, is normally stimulated by multiple motor nerves to several regions within the muscle mass. These muscles do not exhibit spontaneous contractile activity, nor do they respond to stretch by contracting. Multiunit muscles are found in the vas deferens, ciliary muscles, iris, and larger blood vessels, and they are associated with hair (pilomotor muscles). The musculature of the urinary bladder is intermediate in that it exhibits properties of both types (Chap. 6).

Neuron as an integrator

The totality of the influences (excitatory and inhibitory) exerted by other nerve cells at any instant of time determines the state of excitability of the neuron; its somadendritic membrane can be regarded as an integrating mechanism that serves to sum these influences. Each neuron is a complex receptor and processor of a mosaic of numerous inputs. After integrating the stimuli from these inputs, the neurons may relay this information, which, in turn, is part of the input to other neurons, muscle fibers, or glandular cells. The synaptic receptor sites for the stimuli from other neurons are primarily located on the dendrites and cell body of a neuron. Quantitatively the dendrites generally contain more synapses than the cell body. In the motor neurons of the spinal cord in the cat, the surface area of dendrites is about 14 times that of the soma. About one-fifth of the thousands of synapses of each motor neuron are located on the soma and proximal 100 μm of the dendrites; about three-tenths are located on the dendrites between 100 to 300 μm from the soma; and the remaining half are associated with the dendrites more than 300 μm distal from the soma. The density of synapses on the axon hillock (close to the initial segment) is the same as on the soma.

In both the developing and the mature neuron, the cell membrane is not static but rather is a dynamic bilaminar membrane. The dynamism at its molecular level is presumed to be critical to the variety of physiologic activities expressed by this membrane of each neuron. These expressions include those bioelectrical properties associated with chemical synapses, electrical synapses, excitation and inhibition, decremental nonpropagated potentials, and nondecremental propagated potentials. Molecular recognition of plasma-bound molecules is considered to have a significant role in the development of the precise, complex, and intricate neuronal circuitry of the central nervous system and peripheral nervous system during prenatal and postnatal life. Similar cell-to-cell molecular interactions between regenerating neuronal processes and neurolemma cells occur during terminal and collateral nerve regeneration. Molecular-level activity associated with the plasma membrane has been presumed to be involved in some way with memory and learning processes.

Some of the receptor sites on the postsynaptic membrane of the dendrites and cell body are excitatory and some are inhibitory. In *excitatory depolarizing activity* the membrane channels at the receptor sites favor the transmembrane movements of sodium and potassium cations. In *inhibitory hyperpolarizing activity* the membrane channels at the receptor sites presumably favor the transmembrane movements of potassium cations and chloride anions. Interneurons which synapse with excitatory receptor sites are often called *excitatory interneurons;* those which synapse with inhibitory receptor sites are called *inhibitory interneurons.* The nondecremental action potential of either an excitatory or an inhibitory interneuron is "changed" at the synapse to the local decremental event. The dendritic activity is often called a *dendritic potential.*

In other words, each neuron may be influenced by hundreds or thousands of stimuli on its excitatory and inhibitory receptive sites. The complex interplay of the subliminal excitatory postsynaptic potentials (EPSP) and subliminal inhibitory postsynaptic potentials (IPSP) on each neuron endows the neuron with a variety of inputs; this provides the basis for the great plasticity of activity. Neurons are under continual "synaptic bombardment." In this battleground of activity, the neuron reacts and responds. If the algebraic summation of the polarizing EPSPs and hyperpolarizing IPSPs results in a depolarizing event at the low-resistance, low-threshold axon hillock, an action potential is generated and conducted along the axon. On the other hand, if the algebraic summation of the graded subliminal potentials is not enough to stimulate the *initial segment* sufficiently, an action potential is not generated in the axon. Two EPSPs (or IPSPs) of equal size may not be equally effective. One may be more effective than the other because it is located closer to the initial segment. Those EPSPs (or IPSPs) generated on the dendrites are less effective in exciting (or inhibiting) the neuron than those generated on the cell body or axon. Those graded postsynaptic potentials on the dendrites cannot reach the initial segment except by summating with other postsynaptic potentials (refer to "Spatial Summation" and "Temporal Summation" later on in chapter). In many neurons, synapses producing IPSPs are located on the axon hillock or on the initial segment; these synapses can be effective in throttling or blocking the generation of an action potential because they are located at a critical site.

In summary, each neuron is a miniature "integration" center where the confluences and algebraic summation of all the decremental spreads of EPSPs and IPSPs take place on the dendrites and cell body in relation to their geometric distribution and locations on the neuron (Figs. 3-2, 3-9, and 3-10). We are dealing, in these central nervous system cells, with a brain in miniature. The resulting action potential is, in effect, a code message conveying information about graded events in the dendrites and cell body of one neuron to a distant location where a

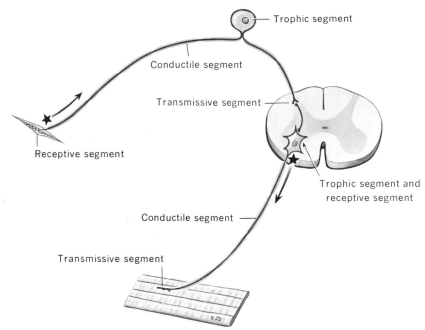

FIGURE 3-9 A structural and functional schema of a neuron. A neuron may be parceled into segments other than the classical dendrite, cell body, axon, and nerve endings. The sensory neuron may be parceled as follows: The receptive segment, which conducts with decrement, is the nerve ending; the initial segment (star) is the nodal site where the decremental conduction becomes the nondecremental (all-or-none) conduction of the conductile segment; the conductile segment, which conducts without decrement (all-or-none), extends from the initial segment to the synaptic endings within the spinal cord; the terminal (transmissive) segment includes the synaptic endings. In this neuron, the cell body is located within the conductile segment. The motor neuron may be subdivided as follows: the receptive segment includes the dendrites and cell body; the initial segment (star) is located just distal to the cell body; the conductile segment extends from the initial segment to the motor end plates; and the terminal segment is located within the motor end plates. In this neuron the cell body is located within the receptive segment.

graded event can be initiated on another neuron. Because the action potential evokes a graded response, the action potential in the central nervous system is said to be *optional*; it is not obligatory. In contrast, the action potential of a motor neuron on the voluntary muscle is *obligatory*.

In addition, a nerve cell fires periodically (ticks like a clock). The basis for this continued background activity is unknown; in effect, this firing is probably determined by some intrinsic mechanism within the neuron. Pacemaker loci may have a role in triggering these spontaneous rhythms.

Physiology of peripheral receptors

The afferent (sensory) neurons conveying information from the internal and external environment to the central nervous system are the uni-

polar and bipolar cells associated with the cranial and spinal nerves. The short peripheral segments of these nerves are associated with nerve endings, or peripheral receptors. According to one system, there are three anatomic forms of peripheral receptor. (1) Some nerve fibers actually end at the body surface and are in direct contact with the external environment. The olfactory nerves are the one example in human beings; these nerve terminals of the olfactory nerve are surrounded only by glandular secretions of the olfactory mucosal surface. (2) The actual nerve endings are in the tissues either as naked nerve endings or as encapsulated endings. (3) The nerve endings may have synaptic contact with a specialized neuroepithelial cell. The hair cells of the vestibular and cochlear system, the rods and cones of the eye, and the "taste cells" of the tongue are neuroepithelial cells.

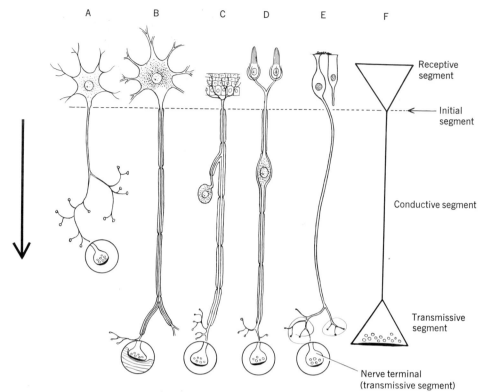

FIGURE 3-10 Structural and functional organization of representative neurons. Most neurons are composed of a receptive segment, an initial segment, a conductile segment, and a transmission segment. The transmission segment of each neuron is encircled. Arrow indicates normal direction of conduction of nerve impulse. *A.* Interneuron. *B.* Lower motor neuron. *C.* Sensory neuron with cell body in spinal ganglion. *D.* Neuron of vestibulocochlear nerve. *E.* Neuron of olfactory nerve. *F.* Functional organization of a neuron. Note that the cell body may be located within the receptive segment (*A*, *B*, and *E*) or within the conductile segment (*C* and *D*). The neuron of the vestibulocochlear nerve is associated with a hair cell in the upper part of figure. (*Adapted from Bodian*).

All receptors are biologic transducers which utilize the stimulus of one form of energy to initiate the "electric" energy of the nerve impulse. Mechanoreceptors utilize mechanical forms of energy that result in sonic sensations in humans, in ultrasonic sensations in dogs and bats, in muscle tension, in sensing movement and body position, in touch and pain, and in information on the blood pressure (pressoreceptors). Chemoreceptors utilize chemical energy that results in taste, in smell, and in evaluating the carbon dioxide content of the blood (chemoreceptors of the carotid body). Light receptors utilize light energy that results in sight. There is some infrared light sensitivity in receptor endings of the rattlesnake. Thermal receptors utilize the temperature gradients that produce the sensations

of cold and warmth. The external energies applied to these receptors act only as triggers to release the energy stored across the plasma membrane. Sensory receptors can be stimulated by more than one form of energy. However, each receptor is especially sensitive to a particular form of energy (as the ear is sensitive to sound waves); this form of energy—actually the lowest intensity stimulus to which a receptor will respond— is known as the *adequate stimulus.*

The result of an effective transduction by the adequate stimulus is the production of a receptor potential (generator potential, generator current) in the nerve terminal. It is called the *generator potential* because it may generate an action potential. This generator potential is actually an **EPSP** because it is a standing potential, is graded, lacks refractoriness, can be summated as the postsynaptic membrane, and spreads passively with decrement for 1 or 2 mm. A short distance from the nerve ending the fiber is ensheathed by a neurolemma cell and in some cases by a myelin sheath. The generator current may spread along the receptor to a site on the nerve with a low threshold for generating an all-or-none action potential. In the case of a myelinated fiber, this site might be located at the first node of Ranvier (see Fig. 3-11). The resulting digital impulse propagates along the nerve fiber to the central nervous system. The neurons through their telodendria have several receptors (a receptor field), each capable of producing a generator potential.

The Pacinian corpuscle serves to illustrate some basic principles of receptor activity (see Fig. 3-11). Within the lamellar capsule are an unmyelinated segment and a myelinated segment of the nerve ending. In the "resting" state the afferent neuron, including the unmyelinated segment, has a potential of 70 mV, the resting potential. Displacement and movement, not

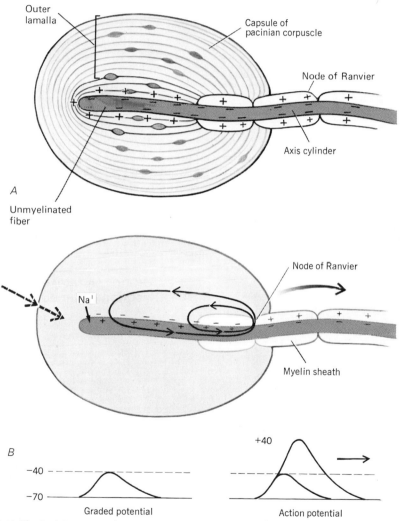

FIGURE 3-11 The Pacinian corpuscle as a receptive segment. *A.* The Pacinian corpuscle prior to stimulation has an axis cylinder with a resting potential. *B.* The stimulated corpuscle (dashed arrow) evokes a graded potential, which, in turn, triggers the generation of an action potential at the first node of Ranvier.

pressure, on the Pacinian corpuscle provide the stimulus which produces changes in the molecular structure of the plasma membrane. This is followed by local changes in the permeability of the unmyelinated portion.

Stimulation changes the low conductance state of the nerve terminal to a state of high conductance to sodium ions. Thus, the extracellular sodium ions are mainly responsible for the depolarization. The *local, graded depolarizing potential* is the generator potential. When the depolarization reaches the electrically excitable membrane at the first node of Ranvier, an action potential is generated in the afferent fiber (see Fig. 3-7).

When the stimulus at the receptor is weak, no action potential develops; when stimulus is strong but brief, several action potentials develop; and when stimulus is strong and sustained, a train of many impulses follows. The digital pulses of the action potentials are the means by which the coded data from the receptors are transmitted to the central nervous system. In another context the code resides in the chemical events of the sodium and potassium ions. This axonal transmission is analogous to a system utilizing only dots, not both dots and dashes. The frequency of the digital pulses transmitted varies. The greater the stimulus, the greater the frequency of the nerve impulses. In this analogy the afferent neurons utilize frequency modulation (FM), not amplitude modulation (AM).

A STRUCTURAL AND FUNCTIONAL CONCEPT OF THE NEURON

The neuron may be thought of as a cell with (1) a receptive segment, (2) an initial segment, (3) a conductile segment, (4) a terminal transmissive synaptic segment, and (5) a trophic segment (see Figs. 3-9 and 3-10). The receptive segment is specialized for the reception of stimuli and for the propagation of decrementally propagated responses. In a sense, the receptive segment monitors and integrates neural information. The initial segment is the junctional or trigger zone between the receptive segment and the conductile segment. It is the site at which the initiation of all-or-none action potential in any neuron is triggered. The conductile segment is specialized

for the conduction of information for long distances from the receptive segment to the terminal transmissive synaptic segment. To perform this function, the conductile segment conducts the nondecremental all-or-none action potentials. The synaptic terminal segment is incorporated in a synapse. The trophic center is the cell body, which is the metabolic center essential to the maintenance of the viability of the neuron. Note that the trophic segment may be located within the receptive segment or within the conductile segment.

In a peripheral sensory myelinated unipolar neuron the receptive portion is the telodendria, the initial segment is the first node of Ranvier between the telodendria and the myelinated fiber, and the conductile segment includes the remaining cell processes, the axon and dendrite (see Figs. 3-10 and 3-11). The trophic segment is located within the conductile segment in the spinal ganglion.

In the typical somatic motor neuron (see Figs. 3-9 and 3-10) the receptive segment includes the dendrites and the cell body; the junctional zone is the initial segment of the axon just distal to the cell body; the conductile segment is the axon; and the synaptic segment is incorporated into the motor end plate. In this motor neuron the trophic segment is within the receptive segment.

Membrane proteins and the functional organization of a neuron (Fig. 2-5)

The proteins within the plasma membrane have been classified into five types: pump, channel, receptor, enzyme, and structural proteins. These membrane proteins that are embedded in the lipid bilayer are called intrinsic proteins. Those that are attached to the membrane surface are called peripheral proteins. Although some proteins are firmly fastened within the plasma membrane, the intrinsic proteins are often free to diffuse within the membrane. The membrane proteins are not distributed uniformly over the entire plasma membrane nor are they present in equal amounts in all neurons. Depending upon the functional demands and requirements, the types and density of the proteins vary in different regions of the neuron. The pump proteins have roles in moving ions across the membrane, as, for example, the sodium pump. The channel proteins form the channels for the passage of ions across the plasma membrane. Receptor proteins are characterized by having specific binding sites with high affinity for certain substances. For example, the neurotransmitter acetylcholine is attracted to a specific binding site on the postsynaptic membrane. Enzyme proteins facilitate certain chemical reactions at the membrane surface. Structural proteins help to interconnect cells (e.g., at gap junctions) and to maintain the subcellular structure of a neuron. An intrinsic protein may act in more than one capacity; for example, it may function as a receptor, an enzyme, and a pump at the same time (see Figs. 2-5 and 2-12).

Pumps are intrinsic membrane proteins that expend metabolic energy to shift ions against concentration gradients in and out of the neuron. The sodium pump is such a protein; more specifically it is called the sodium-potassium adenosine triphosphate pump. It harnesses the energy stored in the phosphate bond of the adenosine triphosphate (ATP); the pump mediates the exchange of three sodium ions on the inside of the neuron for two potassium ions on the inside. The total amount pumped is regulated to the physiological requirements of the neuron. An average small interneuron is calculated to have 1 million sodium pumps with the capacity to transport about 200 million sodium ions per second. Each pump can maximally move about 200 sodium ions and 120 potassium ions across the plasma membrane per second.

Channel proteins are selective and can gate —selective in that the channels are selectively permeable to different ions. The gating is achieved by a mechanism regulating the opening and closing of the membrane channels. With respect to sodium and potassium ions, one type of channel is quite selective by permitting the passage of sodium ions primarily and only slightly of potassium ions. Another channel type is primarily selective for the passage of potassium ions. Another channel type is essentially nonselective in that relatively equal amounts of sodium and potassium ions can pass through each channel.

Two types of channels are recognized on the basis of the gating mechanism. One channel type opens and closes in response to the voltage dif-

ference on either side of the cell membrane. This type is said to be voltage-gated. The voltage-gated channels are usually designated for the ion that passes through the channel most readily (e.g., sodium channel). Other channel types respond by opening when a certain molecule (a neurotransmitter or drug) binds to the receptor site on the channel protein. This type is said to be chemically gated (e.g., acetylcholine-activated channel or GABA-activated channel).

The plasma membrane of an axon (conductile segment of a neuron) has voltage-dependent channels almost exclusively with few, if any, chemically gated channels. In contrast, the plasma membrane of a dendrite and cell body of a neuron (receptive segment of a neuron) have chemically gated channels with only a few voltage-gated channels.

GENERAL PRINCIPLES OF INTERNEURONAL ACTIVITY

The neurons of the nervous system interact in a matrix of organized complexity which is far from being completely unraveled. Several basic principles of the structure and function operative in the nervous system will be described.

Neuronal circuits

The neurons of the nervous sytem are organized in sequences of cells called *neuron circuits*. Some are shown in Figs. 3-12 and 3-13. Although the examples used below are found in the spinal cord (Chap. 5), these circuits are found in all levels of the central nervous system.

1. The simplest circuit, the two-neuron (monosynaptic) chain, as found in the stretch extensor reflex, consists of an afferent neuron, an intermediary synapse, and an efferent neuron (Chap. 5).
2. The three-neuron (disynaptic) open circuit is formed by the intercalation of an interneuron between an afferent neuron and an efferent neuron. An example of this open circuit is the withdrawal flexor reflex (Chap. 5). An open circuit is a chain of neurons connected with other neurons, none of which connects (either directly or indirectly) through an axon with a prior neuron in the chain.

3. The simple closed circuit is formed by the intercalation of an interneuron between the recurrent axon collateral branch of an efferent neuron and the original efferent neuron. A closed circuit contains an interneuron that connects (feeds back) to a prior neuron in the chain (see Fig. 3-12). This is a simple feedback circuit whereby the efferent neuron may influence itself. An example of the closed feedback circuit is found in the anterior horn of the spinal cord in the circuit of the (alpha) motor neuron and the interneuron neuron (Renshaw cell, Chap. 5).

4. The open multiple-chain circuit is formed by many interneurons, all linked through collateral branches and arranged in parallel chains. The synaptic delays and the variability of conduction times in the links of these chains are features of this circuit system. A functional consequence of such a chain is that the neurons at the end of these circuits can be subjected to prolonged and variable stimulation.

5. The closed multiple-chain circuit is formed by many interneurons intercalated between the recurrent axon collateral branch of an efferent neuron and the original efferent neuron. These closed multisynaptic chains form feedback circuits that apparently permit the reverberation of impulses which can thereby raise or lower the excitability of various neurons in the chain.

Principle of divergence

Each neuron synapses with many other neurons. An afferent nerve cell that is stimulated by peripheral receptors terminates in the central nervous system by arborizing into many branches (telodendria), each branch having synaptic con-

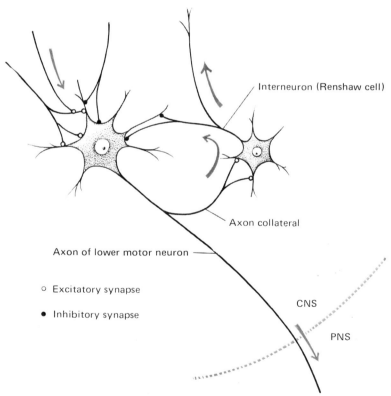

Interneuron (Renshaw cell)

Axon collateral

Axon of lower motor neuron

○ Excitatory synapse

● Inhibitory synapse

CNS

PNS

FIGURE 3-12 The neuron as an integrator. Arrows indicate the direction in which nerve impulses are propagated. Neurons from many sources in the brain, spinal cord, and body convey influences to each lower motor neuron (Chap. 5), which in turn innervates some voluntary-muscle fibers.

tact with the receptive portion of many other neurons (see Fig. 3-13A). The axons of some neurons of the central nervous system are estimated to branch sufficiently to synapse with up to 25,000 or more other neurons. The opportunity of a neuron to excite (or to inhibit) numerous other neurons by the divergence of its axonal terminal branches is a fundamental principle underlying the activity of the central nervous system.

Principle of convergence

Each neuron of the central nervous system is excited and inhibited by the synaptic activity of many other neurons on its dendrites and cell body (see Fig. 3-13B). This receptive portion of the neuron is the focus for the convergence of the activity of, in many cases, literally thousands of other neurons. The integrated reactivity of the excitatory and inhibitory synapses on the receptor portion of the neuron may result in the generation of an action potential in the axon of the neuron.

Principle of afterdischarge

A stimulus such as a pinprick on a finger will evoke a response, the reflex withdrawal of the finger. Theoretically the time interval from stimulus to response in this three-neuron flexor reflex arc is equal to the time of conduction through the three neurons plus the synaptic delays. However, the muscle may continue to contract for many milliseconds after the withdrawal of the stimulus (i.e., the contraction outlasts the stimulus). This is because of "after discharge," which results from the activity of other circuits in addition to the three-neuron reflex arc. The multiple open- and closed-chain circuits provide a succession of discharges which arrive to excite the motor neuron after a slight delay. The neural activity transmitted through the longer multineuronal circuits arrives at the motor neurons later than that transmitted through the short pathway circuits. These multisynaptic systems "recirculate" the neural activity through interneurons, and this results in the sustained excitation of the motor neurons. The (after) discharge, which occurs after the stimulus is off, prolongs the reflex response.

Facilitation

Facilitation (literally, "making easy") is the phenomenon wherein a normally subliminal (subthreshold) stimulus from a presynaptic neuron "primes" a postsynaptic neuron so that another subliminal stimulus can evoke a discharge of the postsynaptic neuron. In brief, the first stimulus has facilitated the postsynaptic neuron. The start of a sprint race offers an analogy. The starter's instruction of "Get set" is the stimulus that "facilitates" the sprinters for the final stimulus of "Go." Many interactions of the central nervous system involve facilitation.

Disinhibition

Facilitation may be produced in one of two ways: by the direct activity of excitatory synapses, or by prevention of the action of inhibitory synapses. The latter is known as *disinhibition*. Disinhibition is functionally expressed in such a circuit as the sequence of a collateral branch of a motor neuron, to a chain of several interneurons, terminating on a motor neuron. In such a circuit, the collateral branch of a motor neuron (neuron 1) synapses and may excite an interneuron (neuron 2) with inhibitory synaptic endings; these endings stimulate an interneuron (neuron 3) with inhibitory synaptic endings, which, in turn, synapse with the postsynaptic membrane of a motor neuron (neuron 4). When neuron 3 is inhibited from firing by neuron 2, motor neuron 4 is actively inhibited. When this circuit is active, the motor neuron (neuron 4) may be temporarily released from this inhibitory stimulation; this release is an expression of disinhibition. This sequence commences with the facilitatory activity of the recurrent collateral branch of neuron 1 and terminates with active inhibition of the inhibitory interneuron (neuron 3). This recurrent facilitatory activity results in disinhibition (a release phenomenon, Chap. 9) of the motor neuron (neuron 4). Recurrent facilitation (disinhibition) and recurrent inhibition (active inhibition of postsynaptic membrane) are important to the organized circuitry of the nervous system.

The inhibition of an inhibitory pool (or an inhibitory pathway) is also called disinhibition.

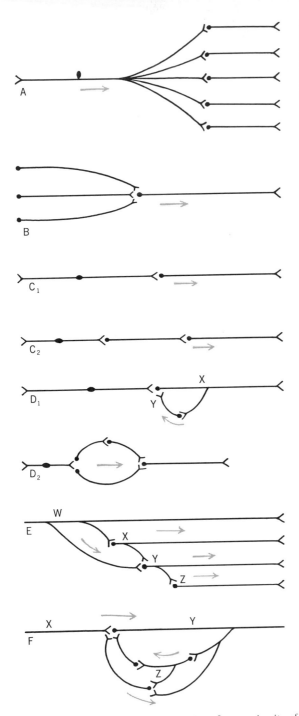

Spatial summation

Summation is an expression of the cumulative effects of a number of stimuli upon a neuron. Spatial summation is the summation (integration) of many EPSPs received almost simultaneously at different sites on the receptive portion of the neuron from several other neurons. This summation may (or may not) produce an action potential. Facilitation depends on spatial summation. The presynaptic neuron activity lowers the threshold of excitation of the postsynaptic neurons (EPSP), thereby facilitating or aiding the stimuli of other neurons to fire the postsynaptic neuron. Spatial summation of the postsynaptic potentials is the rule in the central nervous system.

Temporal summation

Temporal summation is a form of summation whereby the cumulative effects of repetitive subliminal EPSPs from a single presynaptic neuron on the receptive membrane of a postsynaptic neuron may summate in time to excite the neuron. Because of the short excitable period of the synapse, temporal summation is not considered to be as important as spatial summation.

Recruitment

Recruitment (the recruiting of neurons) is a neurophysiologic phenomenon in which a response (action potential) is obtained only after a rapid succession of afferent stimuli is delivered (see Fig. 3-13D). The complex of multiple chains

FIGURE 3-13 Schematic representation of some circuits of neurons. Arrows indicate direction in which nerve impulses are propagated. *A.* Principle of divergence. One presynaptic neuron branches and synapses with several postsynaptic neurons. *B.* Principle of convergence. Several presynaptic neurons synapse with one postsynaptic neuron. *C.* Simple open-type circuits. (*C-1*) Two-neuron sequence of afferent neuron synapsing with efferent neuron, found in a two-neuron reflex. (*C-2*) Three-neuron sequence of afferent neuron, interneuron, and efferent neuron, found in a three-neuron reflex. *D.* Simple closed-type circuits. (*D-1*) Simple feedback circuit, in which the axon collateral branch of neuron X synapses with interneuron Y, which, in turn, synapses with neuron X. Refer to Fig. 3-12. (*D-2*) Simple feed-forward circuit, basic to recruitment and after-discharge, as discussed in text. *E.* Open multiple-neuronal chain circuit. In this circuit, neuron W through a collateral branch, may influence neuron X and, through another collateral branch, may influence neuron Y. In turn neuron X, through a collateral branch, may influence neuron Y, and, in turn, neuron Y, through a collateral branch, may influence neuron Z. In essence the stimulation of neuron W may influence the activity of three other neurons. This is a form of divergence. *F.* Closed multiple-neuronal chain circuit (feedback circuit). In this circuit neuron Y, through a collateral branch, may influence a complex of neurons Z, which in turn may influence (feedback) neurons X and Y.

intercalated between the stimulated sites (afferent neurons) and the responsive sites (efferent neurons) is critical to the phenomenon of recruitment. Recruitment is a form of facilitation primarily utilizing closed multineuronal circuits. The following is a simplified explanation of this complex activity. The impulses resulting from the first afferent volleys travel via short circuits (an open loop) to the motor pool. These initial volleys are subliminal and thus not sufficient by themselves to elicit action potentials in the motor neurons of the motor pool. These initial volleys also activate closed multiple-chain circuits, but the resulting impulses arrive at the motor pool too late to summate with those traveling over the short circuits. However, these initial volleys transmitted through the closed multiple circuits arrive at the same time as the subsequent volleys transmitted with the short circuits. The resulting summation facilitates a response from the motor neurons in the motor pool. Recruitment is a form of facilitation obtained by repetitive stimulation. The complexities of the circuits capable of eliciting recruitment stagger the imagination.

Spontaneous activity in the central nervous system

The nervous system always shows evidence of activity. It is never quiescent. The continuous input from the peripheral receptors and their afferent nerve contributes to this activity. The intrinsic mechanism that keeps the units of the nervous system activated is unknown. It is theorized that without such an intrinsic mechanism (or mechanisms) the central nervous system could not sustain its activity.

One source might be active pacemaker sites. These sites might resemble the *pacemaker cells of the heart.* The pacemakers of the sinoatrial (SA) node, specialized atrial cells, atrioventricular (AV) node, bundle of His, and peripheral Purkinje fibers are automatic in that they can spontaneously excite themselves regularly. These pacemaker cells cycle. They cannot maintain their resting potential. After reaching the resting potential, the potential drifts toward the critical threshold that generates a return to the resting potential. At this point the cycle repeats. In the heart the SA node cycles about 70 to 90 times per minute, the AV node and bundle of His about 40 to 60 cycles per minute, and the Purkinje fibers about 25 to 30 cycles per minute. The SA node is *the* pacemaker because it has the faster cycles, and through these cycles, the SA node synchronizes the cycles of the other pacemaker cells.

The background of continuous and rhythmic spike discharge of neurons in the absence of known stimulation may be accounted for by similar activity. In a *neuronal pacemaker cycle,* the locally produced generator potential constantly drifts to the critical potential at a critical site of the neuron. At this moment, the neuron fires and the new generator potential repeats. These sites might resemble the pacemaker of the heart. The cells of a pacemaker form locally produced generator potentials that drift slowly toward the critical threshold that initiates and results in an action potential. This is followed immediately by a return to the resting or generator potential, which again commences to drift toward the critical threshold. This may account for the background of continuous spike discharge in the absence of known stimulation, or, in part, for rhythmic discharge (Chap. 13).

AUTOMATIC CONTROL SYSTEMS AND FEEDBACK

An understanding of the automatic control systems (servomechanisms) used by mathematicians and engineers is useful for gaining some conceptual insight into the operation of certain activities of the nervous system.

Biologic analogues exist with both the open-loop and the closed-loop control systems. These systems are designed to maintain some predetermined constant state, such as temperature, position, or speed. The open-loop control systems do not utilize feedback in their operation, whereas the closed-loop control systems do. Feedback is the return of a portion of the output of a system to the system proper for the purpose of influencing and automatically regulating the further operation of the system.

Open-loop control system

An example of this type of automatic system is the operation of a dam in the watershed. The dam in the reservoir is an automatic control which acts to prevent the water from rising above a certain predetermined level. However, the height of the dam is not regulated automatically by the amount of water drained out of the reservoir. Also when rainfall is low, the water level in the reservoir fluctuates below the dam level. The pertinent features of this system for this discussion are (1) the fact that the system does not utilize its output to effect its operation (the level of the dam) and (2) the degree of inherent instability (fluctuating water level).

A biologic open-loop system is the body temperature control of some cold-blooded (poikilothermic) animals. These animals apparently possess no feedback mechanism for the fine regulation of heat production and conservation. As a result their body temperature fluctuates widely. The environmental heat which influences the animal's body temperature is analogous to the watershed, and the ability of the animal to lose heat is analogous to the floodgate of the dam. When the environmental heat increases (or decreases) the temperature of the animal rises (or drops). The analogue is the rise (or fall) of the water in the reservoir.

Closed-loop control system

The closed-loop (cycle) systems utilize feedback, in which a fraction of the output of the system is (1) fed back into the system and (2) utilized in the further performance of the system. In brief, output can control or regulate input. The closed-loop system may utilize negative (degenerative) or positive (regenerative) feedback.

Control system utilizing negative feedback

This servomechanism utilizes negative feedback to maintain a predetermined performance (or goal) of the control system. This performance is obtained by making a series of self-correcting adjustments which are based on the feedback of the immediately prior performance (output) of the system to a control box (comparator). The feedback is called negative when the correction is in the opposite (negative) direction of the positive divergence from the predetermined performance. For example, the thermostat (control box) of a heating system (closed-loop control system) directs the maintenance of a constant temperature in a room by utilizing some of the heat (i.e., a feedback of a fraction of the output or controlled quality) to activate the thermostat, which, in turn, attempts to maintain the preset temperature by regulating the heat output of the furnace. In practice, the actual temperature fluctuates about the preset temperature of the thermostat. The system is goal-seeking in its attempt to match the predetermined reference. Information of the actual temperature is fed into the thermostat and compared to the preset temperature control. The sequence of feedback of the actual temperature (output of furnace), comparison of preset temperature (in thermostat), and adjustment (instructions relayed to furnace) is a continuous repetitive sequence. The feedback is a negative because an increase in the room temperature is followed by a reduced activity in the furnace with a subsequent decrease in heat production, while a decrease in the room temperature results in a subsequent increase of heat production. In effect, the negative feedback operates to maintain a relatively constant room temperature.

Control systems that utilize negative feedback act to compensate for the difference between the actual and the predetermined quality. They are self-correcting, error-correcting systems operating to maintain a goal. These systems ensure *stability* and *regulation*. Unless otherwise specified, feedback systems generally utilize negative feedback. Negative feedback subtracts from the input to the control center box. Biologic control systems are largely of this type.

The biologic implications of closed-loop control systems utilizing negative feedback are significant and widespread. Actually the control system concept is embodied in a phrase of Claude Bernard's, "constancy of the internal milieu" (internal environment), and in Walter B. Cannon's principle of homeostasis. Homeostasis represents the preset norm; when the homeostatic condition is upset, the organism utilizes its resources to restore the equilibrium (Chap. 6). Homeostasis is crucial to an animal's freedom of action, permitting the animal to function regardless of changes in the external environment. Homeostasis decreases the organism's dependence on the vagaries of the environment.

Examples of activities with negative feedback include the regulation of (1) visceral activities, (2) somatic activities, and (3) learning processes.

1. Maintenance of a relatively constant body temperature with narrow fluctuations is an expression of homeostasis utilizing the nervous system (Chap. 11). Regulation of the water balance in the body and that of the general hormonal levels are expressions of homeostasis which utilize both the nervous system (feedback through nerve cells) and the endocrine system (feedback through circulatory system) (Chap. 11).

2. Coordination and smooth integration among voluntary muscles are effected through complex feedback control systems in the spinal cord (see "Gamma Reflex Loop," in Chap. 5) and the cerebellum (Chap. 9).

3. In the higher neural processes of learning, negative feedback is used, as, for example, in maze learning. The initial trials in this form of learning are relatively random attempts with numerous oscillations from the preset goal. In subsequent trials, the randomness is reduced and the oscillations are less marked.

Many diseases in humans involve interferences, malfunction, and change in the efficiency of the feedback regulatory systems.

Control system utilizing positive feedback

A servomechanism which utilizes positive feedback returns part of the output to the control box to increase the output. This is a regenerative (or vicious) cycle system. It is unstable. It tends to explode or "run away." In a positive-feedback heating system, an increase in temperature results in a continuous spiraling increase in heat production until the furnace operates at full capacity, breaks down, or explodes.

The initial stages in the generation of an all-or-none action potential utilize the principle of positive feedback. The decrease in the resting potential (receptor potential or postsynaptic excitatory potential, EPSP) may be followed by the sequence of increased sodium conductance, some depolarization, further increase in sodium conductance, etc., until the threshold is reached. The positive feedback results in regeneration until the explosion of the all-or-none action potential. Positive feedback adds to the input to the control center box.

INTEGRATION CENTER AND MODULATION CENTER

Portions of the nervous system operate in feedback systems either as integration centers or as modulators. In a biologic feedback system the integration center is the crucial control center, for it regulates the goal-seeking performance of the system. It is the equivalent of the thermostat in a temperature control system. Without the integrative center the feedback system is essentially uncontrolled.

The hypothalamus acts as the integration center for the regulation of temperature (the controlled quality). When this temperature-regulating region of the hypothalamus is impaired or damaged, temperature control can be so altered that death may result. This feedback system utilizes the temperature of the blood to stimulate the temperature integrative center in the hypothalamus. This activates the nervous system and the organism to set in motion those processes that return the temperature to normal (Chap. 11).

A modulation center or higher control center is a region that may influence the integration center. It is not essential to the operation of the feedback cycle. For example, a timer that changes the setting on a thermostat is a modulator. The timer may raise the setting early in the morning, so that the room may be warm during the day, and lower the setting later in the day, so that the room is cool at night. The essential relation of the thermostat to the furnace is unchanged.

The hypothalamus acts as a modulator of the blood pressure *integration centers* in the lower medulla. Hypothalamic activity can affect the medullary cardiovascular center, causing it to raise (sympathetic effect) or lower (parasympathetic effect) the blood pressure (Chap. 8). It does not have a direct role in the vital feedback mechanism of blood pressure control.

The internal and external environments of

the organism are the sources of the stimuli that trigger the sensors in the body to initiate the transmissions of coded input to the central nervous system. This input is subsequently processed in the nuclear stations of the nervous system. Much of this information is utilized at subconscious levels in a variety of reflex activities. Some of this input may eventually lead to the formulation of a representation of the environment by the mind. In this way, individuals create their own worlds, worlds that are not stereotyped duplications of nature. These copies are biased, rather than faithful, reproductions. In fact, an animal is actually aware only of its own senses and their effects on the nervous system. For example, the physical movements of molecules in the air are vibrations, not sounds. The concert pianist generates air vibrations, not music as such. It is the ear and the brain that transform the vibrations into sounds and music. The air vibrations are transformed by the ear into the coded messages of nerve impulses. These messages are transmitted and processed in the auditory pathways and the higher brain centers, where the air vibrations are subjectively heard and interpreted as sounds or music.

CODING AND PROCESSING IN THE NERVOUS SYSTEM

Sensory endings and environmental energies

The sensory endings are the sources of information for the nervous system. These sensors are stimulated by a limited spectrum of the multitude of specific energies which impinge upon us. We cannot directly sense cosmic rays, radio waves, ultrasonic waves, and many other environmental energies, but we can sense "light" waves, "sound" waves, contact, and certain chemicals, among other forms of energy.

Information about the outer world is differentially sensed by an organism, because the threshold levels of its sensory receptors are different. This is used to advantage. For example, if the eyes were stimulated by all the radiations emanating from the sky at night, the sky would appear as an intensely "lighted" expanse. Since the eyes are sensitive to only a narrow band of

radiation, the stars are visible against the dark background of space.

In addition, humans and other organisms can sense similar stimuli as different perceptions. For example, the retina is sensitive to energies perceived as light in the range of 4×10^{14} to 8×10^{14} vibrations per second, while the skin is sensitive to radiant heat ranging from 3×10^{14} to 8×10^{14} vibrations per second. Note the overlap; i.e., some vibration frequencies are both seen and felt. A gradation of mechanically induced vibrations from 1 to about 20,000 Hz, transmitted through various media, can be sensed by human beings. The lowest frequencies are felt as touch. The frequencies up to 1500 Hz are perceived as vibrations (tested with the base of a tuning fork on a joint). The range of vibrations of from 30 to over 20,000 Hz are sensed as sound. Again note the overlap.

Each sensory receptor responds when adequately stimulated, quite specifically and regardless of the stimulus. For example, retinal stimulation results in the perception of light, whether the source of stimulation consists of "light" waves, electric shocks, or a blow on the eye. A specific energy which is capable of stimulating different types of receptors will evoke the perception of a different sensation from each sensor. For example, when electrical stimulation is applied to taste buds, taste may be sensed; when such stimulation is applied to the spiral organ of Corti of the inner ear, a sound may be sensed; or when it is applied to the retina, light may be sensed.

Receptor membrane, transduction, and receptor potential

The subjective sensation felt by the organism is not due to any known uniqueness in the basic neurophysiology of the neurons but is rather a function of the regions of the brain stimulated. Apparently all neurons are fundamentally similar; they all seem to exhibit similar neurophysiologic properties. Sensory neurons may differ only in that the various neurons are stimulated by different specific energies. However, these differences end at the receptor membrane of the neuron. The sequence of neurophysiologic events exhibited by a sensory neuron, commencing with its stimulation, includes the transduction, formation, and conduction of the code to the synaptic effector site. The code may exert a role in generating a new code in the postsynaptic neuron.

Transduction is the process of converting the signal of the environmental energy into the receptor (generator) potential at the nerve ending (Chap. 3). The receptor potential is graded in some proportion to the intensity of the stimulus. In a sense the receptor membrane corresponds to amplitude modulation (AM). The receptor can be enhanced by both spatial summation and temporal summation. The simultaneous stimulation of many of the arborizing endings of one nerve fiber can summate spatially to create a receptor potential of sufficient magnitude to trigger an action potential (Chap. 3), whereas an increase in the frequency of stimulation of a nerve ending can summate temporally to increase the magnitude of the receptor potential.

Coding in the nervous system

At the present time only a start has been made in the identification and evaluation of the codes employed by the nervous system to transmit information. Only a few aspects of coding are indicated in this account.

Each stimulus, which may be eventually comprehended as a modality, is a composite of several components. Presumably each of these components evokes several codes and even subcodes which are transmitted to the nuclear processing centers in the central nervous system. These components include intensity (a quantitative function), duration (a temporal function), location of stimulus either within or outside the organism, frequency (number of stimuli per unit time), and the dimensions of shape and motion.

The generator potentials evoked by a stimulus in a nerve receptor trigger an all-or-none action potential (digital pulse, spike) at the nodal point in a neuron (Chap. 3). The spike transmitted along the conductile segment (axon channel) is an expression of a code. The frequency of the spike (or of the interval between spikes) forms a basis for coding information; it may be utilized for evaluating gradations in the intensity of a given modality. The more intense the stimulus, the greater the number of impulses transmitted to the central nervous system per unit of time. The number of fibers stimulated is also significant. According to the pattern theory (Chap. 5), information as to the quality of a modality is transmitted via combinations of nerve fibers. This information is conveyed in these various axon channels as a spectrum of velocities ranging from the slow speeds in unmyelinated fibers to the fast speeds of heavily myelinated fibers. The pulse signals traveling in the various temporal patterns and velocities in a number of axon channels are organized into the coded data to which a nucleus is "listening" and from which a nucleus abstracts and processes information before transmitting its output code to other nuclei.

Transfer of information from one neuron to another

The transfer of coded information from one neuron to another occurs at the synapses by the secretion of neurotransmitter substances through each presynaptic membrane into the synaptic cleft where the secretion can influence the postsynaptic membrane of the receptive segment of the neuron. A new code-carrying signal is generated in the postsynaptic neuron. In effect, *each synapse performs a transformation function.*

Processing in the nervous system

The ascending (and descending) pathways function both as processors and as transmitters of coded information. *The processing within the nuclear stations of the pathways is information-linked, not energy-linked.* For example, as noted above, stimulation of the optic system evokes sensations related to visions, regardless of whether the stimulus is light, an electrical shock, or blow on the eye. One critical unsolved problem is: How are the signals selected in the presence of noise? Comparators and information generators may be present in the nervous system. The novelty of the stimulus and the degree of the deviation from random background activity in the nervous system may contribute.

Because of neuron may have numerous synaptic connections with many other neurons (divergence) and each neuron may be stimulated by many other neurons (convergence), the possibilities for interactions among neurons are great. The interactions of the impulses generated in neurons produce excitatory postsynaptic potentials (EPSPs) and inhibitory postsynaptic potentials (IPSPs) which are resolved in each of the neurons of the ascending pathways. One EPSP alone is not able to stimulate a neuron sufficiently to trigger an action potential; hence the importance of algebraic summation of the EPSPs and IPSPs on the receptive membrane of a neuron (Chap. 3).

A pathway does not merely comprise a series of "relay" processing stations receiving input and relaying output like a bucket brigade. The relay or nuclear stations are the sites which alter the characteristics of the transmitted code. For example, the number of neuron channels delivering input into a nucleus, as the result of a stimulus, does not necessarily equal the number of neuron channels discharging output from the

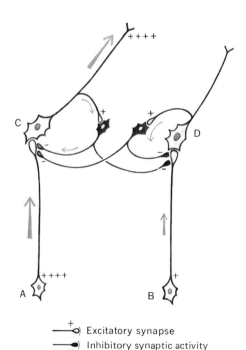

—○) Excitatory synapse
—●) Inhibitory synaptic activity

FIGURE 3-14 Neural processing utilizing presynaptic inhibition. The strong input from neuron A and weak input from neuron B can stimulate discharge in neurons C and D, respectively. This same discharge traveling along recurrent collateral branches of C and D excites "inhibitory neurons" which feed back inhibitory stimuli to the presynaptic terminals of A and B. The stimuli are sufficient to prevent D from firing but insufficient to prevent C from firing.

nucleus. Actually reassessments are made and new codes are generated in each nucleus.

The influences arriving at each nuclear processing station via the multiple axonal channels are biased, enhanced, or dampened within the nucleus or cortex. In effect, each nucleus or cortex acts as an editor. The shaping or sharpening effects of inhibition can occur in three general ways:

1. *Feed-forward inhibition.* The feed-forward neuronal circuits consist of the branches of axons of relay neurons (Golgi type I) entering a nucleus and terminating by synapsing with local circuit neurons. In turn, these neurons exert inhibitory influences upon relay neurons via either presynaptic or postsynaptic inhibition (see Figs. 3-14 and 3-15). *Presynaptic inhibition* occurs when the axons entering a relay nucleus synapse with excitatory local circuit neurons that, in turn, synapse with the terminals of neighboring entering axons (see Figs. 3-14 and 3-15). *Postsynaptic inhibition* occurs when the entering axons synapse with local circuit neurons that, in turn, synapse with the cell bodies of adjacent relay neurons (see Figs. 3-14 and 3-15). Because these inhibitory circuits utilize the interaction between ascending or afferent neurons, their action is referred to as *afferent inhibition.* A *feed-forward inhibitory circuit* is characterized by having one or more inhibitory interneurons within the circuit; these interneurons convey influences in a forward direction toward the more distal levels of the pathway. In such a circuit, the axons of the excitatory neurons have some axon collaterals which excite one or more inhibitory neurons. In turn, these neurons exert inhibitory influences upon other neurons in a forward direction. Feed-forward inhibitory circuits are illustrated in Figs. 3-15, 5-20, and 5-23.

The afferent fiber from the neuromuscular spindle receptors within a muscle excites, among others, an inhibitory interneuron which exerts inhibitory influences upon the alpha motor neuron innervating a voluntary muscle (see Figs. 5-20 and 5-23). Neuron C excites interneuron F, which excites inhibitory neuron I_4 to inhibit neuron E postsynaptically (see Fig. 3-15).

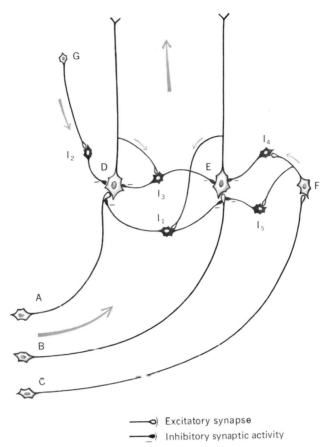

	Excitatory synapse
	Inhibitory synaptic activity

FIGURE 3-15 Neural processing utilizing presynaptic and postsynaptic inhibition. Normally neurons A and B can excite neurons D and E to fire. However, inhibitory influences can modify the receptivity of neurons D and E. The recurrent collateral branch from neuron E can excite interneuron I_1, which exerts presynaptic inhibitory influences on the terminal ending of neurons A and B. The recurrent collateral branch from neuron D can stimulate interneuron I_3, which exerts postsynaptic inhibitory influences on neurons D and E. The descending efferent neuron G (reflected fiber) can stimulate interneuron I_2, which exerts postsynaptic inhibitory influences on neuron D. Excitatory stimuli from neuron C can exert through interneurons F, I_4, and I_5 presynaptic inhibitory influences on the terminal ending of neuron B and postsynaptic inhibitory influences on neuron E.

2. *Local feedback inhibition* (feedback inhibition). The local feedback neuronal circuits consist of collaterals of axons of the relay neurons projecting from the nucleus, synapsing with either excitatory or inhibitory local circuit neurons. These local circuit neurons exert their influences on relay neurons via either presynaptic or postsynaptic inhibition (see Figs. 3-14 and 3-15). For example, the axon collateral of a lower motor neuron excites the inhibitory Renshaw cell that feedback back to inhibit postsynaptically the lower motor neuron (see Fig. 3-12).

3. *Feedback inhibition.* A *feedback inhibitory circuit* is characterized by having one or more inhibitory interneurons which convey inhibitory influences back (feedback) to the original output neuron. A feedback inhibitory control circuit performs its role through both presynaptic and postsynaptic inhibition (Chap. 3). Feedback inhibitory circuits utilizing postsynaptic inhibition are illustrated in Figs. 3-12 and 3-15. The axon collateral of the lower motor neuron excites the inhibitory interneuron (Renshaw cell), which feeds back to inhibit the lower motor neuron (see Fig. 3-12).

The axon collateral of neuron D excites interneuron I_3, which feeds back to inhibit output neuron D (see Fig. 3-15). Feedback inhibitory circuits utilizing presynaptic inhibition are illustrated in Figs. 3-14 and 3-15. The axon collaterals of neurons C and D excite inhibitory neurons, which feed back to inhibit neurons A and B by presynaptic inhibition (see Fig. 3-14). Recall that presynaptic inhibition is exerted via an interneuron which excites (Chap. 3). The axon collateral of neuron E excites interneuron I, which feeds back to inhibit neuron E by presynaptic inhibition (see Fig. 3-15).

4. *Reflected feedback inhibition (or excitation).* This consists of descending centrifugal fibers (reflected descending fibers) originating from rostrally located centers (cortex and nuclei) to more caudally located nuclei or receptors of the ascending pathways (see Fig. 3-15). Nerve fibers may project from the brain stem or spinal cord via fibers known as efferents to some sensory receptors. Descending fibers are usually inhibitory in their activity, but some may be excitatory. The inhibitory effects can be expressed as either presynaptic or postsynaptic inhibition (see Fig. 3-15). Many receptors are under the influence of efferent neurons of reflected feedback circuits. These efferent neurons with their cell bodies in the neuraxis may facilitate or inhibit, thereby making the sensory endings more or less receptive. The gamma efferent fibers to neuromuscular spindles (Chap. 5) and the cochlear efferent fibers to the spiral organ of Corti (Chap. 10) are two examples of such neurons.

In part owing to divergence, channels within the pathways tend to overlap within the relay nuclei. Inhibition in the forms of feed-forward, local feedback, and reflected feedback circuits are processing mechanisms utilized to limit the effects of divergence and suppress smearing overlap. The general principle is that inhibition is exerted through the local circuit neurons through both presynaptic and postsynaptic inhibition. The negative feedback limits the spatial spread of the overlap and thereby preserves the individual channels. Because the inhibitory field surrounds (surround) the channel (center) which is excitatory, the term *afferent or surround inhibition* is used. The descending centrifugal fibers from higher centers (e.g., corticonuclear fibers, Chap. 16) to the nuclei of the ascending pathways incorporate inhibitory interneurons. This is illustrated in Fig. 3-15. The descending fibers of neuron G excite inhibitory neuron I_2, which inhibits neuron D postsynaptically.

In the posterior column, medial lemniscus, thalamocortical pathway, there are no relay neurons with long axons that exert inhibition by direct monosynaptic activity; this applies to both ascending and descending fibers within the system (Chap. 5). Presynaptic inhibition is the prevalent form of inhibition in the nucleus gracilis and nucleus cuneatus, whereas postsynaptic inhibition is utilized in the ventral posterior thalamic nucleus and in the cortex (Chap. 5). In a reflected feedback circuit (1) the inhibitory influences may limit the spatial spread by inhibiting the surround of each channel while (2) the facilitatory influences (positive feedback) to the center of an active zone (channel) in the nucleus can act to facilitate (enhance) the activity in the center. A discussion of center-surround in the visual system is presented in Chap. 12. In brief, the descending fibers can both inhibit or excite activity in the relay nuclei.

In the anterolateral ascending pathway, afferent (surround, lateral) inhibition does not occur in the relay nuclei (Chap. 5). Reflected inhibition through the descending pathways from the somatosensory cortex does occur in the relay nuclei (posterior horn and thalamic nuclei).

These inhibitory circuits exert their effects in the nuclei of both the ascending reticular and the ascending lemniscal systems. The modulating influences act to suppress some of the input channels, possibly those which are transmitting noise. The effectively inhibited channels surround excitatory foci which serve to stimulate the output channels; these output channels transmit the signals with less noise. For example, the inhibitory ring of *off* sets surrounding an excitatory focus of an *on* set, as found in the visual pathways, illustrates the interaction of inhibitory activity in nuclear processing. A negative feedback inhibitory circuit tends to prevent those neurons with relatively weak excitatory input from firing (filters out the noise); it may modify but not prevent those neurons with relatively strong facilitatory input from firing (contain the coded signals). This is an example of lateral (mutual, afferent contrast, Chap. 12) inhibition. Some information being transmitted in a coded pattern is lost at synaptic relays. The critical significance of inhibition is that it lowers the background activity so that the message can come through. Inhibition acts "to clear the addresses of the computer." *In a sense, the signals are strengthened and the noise is suppressed.*

BIBLIOGRAPHY

Bodian, D.: The generalized vertebrate neuron. Science, 137:323–326, 1962.

Cooper, J. R., F. E. Bloom, and R. H. Roth: *The Biochemical Basis of Neuropharmacology*, Oxford University Press, New York, 1978.

Eccles, J. C.: *The Physiology of Synapses*, Academic Press, Inc., New York, 1973.

Florey, E.: *An Introduction to General and Comparative Animal Physiology*, W. B. Saunders Company, Philadelphia, 1966.

Guyton, A. C.: *Structure and Function of the Nervous System*, W. B. Saunders Company, Philadelphia, 1976.

Heuser, J., and T. S. Reese: Stimulation induced uptake and release of peroxidase from synaptic vesicles in frog neuromuscular junctions. Anat Rec, 172:329–240, 1972.

———— and ————: Evidence for recycling of synaptic vesicle membrane during transmitter release at the frog neurotransmitter junction. J Cell Biol, 57:315–344, 1973.

Hoar, W. S.: *General and Comparative Physiology*, Prentice-Hall, Inc., Englewood Cliffs, N.J., 1975.

Katz, B.: *Nerve, Muscle and Synapse*, McGraw-Hill Book Company, New York, 1966.

Kuffler, S. W., and J. G. Nicholls: *From Neuron to Brain: A Cellular Approach to the Function of the Nervous System*, Sinauer Associates, Sunderland, Mass., 1976.

Loewenstein, W. R. (ed.): "Principles of Receptor Physiology," in *Handbook of Sensory Physiology*, vol. 1, Springer-Verlag, Berlin and New York, 1971, pp. 1–600.

McLennan, H.: *Synaptic Transmission*, W. B. Saunders Company, Philadelphia, 1970.

Mountcastle, V. B.: *Medical Physiology*, The C. V. Mosby Company, St. Louis, 1974.

Quarton, G. C., T. Melnechuk, and F. O. Schmitt: *The Neurosciences*, Rockefeller University Press, New York, 1967.

Ruch, T. C., and H. D. Patton (eds.): *Neurophsiology*, W. B. Saunders Company, Philadelphia, 1974.

Schmitt, F. O. (ed.): *The Neurosciences—Third Study Program*. The M.I.T. Press, Cambridge, Mass, 1974.

————, G. C. Quarton, T. Melnechuk, and G. Adelman (eds.): *The Neurosciences—Second Study Program*, Rockefeller University Press, New York, 1970.

———— et al. (eds.): *Neurosciences Research Program*, The M.I.T. Press, Cambridge, Mass., 1966 to date.

Schmitt, F. O., and F. G. Worden (eds.): *The Neurosciences—Fourth Study Program*, The M.I.T. Press, Cambridge, Mass., 1978.

Shepherd, G. M.: *The Synaptic Organization of the Brain*, Oxford University Press, New York, 1979.

Stevens, C. F.: The neuron. Sci Am, 241:54–65, 1979.

Tamar, H.: *Principles of Sensory Physiology*, Charles C Thomas, Publisher, Springfield, Ill., 1972.

Varon, S. S., and G. G. Somjen: *Neuron-Glia Interactions*, Neurosciences Research Program Bulletin, The M.I.T. Press, Cambridge, Mass., 1979.

Watson, W. E.: *Cell Biology of the Brain*. John Wiley & Sons, Inc., New York, 1976.

CHAPTER FOUR

DEVELOPMENT AND GROWTH OF THE NERVOUS SYSTEM

The cardiovascular system and the nervous system are the first organ systems to function during embryonic life. In humans, the heart begins to beat late in the third week after fertilization. Before the heart beats, the nervous system commences to differentiate and to change in shape into the *plate stage* (Fig. 4-1). To attain this stage, the neural plate does not increase in size. Growth in size occurs after the heart commences to beat and blood slowly circulates to bring oxygen and essential nutrients to the developing nervous system. During the second month, an avoidance reflex in the human embryo evokes withdrawal of the head by contraction of the neck muscles when stimuli are applied to the upper lip. A mother may feel life as early as the twelfth prenatal week.

The nervous system is actually a highly specialized epithelium. Embryologically it is derived from the ectodermal epithelial layer. Like other epithelial tissues, the neurons and glial cells exhibit many features of other epithelial tissues as, for example, typical junctional complexes of cell-to-cell contacts.

Differentiation and cell multiplication characterize development during early prenatal life, whereas growth (increase in size) is more prominent during late fetal and postnatal life. The formation of new neurons by mitosis normally ceases during late prenatal life and probably does not occur after birth in humans. To generate a human brain containing up to 100 billion neurons requires the production and differentiation of an average of about 200,000 neurons per minute throughout the entire length of prenatal life. There are roughly 10 to 15 billion neurons in the cerebral cortex and up to 50 to 100 billion neurons in the cerebellar cortex. Growth of the nervous tissues continues postnatally, especially during the first 3 years after birth, by the increase in size of neurons and glia, and by myelination.

FIRST PRENATAL MONTH

When the human embryo is but 1.5 mm long (18 days old), the ectoderm, or the outer germ layer, differentiates and thickens along the future midline of the back to form the *neural plate* or *flat plate stage* (see Fig. 4-1). This neural plate is exposed to the surface and to the amniotic fluid; it is continuous laterally with the future skin. Certain portions of the ectoderm differentiate and thicken in the head region to form the placodes (thickened ectodermal anlagen) or organs of special sense such as the eyes (optic placode), ears (auditory placode), and nose (nasal placode). In fact, the neural plate is a giant placode. The neural plate elongates, and its lateral edges are raised to form the neural folds or keyhole stage (Fig. 4-1). The anterior end of the neural plate enlarges and will develop into the brain. The lateral edges, or lips, continue to rise and grow medially until they meet and unite in the midline to form the neural tube. This midline union commences in the cervical region and progresses both cephalically and caudally until the entire plate is converted into the neural tube (in 25 days) or neural tube stage (see Fig. 4-1). The tube becomes detached from the skin and sinks beneath the surface (see Fig. 4-2). The cavity of the

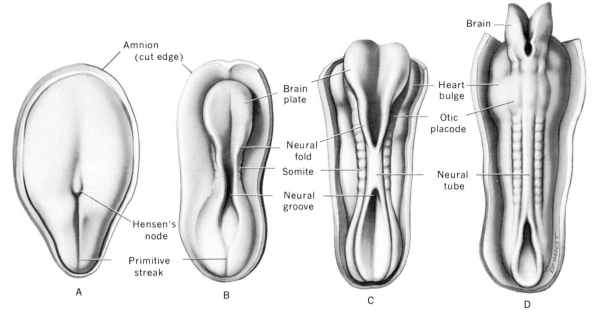

FIGURE 4-1 Dorsal aspect of human embryo. *A.* Primitive-streak plate stage of 16-day presomite embryo. *B.* Two-somite keyhole stage of approximately 20-day embryo. Note first somites, neural fold, and neural groove. *C.* Seven-somite stage of approximately 22-day embryo. *D.* Ten-somite neural tube stage of approximately 23-day embryo. (*Adapted from Scammon.*)

neural tube persists in the adult as the ventricular system of the brain and the central canal of the spinal cord. The nasal (olfactory) placode develops into the olfactory pit, and the optic and the otic placodes develop into the optic and the otic vesicles, respectively. These vesicles differentiate into various structures associated with the nose, eyes, and ears (Fig. 4-8).

The cephalic end of the neural tube differentiates and enlarges into three dilations called the "primary brain vesicles." Rostrally to caudally, the three divisions are the prosencephalon or forebrain, the mesencephalon or midbrain, and the rhombencephalon or hindbrain (Table 4-1). A bilateral column of cells differentiates from the neural ectoderm at the original junction of the skin ectoderm and the rolled edges of the neural plate. These two columns of cells become the neural crests (see the accompanying Figs. 4-2 and 4-3).

The three-vesicle stage of the brain, the remainder of the neural tube (which will develop into the spinal cord), several placodes, and neural crests constitute the embryonic nervous system at the stage attained by the end of the first

month after fertilization in humans. Thus, basically the nervous system originates as a surface structure and then sinks beneath the body surface.

The neural tube, placodes, and neural crests are derived from ectoderm. The neural tube is the primordial structure for the central nervous system (brain and spinal cord), including all neurons in the central nervous system, oligodendroglia, and astroglia. The neural crest gives rise to a number of neural and nonneural derivatives. The neural derivatives include (1) neurons in all the sensory, autonomic, and enteric ganglia, (2) cells of the pia mater and arachnoid and the sclera and choroid coats of the eye, (3) neurolemma (Schwann) cells and satellite cells of the ganglia, (4) adrenal medullary cells, and (5) receptor cells of the carotid body. Some neurons of sensory ganglia of cranial nerves V, VII, IX, and X are derived from cells of the otic placode. Some cells of the parasympathetic ganglia are derived from cells of the neural tube. Nonneural derivatives include (1) pigment-producing cells (melanophores) of the skin and connective tissues; (2) odontoblasts of tooth pulp; (3) much of

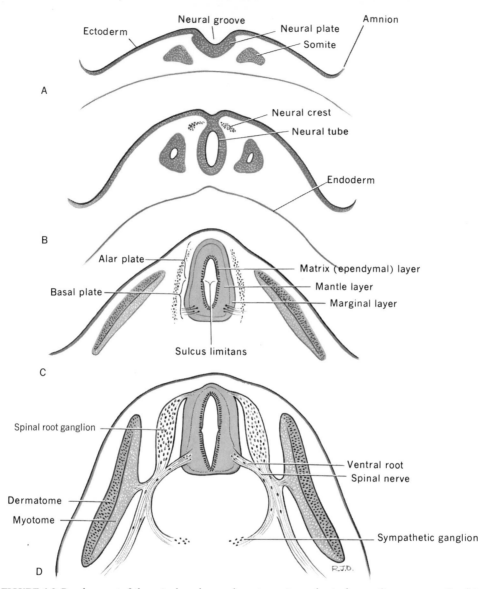

FIGURE 4-2 Development of the spinal cord, neural crest, somite, and spinal nerve (transverse sections) in human embryo of the following ages: *A*. Approximately 19 days. *B*. Approximately 20 days. *C*. Approximately 26 days. *D*. After 1 month of age.

the skull and cartilage, connective tissues, and muscles of the face and branchial arches; and (4) chromaffin cells.

Several mesodermally derived elements are associated with the nervous system. Those that secondarily invade the central nervous system include the blood vessels and microglial cells.

Surrounding the central nervous system is the dura mater. The extraneural mesodermal elements of the peripheral nervous system include the outer satellite cells of the peripheral ganglia; the epineurium, perineurium, and endoneurium of the peripheral nerves; and the capsules of some peripheral sensory endings.

Table 4-1
The derivatives of the neural tube

Primary vesicles	Subdivisions	Derivatives	Lumina or cavities
Brain			
Prosencephalon (forebrain)	Telencephalon (endbrain)	Cerebral cortex Corpora striata Rhinencephalon Rostral hypothalamus	Lateral ventricles Rostral part of third ventricle
	Diencephalon (twixt-brain; between-brain)	Epithalamus Thalamus Hypothalamus Ventral thalamus	Most of third ventricle
Mesencephalon (midbrain)	Mesencephalon (midbrain)	Corpora quadrigemina Tegmentum Crura cerebri	Cerebral aqueduct of Sylvius (liter)
Rhombencephalon (hindbrain)	Metencephalon (afterbrain)	Cerebellum Pons	
	Myelencephalon (spinal brain)	Medulla oblongata	Fourth ventricle
Spinal cord	Spinal cord	Spinal cord	Central canal

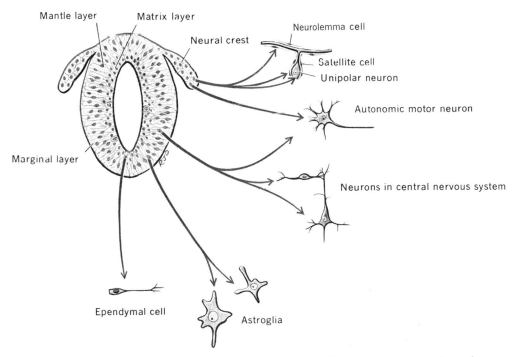

FIGURE 4-3 Schematic diagram illustrating some of the cells derived from the neural tube and neural crest. Note that mitotic activity is restricted to the cells of the matrix layer adjacent to the central canal.

EMBRYONIC CENTRAL NERVOUS SYSTEM

The embryonic central nervous system (neural plate) comprises four concentric zones: ventricular, subventricular, intermediate (mantle) and marginal (see Fig. 4-4). The adult nervous system is derived from these basic zones, but none of the four corresponds directly to any adult component.

The *ventricular zone* (germinal epithelium, neuroepithelium, matrix layer, and ventricular layer) comprises one type of cell—the ventricular cell. Recent studies indicate that the apparent differences among the cells of this lamina are actually differences in the stages of the mitotic cycle of each cell of the pseudostratified columnar epithelia ventricular zone. The nucleus of each ventricular cell migrates to the luminal end of the cell (adjacent to the central canal), rounds up, and undergoes a mitotic division; after dividing, the nuclei of the daughter cells migrate to the apical portions of their respective cells, where the replication of its deoxyribonucleoproteins occurs. Thus the ventricular zone is known as the lamina of the *to-and-fro nuclear movement*. The mitotic and nuclear migration cycle lasts from 5 to 24 h. Ventricular cells are the progenitors of all neurons and macroglia of the central nervous system. This zone will attenuate and eventually disappear after all its cells differentiate.

The *subventricular zone* is located adjacent to the ventricular zone. The subventricular cells are small cells which proliferate by mitosis. They do not exhibit the to-and-fro nuclear movements during their mitotic cycles. The subventricular zone persists from only a few days in the spinal cord to many months or even years in the cerebral hemisphere. This zone generates certain classes of neurons and all macroglia (astrocytes and oligodendroglia) of the central nervous system. In the spinal cord, the ventricular layer gives rise to the neurons, while the subventricular layer generates all spinal macroglia. Those progenitor cells (neuroblasts) destined to form neurons migrate from the ventricular and subventricular zones during development before those subventricular cells destined to form macroglia.

Once neuroblasts move out of the generator zones, they are postmitotic cells. With the possible exception of some microneurons, which differentiate in the subventricular zones of the brain (rhombic lip and ganglionic eminence, see below), in humans all neurons appear during prenatal life, whereas macroglia are generated during prenatal and postnatal life. In fact, glial cells may proliferate at a low rate throughout life. Once neuroblasts migrate from the ventricular zone, they lose their capacity to divide—they are postmitotic cells. Neuroblasts migrating out of the subventricular zone may be either postmitotic cells or mitotically capable cells. Those subventricular cells invading cortex may continue to divide.

There are two important specialized areas composed of subventricular cells: the rhombic lip and the ganglionic eminence. The *rhombic lips*, located at the lateral margins of the fourth ventricle, give rise to many cells of the cerebellum (granule, stellate, and basket cells) and the brainstem (neurons of the inferior olivary, reticularis pontine, and pontine nuclei, see Fig. 4-6). The *ganglionic eminence*, located in the floor of the lateral ventricle near the future caudate nucleus, is the site of origin of cells of the basal ganglia and pulvinar, and possibly of some cells of the association cortical areas. This eminence and primordial nests of cells in the hippocampal region may be the source, in human beings, for the differentiation of microneurons postnatally in the adult. Recall that some authorities claim that new neurons do not differentiate postnatally in humans.

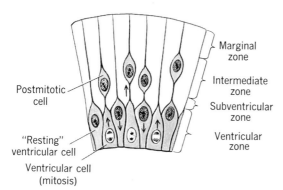

FIGURE 4-4 The four zones of the embryonic central nervous system. The arrows within the ventricular cells indicate the direction in which their nuclei migrate during a mitotic cycle. The arrow outside the cells indicates the direction in which the postmitotic neuroblasts migrate.

The *intermediate (mantle) zone* is the lamina immediately external to the subventricular zone. The postmitotic neurons migrate to this zone, aggregate into cell groups, and differentiate their cell processes. Macroglial cells also occupy this zone. In general the intermediate zone seems to evolve into the gray matter of the central nervous system with its complex neural organizations. In the potential cerebral and cerebellar areas, other neurons migrate and collect to form the *cortical plate;* these neurons form efferent axons that course inward (these are the future cortical neurons) to and through the intermediate layer. Later other neurons and macroglia migrate in the cortical plate from the subventricular zone (see Fig. 4-5). Considerations of the development of the cerebral and cerebellar cortex will be outlined below.

The *marginal zone* is the cell-sparse layer with no primary cells of its own. In the early stages the ventricular cells have processes which extend to the outer margin of the zone. Eventually the marginal layer forms much of the white matter as it is replaced by ingrowing axons, dendrites, synaptic terminals, and macroglia.

The following are some generalities. The first neurons and first glial cells probably differentiate at the same time in most regions of the developing nervous system. All neurons are formed by early infancy and are postmitotic, whereas it is likely that glial cells retain their capacity to divide throughout the life of human beings. As a rule the larger (Golgi type I) neurons differentiate before the small (local circuit neurons) neurons do. The neurons and many associated cells are derived from the ventricular zone, subventricular zone, ganglionic eminence, rhombic lip, and neural crest.

Glycogen is present in the neurons, glia, and cells of the tela choroidea during embryonic and fetal life. In the adult these cells do not contain any histochemically detectable amounts of glycogen.

Individuals are as old as their neurons, in the sense that all neurons are generated during prenatal and early postnatal life and are not replaced by new neurons during a given lifetime. The specific patterns of connectivity within the nervous system assumed by any neuron are the exquisite product of numerous events

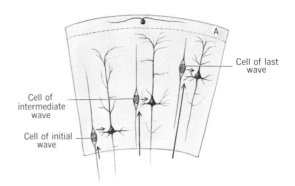

FIGURE 4-5 The "inside-out" migration of cells forming the cerebral cortex. The cells migrate (arrows) into the cortical plate to form the cortical laminae sequentially from the deepest (lamina VI) to the most superficial lamina. Lamina I (A) is a derivative of the marginal zone.

throughout the life of the neuron. The structural organization and functional expression exhibited by each neuron at any time results from the continual interactions between intrinsic influences from within the neuron—largely of genetic origin—and extrinsic influences from environmental sources. The predictability of the form and connections of a neuron has been called *neural specificity;* this is presumably determined genetically. Variation from the predictable pattern under certain conditions has been called *neural plasticity* (Lund); this is presumed to be largely determined by environmental factors. The variants are more marked if the environmental influences occur during development rather than during later life.

In the following account, the life history of a neuron is outlined on the basis of four periods, among which there is considerable overlapping.

Period of genesis until the postmitotic neuron commences to migrate During this period, prospective neurons are generated in the ventricular zone, rhombic lip, and ganglionic eminence. The full complement of genetic information has been incorporated within the immature neuron with the instructions for expressing *neuronal specificity:* namely, (1) to migrate to its designated locale in the nervous system, (2) to assume the complete structural identity characteristic of that neuron; and (3) to develop those physiologic properties normally exhibited by that neuron. In order to find its way during its migration to its destination, the young postmitotic neuron is equipped with "built-in" recognition macromolecules—probably glycoproteins—incorporated within its plasma membrane (Fig. 2-5). In addition to their critical role in the guidance of the cell during its migration, these macromolecules may be significant in some aspects of the growth and maturation of the cell and in some of the adjustments the neuron makes to the environment in which it migrates and develops.

Period from becoming a postmitotic cell to the formation of its synaptic connections During this period (1) the neuron migrates from its source; (2) its axon and dendrites differentiate and grow; and (3) synapses with other neurons are formed.

The genesis, migration, initial differentiation, and outgrowth of axons depend on a developmental timetable that is intrinsic to the developing neurons; it is unaffected by sensory input or by transynaptic stimulation (Jacobson).

This is the interval when *neural specificity* may be modified by environmental influences expressed as *neural plasticity*. The plasticity can be gauged by slight alterations in the position of the cell body, in the arborization pattern of the dendritic tree, and in the course of the axon and distribution pattern of its terminals. The environmental influences exerted during this period can result in various structural and functional alterations, some of which can be severe (see "Critical Periods" later on). With the formation of input synapses from other neurons, the neuron is integrated as a functional entity within the nervous system.

Each postmitotic cell migrates to its definitive location, where it is incorporated into "nuclear groups" or laminae. This migration is ameboid, with the cell body moving in the preferred direction and its axon extending behind in the so-called axon-trailing method. The cell body is motile and the axon spins out in the wake. During this migration guidance through the developing nervous system makes use of the recognition macromolecules. After the cell body reaches its nucleus or lamina, the growth of the dendrites and axons also makes use of these macromolecules of the plasma membranes located on both the probing cell processes and the target cells. The specificity of the chemotactic influences of these macromolecules is demonstrated in the restitution and functional recovery of severed visual pathways in the frog (Sperry) and other vertebrates. The severed fibers projecting from the retina regenerate and then unerringly grow to the visual regions in these animals (tectum). Each fiber grows along the correct route through the optic chiasm, bypasses denervated neurons (those which were not originally innervated by the fiber in question), and seeks out and makes synaptic connections with the precise visual neurons to which its retinal neurons originally synapsed.

The functional (physiological and biochemical) maturation of each neuron proceeds along with its morphological development. One of these maturational processes consists of the biochemical specializations within the plasma membranes which enable the axon terminals to recognize the appropriate target sites in order to form the "correct" synaptic connections. Another is the development of the biochemical apparatus to elaborate (1) the neurotransmitter characteristic of each neuron and (2) the elusive neurotrophic factors (see Chap. 6).

Evidence indicates that, at least for some neurons, the neurotransmitter synthesized and released by a neuron is determined following the interaction of genetic influences (neural specificity) and environmental influences (neural plasticity). This interaction is illustrated in the development of postganglionic sympathetic neurons of the autonomic nervous system (Chap. 6).

The postganglionic sympathetic neurons originate from a common source—namely, the neural crest. Of these neurons, most become adrenergic while some become cholinergic (Chap. 6). During their migration from the neural crest to their appropriate peripheral location, all these immature sympathetic neurons differentiate biochemically into adrenergic neurons. It can be demonstrated that they show adrenergic functions (Patterson et al.), a genetic expression of "neuronal specificity." At some interval during maturation, certain environmental influences affect the cell's further development to determine whether it (1) continues to evolve into a mature adrenergic neuron or (2) changes direction to become a mature cholinergic neuron. Thus, during this interval the immature sympathetic neurons are transiently plastic with respect to their choice of neurotransmitter.

Two sources are thought to affect the sympathetic neurons choice of neurotransmitter (1) electrical activity derived from the spinal cord and (2) environmental factors, probably of a chemical nature, from the nonneural cells—especially the target organs (muscle or glandular cells). To summarize a complex subject, the peripheral structures apparently do have a role in determining the biochemical characteristics of neurons by nurturing their differentiation into adrenergic or cholinergic neurons (Bunge et al.).

The advancing tip of a growing process (axon and dendrite) is a bulbous enlargement known as a growth cone, which, in turn, sends out slender, fine, spinelike projections called filopodia. These filopodia act as probes sensing the environment. Once the decision to advance is made, many filopodia retract and disappear, the growth cone advances into a filopodia, and the vents are repeated. If two filopodia persist, then the cell process divides into two processes. Ultimately, synaptic connections are consummated. The growth cones and the substrate in which they grow retain "contact" by matching chemical affinities. During this period, the plasma membrane of the dendrites and cell body typically becomes a receptive membrane with receptor site macromolecules specialized to act as targets for the reception of cell processes of other neurons seeking to make synaptic connections. The plasma membrane of each growing axon terminal acquires recognition macromolecules that seek out the receptive sites on target neurons.

The migration and guidance of differentiating and growing axons are expressed in the *blueprint hypothesis* of Singer, Woodlander, and Egar. It asserts that inherent in the primitive germinal neuroepithelium and its derivative primitive glia (radial glia) is the pattern of the primary neuronal pathways which is expressed in neurogenesis as formed channels or spaces between the processes of the radial glia, the surfaces of which contain trace pathways which the growing nerve processes follow toward destination. The trace pathways are envisioned as mechanical-chemical itineraries which the nerve processes follow according to their individual affinities.

Period of consolidation and maturity During this period the neuron adjusts, establishes, and consolidates its structural and functional interconnections so that it can perform its role throughout adult life. The adjustments are in the enhancement of essential connections (input and output) and in the elimination of "nonessential" connections. These anatomical, physiological, and biochemical adaptations can be considered in the context of learning, both in the sensory and motor spheres at the conscious as well as at the subconscious levels. The wide spectrum of behavioral activities includes the evaluation of sensory inputs and of the reactions to them by the somatic and the visceral systems. Among these are the appreciation of the vast array of sensory stimuli and the motor expressions of balancing, walking, manual dexterity, and talking.

The basic theory is that the nervous system is essentially prewired and that small but significant portions are constantly reforming. The brain is never still; it forever changes its structural and biochemical constitution to cope with new demands and perceptions. Isotope studies reveal that the biochemical turnover within the nervous system is rapid. For example, on the basis of half-life, free amino acids in the brain are used up within half an hour. Depending upon the substance, the rate of turnover ranges from "fast turnover" of a few hours to "slow turnover" measured in days. In the case of myelin, the half-life of one of its constituents, lecithin, is about 16 days. Protein, considered to be a most stable entity, also turns over to an astonishing degree. Every 30 days a rat retains only about 25 percent of its brain protein and replaces the rest, so that 6 months later only about 1 to 2 percent of the original protein remains as such.

The concept of the reorganization of synaptic connections is consistent with the recovery of patients following certain types of lesions or in the ontogeny of cerebral dominance (Chap. 16). For example, the dendritic tree is fairly rigidly set in each neuron, but its spines cannot be maintained without afferent input. The primary dendritic arborization is genetically determined while the dendritic spines are sustained by environmental (trophic) influences. It is known that spines may disappear after deafferentation or sensory deprivation, and even with increasing age. The turnover of dendritic spines and collateral sprouting by axons of the central nervous system are indications of the plasticity of neurons.

Period associated with aging Few, if any, new neurons are formed after birth in humans. The number of neurons tends to decrease with age, for as neurons die they are not replaced. The consequences of a slight loss of neurons are not noticeable because other neurons may compensate for the decreased number of neurons. Of an estimated loss of one-tenth of our neurons in the 50 years from 20 to 70 years of age, an average loss of 50,000 or so cerebral cortical neurons daily is indicated.

The brain is said to decrease gradually in weight over the years, losing as much as 10 to 20 percent of its weight between the ages of 20 and 90 years. It is presumed that this relates to the loss and atrophy of neurons and glia. In general, the number of neurons increases rapidly during early development, it remains relatively unchanged through maturity, and then it declines during senescence. The loss of cells varies from region to region, with the brainstem exhibiting only a slight decline and the cerebral cortex undergoing the greatest loss. Some evidence indicates that the decrease in weight and the degree of cortical atrophy in healthy old subjects who have no pathologic condition of the brain are relatively slight. The brains of such individuals are within normal weight ranges for young adults and have cerebrums exhibiting no apparent cortical atrophy. The data upon which microscopic aging changes in humans are based are not extensive. It has been demonstrated that no noticeable cell loss with aging seems to occur in such brainstem nuclei as the inferior olivary nucleus, the cochlear nuclei, and nuclei of the motor nuclei of cranial nerves III, IV, VI, and VII. As yet, the locus coeruleus is the only brain stem nucleus in which cell loss during aging has been documented. The loss of cells in the cerebral cortex is greatest in the neocortex in the frontal pole, precentral gyrus, cingulate gyrus, and primary visual cortex. The loss occurred in all cortical laminae but especially in layers II and IV (Brody). Evidence does indicate that the number and size of the spines of cerebral cortical cells are reduced in old individuals. It is unlikely that these losses are involved with limiting the life span.

Postnatally, the amount of extracellular space in the brain is reduced from about 20 percent during circumnatal life to about 10 percent at 3 years of age. Neurons undergo senescence. Aging of the neurons is evidenced by change in size (either decrease or increase), by the accumulation of pigment, or by the decrease in amount of Nissl substance. In humans, for example, the quantity of ribonucleoproteins in the alpha motor neurons of the spinal cord increases significantly from birth to 40 years of age, plateaus from 40 to 60 years, and decreases from 60 years on. In elderly people, decrease in the weight of the brain, increase in the size of the ventricles, and calcification in the meninges are all signs of an aging nervous system.

Lipofuscin granules are probably the harmless by-products of lysosomal activity. They increase in amount with aging. In old age, these so-called age pigments can occupy as much as 75 percent of the volume of a cell body in the large neurons of the dentate nucleus of the cerebellum. Iron-containing granules increase with aging in the neurons of the globus pallidus and substantia nigra.

Involutionary changes in the surface structure of the cerebral hemisphere occur in old age. Atrophic changes are found in the following cerebral cortical regions, roughly in the following temporal sequence: (1) limbic lobe structures such as the uncus and cingulate gyrus, (2) the insula, and (3) the orbital gyri of the frontal lobe. These regions appear reduced in surface area and width in the elderly as compared with the young. The last to show such gross objective signs of aging are the gyri of the frontal and parietal lobes, since they may appear normal even in persons in their nineties.

An indication of the degree of the aging process after the prime of life is obtained by comparing several parameters in the 30-year-old age group with those in the 75-year-old age group. In the older group, the reduction in brain weight is about 10 percent; in the blood flow to the brain, about 20 percent; in the number of nerve fibers in large nerves, about one-third; in the number of taste buds, about two-thirds; and in the velocity of nerve conduction, about 10 percent. The latter correlates with the observation that the rate and magnitude of reflex responses to stimulation do decrease with age.

DEVELOPMENT OF REFLEX ARCS

A basic "unit" of neural activity is the simple reflex arc. Stimulation of a receptor and production of a response from an effector indicate the presence of a functional reflex arc. Each component of an arc expresses its functional activity at different times. The sequence for the initiation of activity in the several components is as follows:

1. A muscle cell exhibits intrinsic contractility prior to being innervated.
2. A motor neuron is capable of conducting an action potential and, through the motor end plate, of stimulating a muscle cell to contract. The functional unity of the motor neuron, motor end plate, and muscle cell is thus established.
3. The afferent neuron can be stimulated to conduct an action potential to the central nervous system, but the reflex arc is not active.
4. The reflex arc does not become functional until the interneurons form the final synaptic interconnections between the afferent and efferent neurons. The basic patterns of reflex activity develop without any reference to sensory stimulation.

SULCUS LIMITANS

A longitudinal groove, called the *sulcus limitans,* is present on either side of the inner surface of the neural tube (see Fig. 4-2). The portion of the tube posterior to the sulcus is the *dorsal* or *alar plate;* the portion on the anterior side is the *ventral* or *basal plate.* In the spinal cord, as well as in the brainstem, (1) the sensory (afferent) nuclei associated with the input from the peripheral, spinal, and cranial nerves become differentiated in the gray matter of the alar plate, and (2) the motor (efferent) nuclei of the cranial and spinal nerves differentiate in the basal plate.

SPINAL CORD

Up to about the third fetal month, the spinal cord extends throughout the entire length of the developing vertebral column. At this time the dorsal (sensory) roots and the ventral (motor) roots of the spinal nerves extend laterally at right angles from the spinal cord. The roots unite in the intervertebral foramina to form the spinal nerves. The roots and spinal nerves are products of outgrowths from the spinal cord and neural crests (see Fig. 4-4). Because the spinal cord elongates at a slower rate than the bony vertebral column, the cord becomes relatively shorter than the vertebral column after the third fetal month. At birth the caudal end of the spinal cord is located at the level of the L3 vertebra, and at adolescence, as in the adult, this caudal end is located at the level approximately between the L1 and L2 vertebrae. During the long period of the differential growth of the spinal cord and vertebral column, the root filaments between the spinal cord and the intervertebral foramina elongate. As a result of this disparity in growth, the lumbar, sacral, and coccygeal roots become directed caudally at an acute angle to the spinal cord. The subarachnoid space below the first lumbar vertebra in the adult is occupied by dorsal and ventral roots of spinal nerves (cauda equina) and the filum terminale, not by spinal cord (see Fig. 5-1).

PATTERNED DIFFERENTIATION OF THE CEREBRAL CORTEX AND CEREBELLAR CORTEX

The various regions of the central nervous system evolve during development in an orderly patterned program—probably genetically determined. The general sequences of the states of neuronal migration and maturation in the formation of the cerebral cortex and the cerebellar cortex will be outlined to illustrate the general features of neurogenetic events. The neuronal organization of the adult cerebellar cortex and that of the cerebral cortex are described in Chaps. 9 and 16.

Cerebral cortex

The neurons of the six-layered neocortex are derived from the ventricular and subventricular zones of the telencephalon. The cells migrate from these zones through the intermediate zone to the cortical plate in an *"inside-out" migration* of successive waves of cells which form the deeper layers before those of more superficial layers (see Fig. 4-5). The initial waves of cell migration proceed as far as the cells can go to a location between the marginal layer (which differentiates into lamina 1) and the white matter; these cells form the deepest layers of the adult neocortex. Other waves migrate among and past the cells of the initial migration and come to lie in the middle third of the mature cortex. Other waves of cells migrate among and past the cells of the previous waves and come to lie in the superficial layers of the mature cortex. These migratory patterns of developing neurons passing other developing neurons permit connectivity among neurons which is consistent with the radial columnar organization of the cortex (Chap. 16).

The presumed sequence of differentiation of the major cortical neurons is roughly as follows: pyramidal cells (efferent neurons of cortex), specific thalamic afferent fibers (primary afferent neuron to the cortex), stellate cells (intrinsic interneurons of the major neuronal circuits), horizontal cells and pyramidal axon collaterals (lateral interactions by intrinsic interneurons), and the callosal and association neurons (secondary extrinsic afferent neurons).

The temporal order of development of a pyramidal cell comprises in order: apical dendrite, basilar dendrites, axodendritic synapses, axosomatic synapses, and axodendritic synapses on spines. In humans, the apical dendritic system develops primarily during late prenatal life, while the basilar dendritic system develops during the first postnatal years. Even in their earliest developmental stages, the pyramidal cells are radially oriented neurons, which presage the functional columns of the adult (Chap. 16). The radial axis of apical dendrite and cell body of each pyramidal cell is formed before the laterally directed basilar dendrites.

The cerebral cortical neurons are said to display their basic physiologic properties soon after they differentiate within the cortex. With the differentiation and growth of the neuropil, there is an increase in the number of synapses both of the axosomatic type that predominate at birth and the axodendritic type that predominate in the matured brain. The neuronal complement of most of the cerebral cortex is completed by birth. After birth some neurons are generated in the ganglionic eminence and migrate to the hippocampus, and other new cells migrate to the olfactory bulb.

Cerebellar cortex

The histogenesis of the cerebellum, especially the cortex, is a dramatic example of the migration of germinal cells from two sources in two directions to mesh finally into the functionally integrated unit (see Fig. 4-6). Only the most general outlines of a precisely timed and integrated sequence of events will be presented. The two sources are (1) the ventricular and subventricular zones and (2) the rhombic lip. The two directions are (1) the direct migration of germinal cells from the zones to the cerebellar plate (rudiment of the cerebellum) and (2) the migration of germinal cells from the rhombic lip (subventricular derivative) along the outer surface of the cerebellar plate (external granular layer) and then deep into the cerebellar plate to mesh with the neurons of the direct migration. After differentiating, neuroblasts migrate from the ventricular and subventricular zones into the mantle layer of the cerebellar plate. The mantle layer evolves into two strata: the young neurons of the deep stratum differentiate into the neurons of the deep cerebellar nuclei (fastigii, globose, emboliform, and dentate nuclei), while the young neurons of the more superficial stratum differentiate into the Purkinje cells and the Golgi cells. Germinal cells from the rhombic lip migrate over the surface of the cortical plate to form another germinal zone, called the external granular layer. This layer gives rise to granule cells, basket cells, and stellate cells of the cerebellar cortex. Glial cells of the cerebellum are derived from the same sources as the neurons. In addition to being the source of certain cerebellar neurons, cells from the rhombic lip migrate to form the neurons of the pontine nuclei and inferior olivary nucleus of the brainstem.

The tumor cells of a medulloblastoma—a brainstem tumor in children—is said to be formed from the cells of the rhombic lip that have failed to stop dividing.

The following complex events are thought to be causally related; this comprises the meshing

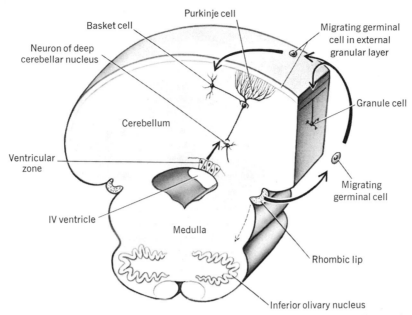

FIGURE 4-6 The routes (arrows) of migration of cells during the histogenesis of the cerebellum. (*Adapted from Sidman and Rakic.*)

of the zone derivative (Purkinje cells, Golgi cells, and some glial cells) with those of the external granular layer. The Purkinje cells form their dendritic trees within the molecular layer. At the same time the granule cells migrate down from the external granular layer through the molecular layer to the granular layer (deep to cell bodies of Purkinje cells) along the preexisting processes of glial cells (Bergmann glial cells). These processes of Bergmann cells apparently are the guidelines for the migrating granule cells (Rakic). Interactions between the Purkinje cells and the migrating granule cells are presumed to take place within the molecular layer; this results in the formation of the parallel fibers of the granule cells, the complete differentiation of the dendritic trees of the Purkinje cells, and the specific synaptic connections between these two neuron cell types. The development of the cerebellum is further integrated into sequences involving the differentiation and growth of the Golgi cells, stellate cells, basket cells, climbing fibers, and mossy fibers.

Although most of the cerebellar neurons are present at birth, there is considerable multiplication of cerebellar granule cells during infancy.

Thus, the cerebellum is especially vulnerable to postnatal insults that interfere with cell division.

PERIPHERAL NERVOUS SYSTEM

Adjacent to the neural tube are 31 pairs of somites. These are the structures that differentiate into muscles, skeleton (including the vertebral column), and connective tissues (see Figs. 4-2 and 4-7). The somites are segmental (metameric) structures arranged in sequence from the first cervical level through the coccygeal levels (see Fig. 4-7). They form the basis for the segmental innervation pattern of the spinal nerves, in that a pair of nerves is developed in association with each pair of somites (see "Spinal Cord," earlier in this chapter). The apparent segmentation of the spinal cord is dependent on the development of paired segmental nerves. The continuous bilateral neural crest becomes segmented into paired units, one pair for each future sensory ganglion of the spinal and cranial nerves (see Fig. 4-3).

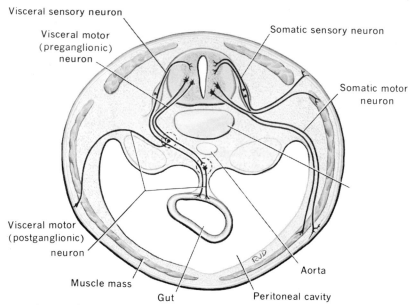

Visceral sensory neuron

Visceral motor (preganglionic) neuron

Somatic sensory neuron

Somatic motor neuron

Visceral motor (postganglionic) neuron

Muscle mass

Gut

Aorta

Peritoneal cavity

FIGURE 4-7 Schematic diagram (transverse section) illustrating the functional components of a typical spinal nerve. Somatic components on the right of figure, visceral components on the left. (Refer to Figs. 5-4 and 6-4.)

The peripheral nervous system develops from the following primordial sources (see Figs. 4-2 and 4-3):

1. Neuroblasts of the neural crest differentiate into the sensory ganglionic (dorsal root) neurons and their processes.
2. Neuroblasts of the basal plate differentiate into the lower motor neurons. Their axons emerge from the neural tube to the ventral root and innervate the muscles and many glands.
3. Neuroblasts of the neural crest and of the basal plate migrate peripherally to form the ganglia of the autonomic nervous system.
4. Cells of the neural crest differentiate into the satellite cells of the ganglia and the neurolemma (Schwann) cells of the peripheral nerves.
5. Mesodermal cells differentiate into the connective tissue elements such as the endoneurium, perineurium, epineurium, and blood vessels.

An axon has its full complement of neurolemma cells by the time it innervates an end organ (either sensory or motor). Myelination commences when the axon reaches 1 to 2 μm in diameter. During the subsequent growth in length, the internode elongates. Those axons which have the largest diameters when mature are those which commence to myelinate first. Within the same general region of the nervous system, the motor nerves tend to develop before the sensory pathways (e.g., somatosensory, auditory, and optic), the neurons tend to mature in an ascending order, commencing with those closest to the peripheral receptors and ending with those neurons of the highest order at the most rostral levels of the neuraxis.

The precise mechanisms by which the peripheral nervous system is organized into complex patterns that are basically similar in different individuals are not really understood. Some observations are instructive. The outgrowths from the neural crest and the basal plate occur early in development and invade the adjacent somites. As the somites differentiate and their subdivisions migrate to their respective locations in the body, they maintain their connections with nerve fibers. In effect, the elongating nerve processes are "towed" along to the periphery by developing nonneural tissues such as muscle cells. Subsequent outgrowths of other nerve fibers follow their predecessors and form nerve fascicles and future nerves. Neurolemma cells accompany the processes, and subsequently myelination occurs.

The number of nodes of Ranvier is fixed at an early state of development. As a result, the length of the internodal segments increases as the nerve elongates. An example of the consequence of the towing of nerve fibers by the primordial muscle cells is found in the innervation of the diaphragm, a voluntary respiratory muscle forming a septum between the thorax and the abdomen. The diphragmatic muscles are derived from somites of the third, fourth and fifth cervical segments. After these somites are innervated, the primordial muscle cells that will form the diaphragm migrate and tow their innervation with them to the site of the future diaphragm in the lower thoracic region. Other portions of these same somites remain in the vicinity of the midcervical regions. Hence, some fibers of the third, fourth, and fifth cervical nerves innervate the diaphragm via the long phrenic nerve, and other fibers innervate neck muscles by shorter cervical nerves.

A reciprocal relation exists between the peripheral nerves and the peripheral tissues. An uninnervated muscle cell is receptive to becoming innervated, but once innervated it will usually reject further innervation. (This is similar to the fertilization of an egg; immediately after an egg is fertilized by a sperm, no other sperm can penetrate the fertilized egg.) In the terminology of communication engineers, the peripheral nerves are programmed by peripheral structures. This mechanism may help to ensure that all muscle fibers become innervated.

Nerve fibers possess the capacity to branch. Hence several uninnervated muscle cells may become innervated by a single axon. This is another mechanism to ensure the innervation of all voluntary muscle cells. This potential of a nerve fiber to branch is retained throughout life, as is the potential of a nerve process to grow in length. Later in life this is expressed in nerve regeneration and in collateral nerve sprouting (Chap. 2). The inability of neurons to multiply by mitosis after birth may be a liability, but the nervous system compensates for this by having the nerve cells retain the capacity to grow and branch. These capacities are, in effect, the retention of an embryonic potential.

CRITICAL PERIODS: EFFECTS OF GENETIC AND ENVIRONMENTAL FACTORS ON THE DEVELOPMENT OF THE NERVOUS SYSTEM

Although the entire nervous system develops as an integrated organ system, its various parts and subparts mature at different rates and tempos. During its ontogeny, each structure passes through one or more critical or sensitive periods, during which it is sensitive to various influences. These periods are generally times of rapid biochemical differentiation. At such a period, the proper influences have a significant role in advancing normal development. Subsequent normal development is often impaired when these influences are wanting or when abnormal influences are exerted at these critical times. When the impaired development results in anatomic abnormalities which are present at birth, they are called congenital malformations. These abnormalities are usually caused by *genetic factors*–chromosomal abnormalities or mutant genes, and *environmental factors*.

Genetic factors

Many cases of congenital mental deficiency and retardation are the result of trisomy of autosomes (three chromosomes instead of the usual pair). *Down's syndrome* (*mongolism*) is a genetic condition in which there are three of the No. 21 chromosome.

Another genetic disease, *phenylketonuria (PKU)*, is a clinical syndrome of marked mental retardation associated with irritability and abnormal EEG patterns. This condition is due to an inherited inborn error of phenylalanine metabolism (transmitted by an autosomal recessive gene) that results in an excessive accumulation of the amino acid phenylalanine and its metabolites. The basic defect is a deficiency of the enzyme phenylalanine hydroxylase in the liver; it is essential for the conversion of phenylalanine to tyrosine. Treatment consists of placing PKU patients on a low-phenylalanine diet commencing in the first year of life; this must be done at this time because the brain damage caused by this condition is due to the accumulation of excess phenylalanine, which reaches its peak between the second and third years of life.

Environmental factors

Environmental factors have a significant role in the normal ontogeny of the nervous system during prenatal life and infancy. Among these factors, which will be discussed briefly, are nutrition, hormones, external stimulation, and oxygen levels in the circulation. Other causal factors associated with anomalies, mental retardation, and functional disabilities include: infections such as German measles (rubella) and syphilis; excessive irradiation of the developing organism; birth trauma and injuries; and various chemical substances.

Nutrition

Malnutrition and undernutrition during fetal life, infancy, and childhood do have an effect on the developing nervous system. Certain nutritional deficiencies, especially those occurring at the critical early rapid period of maturation, can result in permanent damage.

In humans, this critical period extends from the second trimester of pregnancy through most of the first year after birth. During this interval many neurons and macroglia are being replicated and much of the brain growth is taking place. The evidence indicated that under severe protein malnutrition, the rates of proliferation of new neurons and glial cells are reduced. This reduction occurs during fetal life because even the fetus is *not* protected from maternal malnutrition. The developing brain is vulnerable during the remainder of this critical period of postnatal life; the formation of glial cells is impaired, and myelination is inefficient. Malnutrition during this period in human infants is known as *marasmus*. If the child is fed a nutritionally adequate diet after this period, the damage is not completely repaired, even though normal appearance may be achieved in some subjects. Those who appear to be healthy have brains which may be damaged by the protein deficiency. The functional abnormalities in children reared on nutritionally inadequate diets may consist of transient apathy, lethargy, or hyperirritability, together with a lesser intellectual development as measured by a decrease of some 10 to 20 percent of mental capacity.

Prolonged protein deficiency in children from 1 to 2 years of age may result in *kwashiorkor*. In this condition, the number of neurons is not reduced, because the deficiency occurs after the full complement of neurons is formed; however, the complete differentiation and connectivity of these cortical cells may be impaired. If, after being subjected to prolonged, severe malnutrition, children with kwashiorkor are fed a normal diet, their IQ test scores are still below those of other children in the same population, even siblings, who were not subjected to severe malnutrition.

The timing of nutritional deprivation is a critical factor in determining whether or not subsequent recovery from the effects of such deficiencies is possible. In contrast to brains of fetuses and young children, the brains of adolescents and adults are most resistant to permanent effects of malnutrition. The young and mature adult victims of starvation during World War II did not show any loss of intelligence after their nutritional rehabilitation.

Although the most serious effects of subnormal physical and mental development result from the prolonged intake of diets deficient in proteins with the essential amino acids, mental and neurologic maturation may be slowed down by deficiencies in vitamins, minerals, and calories during prenatal and circumnatal life.

The effects of malnutrition assume gigantic proportions in the world today. Roughly 60 percent of the world's preschool population—over 300 million children—is exposed to varying degrees of undernutrition. These children live primarily in underdeveloped lands on diets low in proteins and calories. Malnutrition is contributory to the early death of many of them. Survivors grow up in poverty and become adults with physical and mental handicaps. Thus these poverty (nongenetic) conditions are perpetuated through their children—to be passed on from one generation to the next.

Hormones and behavioral patterns

Adult male sexual patterns of behavior are largely determined by the action of steroid hormones on certain neurons in the brain at a critical period during development. This period apparently occurs only during the fourth to seventh fetal months in the human and only during the first few days after birth in the rat. Hormonal influences at this critical state can impose a permanent change, which is eventually expressed months and years later in juvenile and adult male behavioral patterns. The absence of the action of steroid hormones in these neurons in the brain at this critical period is eventually expressed in juvenile and adult female behavior patterns in genetic males and females.

The explanation for this phenomenon has been established through experimental studies in rats and, in part, in rhesus monkeys (McEwen et al.). Presumably many behavioral patterns in the human have a similar basis.

It is the estrogen hormone estradiol that actually evokes the neural patterns in the immature brain that ultimately result in producing male sexual behavior. A special biochemical condition acts to prevent the estradiol from being able to produce a similar result in the female. Most paradoxical is the observation that testosterone released from the newborn rat's testis is the precursor from which the estradiol is formed. The following is the explanation for these statements.

The key biochemical events occur in specific target neurons located in the preoptic area, hypothalamus, and amygdaloid body; these cells have the metabolic mechanisms essential to converting the testosterone obtained from the bloodstream into estradiol. These target neurons (1) contain specific receptor proteins within their cytoplasm and (2) convert the testosterone into estradiol. The brain of the rhesus monkey has the same pattern of estradiol concentrating neurons as does the rat brain. Presumably estradiol is the agent responsible for the brain differentiation associated with male sexual behavior. The receptor estradiol complexes pass through the nuclear membrane and interact with specific genes on the chromosomes. The resultant messenger RNA migrates from the nucleus to the cytoplasm where it presides over the sythesis of protein by the endoplasmic reticulum. In essence, the steroid hormones affect the genetic substrates and, in turn, produce a permanent change in the structural and functional makeup of these hormonally sensitive differen-

tiating nerve cells. It is still a matter of conjecture as to how the neurons influence male behavior.

In brief, if the hormones testosterone and estradiol are available to certain neurons in the brain at this critical period of development, the result is an animal, including a human, expressing the juvenile and adult male type of behavioral patterns.

The relation of these steroid hormones to the brains of females is instructive. The adult female sexual behavioral pattern results if these steroid hormones are *not* made available to these hormone-sensitive target cells during the critical period. This access is prevented in the female newborn rat by a blood protein called alpha-fetoprotein. This protein binds circulating estradiol and thereby keeps it from reaching the target neurons. Thus, these neurons express their natural role of influencing the development of female behavioral patterns. In contrast, this alpha-fetoprotein does *not* bind testosterone. This nonbinding property explains why the administration of testosterone directly to newborn female rats produces adult female rats that express adult male behavioral patterns. This is consistent with the observation that male rats castrated prior to the critical period ultimately exhibit female patterns of behavior. Of clinical significance in humans is the occurrence of adult male behavioral patterns in human females whose mothers were therapeutically treated with excessive doses of androgens during pregnancy. These prenatally androgenized females typically identify themselves during and following adolescence as "tomboys."

The mental retardation associated with *cretinism* in humans is due to a thyroid hormone deficiency at a critical period during the late stages of in utero development (estimated to begin at the seventh fetal month). The cerebral cortex of cretinoid individuals is poorly developed. There is a reduction in number and size of the cell bodies of the neurons, as well as hypoplasia of both their axons and dendrites. Axodendritic synaptic connections are reduced in number. The electrical activity of the cortex is altered, and protein and nucleic acid metabolism in the neurons is impaired. In contrast to the drastic effects from hypothyroidism in the prenatal human fetus, hypothroidism in children, juveniles, and adults does not seem to produce any adverse effects on the brain or the capacity for learning. Mental retardation of the cretinoid human being can be prevented or effectively remedied if adequate doses of thyroid hormones are given during the first year of life.

External stimulation during ontogeny of the visual system The development of each pathway system in its full anatomic, physiologic, and functional complexities is the expression of the organism's genetic potential supplemented and reinforced by environmental stimuli exerted upon the system during ontogeny. In a sensory pathway such as the visual system, the stimuli are a variety of visual experiences. In the motor sphere responses to stimuli are expressed by varied motor activities. The absence or a minimal amount of stimulation at critical periods hampers or even prevents the normal development of a system. The exact age at which a critical period occurs and the precise duration of each critical period in humans are not known. Some aspects of the concept of critical periods will be outlined in relation to the visual system.

The differentiation, growth, and precise synaptic connectivity of the visual pathways are primarily predetermined genetically. It appears that the neurons of the visual pathways from both retinas to the visual cortices are instructed and programmed genetically to construct this binocular, topographically organized system. This complex neural connectivity is established before the eyes have received any photic stimulation. Except for a few slight neurophysiologic differences, all types of visual responses of neurons in the optic pathways of visually inexperienced kittens are strikingly similar to those of the adult cat. This indicated that complex neural connections do develop without the benefit of visual experiences.

Drastic reduction and complete deprivation of light stimulation result in morphologic, neurophysiologic, and behavioral deficits in the visual system. The degree to which the visual system is altered is related to the age of the animal and to the length of time the animal is subjected to visual deprivation. If the deprivation occurs only before the critical period, the visual system remains normal. If the deprivation occurs after the critical period, the visual system also remains normal. If the deprivation occurs for a long stretch of the critical period, abnormalities in the visual system occur (e.g., alterations in pattern discrimination, difficulty in fixating objects). The longer the animal has been visually deprived during this critical period, the more severe the effects to the visual system. In the kitten, the critical period is estimated to last from the fourth to the tenth or twelfth week postnatally. The following experiment is illustrative. During the critical period, the right eye of a kitten is exposed only to vertical lines and the left eye of the same kitten is exposed only to horizontal lines; later in life the right eye responds to vertical lines and is indifferent to horizontal lines, while the left eye responds to horizontal lines and is indifferent to vertical lines. This can be demonstrated by behavioral responses of the cat.

Amblyopia, or lazy-eye, in humans is presumed to be caused by inadequate stimulation by formed objects of the macula of one eye during the critical stages, probably between the second and fourth years of age. The slightly crossed-eyed child favors one eye over the other (to avoid seeing double), with the result that the visual pathway from the macula of one eye is not adequately stimulated and hence fails to maintain normal connections.

This concept of the critical period during childhood is the basis of the suggestion that young children should be exposed to rich visual experiences, even more than they can handle intelligently. This should help to ensure the optimal maturation of the child's visual pathways.

The person who is congenitally blind (from *cataracts*) and whose capacity to receive environmental visual stimuli is surgically restored after several years will never see "normally" because the inadequately developed optic system cannot compensate effectively. Upon reacquiring sight such a person first obtains impressions of brightness and color. Gross differences in the perception of depth eventually develop into the ability to estimate depth. The idea of shape, determined visually, is secondarily acquired, after shape has been consciously interpreted. The functional return is generally limited to crude discriminations, gross depth perceptions, and identifications of large objects. Recognition of large letters is possible, but that of small letters is unlikely. Again, the absence of adequate visual stimulation during the critical period prevented a normal visual pathway from sustaining itself.

Many neurons differentiating prenatally are integrated into neuronal circuits that express a remarkable degree of sophistication prior to receiving active environmental stimulation. For example, the visually naive newborn kitten elicits essentially the same types of electrically recorded responses that are obtained in the visual cortex of the adult cat. This indicates that the basic intrinsic visual pathways are prewired with a functionally highly advanced circuitry prior to the advent of external environmental stimulation. An expression of functional circuitry is the remarkable repertoire of limb movements exhibited by newborn monkeys. Experimental studies of the movements utilizing prenatal and newborn monkeys yield some pertinent information relative to the question, "Did the newborn monkeys 'learn' the dexterous limb movements in utero utilizing sensory feedback from their own fetal movements?" Apparently, the newborn monkeys had "learned" to use their limbs without any input from sensory feedback generated from the movement (Taub et al.). Newborn monkeys in whom a number of consecutive dorsal roots had been severed two-fifths of the way through the prenatal period exhibited precisely normal movements in those limbs lacking dorsal root innervation. Presumably many motor programs are genetically determined by circuits restricted to the central nervous system. The basic repertoire of limb movements develops without the need of sensory feedback or the afferent limb of reflex loops. Sensory feedback is essential for the "fine tuning" needed to correct and to smooth out the roughness from the relatively clumsy movements of the newborn monkey during early postnatal development.

Oxygen levels and perinatal brain damage The brain is so dependent upon continuous supplies of oxygen and glucose that the deprivation of either for even a few minutes may result in irreversible brain damage. Depending upon degree and duration, hypoxia during the perinatal period (i.e., the last half of pregnancy and the first month after birth) may lead to pathologic changes, cerebral palsy, and certain types of mental retardation. This *hypoxia* of the fetal circulation to the developing brain may be due to impairment of placental functional activity or to an oxygen deficiency in the maternal blood associated with toxemia, anemia, or cardiac disorders. Experimental studies indicate that several episodes of prolonged partial asphyxia of full-term monkey fetuses lead to cerebral hemispheric damage—including various degrees of cortical atrophy, sclerosis of the white matter, and pathologic changes in the basal ganglia (Myers). This damage is similar to that described in the brains of human beings with perinatal injury, cerebral palsy, or mental retardation. In contrast, a single episode of acute total asphyxia, when of sufficient length, leads to damage restricted to the brainstem; this has little resemblance to the more common pattern noticed in perinatal injury in human infants (Myers).

Prenatal motor activity The early ontogenesis of the neuronal circuits involved with the motor innervation of the somatic musculature has an essential role in the regulation of the muscular contractions which are common during prenatal life. These somatic movements of the fetus are more than the expression of casual contractions. They are activities which are essential to the development of normal musculature. Experimental evidence indicates that in the absence of such movements muscles are small and poorly developed.

The effect of an injury to the central nervous system in the fetal brain is most serious when the lesion is associated with a structure that is in an early stage of a critical developmental sequence. This is contrary to the general rule which states that in humans and primates the effects of brain injury are usually less severe if the lesion occurs when the subject is young than when it is mature. The usual explanations are (1) that the young brain is more resilient than the mature brain of an adult and (2) that compensatory mechanisms are more apt to rectify the effects during subsequent development. For example, it is probable that alternative pathways or circuits can develop to alleviate the deficiency in the younger brain.

BRAIN

Prenatal development

Early in the second fetal month, the "three-vesicle brain" differentiates into the "five-vesicle brain" (see Fig. 4-8). The prosencephalic vesicle is subdivided into the telencephalon, or endbrain, and the diencephalon, or between (twixt) brain. The mesencephalic vesicle remains as the midbrain; the rhombencephalic vesicle is subdivided into the metencephalon, or afterbrain, and the myelencephalon, or spinal brain. The derivatives of the neural tube and its vesicles are outlined in Table 4-1.

The development of the "contorted" brain from the tubelike structure is the result of the complex integration of several processes: (1) three bends known as flexures, (2) differential enlargements of the different regions, (3) growth of portions of the cerebral hemispheres over the diencephalon, midbrain, and cerebellum, and (4) the formation of sulci and gyri in the cerebral and cerebellar cortices (see Fig. 4-9). The flexures are the mesencephalic (midbrain) flexure (forming an acute angle on the anterior surface of the brain), the pontine flexure (forming an acute angle on the posterior surface), and the cervical flexure at the lower medulla (forming an acute angle on the anterior surface). The posterolateral margin of the rhombencephalon is the rhombic lip, which develops into the cerebellum. The differential enlargement is most pronounced in the

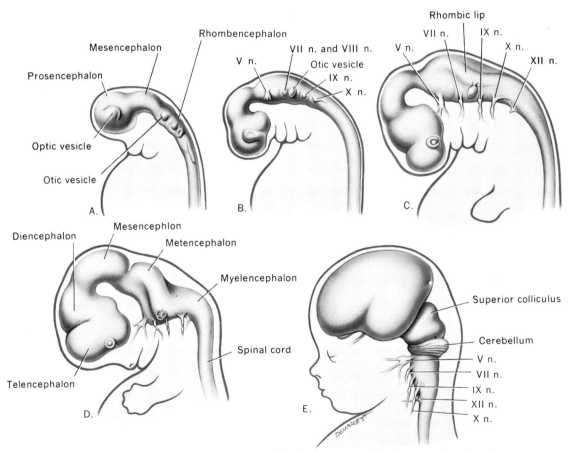

FIGURE 4-8 Human brain (lateral view). *A.* In 3-week embryo. *B.* In 4-week embryo. *C.* In 5-week embryo. *D.* In 7-week embryo. *E.* In 11-week fetus. n., cranial nerve. (*Adapted from Corliss*).

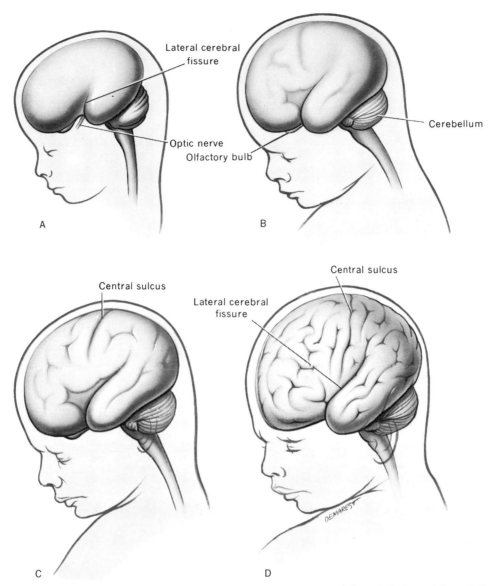

FIGURE 4-9 Human brain (lateral view). *A.* In 4-month fetus. *B.* In 6-month fetus. *C.* In 8-month fetus. *D.* In newborn infant. (*Adapted from Corliss*).

cerebral and cerebellar hemispheres. The telencephalon during development surrounds most of the diencephalon; there is an intussusception of the diencephalon into the telencephalon. As the result of a partial intussusception of the upper midbrain into the diencephalon, the substantia nigra, nucleus ruber, and surrounding tegmentum protrude rostrally into the diencephalon.

Three placodes give rise to important recep-

tor elements of the olfactory, optic, and auditory systems. Each nasal placode gives rise to the olfactory pit in which are differentiated the olfactory receptor neurons and associated epithelial cells of the olfactory mucosa (Chap. 15). The optic placode and vesicle contain the progenitors of the neurons and cells of the pigment layer of the retina and cells and processes of the neurons and cells of the neuroretina (see Figs. 4-8

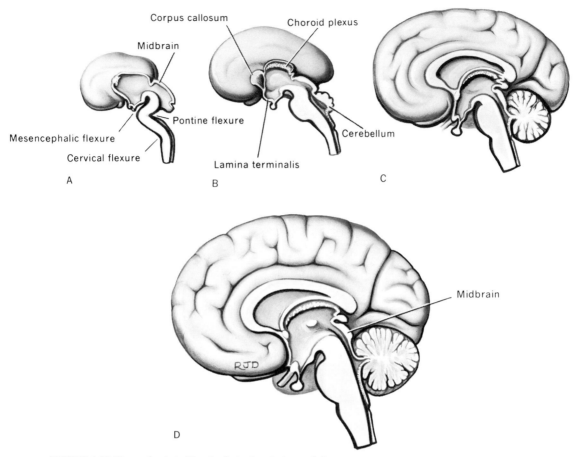

FIGURE 4-10 Human brain (midsagittal view). *A.* In 3-month fetus. *B.* In 4-month fetus. *C.* In 8-month fetus. *D.* In newborn infant. (*Adapted from Corliss*).

and 12-5 and Chap. 12). The otic (acousticovestibular) placode and vesicle are composed of cells that develop into the sensory epithelial cells of the cochlea, semicircular canals, utricle, and saccule, and the bipolar cells in the cochlear (spiral) and vestibular ganglia (see Figs. 4-1 and 4-8 and Chap. 10). Some cells of cranial nerve V, VII, IX, and X are derived from the otic vesicle.

The main outlines of the form of the brain are recognizable and the external surface of the brain is still smooth at the end of the third fetal month. Fissuration commences in the fourth fetal month with the appearance of the lateral sulcus of the cerebrum and posterolateral sulcus of the cerebellum separating the nodulus and flocculi from the vermis. The central sulcus, calcarine sulcus, and parietooccipital sulcus are indicated by the fifth fetal month; all the main gyri and sulci of the cerebral cortex are present by the seventh fetal month. The external structure of the cerebral hemisphere of the 8-month fetus is characterized by the prominence of the precentral and postcentral gyri, by a wide-open lateral sulcus exping the insula, and by the presence of all primary and secondary sulci and a few tertiary sulci. The occipital lobe overrides the cerebellum. During the last month of fetal life the frontal and temporal lobes are stubby, the insula is still exposed to the surface, and the occipital poles are blunt. The cortical gyri are broad and plump, and the fissures are shallow. The patterns of the primary and secondary sulci are simple and present a diagrammatic appearance (Figs. 4-9 and 4-10).

The cerebrum of the full-term neonate is more fully developed in the regions posterior to the central sulcus than in the anterior regions. The frontal pole and the temporal pole are relatively short, and the insula is almost completely covered by the adjacent lobes. The number of tertiary sulci is still small. The leptomeninges are not completely adherent to the brain, and they do not dip into all the sulci. The superficial blood vessels are straight. The brain has a gelatinous consistency because except for some somatic afferent tracts (general somatic, auditory, and visual systems), the subcortical white matter is unmyelinated. As a result, the cortex is poorly demarcated from the white matter. By the end of infancy, at 2 years of age, the relative size and proportions of the brain and its subdivisions are essentially similar to those of the adult brain. The brain is firmer. The gray cortex is demarcated from the subcortical white matter, which is now myelinated. The superficial cortical blood vessels are predominately tucked into the fissures and sulci. After the end of the second year the tertiary sulci dominate the topographic pattern of the cerebral surface. These sulci are variable from brain to brain and thereby put the stamp of individuality on each brain. Tertiary sulcation may continue throughout life.

Postnatal growth

The large brain in the newborn infant exceeds 10 percent of the entire body weight; in the adult the brain constitutes only approximately 2 percent of the total body weight. The postnatal growth of the brain is rapid, especially during the first 2 years after birth (see Fig. 4-11). The brain weighs about 350 g in the full-term infant and about 1000 g at the end of the first year. The rate of growth slows down after this, and by puberty the brain weighs about 1250 g in girls and 1375 g in boys. It appears that the brain of a girl grows more rapidly than that of a boy up to the third year, but the brains of boys grow more rapidly after that. This brain size is reflected in the growth of the cranial skeleton. In contrast to the adult, the young child has a large cranium in relation to the face. Head circumference is a measure of the growth of the brain. The head circumference is 34 cm at birth, 46 cm at the end of the first year, 48 cm at the end of the second year,

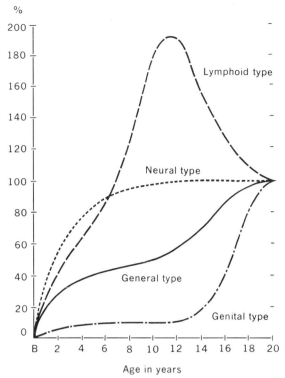

FIGURE 4-11 Graph illustrating the postnatal growth of the major organ systems and general body size. Note that relative to the other organ systems and general body growth, the nervous system grows most rapidly during the first years after birth. In this graph, the end of each curve in the upper right represents the weight of each organ system at 20 years of age, expressed as 100 percent. Other points in the curves represent weight of each organ system at different ages as the percentage of the weight at 20 years of age. (*After Scammon.*)

52 cm at 10 years, and only slightly larger at puberty and in the adult.

Humans are unusual among mammals in at least two ways. (1) Of all the large-brained mammals, humans have the largest brain relative to total body weight. They do not have the largest brain—several large-brained mammals, such as elephants and whales, have brains which are larger than human brains but smaller relative to total body weight. There are several monkeys, all small, with brains which are larger, relative to their body weights, than human brains. (2) The major increase in the absolute size of the human brain occurs during postnatal life. The 2½- to 3-fold increase in human brains during the first year after birth is unique among mammals (see Fig. 4-11). The human being might not have survived as a species but for the evolution of a brain that grows considerably during postnatal life. An infant whose brain at birth was the size of that of a year-old infant could not have been delivered naturally through the human female pelvis.

PRENATAL AND POSTNATAL ACTIVITY IN HUMANS

Motor activity

The initial reflex activity in response to external stimuli, as noted above, is the withdrawal of the head from an irritation of the upper lip during the seventh week after fertilization. The area of sensitivity expands until by the fourteenth week tactile stimulation of the face will evoke responses that include rotation of the head, contraction of the contralateral trunk musculature, extension of the trunk, extension of the upper extremities at the shoulder, and rotation of the pelvis to the opposite side. Reactions of the early fetus to tactile stimulation of the lips include swallowing movements ($10\frac{1}{2}$ weeks), protrusion and pursing of both lips (22 weeks), and audible sucking (twenty-ninth week). In the realm of respiratory activities, the chest musculature contractions can be evoked at the thirteenth week, contractions of the diaphragm have been noted at the twenty-second week, and continuous respiratory movements have been observed at the twenty-seventh week, long before the date of normal delivery. The fetal respiratory movements result in the aspiration of amniotic fluid. Local trunk reflexes and local reflexes of the extremities have been evoked in the third fetal month.

The newborn infant retains many of the fetal flexor attitudes, such as flexed limbs, closed hands, and adducted thumbs. The reaction to a sudden noise is characterized by intense simple and stereotyped motions. The primitive reflexes involve the overall response of the entire body and limbs. Many visceral activities, although well developed, are not fully differentiated. Respiration is irregular, the body temperature fluctuates, and swallowing and peristaltic activities are not fully coordinated. The reflexes that are easily evoked include hiccupping, urination, and sweating. The newborn infant's activities are not dependent on the cerebral cortex, since similar reactions are exhibited by the anencephalic monster, i.e., one with essentially no forebrain. For all intents, the newborn infant is a reflex animal with all motor activity operating through subcortical influences.

The typical neonatal infant's mass movements are gradually modified in the early months of life. By the third month, isolated movements and conscious motor activity are in evidence. Mastery of the volitional motor movements is expressed first in the proximal joints of the limb and later by the movements of the more distal joints. The movements of the head, spine, and legs are perfected before a child assumes the upright posture and ambulates. The coordinated movements of the shoulders, the flexor-extensor activities of the elbow and wrists, the primitive palm graspings, all precede the coordinated movements of the fingers. Individuation of the skilled movements out of the previous generalized movements is indicated.

Progress in motor coordination during the child's first year is expressed, in general, as follows: first month, smiles in response to an adult; second month, vocalizes with such sounds as "ah" and "uh"; third month, head control indicated when infant is raised by his hands from supine to sitting position, the head coming forward with the body instead of lagging; fourth month, hand control, indicated by grasping for object held within sight and reach; fifth month, rolls body from supine to prone; sixth month, sits without support for several seconds; seventh month, crawls voluntarily by pushing with legs, rolling, and hitching; eighth month, picks up small objects by opposing the thumb and index finger; ninth month, pulses self up to standing position; tenth month, walks without support but by holding on to adult's hand or stable object; eleventh month, stands alone and without support for several seconds; and twelfth month, walks alone without support for several seconds.

Sensory activity

The newborn infant's initial impressions of the external world come through the touch receptors. Touch is apparently highly evolved. Contact with mother, nipple, and clothes is a primary source of information. The protopathic senses of pain, temperature, and touch; kinesthetic sense, and visceral senses are all present at birth but are poorly localized. The tolerance of pain, especially if the child's attention is diverted by sucking a nipple, suggests that the sensitivity to pain is less than in an older child.

The development of visual perception progresses from birth through the first decade of life. During the first few weeks of life, the infant distinguishes light from dark but probably perceives only vague visual images. The baby's eyes move without fixing upon specific objects. A bright light causes the pupil to contract and the eyelids to close. From 1 month after birth, the eye can fix on a bright object and follow the object for a few seconds. During the third and fourth months, the infant commences to fix upon and recognize the mother and such objects as the bottle and is able to follow objects well. The child is normally farsighted. By the sixth month, recognition of familiar faces and objects is well developed. Strange objects may evoke crying spells. The eyes and the visual system continue to develop during the first decade. Objects should be large when a child is learning from visual cues.

The newborn infant is actually deaf at birth, mainly because of the absence of air in the eustachian tube and the presence of embryonic tissue in the middle ear. Several days after birth, hearing becomes acute, especially to a high-pitched voice. At 1 month the infant can respond by turning in the direction of a sound, especially an unusual one.

The senses of smell and taste are present at birth. They are well-developed by the second and third months.

CONGENITAL DEFECTS AND ABNORMAL DEVELOPMENT

Of all the malformations and congenital defects in human beings, ranging from minor observable variations from the norm to lethal abnormalities, as many as one-half are estimated to involve the nervous system. Slight decrease in intelligence due to a defect in development is hard to establish. Striking abnormalities definitely attributable to ontogenetic defects include the absence of a brain (anencephalus), extremely small brain (microcephalus), excessive enlargement of the ventricular cavities (hydrocephalus), and the absence of a head (acrania).

Theoretically most of the anomalies of the nervous system arise in one of two ways. (1) Ballooning defects. Pressure develops in the ventricular system. In turn, ballooning may occur in a specific "weak" part of the nervous system, or a generalized increase in pressure may result in excessive enlargement of the ventricles, producing hydrocephalus (water in the brain). In the latter, the brain is compressed between the high ventricular pressure and the unexpandable skull, with the result that severe brain damage occurs unless the pressure is relieved. (2) Lip defects in the neural folds. The lips of the neural folds exhibit developmental flaws that result in variable defects, the most extreme being the nonfusion of lips leading to the formation of an abnormal open neural tube. These two ways by which anomalies are formed are not causal but mechanistic. The causes of anomalies are not fully known. They have genetic and environmental bases. The environmental causes include the lack of an important metabolite (e.g., oxygen) at a critical stage or the presence of a noxious substance (e.g., a poison) which might inhibit a vital metabolic action at a critical time.

Spina bifida is one of the more common examples of defects; the term is used to cover a wide range of closure defects, usually located in the lower lumbar region (see Fig. 4-12). The most extreme version occurs when the neural plate in the lumbar region remains as a plate exposed to the outside. An infant with this defect has bladder and bowel incontinence, sensory loss, and motor paralysis of the lower extremities. In less severe cases the meninges or the meninges along with the spinal cord, though displaced backward, are still covered by the skin. In a minor form, only the bony vertebral arches may be defective. The persistence of an attachment of the caudal end of the spinal cord in a minor form of spina bifida results in the stretching of the spinal cord as far caudad as the fifth lumbar vertebra. The degenerative changes associated with this *tethering of the spinal cord* are accompanied by some motor deficits. Severing the attachment

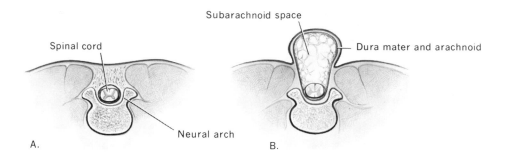

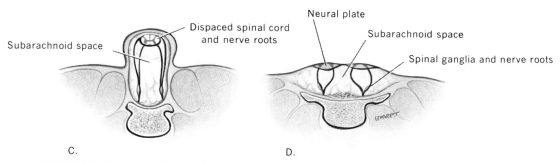

FIGURE 4-12 Some anomalies which may occur in the lumbosacral region. *A.* Spina bifida occulta results from the failure of the neural arches of the vertebrae to fuse dorsally. *B.* Spina bifida with meningocele is a defect with a subarachnoid fluid-filled meningeal cyst bulging through unfused neural arches. Cyst is covered with skin. *C.* Spina bifida with myelomeningocele is a defect with meningeal cyst containing spinal cord and nerve roots. *D.* Spina bifida with myeloschisis is a defect in which neural plate (having failed to close) is exposed to surface. (*Adapted from Corliss*).

by surgery will relieve the stretch and can arrest any further degenerative changes.

BIBLIOGRAPHY

Altman, J.: Autoradiographic and histological studies of postnatal neurogenesis. J Comp Neurol, 128:431–474, 1966.

Angevine, J. B., Jr., et al.: Embryonic vertebrate central nervous system: revised terminology. Anat Rec, 166:257–261, 1970.

Berrill, N. J., and G. Karp: *Development*, McGraw-Hill Book Company, New York, 1976.

Brazier, M. A. B. (ed.): *Growth and Development of the Brain: Nutritional, Genetic, and Environmental Factors*, Raven Press, New York, 1975.

Brody, H.: "Structural Changes in the Aging Nervous System," in H. Blumenthal (ed.), *Interdisciplinary Topics in Gerontology*, Karger, Basel, 1970, chap. 1, pp. 1–12.

Bunge, R., M. Johnson, and C. D. Ross: Nature and nurture in development of the autonomic nervous system. Science, 199:1409–1416, 1978.

Corliss, C. E.: *Patten's Human Embryology*, McGraw-Hill Book Company, New York, 1976.

Cowan, W. M.: The development of the brain. Sci Am, 241:112–133, 1979.

Dodge, P. R., A. L. Prensky, and R. D. Feigin: *Nutrition and the Developing Nervous System*, The C. V. Mosby Company, St. Louis, 1975.

Edds, M. V., Jr., et al.: "Development of the Nervous System," in F. O. Schmitt (ed.), *The Neurosciences*, Rockefeller University Press, New York, 1970.

Grenell, R. G., and R. E. Scammon: An iconometrographic representation of the growth of the central nervous system in man. J Comp Neurol, 79:329–354, 1943.

Hamilton, W. J., and H. W. Mossman: *Human Embryology*, W. Heffer and Sons, Ltd., Cambridge, England, 1972.

Hess, A.: The experimental embryology of the foetal nervous system. Biol Rev, 32:231–260, 1957.

Jacobson, M.: *Developmental Neurobiology*, Plenum Press, New York, 1978.

Kalter, H.: *Teratology of the Central Nervous System,* University of Chicago Press, Chicago, 1968.

Langman, J.: *Medical Embryology, Human Development, Normal and Abnormal,* The Williams and Wilkins Company, Baltimore, 1975.

Lemire, R. J., J. D. Loeser, R. W. Leech, and E. C. Alvord, Jr.: *Normal and Abnormal Development of the Human Nervous System,* Harper and Row, New York, 1975.

Lund, R. D.: *Development and Plasticity of the Brain,* Oxford University Press, New York, 1978.

McEwen, B., L. Krey, and V. Luine: Steroid hormone action in the neuroendocrine system: where is the genome involved? Res Publ Assoc Res Nerv Ment Dis, 56:255–268, 1978.

Moore, K. L.: *The Developing Human,* W. B. Saunders Company, Philadelphia, 1977.

Munger, B. L.: Neural-epithelial interactions in sensory receptors. J Invest Dermatol, 69:27–40, 1977.

Myers, R. E.: Two patterns of perinatal brain damage and their conditions of occurrence. Am J Obstet Gynecol, 112:246–276, 1972.

O'Rahilly, R., and E. Gardner: The timing and sequence of events in the development of the human nervous system during the embryonic period proper. Z Anat Entwicklungsgesch, 134:1–12, 1971.

Patterson, P., D. Potter, and E. Furshpan: The chemical differentiation of nerve cells. Sci Am, 239:50–59, 1978.

Pfenninger, K. H., and R. P. Rees: "From the Growth Cone to the Synapse. Properties of Membranes Involved in Synapse Formation," in S. Barondes (ed.), *Neuronal Recognition,* Plenum Press, New York, 1976, pp. 131–178.

Rakic, P.: Kinetics of proliferation and latency between final cell division and onset of differentiation of cerebellar stellate and basket neurons. J Comp Neurol, 147:523–546, 1973.

Rockstein, M. (ed.): *Development and Aging in the Nervous System,* Academic Press, Inc., New York, 1973.

Scammon, R. E.: "Developmental Anatomy," in J. P. Schaeffer (ed.) *Morris' Human Anatomy,* McGraw-Hill Book Company, New York, 1953.

Sidman, R. L.: "Cell–Cell Recognition in the Developing Central Nervous System," in F. O. Schmitt and F. G. Worden (eds.), *The Neurosciences—Third Study Program,* M. I. T. Press, Cambridge, Mass., 1974, chap. 65, pp. 743–758.

Singer, M., R. Woodlander, and M. Egar: Axonal guidance during embryogenesis and regeneration in the spinal cord of the newt. The blueprint hypophysis of neuronal pathway patterning. J Comp Neurol, 185:1–22, 1979.

Sperry, R. W.: "Physiological Plasticity and Brain Circuit Theory," in H. Harlow and C. Woolsey (eds.), *Biological and Biochemical Bases of Behavior,* Univ. of Wisconsin Press, Madison, Wis., 1958, pp. 401–424.

Taub, E., G. Barro, R. Heitmann, H. C. Grier, and D. P. Martin: "Effect of Forelimb Deafferentation During the Mid-prenatal Period on Motor Development in Monkeys," in E. Asmussen and K. Jorgenson (eds.), *Biomechanics VI-A,* University Park Press, Baltimore, 1978, pp. 125–129.

Timiras, P. S.: *Developmental Physiology and Aging,* The Macmillan Company, New York, 1972.

Winick, M.: *Malnutrition and Brain Development,* Oxford University Press, New York, 1976.

CHAPTER FIVE

THE SPINAL CORD

GROSS ANATOMY

The *spinal cord* is that portion of the central nervous system which is surrounded and protected by the vertebral column. The flexible *vertebral column* consists of a series of bony vertebrae, including seven cervical vertebrae, twelve thoracic vertebrae, five lumbar vertebrae, five fused sacral vertebrae (sacrum), and the coccyx. On the sides of the column are located paired openings called *intervertebral foramina;* one pair of foramina is typically located between two successive vertebrae.

The spinal cord, which is continuous with the medulla, is a cylinder that is slightly flattened posterolaterally (i.e., it is wider than it is deep) and surrounded by the three meninges: pia mater, arachnoid, and dura mater (see Fig. 5-1). It lies within the upper two-thirds of the vertebral canal (the cavity within the vertebral column) and terminates caudally as the cone-shaped *conus medullaris*, at the level between the first and second lumbar vertebrae (the upper small of the back). The pia mater continues caudally from the tip of the conus as a nonneural thread, the *filum terminale*, to the end of the bony vertebral column, where it is anchored into the ligament on the posterior side of the coccyx. The piarachnoid and the dura mater continue as tubular sheaths to the level of the second sacral vertebra, where they fuse with the filum terminale. Note that the subarachnoid space with its cerebrospinal fluid extends below the level of the spinal cord to the second sacral vertebral level.

The spinal cord is suspended from the dura mater by a series of 20 to 22 pairs of *denticulate ligaments*, which are flanges of epipial tissue (outer layer of pia mater which is continuous with the arachnoid trabeculae) extending laterally from the pia mater to the dura mater. These collagenous ligaments of epipeal pial tissue are attached medially to a continuous line on either side of the entire spinal cord from the medulla to the conus medullaris midway between the dorsal and ventral roots. The lateral, free edges of the denticulate ligaments are scalloped (see Fig. 5-2). Each ligament extends laterally to a pointed process, which passes through the arachnoid, and then it attaches to the dura mater; this point of attachment is located between sites of the emergence of two successive spinal nerve roots. In general, denticulate ligament is found above the first cervical roots and between all successive roots through the first lumbar; at the latter site the ligament is continuous with the filum terminale.

SPINAL NERVES

General relations

An almost continuous series of *spinal nerve rootlets* emerges from the posterolateral sulcus and another series emerges from the sulcus on the

FIGURE 5-1 The spinal cord and its relation to the vertebral column (as viewed from behind). The first cervical dorsal root and spinal ganglion are absent. Each spinal ganglion is located in the region of an intervertebral foramen. The length and caudally directed slant of the spinal roots increase progressively from cervical to coccygeal levels.

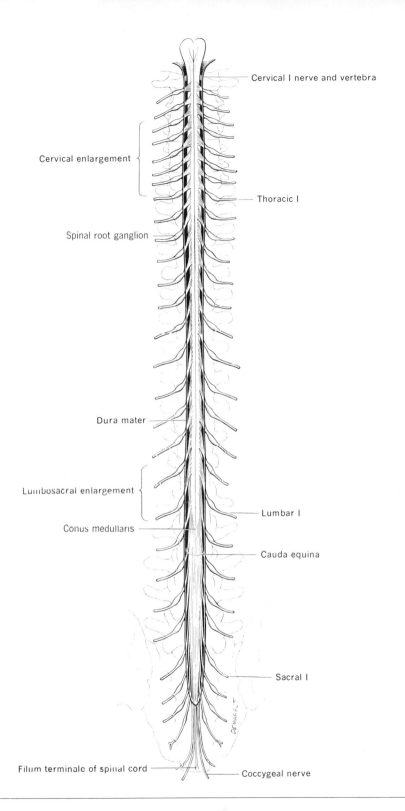

Cervical I nerve and vertebra

Cervical enlargement

Thoracic I

Spinal root ganglion

Dura mater

Lumbosacral enlargement

Lumbar I

Conus medullaris

Cauda equina

Sacral I

Filum terminale of spinal cord

Coccygeal nerve

THE SPINAL CORD

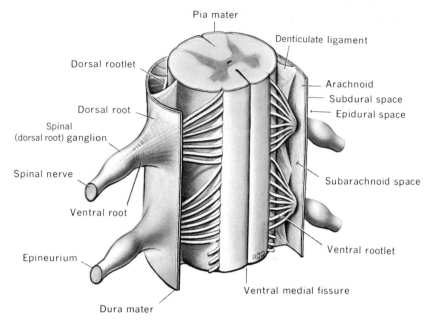

Pia mater

Denticulate ligament

Dorsal rootlet

Dorsal root

Spinal
(dorsal root) ganglion

Spinal nerve

Ventral root

Epineurium

Dura mater

Arachnoid

Subdural space

Epidural space

Subarachnoid space

Ventral rootlet

Ventral medial fissure

FIGURE 5-2 Two segments of the spinal cord and its meningeal coverings. Note that (1) several rootlets merge to form one spinal nerve; (2) the dura mater and arachnoid, as the dural sleeve, are continuous with the spineurium of each spinal nerve; (3) the pia mater is continuous with the denticulate ligament; and (4) the subarachnoid space extends within the dural sleeve into the region of the spinal ganglion.

anterolateral sulcus of the spinal cord (see Figs. 5-1, 5-2, and 5-9). These rootlets collect laterally as *spinal roots* and finally form the 31 pairs of spinal nerves (see Figs. 5-2 and 5-3). A typical spinal nerve passes through an intervertebral foramen and is then distributed to a segment of the body. (The first cervical nerve, an exception, passes between occipital bone and the first cervi-

Table 5-1
Levels of spinal cord segments

Spinous process of vertebra	Interspace between vertebral bodies*	Spinal cord segment
C1		C1–2
C6	C6	T1
T10	T10	L1
T12	T12	S1
	T12–L1	All sacral and coccygeal levels
	S2 or S3	Caudal termination of subarachnoid space
	Coccyx	Termination of filum terminale

Named from centrum of vertebra above interspace.

cal vertebra.) There are eight pairs of cervical, twelve pairs of thoracic, five pairs of lumbar, five pairs of sacral, and one pair of coccygeal spinal nerves. Each of the first seven cervical nerves is named from the bony vertebra immediately below its exit through the intervertebral foramen (e.g., the third cervical nerve passes through the intervertebral foramen located between the second and the third cervical vertebrae). The eighth cervical nerve passes through the intervertebral foramen between the seventh cervical and the first thoracic vertebrae. Each of the other spinal nerves is named after the vertebra above its exit from the vertebral column. In this conventional system, the nerve is named in relation to the level of its exit from the bony vertebral column. Because the spinal cord is shorter than the vertebral column, the level for the exit of a specific spinal nerve from the cord is usually different from the level of its exit from the vertebral column (see Fig. 5-1 and Table 5-1). For example, the rootlets of the first cervical nerve exit from the spinal cord at the level of the first cervical vertebra; the rootlets of the first thoracic nerve exit at the level of the seventh cervical ver-

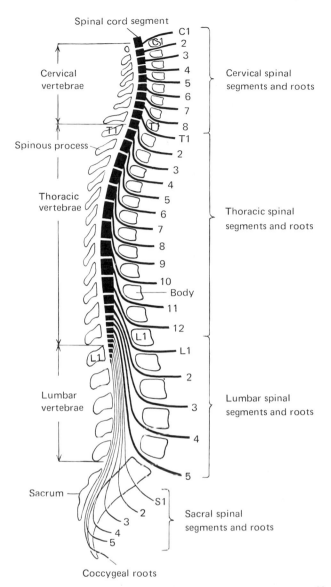

FIGURE 5-3 The topographic relations of the spinal cord segments, spinous processes, and bodies of the vertebrae, intervertebral foramina, and spinal nerves. Refer to Table 5.1. Each spinal cord segment (except upper cervical segments) is located at a higher vertebral level than the spinal nerve emerging through its intervertebral foramen. (*Adapted from Haymaker, Bing's Local Diagnosis in Neurological Diseases, The C. V. Mosby Company, St. Louis.*)

tebra; the rootlets of the first lumbar spinal nerve emerge at the level of the twelfth thoracic vertebra; and the rootlets of all sacral nerves exit at the level of the first lumbar vertebra.

The spinal cord is actually a nonsegmented structure; this is indicated by the presence of a continuous series of emerging rootlets and the gradual changes in the internal structure of the spinal cord. Its apparent segmentation into 31 spinal segments (see Fig. 5-3) is an expression of 31 pairs of spinal nerves, which develop embryologically in relation to the segmented somites. On the posterior aspect of the cord are three longitudinal grooves (Fig. 5-9)—the *posterior me-*

dian sulcus, posterior intermediate sulcus, and posterolateral sulcus; on the anterior aspect are two longitudinal grooves—the anterior median fissure and anterolateral sulcus. Except for the posterior intermediate sulcus, which extends through the cervical and upper half of the thoracic spinal levels, all these grooves extend throughout the entire length of the spinal cord. The posterior medial sulcus and anterior median fissure are located in the midsagittal plane. The posterolateral sulci and anterolateral sulci are paired grooves located at the emergence of the posterior and anterior spinal rootlets, respectively. The posterior intermediate sulci are paired grooves located between the posterior median sulcus and the posterolateral sulci.

All rootlets pass through the subarachnoid space and the cerebrospinal fluid surrounding the spinal cord before joining the arachnoid and dural meningeal layers which form the *dural sleeve* around the emerging roots before they unite to form the spinal nerves (see Fig. 5-2). The dural sleeve is continuous distally with the epineurium of the peripheral nerves. The piarachnoid is said to be continuous with the perineural epithelial sheath of the peripheral nerve. The subarachnoid space caudal to the conus medullaris contains cerebrospinal fluid and the cauda equina (horse's tail). The cauda equina is composed of the roots of the lower lumbar, sacral, and coccygeal nerves. The lower lumbar approach of inserting a hypodermic needle between the neural arches of the third and fourth lumbar vertebrae into the subarachnoid space

(*spinal puncture or tap*) is used to obtain samples of cerebrospinal fluid. In this procedure, the spinal cord cannot be injured and the occasional nicking of a root by the needle in the cauda equina is of minor consequence. Between the dura and the vertebrae is the epidural space, which is filled with blood vessels and fat. The anesthetic that produces caudal (sacral) anesthesia (as for painless childbirth) is introduced into the epidural space below the second sacral vertebral level, so that it reaches the sacral nerves and avoids the subarachnoid space with its circulating cerebrospinal fluid.

Roots, rami, and plexuses

Each *spinal nerve* has a dorsal root and a ventral root (see Figs. 5-2 and 5-4). The *dorsal, or sensory, root* consists of the sensory or afferent fibers that transmit impulses (input) from sensory receptors in the body to the spinal cord. This root contains a *spinal (sensory dorsal root) ganglion* that is located within the intervertebral foramen. This ganglion contains the cell bodies of the sensory neurons. The *ventral*, or *motor*, *root* consists of the motor or efferent nerve fibers whose cell bodies are located within the gray matter of the spinal cord. The motor fibers transmit impulses (output) from the spinal cord via motor roots and spinal nerves to the muscles and glands of the body.

Recent evidence indicates that afferent (sensory) fibers are also present in the ventral roots of spinal nerves (Coggeshall). Apparently, numerous fine unmyelinated fibers in the ventral roots have their cell bodies in the dorsal root ganglia and not elsewhere (in the cat). In effect, the centrally directed axons of these ganglion cells course distally through the dorsal root to the site where the dorsal and ventral roots meet and then recurve and pass through the ventral root and enter the spinal cord (see Fig. 5-13).

Distal to its emergence through the vertebral column, a spinal nerve divides into four rami (see Fig. 5-4). The large *dorsal ramus (division)* branches into the nerves that innervate the general region and intrinsic muscles of the back. The large *ventral ramus (division)* branches into the nerves and plexuses (in combination with branches of other ventral divisions) that innervate (1) the region and muscles of the body wall

Table 5-2
Innervation of dermatomes by dorsal spinal roots

Dorsal spinal root	Body region innervated*
C2	Occiput
C4	Neck and upper shoulder
T1	Upper thorax and inner side of arm
T4	Nipple zone
T10	Umbilical girdle zone
L1	Inguinal region
L4	Great toe, lateral thigh, and medial leg
S3	Medial thigh
S5	Perianal region

* Dermatome and region to which radicular pain is referred.

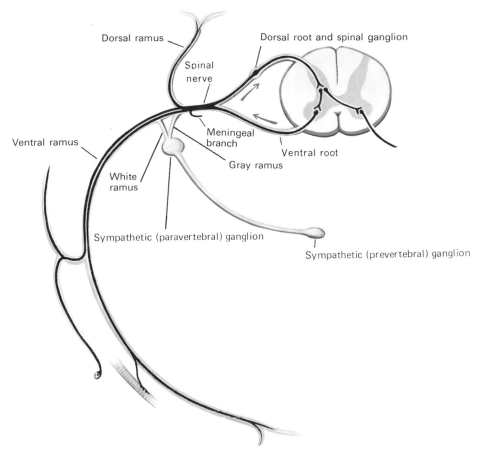

FIGURE 5-4 Diagram of a typical thoracic spinal nerve. The union of the dorsal and ventral roots forms a spinal nerve. The nerve divides into a posterior primary ramus, an anterior primary ramus, a meningeal ramus, and white and gray rami communicantes (see Fig. 6-4 and Chap. 6).

(neck, chest, and abdominal wall), (2) the limbs, and (3) the "perineal" region. The small rami communicantes are connected to the sympathetic trunk. The small recurrent meningeal branches innervate the meningeal membranes and blood vessels of the spinal cord.

The ventral rami of the spinal nerves form *plexuses*, which are located just distal to the sites where the nerves emerge from the intervertebral foramina. These plexuses give rise to peripheral nerves. By convention, C indicates cervical; T, thoracic; L, lumbar; S, sacral; and Co, coccygeal spinal levels or nerves. The *cervical plexus* is derived from the anterior rami of spinal nerves C1 through C4; these innervate the neck and back of the head. The *brachial plexus*, derived

from spinal nerves C5 through T1 or T2, gives rise to the nerves innervating the upper extremity. Except for the contribution of T1 and T2 to the brachial plexus and of T12 to the lumbar plexus, the thoracic nerves (T3 through T11) are simple in their course and distribution; they do not form plexuses. The *lumbar plexus* is derived from spinal levels T12 through L4; the *sacral plexus* from L4 through S4; and the *coccygeal plexus* from spinal nerves S4 through Co. T12 does not always join the lumbar plexus. L4 and S4 contribute branches to both the lumbar and sacral plexuses. The nerves innervating the lower extremity are derived primarily from L2 through S3 of the lumbar and sacral plexuses. Nerves from the upper lumbar levels of the lumbar plexuses innervate the lower trunk above the level of the lower extremity, while nerves from the lower sacral levels of the sacral plexus and from the coccygeal plexus innervate the perineum.

The spinal cord has two enlargements (see Figs. 5-1 and 5-7): the cervical enlargement includes the fifth cervical through the first thoracic cord levels; and the lumbosacral enlargement includes the L2 or L3 through the S3 spinal cord levels. The cervical enlargement contributes the innervation to the upper extremities; the lumbosacral enlargement contributes the innervation to the lower extremities.

The nerve fibers in the spinal nerves include two afferent and two efferent components. The *general somatic afferent fibers* are those sensory components innervating the entire body exclusive of the visceral organs (see Fig. 7-2). The *general visceral afferent fibers* are those sensory components innervating the visceral organs (digestive system, circulatory system) (see Fig. 6-4). The *general somatic efferent fibers* are those motor components innervating the voluntary skeletal (striated) muscles. The *general visceral efferent fibers* are those motor components innervating the involuntary smooth (nonstriated) muscles, cardiac muscle, and glands (see Chap. 6 and Fig. 6-4). All spinal nerve components are in the general categories because they are widely distributed throughout the body.

Dermatomes

Each spinal nerve is distributed to a specific segment or region of the body. The dorsal root of each spinal nerve supplies the sensory innervation to a body segment known as a *dermatome* (see Figs. 5-5 and 5-6). Theoretically there are 31 pairs of dermatomes, one pair for each spinal nerve. Actually there are 30 dermatomes, for the first cervical nerve has either no dorsal roots, or a tiny one; it does not directly innervate a dermatome. The minute dorsal root of the coccygeal nerve joins the fifth sacral nerve. The second dermatome is located in the back of the head behind the ears and upper part of the neck; the third and fourth dermatomes are in the neck; the fifth through eighth cervical and first thoracic dermatomes are in the upper extremity; the second through twelfth thoracic and the first lumbar

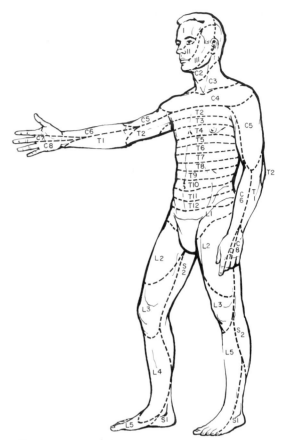

FIGURE 5-5 Segmental innervation of the skin (dermatome). Each dorsal (sensory) spinal root innervates one dermatome. The first cervical nerve usually has no cutaneous distribution. The trigeminal nerve supplies most of the general somatic sensory innervation to the anterior aspect of the head (ophthalmic division V1, maxillary division V2, and mandibular division V3).

dermatomes are in the thoracic and abdominal walls, and the other dermatomes are located in the lower extremity and the gluteal and coccygeal regions (see Table 5-2).

The dermatomes are not exactly distinct and separate segments. There is considerable overlapping between any two adjacent dermatomes. A dermatome will often overlap with about half the dermatome more rostrally located and about half the dermatome more caudally located. As a consequence, if one spinal nerve were completely nonfunctional, no area of complete anesthesia on the skin would be found, for the nerve fibers from the two adjacent dermatomes would pick up the sensory stimuli. On the other hand, if a dorsal root of one spinal nerve is irritated, as in herpes zoster (shingles, a viral infection of a spinal ganglion), the noxious stimuli would be felt subjectively from the entire dermatome, including the overlap. The dermatomal area associated with pain and thermal sense is larger than that associated with the tactile sensations.

Distribution of ventral roots

The ventral root of each spinal nerve is composed of nerve fibers from one spinal segment. These fibers supply somatic motor innervation to several voluntary muscles. The following is a list of representative muscles and spinal segments involved with their innervation (Table 5-3):

1. Biceps brachii muscle (flexes elbow and supinates forearm), by segments C5 and C6
2. Triceps muscle (extends elbow), by C6 through C8
3. Brachialis muscle (flexes elbow), by C6 and C7
4. Intrinsic muscles of the hand, by C8 and T1; wrist tendon reflex, C8 and T1
5. Thoracic musculature, by T1 through T8
6. Abdominal musculature, by T6 through T12
7. Cremasteric reflex, by T12 to L2
8. Quadriceps femoris muscle (knee jerk), by L2 through L4
9. Gastrocnemius muscle (ankle jerk for plantar flexion of foot), by L5 through S2 (see Table 5-3)
10. Plantar reflex, by L5 through S2
11. Anal reflex, by S4 through Co

SIMPLE REFLEX ARC

The circuit known as a *simple reflex arc* includes (see Fig. 2-2) (1) a sensory receptor (e.g., a neuromuscular spindle or a Meissner's corpuscle), (2) a sensory or afferent neuron (a unipolar neuron with cell body in the spinal ganglion) which enters the posterior gray column of the spinal cord, (3) interneurons (association, intercalated, or internuncial neurons) that lie wholly within the gray matter of the spinal cord, (4) a motor or efferent neuron in the anterior (ventral) horn of

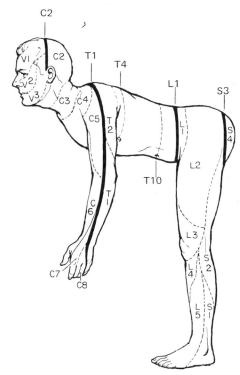

FIGURE 5-6 Dermatomes of the skin. (Refer to Table 5-2.) The trigeminal nerve is represented by the ophthalmic division (V1), maxillary division (V2), and mandibular division (V3). (*Adapted from Haymaker, Bing's Local Diagnosis in Neurological Diseases, The C. V. Mosby Company, St. Louis.*)

the gray matter, and (5) an effector (muscle cell). This three-neuron reflex arc (comprises an afferent neuron, interneuron, and efferent neuron) is typical of a flexor reflex such as the elbow flexing. The simple spinal reflex arcs are actually "abstractions" out of the complex neural circuitry.

Table 5-3
Innervation of voluntary muscles by ventral spinal roots

Ventral spinal root	Muscles innervated
C5–6	Biceps brachii (flexes elbow)
C6–8	Triceps brachii (extends elbow)
T1–8	Thoracic musculature
T6–12	Abdominal musculature
L2–4	Quadriceps femoris (knee jerk, patellar tendon reflex)
L5–S1 or S2	Gastrocnemius [Achilles tendon reflex (ankle jerk)]

Reflexes can be named by the number of neurons in the sequence from receptor to effector. *Monosynaptic reflexes* comprise the sequence of afferent neuron and efferent neuron. *Disynaptic reflexes* comprise the sequence of afferent neuron, interneuron, and efferent neuron. *Polysnaptic reflexes* include the sequence of afferent neuron, several interneurons, and efferent neurons. The afferent limbs of these reflexes include afferent fibers Ia, Ib, II, and III from muscle receptors and afferent fibers II, III, and IV from cutaneous receptors. (See "Classification of Nerve Fibers," page 165).

SENSORY UNIT AND MOTOR UNIT

One sensory neuron, its processes, and its sensory receptors form a *sensory unit*. One sensory unit may terminate peripherally as one process, as the neuron associated with one Pacinian corpuscle. Another unit may terminate in many branches over an area as great as a square millimeter. In functional terms, the spatial region or area from which stimuli can influence the firing of the one neuron is known as the *receptive field* of that neuron. These stimuli should be of adequate intensity and proper quality. The receptive area of a "light-touch neuron" is that area of the skin the touching of which provokes an action potential in that neuron. In brief, some receptive fields may be diffuse and others located precisely in a limited area. Extensive overlapping among receptive fields occurs.

Fine discrimination is characteristic of those regions such as the lips or fingertips where high densities of small receptive fields are present. In contrast, gross discrimination is associated with regions such as the small of the back with large receptive fields. A receptive field is an expression of a small locus of sensory localization; a dermatome or the sensory distribution of a nerve is a large locus of localization.

One motor neuron and the muscle fibers it innervates form a *motor unit*. This comprises the *anterior horn neuron* (sometimes called the *motoneurons*, *alpha motor neuron*, or *lower motor neuron*), its axon, and all terminal branches, motor end plates, innervating muscle fibers. In humans, a motor unit is composed of from 6 to over 2000 muscle fibers. Muscles under delicate control have small motor units; in such muscles the number of muscle fibers in each motor unit is stated to be 13 for the opponens pollicis, 3 to 6 for the extraocular muscles, and 25 for the platysma muscles. The sartorius, rectus femoris, and first dorsal interosseous muscles have motor units, each composed of about 300 muscle fibers. The powerful major limb muscles such as the gastrocnemius has motor units of just over 2000 muscle fibers. The average motor unit may be taken to consist of about 200 muscle fibers. In general, each muscle fiber of human beings is innervated by one or occasionally by two motor end plates. Multiple innervations of some muscle fibers have been reported. The motor end plate is most often located in the middle of a muscle fiber. When the motor neuron is stimulated, all the muscle cells of the motor unit contract. The nerve impulse of a motor fiber results in excitatory activity in the synapse at the motor end plate—hence an *obligatory contraction* is elicited from the stimulation of its innervating nerve fiber. The muscle fibers in each motor unit are not necessarily adjacent but are usually interspersed among muscle fibers of other motor units.

Under certain conditions some motor units may innervate up to 10 times as many muscle fibers as normally. These so-called macromotor units are formed by the addition of more muscle fibers to the normal motor unit through collateral sprouting (Chap. 2). In some cases of poliomyelitis, for example, many, but not all, the motor nerve fibers to a skeletal muscle may degenerate and form neurolemma bands (Chap. 2). In turn, an axon of a normal motor unit regenerates preterminal sprouts, which invade the neurolemma bands of adjacent degenerated axons. These sprouts elongate within the cords until they reinnervate the denervated muscle fibers. With these macromotor units, the muscle regains much lost function. The degree of control over that muscle is less than that over the normally innervated muscle.

The nerve terminals of a trunk fiber of a motor unit do not necessarily innervate adjacent muscle fibers. Rather, the terminals of each unit innervate some but not all of the muscle fibers of many muscle fasicles. Thus, motor units overlap in their distribution.

Small motor units are found in those muscles where precise, delicate, and fine control occurs (extraocular muscles and intrinsic muscles of the hand). Large motor units are found in those muscles where gross actions are generated (postural muscles of the extremities). As a consequence, the force generated by a motor unit is inversely related to the precision of control.

Muscles of the motor units do differ in their susceptibility to fatigue and in the tension generated. At one end of the spectrum are the so-called *slow-twitch motor units* that have a great resistance to fatigue but generate relatively little muscle tension. Each unit can be stimulated to remain active for relatively long periods of time. A twitch is the response of the output of a motor unit following the release of neurotransmitter of a single motor unit. At the other end are the so-called *fast-twist motor units* that fatigue rapidly but generate large peak muscle tension. In a movement motor units are sequentially recruited. By selectively mobilizing varying numbers of small motor units, small motor tensions are generated and can be precisely controlled (Henneman). To increase the total muscle activity in the movement, the large motor units are recruited with the resulting increased increments in muscle tension. More specifically, the slow-twitch motor units are first to be recruited. This is followed by the recruitment of fast-twitch motor units.

Actually three types of mammalian muscle fibers are recognized on the basis of certain structural and functional criteria. There are white fibers and two types of red fibers. (1) *White fibers* are called *fast-twitch glycolytic* ((or *fast-contracting*, *fast-fatiguing*) fibers. They have a high glycogen content, are poorly vascularized, belong to large motor units and are fast-fatiguing. These muscle fibers relax and contract at fast rates. (2) *Some red fibers* are called *fast-twitch, oxidative-glycolytic* (or *fast-contracting, fatigue-resistant*) fibers. They have a high glycogen content, are richly vascularized, belong to intermediate-sized motor units, and fatigue at an intermediate rate. These muscles relax and contract at intermediate rates. (3) Other red fibers are called *slow-twitch oxidative* (or *slow-contracting*) fibers. They have a low glycogen content, are richly vascularized, belong to small motor units and are slow-fatiguing. These muscles relax and contract at slow rates.

ORGANIZATION OF GRAY MATTER AND WHITE MATTER OF SPINAL CORD

The spinal cord is organized as white matter surrounding the butterfly-shaped (Figs. 5-7 and 5-8) gray matter. The white matter consists of both lightly myelinated and unmyelinated fibers oriented parallel to the long axis of the spinal cord; cell bodies are absent. The gray matter consists of cell bodies and many unmyelinated and some lightly myelinated fibers oriented at right angles to the long axis of the spinal cord. A *nucleus* is an anatomically defined group or column of cell bodies within the central nervous system; each has a more or less specific function. A *lamina* is an anatomically defined group or column of cell bodies; 10 laminae are recognized (see Fig. 5-11). A *neuron pool* is a physiologically defined group of functionally similar cell bodies; each cell body tends to funtion together with the others when stimulated. Glial cells and blood vessels are found throughout the entire spinal cord. The rich vascularity and the unmyelinated fibers produce the color of the gray matter, whereas the white myelinated fibers produce the color of the white matter.

The *white matter* in each half of the spinal cord is arranged into three *funiculi* (*columns*): the *posterior funiculus*, located between the posterior median septum and posterior horn; the *lateral funiculus*, located between the posterior and anterior horns; and the *anterior funiculus*, located between the anterior horn and the anterior median fissure (see Fig. 5-9). The funiculi are subdivided into bundles of fibers called tracts or fasciculi, which will be analyzed further on with the pathways. The *gray matter* is subdivided into the posterior horn, the intermediate zone with a lateral horn, and the anterior horn (see Fig. 5-9).

Regional differences are present at various levels of the spinal cord (Figs. 5-7, 5-8). The amount of gray matter at any spinal level is largely related to the richness of the peripheral innervation. Hence the gray matter is largest in the spinal segments of the cervical and lumbosacral enlargements innervating the upper and lower extremities; such large structures require a massive innervation. The thoracic and upper lumbar levels have relatively small amounts of gray matter because they innervate the thoracic and abdominal regions.

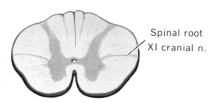

Spinal root
XI cranial n.

High cervical segment

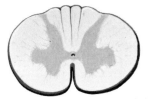

Cervical enlargement segment

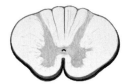

Thoracic segment

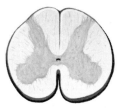

Lumbar segment

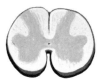

High sacral segment

FIGURE 5-7 Segments of the human spinal cord. The cross-sectional area of the white matter increases as the cord is ascended. The gray matter is larger at the levels innervating the extremities.

The absolute number of nerve fibers in the white matter increases at each successive higher spinal segment. Stated otherwise, the white matter of a spinal level caudal to another level contains fewer fibers. This difference results because (1) additional fibers of the ascending sensory pathways join the white matter at each higher spinal level and (2) fibers of the descending pathways from the brain leave the white matter before terminating in the gray matter at each successive spinal level.

The cell bodies in the gray matter are grouped into clusters of *nuclei* or *laminae*, which extend through the long axis of the spinal cord (see Figs. 5-10 and 5-11). These nuclei and laminae are characterized by microscopic criteria. On the basis of the course of their axons, two types of neurons are recognized: *root neurons* (*cells*) and *column neurons* (*cells*). The cell bodies of the root neurons give rise to the axons which emerge from the spinal cord through the ventral roots; these are neurons with cell bodies in the central nervous system and axons terminating in the periphery outside the central nervous system. They include the alpha and gamma motor neurons of the somatic nervous system and preganglionic neurons of the autonomic nervous system (see Fig. 5-12).

The *column neurons* have axons which terminate within the central nervous system, both in the spinal cord and in the brain. These include (1) *intrasegmental neurons*—those with axons which arborize and terminate within the gray matter of the spinal segment in which the cell body is located; (2) *intersegmental neurons*—those with axons which bifurcate into branches which ascend or descend in the white matter before arborizing and terminating in the gray matter of many spinal segments; (3) *commissural neurons*—those with axons which cross over (decussate) from one side of the spinal cord to the other side before bifurcating, arborizing, and terminating in the gray matter of the same and other spinal segments on the opposite side from the location of the cell bodies; and (4) *suprasegmental neurons*—those with axons which ascend on the same side (ipsilaterally) or decussate and ascend on the opposite side (contralaterally) before terminating in the brain (see Fig. 5-12).

According to the *schema of nuclei,* the gray matter comprises a number of nuclei (see Fig. 5-10). The more important include the postero-marginal nucleus, substantia gelatinosa, and proper sensory nucleus (nucleus proprius) of the posterior horn; the dorsal (thoracic) nucleus of Clarke; the intermediomedial nucleus and intermediolateral nucleus of the zona intermedia;

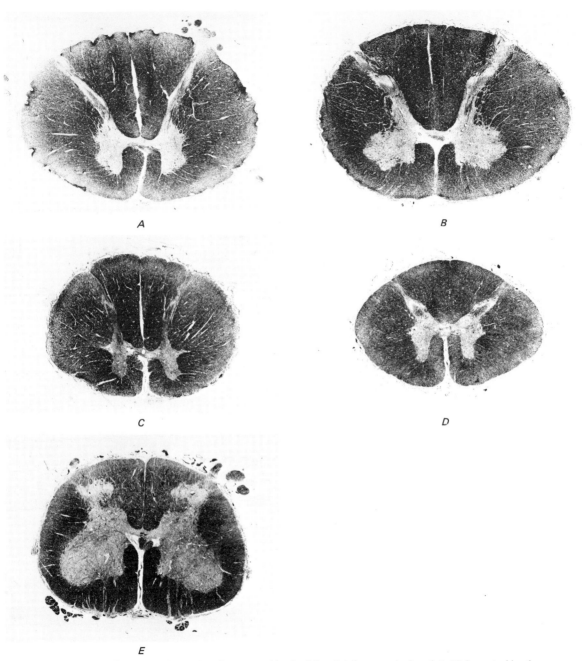

FIGURE 5-8 Representative sections from several levels of the adult human spinal cord. *A.* High cervical level. *B.* Cervical enlargement level. *C.* Midthoracic level. *D.* Low thoracic level. *E.* Lumbar level. All photographs of these Weigert-stained sections are at the same enlargement. (*Courtesy of Dr. Joyce Shriver, Department of Anatomy, Mount Sinai School of Medicine, New York.*)

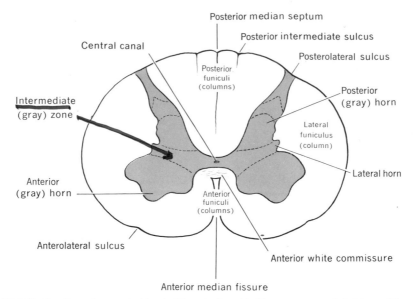

Posterior median septum

Posterior intermediate sulcus

Central canal

Posterolateral sulcus

Posterior funiculi (columns)

Posterior (gray) horn

Intermediate (gray) zone

Lateral funiculus (column)

Anterior (gray) horn

Lateral horn

Anterior funiculi (columns)

Anterolateral sulcus

Anterior white commissure

Anterior median fissure

FIGURE 5-9 Section through a cervical level of the spinal cord to illustrate some subdivisions of the gray matter and white matter. The white matter is composed of three funiculi (columns). The gray matter is divided into two horns and an intermediate zone. The posterior gray commissure and anterior gray commissure are located on either side of the central canal.

and the medial nuclear column and lateral nuclear column of the anterior horn.

According to Rexed's *schema of laminae,* the gray matter comprises 10 laminae (see Fig. 5-11). Laminae I through VI are located in the posterior horn. Lamina VII is coextensive with the zona intermedia, although it may extend into the anterior horn. Laminae VIII and IX are located in the anterior horn, while lamina X is present in the gray matter surrounding the central canal. The laminae and the corresponding nuclei are outlined in Table 5-4.

The *posteromarginal nucleus, substantia gelatinosa,* and *proper sensory nucleus* are found in all levels of the spinal cord. These nuclear columns receive input from the general somatic afferent fibers of the spinal nerves and from some descending fibers from the brain. Just lateral to the posterior horn within the white matter of cervical levels 1 and 2 is a nucleus called the *lateral cervical nucleus.* The *dorsal (thoracic) nucleus of Clarke* is present at all levels from segments T1 through L2 or L3; it is largest in the lower thoracic and lumbar levels. This is the nucleus of origin of the posterior spinocerebellar tract. The *intermediomedial nucleus* probably receives the main input from the general visceral afferent

fibers of the spinal nerves. The *intermediolateral nucleus* is located from T1 through L2 or L3 in the lateral horn. It is the nucleus of origin of most preganglionic sympathetic fibers; some fibers may arise from cell bodies located in the zona intermedia. Cells in the lateral aspect of lamina VII of spinal levels S2 through S4 form the so-called sacral autonomic nuclei. These are the cell bodies of the preganglionic parasympathetic neurons; their axons pass through the

Table 5-4
Laminae and corresponding nuclei

Lamina	Corresponding nucleus
I	Posteromarginal nucleus
II	Substantia gelatinosa
III and IV	Proper sensory nucleus (nucleus proprius)
V	Zone anterior to lamina IV
VI	Zone at base of posterior horn
VII	Zona intermedia (includes intermediomedial nucleus, dorsal nucleus of Clarke, and sacral autonomic nuclei)
VIII	Zone in anterior horn (restricted to medial aspect in cervical and lumbosacral enlargements)
IX	Medial nuclear column and lateral nuclear column

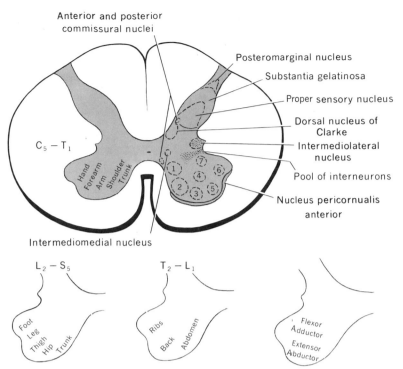

FIGURE 5-10 Composite diagram of a spinal cord segment illustrating the nuclei in the gray matter. The nuclei in the posterior horn and intermediate gray matter are labeled. The intermediolateral nucleus contains visceral efferent neurons (Chap. 6). A neuron pool composed of interneurons is located in the intermediate gray matter. The motor nuclei of alpha and gamma efferent neurons include (1) dorsomedial, (2) ventromedial, (3) anterior, (4) central, (5) ventrolateral, (6) dorsolateral, and (7) retrodorsolateral nuclei. On left of main figure and in the lower diagrams are illustrated the general topographic locations of the muscle groups innervated in the upper extremity (C5 to T1), the lower extremity (L2 to S5), and the thoracoabdominal region (T2 to L1). The nucleus pericornualis anterior is located in the cervical and lumbar segments.

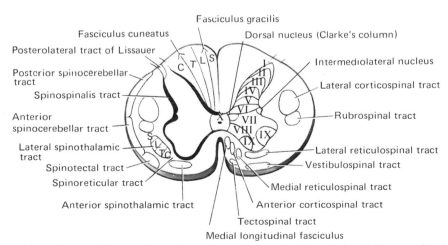

FIGURE 5-11 Composite diagram of Rexed's laminae and the tracts of the spinal cord. The ascending tracts are represented on the left, and the descending tracts on the right. The lamination of the posterior columns and the lateral spinothalamic tract is indicated: C, cervical; T, thoracic; L, lumbar; S, sacral.

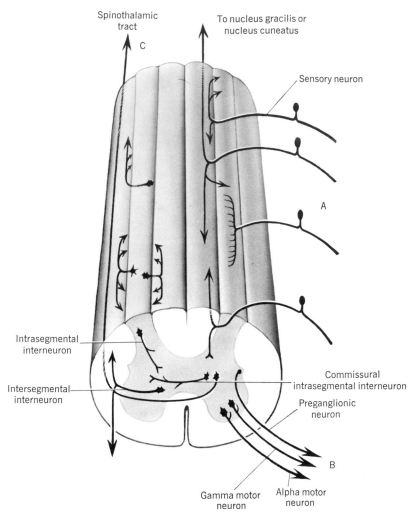

Spinothalamic tract

C

To nucleus gracilis or nucleus cuneatus

Sensory neuron

A

Intrasegmental interneuron

Intersegmental interneuron

Commissural intrasegmental interneuron

Preganglionic neuron

B

Gamma motor neuron

Alpha motor neuron

FIGURE 5-12 Typical neurons found within the spinal cord. The axons of the sensory neurons (*A* on right) enter the posterior horn. The collateral branches may terminate there in the gray matter or may ascend or descend in the white matter (fasciculi proprii or posterolateral fasciculus) and terminate at other spinal levels. The axons of the three types of motor neurons pass via the ventral spinal roots (*B* on lower right). The intrinsic spinal interneurons (mainly on left side of figure) have main branches and collaterals which (1) terminate at once within the gray matter or (2) ascend and descend for many spinal levels before terminating in the gray matter of other spinal levels. Some main axons ascend to the brain (*C*).

ventral roots of the sacral nerves and join the "pelvic nerves." The nuclear columns of the anterior horn contain the cell bodies of the lower motor neurons (alpha and gamma motor neurons) of the general somatic efferent system. The *medial nuclear column* (ventromedial and dorsomedial nuclei) contains the cell bodies of neurons innervating the neck, back, intercostal, and abdominal musculature. Some of the intercostal and abdominal musculature may be innervated

by neurons located in the lateral nuclear column. The medial column is found at all spinal levels. The *lateral nuclear column* (ventrolateral, dorsolateral, and retrodorsal nuclei) contains the cell bodies of neurons innervating the musculature of the extremities. Hence this lateral column is prominent in the *cervical enlargement* (C5 through T1), which innervates the upper extremity, and in the *lumbosacral enlargement* (L2 through S3), which innervates the lower extremity. The nucleus of origin of the neurons innervating the diaphragm via the phrenic nerve is located in the lateral aspect of lamina IX in the midcervical segments, especially C4. The cells of origin of the fibers of the *spinal accessory cranial nucleus* are located in the lateral aspect of lamina IX in spinal levels C1 through C6.

Except for lamina VI, which is absent from levels T4 through L2, all laminae are located at all spinal cord levels. Laminae V and VI are often divided into medial and lateral regions. Lamina VI is well developed in the cervical and lumbosacral enlargements. Lamina VIII is located on the medial aspect of the anterior horn in the cervical and lumbosacral enlargements; in the other levels this lamina extends laterally across the anterior horn ventral to lamina VII.

CLASSIFICATION OF NERVE FIBERS

The peripheral nerves and their spinal roots are a composite of populations of different types of fibers. On the basis of several criteria, the nerve fibers of the peripheral nervous system are classified by three different systems. In the *general classification* the fiber types are designated by capital letters (A, B, and C). In the *dorsal root afferent fiber classification* the fibers are designated by Roman numerals (I, II, III, and IV). In the *ventral root efferent fiber classification* the fibers are designated by Greek letters (α, β, and γ). All systems are used.

General classification (Table 5-5)

The range of fiber size and velocity is the criterion upon which this system is based. Conduction velocities are directly related to the diameter of the fiber and to the length of the internode; the larger these dimensions are, the greater the speed of conduction. In the medium to large fibers, the *speed of conduction* in meters per second (m/s) is roughly equal to the diameter of the fiber in micrometers (including myelin sheath) times the conversion factor 6. The conversion factor for fine fibers is 4. Thus a fiber with a diameter of 22 μm should conduct at speeds of 132 m/s. These highest velocities are at about 200 miles per hour, or a little less than one-third the speed of sound.

The *A fibers* are the myelinated somatic afferent and somatic efferent nerve fibers. This group includes those fibers which transmit impulses from such afferent endings as Meissner's corpuscles, Pacinian corpuscles, neuromuscular spindles, and Golgi neurotendinous endings and impulses to the efferent motor end plates.

The *A group* is further divided into four subgroups: alpha (α), beta (β), gamma (γ), and delta (δ) neurons. These range from the alpha neurons, which have the most heavily myelinated axons with the highest conduction velocities, to the delta neurons, which have lightly myelinated fibers with the slowest conduction velocities of the A group.

The *B fibers* are myelinated efferent preganglionic fibers of the autonomic nervous system. These fibers are up to 3 μm in diameter and conduct at speeds of from 3 to 15 m/s.

The *C fibers* are unmyelinated fibers including (1) the postganglionic sympathetic axons of the autonomic nervous system and (2) the unmyelinated afferent fibers of the peripheral nerves and dorsal roots. These fibers are probably associated with the entire spectrum of sensory modalities, as are the A fibers. The postganglionic sympathetic C fibers range from 0.3 to

Table 5-5
Classification of nerve fibers in peripheral nerves

Group	Diameter,* μm	Conduction velocity, m/s	Role
A	1–20 myelinated α, β, γ, δ	5–120	Afferent fibers for pain, temperature, touch, pressure, and vibration; somatic efferent fibers
B	1–3 myelinated	3–15	Visceral afferent fibers; preganglionic visceral efferent fibers
C	0.3–1.3 unmyelinated	0.7–2.3	Afferent fibers for pain and temperature; postganglionic visceral efferent fibers

Including myelin sheath when present.

1.3 μm in diameter and have conduction speeds of from 0.7 to 2.3 m/s. The afferent C fibers range from 0.4 to 1.2 μm in diameter and have conduction speeds of from 0.6 to 2.0 m/s. The afferent C fibers commence as free nerve endings.

Dorsal root classification

All sensory input to the spinal cord enters via nerve fibers of the dorsal roots. These afferent fibers have been classified into groups I, II, III, and IV. As compared with the general classification, groups I and II correspond to A group, alpha subgroup; group II corresponds to A group, delta subgroup; and group IV corresponds to C group.

Group Ia fibers arborize peripherally as the primary sensory endings (annulospinal endings) on the intrafusal fibers of the neuromuscular spindles. *Group Ib fibers* terminate peripherally as the Golgi tendon organs (GTO). Group I fibers range approximately from 12 to 20 (average 16) μm in diameter, with conduction velocities of 70 to 120 m/s (see Fig. 2-20).

Group II fibers are associated with such peripheral nerve endings as the secondary sensory endings (flower spray endings) of the neuromuscular spindle, and with encapsulated receptors such as the cutaneous touch-pressure receptors (Merkel's and Meissner's corpuscles), skin and joint receptors (Pacinian corpuscles), dermal receptors (Ruffini's corpuscles), and some joint receptors (laminated paciniform corpuscle). The group II fibers range from approximately 5 to 14 (average 8) μm in diameter, with conduction velocities of from 30 to 70 m/s (see Fig. 2-19).

Group III and Group IV fibers terminate as nonencapsulated (free) nerve endings; these include the hair receptor endings in the integument and the touch, pressure, and pain-free nerve endings in the skin and blood vessels. The group III fibers range from approximately 2 to 7 μm in diameter, with conduction velocities of 12 to 30 m/s. The group IV fibers range from approximately 0.5 to 1 μm in diameter, with velocities of 0.5 to 2 m/s (see Fig. 2-19).

The terms I, II, III, and IV are usually used in the anatomic sense. The designations Ia, Ib, and secondary spindle group II are used in the physiologic sense. Group I are thickly myelinated, group II are medium myelinated, group III are finely myelinated, and group IV are unmyelinated fibers.

Ventral root classification

Three types of efferent (motor) fibers emerge from the spinal cord and brainstem. The *thickly myelinated α (alpha) fibers* from the alpha motor neurons of somatic motor nuclei terminate as the motor end plates of the extrafusal muscles. The fibers range from 10 to 20 μm in diameter and have conduction velocities of from 15 to 120 m/s. The *finely myelinated γ (gamma) fibers* from the gamma motor neurons of the spinal cord and brainstem are of two types; one type terminates as discrete motor end plates, and the other type terminates as a fine network ("trail" endings) on the intrafusal muscle fibers of the neuromuscular spindles. These gamma fibers range from 2 to 10 μm in diameter, with conduction velocities of from 10 to 45 m/s. The *preganglionic autonomic myelinated fibers (group B fibers)* are less than 3 μm in diameter with velocities of 3 to 15 m/s. The β (beta) fibers are few in number; these fibers innervate both extrafusal and intrafusal fibers (see Fig. 2-20).

GENERAL ASPECTS OF AFFERENT INPUT AND EFFERENT OUTPUT

Classifications of afferent (sensory) input (Table 5-6)

The streams of impulses conveyed by the peripheral nerves from both the external and internal environments are the sources of the information fed into the central nervous system. The number of senses exceeds the proverbial five sensations of touch, sight, sound, smell, and taste. The several classifications outlined below point up various aspects of afferent, or sensory, input. None is wholly satisfactory.

Subjectively, afferent stimuli may produce either unconscious or conscious sensations. The unconscious "sensations" are ultimately expressed in such varied activities as breathing, muscle coordination, and digestion. The conscious sensations encompass a wide spectrum such as pain, sight, and well-being.

Table 5-6
Classification of sensory receptors
(probable functional roles)

I. Receptors of general sensibility (exteroceptive)
   A. Endings in epidermis
      1. Free nerve endings (tactile, pain, thermal sense)
      2. Terminal disks of Merkel (tactile)
      3. Nerve (peritrichial) endings in hair follicle (tactile, movement detector)
   B. Endings in connective tissues (skin and connective tissue throughout body)
      1. Free nerve endings (pain, thermal sense)
      2. Encapsulated nerve endings
         a. End bulbs of Ruffini (touch-pressure, position sense, kinesthesia)
         b. Corpuscles of Meissner (tactile, flutter sense)
         c. Corpuscles of Pacini (vibratory sense, touch-pressure)
   C. Endings in muscles, tendons, and joints (proprioceptive)
      1. Neuromuscular spindles (stretch receptors)
      2. Golgi tendon organs, neurotendinous endings (tension receptors)
      3. End bulbs of Ruffini in joint capsule (touch-pressure, position sense, kinesthesia)
      4. Corpuscles of Pacini (touch-pressure, vibratory sense, kinesthesia)
      5. Free nerve endings (pain)
II. Receptors of special senses
   A. Bipolar neurons of olfactory mucosa (olfaction)
   B. Taste buds (gustatory sense)
   C. Rods and cones in retina (vision)
   D. Hair cells in spiral organ of Corti (audition)
   E. Hair cells in semicircular canals, saccule, and utricle (equilibrium, vestibular sense)
III. Special receptors in viscera (interoceptive)
   A. Pressoreceptors in carotid sinus and aortic arch (monitor arterial pressure)
   B. Chemoreceptors in carotid and aortic bodies and in or on surface of medulla (monitor arterial oxygen and carbon dioxide levels)
   C. Chemoreceptors probably located in supraoptic nucleus of hypothalamus (monitor osmolarity of blood)
   D. Free nerve endings in viscera (pain, fullness)
   E. Receptors in lungs (respiratory and cough reflexes)

The distribution of the sensors is the basis of a widely used classification. The *general afferent receptors* have a widespread distribution over the body and include receptors that result in such sensations as pain, touch, visceral sense, and thermal appreciation, and in unconscious responses such as the reflexes. The *special afferent receptors* are associated with highly special-ized senses and are concentrated in small areas of the body. They include the receptors for such sensations as smell, sight, hearing, and taste. In humans, they are located in the head and are conveyed only by cranial nerves.

The location of the sensors is used as the basis of the classification of afferent input: The *exteroceptive* (cutaneous or superficial) *modalities* are sensed by those receptors which are located in the skin or its derivatives and which respond mainly to external agents and changes in the external environment. Exteroceptive sensations include the classic four cutaneous sensations of pain, warmth, cold, and light touch (tactile sense). Modalities associated with the position and movements of the body and sensed by receptors located deep in the body tissues are called *proprioceptive* by anatomists and physiologists, *kinesthetic* by experimental psychologists, or *deep sensibilities* (all are synonyms). They include such conscious senses as the appreciation of movement or of position of the body and limbs; the judging of weight, shape, and form; and the feeling of vibratory sense (as ascertained by a tuning fork applied to a joint), deep pain, and pressure. The kinesthetic sense is generally limited to the appreciation of movement and position of the body and limbs. The *interoceptive* or *visceral* senses have a role in the visceral activities of digestion, circulation, and others, including such sensations as fullness of the stomach or bladder, pain from excessive distention, and cramps from muscle spasms. These visceral senses are poorly localized and diffuse. Nerve fibers associated with the exteroceptive and propioceptive senses are known as general somatic afferent fibers; those associated with the interoceptive senses are known as general visceral afferent fibers. "Somatic" refers to the body wall and limbs; "visceral" refers to the "vital" organ systems, including the circulatory, digestive, respiratory, and excretory systems.

The terms *protopathic sensations* and *epicritic sensations* have special usages. The protopathic sensations are the poorly localized modalities such as crude touch, crude temperature, and awareness of pain; they are considered to be phylogenetically old. The epicritic sensations are the precise modalities, such as fine temperature and touch discrimination, and are considered to be phylogenetically new. For example, diffuse, dull, nagging pain is protopathic, while sharp, localized pain is epicritic.

Role of peripheral sensory receptors

Our contact with the world—both the internal and external environments—is through our receptors. The relation of the receptors to the subjective senses is controversial. The wide range of subjective expressions includes the sensations of pain, touch, warmth, cold, itching, wetness, tickling, malaise, well-being, and position appreciation. Each of these sensations has many variations, e.g., sharp pain, burning pain, and dull pain. Even the primary sensory modalities of pain, warmth, cold, and touch are actually defined in abstract philosophical terms.

The doctrine of specific nerve energies (specificity theory) implies that the primary modalities are subserved by morphologically specific nerve endings: pain by free nerve endings, light touch by Merkel's disks and flutter sense by Meissner's corpuscles, and vibratory and pressure sense by Pacinian corpuscles. The doctrine states that each sensation is dependent on (1) the nature of the stimulus and (2) the nerve endings stimulated. Each *receptor* may be characterized by its adequate stimulus, which is that form of energy to which the receptor is most sensitive.

Evidence is available that such a simplified correlation between structure and function is not universal. The concept of a specific nerve fiber for each sense has been supplanted by the *pattern theory of sensation,* which implies that groups of nerve endings, each associated with different nerve fibers, form a complex or "spot." Such a group of endings constitutes a cold spot, a warm spot, or a touch spot. A specific stimulus evokes a stream of nerve impulses which are dispersed spatially and temporally and which are conveyed by the various fibers innervating the spot. It is theoretically possible for such sensations as pain, itch, and tingle to arise from the same complex of endings stimulated in different ways and combinations. The peripheral spots are primarily initiators of a train of impulses that may reach and activate these brain centers. The interplay of various combinations of impulses is basic to the intricacy of the input to the central nervous system. Actually, conscious sensations are primarily an expression of the complex interactions in the centers of the brain.

The term *sensory* is used synonymously with *afferent* and does not necessarily imply conscious sensation.

Afferent (sensory) input

The *dorsal roots* are composed of sensory neurons conveying input to the spinal cord. Each of these neurons is a pseudounipolar neuron with its cell body in the spinal (dorsal root) ganglion. Before entering the spinal cord many dorsal root fibers branch (Langford and Coggeshall) and then the fibers segregate into a medial bundle and a lateral bundle. The *medial bundle* is composed of relatively thick myelinated fibers. The myelinated fibers pass through the posterior funiculus adjacent to the gray matter and medial portions of laminae II, III, and IV of the posterior horn. The main fibers branch into collaterals which (1) may extend to, and terminate in, the gray matter at the spinal level of entrance, (2) may ascend or descend within the posterior columns and terminate in the gray matter of other spinal segments, and (3) may ascend to terminate in some nuclei of the medulla (see Figs. 5-12 and 5-13). Many fibers recurve in lamina IV and extend back into laminae II, III, and IV. Many fibers terminate in the medial and central regions of laminae V, VI, and VII, especially in the dorsal nucleus of Clarke and the intermediomedial nucleus (see Fig. 5-17). Other branches terminate (1) in lamina VIII and medial lamina IX and (2) in lateral lamina IX, respectively.

The *lateral bundle,* composed of finely myelinated and unmyelinated fibers, passes into the posterolateral tract of Lissauer, where each fiber bifurcates into an ascending branch, which extends rostrally for from one to three spinal segments, and a descending branch, which extends caudally for a segment or so (see Fig. 5-17). Collaterals from these branches terminate largely in lamina I and to a lesser degree in laminae II and III. In general, the terminal fibers are distributed primarily to the laminae at the segmental level of entrance and to the same laminae, but in lesser numbers, in the segmental levels just above and below the level of entrance (see Fig. 5-13). The intermediomedial nucleus receives direct input from dorsal root fibers; this nucleus

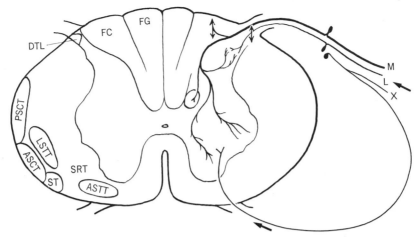

FIGURE 5-13 Schema illustrating (1) the course and termination of dorsal root fibers within the spinal cord (right half of figure) and (2) the major ascending tracts of the spinal cord (left half of figure). Note the sensory fiber (X) with cell body in dorsal root ganglion and central process passing through ventral root. The lateral bundle (L) of lightly myelinated fibers passes into the dorsolateral tract of Lissauer (DTL), and into laminae I, II, and III. The medial bundle (M) of heavily myelinated fibers passes into the posterior column and to many laminae including the anterior horn. The bifurcation of fibers into ascending and descending branches forms the dorsolateral tract and posterior column. The ascending tracts include the fasciculus gracilis (FG), fasciculus cuneatus (FC), posterior spinocerebellar tract (PSCT), anterior spinocerebellar tract (ASCT), anterior spinothalamic tract (ASTT), lateral spinothalamic tract (LSTT), spinotectal tract (ST), and spinoreticular tract (SRT). (*From Noback and Harting, Spinal Cord, S. Karger, Publisher, Basel, 1971.*)

may be the terminal nucleus for visceral afferent fibers. On the other hand, the intermediolateral nucleus does not receive any direct input from dorsal root fibers; this is the nucleus of origin of preganglionic sympathetic neurons (Chap. 6).

Efferent (motor) output

The integrated activity of the central nervous system can be expressed ultimately *only* in terms of the contraction of muscle fibers and the secretion of glands. Through these effectors, the organism responds to internal stimuli and to influences from the external environment. The voluntary (striated) muscles are innervated by the general somatic efferent neurons. These neurons have their cell bodies in the anterior horn of the spinal cord (Fig. 5-12). The large alpha efferent neurons (lower motor neurons) innervate the muscle fibers proper; the small gamma efferent neurons innervate the small muscle fibers of the neuromuscular spindle sensory endings. The involuntary (smooth) muscles, cardiac muscle, and glands are innervated by the general visceral efferent neurons of the autonomic nervous system (Chap. 6).

General aspects of the ascending pathways from the spinal cord to the brain

Environmental energies from both inside and outside the body stimulate sensory receptors, which are located throughout the organism. Following the transduction of these energies at the receptors, coded information is transmitted as nerve impulse patterns (action potentials) via fibers in the spinal nerves to nuclei within the central nervous system for neural processing. Some inputs may be relayed via ascending sensory pathways consisting of groups of nerve fibers (*tracts*) linking *processing centers* (*nuclei*) until information eventually reaches the higher centers in the brain (e.g., the cerebral cortex or cerebellar cortex).

Basic pathways In a general way, the ascending pathway systems of the spinal cord which terminate in the cerebral cortex or cerebellar cortex may be subdivided into *three basic tract systems: anterolateral system, posterior column–medial lemniscal system,* and *spinocerebellar system.* The *anterolateral system,* so called because its compo-

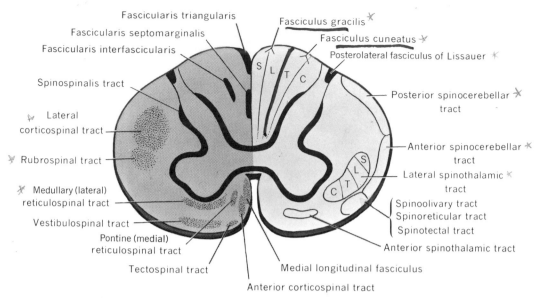

FIGURE 5-14 The spinal cord tracts. The ascending tracts are represented as plain outlines on the right, the descending tracts as stippled outlines on the left, and the intrinsic spinal tracts (composed of descending and/or ascending fibers) as solid outlines. The representation of the tracts is arbitrarily drawn. The lamination of the posterior columns and lateral spinothalamic tracts is indicated (C, cervical; T, thoracic; L, lumbar; S, sacral).

nents ascend through the anterolateral part of the spinal cord, comprises several tracts: (1) lateral spinothalamic tract, (2) anterior spinothalamic tract, (3) indirect spinoreticulothalamic pathway, and (4) the spinotectal tract. The *posterior column–medial lemniscal system* includes the posterior column—medial lemniscal pathway and, in addition, the spinocervicothalamic (spinocervicolemniscal) pathway. The *spinocerebellar system* includes the anterior and posterior spinocerebellar tracts, the cuneocerebellar tract, and the rostral spinocerebellar tract. The first two systems ascend to the cerebral cortex while the third ascends to the cerebellar cortex.

Physiologically, many major ascending pathways are organized in *labeled lines* commencing peripherally in receptors specialized to sense specific environmental energies. Receptors may be specialized neuroepithelial cells (hair cells in the cochlea) or terminal endings of axons (free nerve endings). Modern evidence supports the reality of receptor specificity. The concept of labeled lines is an outgrowth of the doctrine of specific nerve energies; it implies that the message from a receptor or group of similar receptors is conveyed by a sequence of neurons to an

identifiable locus in the higher levels of the brain. Each labeled line (*private line*) within a pathway is involved with a specific class of receptors resulting in a particular sensation. In this concept a peripheral receptor and its sensory nerve are modality-specific, with each responding to one mode of stimulation or sensory quality. The labeled lines are spatially organized within the pathway, so that only minimal crosstalk occurs, if any. This spatial localization within a pathway can take the form of a somatotopic (topographical) organization. This means that a specific route within each pathway is associated with a specific locus in the body.

It must be understood that the spinal cord per se is not primarily concerned with sensations that are associated with consciousness. Rather, the spinal cord is the region of the central nervous system concerned with reflex responses. Sensations and awareness are realized in the higher levels of the brain.

The ascending pathways contain processing centers—called *relay nuclei*—such as the nucleus cuneatus and ventral posterior nucleus of the thalamus. These relay nuclei contain two types of neurons: (1) *relay, principal,* or *transmis-*

sion cells and (2) *local circuit neurons* (*interneurons or intercalated neurons*). Relay cells are Golgi type I neurons with long axons projecting from one nucleus to another nucleus. The local circuit neurons are either *Golgi type II cells* with axons arborizing in the vicinity of the cell body and its dendritic tree or *modified Golgi type II cells* with an axonal spread that extends beyond the confines of the dendritic tree. Some examples of the latter cells are Renshaw cells of the anterior horn and the gelatinosa cells of the posterior horn of the spinal cord (Chap. 5). The processing of the incoming afferent message takes place in the nucleus. This processing utilized (1) feedforward inhibitory circuits, (2) feedback inhibitory circuits, and (3) reflected feedback circuits (see Figs. 3-13, 3-14, and 3-15).

The relay cells in a nucleus are stimulated by influences derived by convergence and divergence from the receptive fields in the periphery. Anatomically it is the receptive field that projects directly or indirectly through local circuit neurons to the relay neuron. Physiologically, it is the receptive field that conveys inputs that will either increase or decrease the firing of the relay neuron.

The fates of the sensory inputs into the central nervous system can vary; they may be phased out, incorporated into one or more of a variety of reflex activities, or embedded in either the conscious or subconscious memory for future use. At the present time, some elements are known concerning some of the mechanisms by which the nervous system rejects or makes use of the barrage of seemingly meaningless "noise" conveyed from the receptors and how the neuronal organization is set up to extract meaningful signals from this noise. Sensory stimuli can be modulated by actions at the periphery such as closing one's eyes or changing the size of pupils in response to the degree of light intensity.

In addition, processing mechanisms exist to preserve and to sharpen the integrity of the channels within a major pathway. For example, the channels conveying information from several distinguishable tactile spots on the ball of the thumb are maintained as separate channels in order to retain the identities of these tactile spots until these separate channels reach the cerebral cortical level. The processing by inhibitory activity acts to prevent smearing overlap that would obscure or destroy the separateness of the channels.

Pain and temperature pathway; anterolateral system
(Figs. 5-15 and 5-16)

Modalities of pain and temperature The pathways concerned with the modalities of pain and thermal senses take parallel courses through the nervous system. Pain is a warning signal alerting the organism. It is inherently a subjective experience with unpleasant qualities, psychologically determined. Emotional and cultural attitudes color its intensity. The Indian fakir and the professional boxer cultivate an emotional detachment which enables them to disregard pain, while a slightly injured child heightens the feeling. On the one hand, pain has an essential role in our survival, but, on the other hand, it can be, when intractable or accompanied by fear, our enemy.

Pain can be initiated in several ways—by mechanical, thermal, electrical, and chemical stimuli. Some types of pain include fast-conducted, sharp, prickling pain; slowly conducted, burning pain; and deep, aching pain (in joints, tendons, and viscera). Some tissues are more likely to exhibit pain than others. A needle inserted into the skin evokes intense pain, while one probed into a muscle produces little pain. An arterial puncture is painful; a venous puncture (venipuncture) is almost painless. The distention of the ureters by a kidney stone produces what is probably the most excruciating of pains. Distention of hollow viscera and muscle spasms (cramps) are painful, yet burning or cutting the intestines evokes scarcely any painful sensation. The tenderness of an inflammation is related to the turgor of the tissues. Slight mechanical traction on the abdominal mesenteries evokes intense pain.

Pain perception may be subdivided into two phases: initial sensation and reaction following that sensation. Soldiers with potentially painful wounds inflicted during intense battle conditions usually experienced minimal pain. To them, the traumatic wounds were secondary to

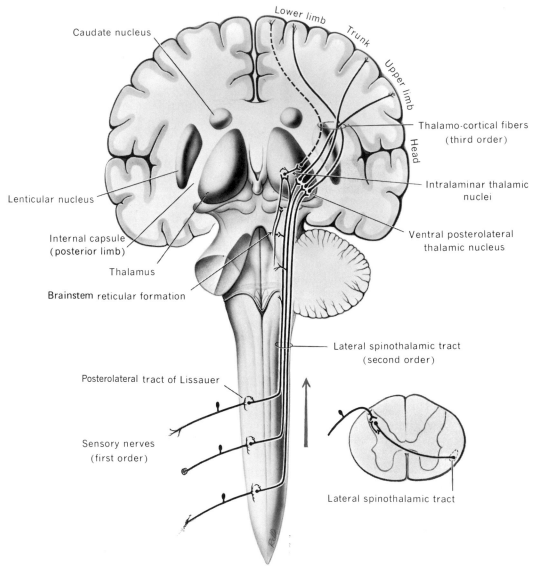

FIGURE 5-15 The spinothalamic pathways. The direct spinothalamic pathway comprises (1) neurons of the first order with cell bodies in the spinal ganglia, (2) neurons of the second order with cell bodies in the posterior horns and with axons that decussate and ascend as the lateral spinothalamic tract to the thalamus, and (3) neurons of the third order with cell bodies in the thalamus and with axons that project to the cerebral cortex.

The indirect spinothalamic pathway is composed of (1) neurons of the first order, (2) sequence of several neurons of the second order that project through the brainstem reticular formation to the intralaminar thalamic nuclei, and (3) neurons of the third order with cell bodies in the thalamus and with axons that project to the cerebral cortex (the latter is represented in broken line because course is not precisely known). Note interneurons in the relay nuclei (see Fig. 3-15).

the knowledge that their war was over. When out of danger at the base hospital or hospital ship, they complained of the severe pain and demanded morphine. This is a demonstration of the powerful modulatory effects of the brain on pain processing through the reflected feedback circuits.

No sensations are evoked when the exposed human brain is cut or cauterized; this is because the brain proper has no sensory receptors.

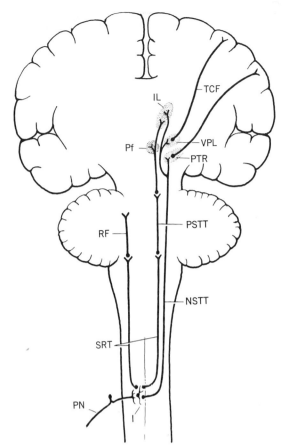

FIGURE 5-16 The spinothalamic pathways. The ascending tracts of the spinothalamic system consist of (1) the lateral spinothalamic tract (neospinothalamic tract, NSTT), (2) the spinoreticulothalamic pathway (paleospinothalamic tract, PSTT), and (3) the anterior spinothalamic tract. Interneurons (I) stand between central terminations of the peripheral nerves (PN) and the ascending tracts, including the spinoreticular tract (SRT) and lateral spinothalamic tract. [The paleospinothalamic tract includes interneurons located in the brainstem reticular formation (RF).] The thalamic nuclei, integrated within the spinothalamic pathways, include the intralaminar nuclei (IL), parafascicular nucleus (Pf), posterior thalamic region (PTR), and ventral posterior lateral nucleus (VPL). Influences from the thalamus are projected by thalamocortical fibers (TCF). (*From Noback and Harting, Spinal Cord, S. Karger, Publisher, Basel.*)

Cold spots and *warm spots* cover the body, with the cold spots being more numerous. For example, the lips have both warm and cold spots, while the tongue is only slightly sensitive to warmth. The rationale of placing a cool wet towel on the forehead on a hot day is valid, because the forehead is more sensitive to cold than

to warmth. The warm receptors respond to normal body temperature. In a warm environment the warm receptors are active, whereas in a cold environment they are turned off. Cold receptors are turned on in a cold environment and off in a warm environment. The identity of specific thermal receptors is not resolved.

Input to the spinal cord

Nociceptors (noxious receptors) are classified into three types; all are probably free nerve endings. Their threshold to natural stimuli is high in comparison to other receptors in the same tissue. In turn, the pain inputs are transmitted via *A delta and C afferent fibers* to the dorsal horn of the spinal cord (see Fig. 5-17). The types comprise (1) receptors responding to mechanical stimuli following cutaneous distortion that does not damage the skin (A delta fibers), (2) receptors responding to intense thermal and mechanical stimuli that are damaging to the skin (A delta fibers), and (3) polymodal receptors responding to a combination of mechanical and thermal stimuli including noxious heat, irritant chemicals applied to the skin, and sunburn inflammation (C fibers). In humans, a great majority of the unmyelinated C fibers are concerned with nociception. This relation of pain with specific peripheral receptors and nerve fibers is consistent with the specificity theory.

It is likely that such chemical substances as histamine, bradykinin, acidity of the tissues, and potassium released by tissue cells are intermediaries that excite nociceptive endings in humans. In this sense, pain receptors may be chemoreceptors. The same receptor and nerve fiber may give rise to different subjective sensations. For example, slight passive distention of the stomach or urinary bladder results in the feeling of fullness, greater distention produces marked discomfort, and extreme distention or contraction gives the feeling of intense pain and cramps.

The A delta afferents convey information that is felt as localized, sharp, stabbing pain which is rapidly evoked (first flush) but soon disappears. The C afferents are involved in less localized, dull, diffuse pain that persists and may have an aching or itching quality. All types of pain can evoke reflex activities.

The large-diameter dorsal root afferents (including the A delta fibers) course along the medial aspect of the posterior horn and toward its base; they then reverse direction and, within the horn, pass through laminae IV and V, giving off collaterals before terminating in laminae II and III (see Fig. 5-17). These fibers end as radially oriented terminal bushes in the gelatinosa glomeruli (see later discussion). The fine-diameter dorsal root afferents enter through the lateral portion of the root and then bifurcate to ascend and to descend one or two spinal levels in the dorsolateral tract of Lissauer. Collaterals from Lissauer's tract extend as terminals in laminae I, II, and III (see Fig. 5-17).

The posterior horn has a most complex circuitry which has not been fully explained. Its diverse neuronal populations receiving input from a large number of sources provide a matrix for the multifaceted synaptic connections of the posterior horn neurons which are the critical links between the periphery and the higher neural centers.

Many neurons are segregated by modalities—some responsive to tactile stimuli, some to pain stimuli, some to thermal stimuli applied to peripheral receptors. Different neurons may respond to different portions of the spectrum from noxious to nonnoxious stimuli. Some neurons respond to stimuli from somatic sources (cutaneous or muscle) and others only to those from visceral sources. Certain neurons respond to convergent input from both somatic and visceral stimulation. These cells where viscerosomatic convergence takes place may be significant in the phenomenon of referred pain (see later discussion). Some neurons respond optimally to small receptive fields and others to large receptive fields.

Posterolateral tract of Lissauer and laminae of the posterior horn

Lissauer's tract is composed of fine axonal fibers from two sources: (1) the dorsal root and (2) gelantinosa cells of laminae II and III. The dorsal root fibers bifurcate in the tract, ascend and descend one or two segmental levels, and send collaterals to laminae I, II, and III (see Fig. 5-7). The axons of the gelatinosa cells pass to Lissauer's tract, bifurcate, and ascend and descend as many as five or six spinal levels and send collaterals to laminae I, II, and III. These axons of gelatinosa cells are feedback fibers to the substantia gelatinosa. Lissauer's tract as a structural and functional entity is continuous at the second cervical level to the spinal tract of the trigeminal nerve (Chaps. 7 and 8).

Lamina I The characteristic *marginal or pericornual neurons* are large cells with their processes largely oriented parallel to the dorsal surface of the spinal cord and spilling over slightly into the substantia gelatinosa (Ralston and Ralston). The axons of these cells project (1) through the anterior commissure to the lateral spinothalamic tract and (2) via the spinospinalis tract to other segmental levels (see Fig. 5-17). Local circuit neurons are present. Lamina I receives input from collaterals of C fibers and from axons of gelatinosa cells.

Laminae II (substantia gelatinosa) The substantia gelatinosa (laminae II) can be conceptually organized around its local circuit neuron called the *gelatinosa cell*. This cell is bipolar by virtue of two dendritic tufts radially oriented parallel to the central axis of the dorsal horn (see Fig. 5-17). The axons of these cells arise from dendrites and meander for long distances in tortuous courses to the spinospinalis tract and Lissauer's tract, where each axon bifurcates and ascends and descends for as many as five or six spinal levels. Along their course each gives off collaterals to lamina I and the substantia gelatinosa. These axons are the routes for intragelatinosa communication.

The dendritic and axonal processes of the gelatinosa cells are integral structures of the *gelatinosa glomeruli*, where the interaction with the axonal and dendritic processes of other cell types occurs. The components of a *glomerulus* are schematically presented in Fig. 5-17. It is probably composed of (1) dendritic branches of gelatinosa cells and relay cells of laminae III, IV, and V and (2) axonal endings of myelinated (presumably A delta) fibers from the medial bundle, C fibers from the lateral bundle, and axon terminals of gelatinosa cells from the same and other spinal segments. The presence of axodendritic, axoaxonic, dendrodendritic, and dendroaxonic synapses within a glomerulus are indicative of

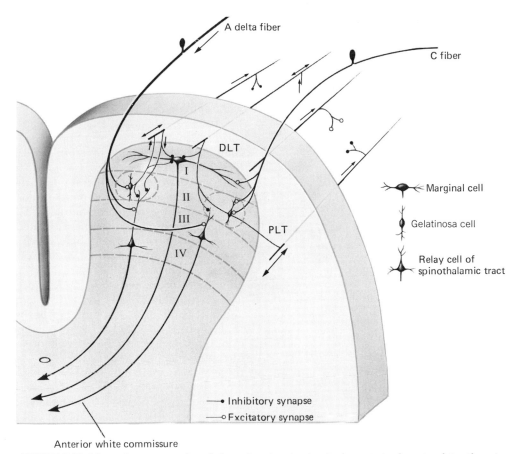

A delta fiber

C fiber

DLT

I

II

III

IV

PLT

Marginal cell

Gelatinosa cell

Relay cell of
spinothalamic tract

→ Inhibitory synapse
—o Excitatory synapse

Anterior white commissure

FIGURE 5-17 Schematic representation of the nociceptive circuitry in the posterior horn involving the primary afferents (A delta and C fibers), intrinsic interneurons (marginal and gelatinosa cells) and relay neurons of the spinothalamic tract. (1) A high threshold nociceptive C fiber from the dorsal root passes through the lateral bundle, its ascending and descending fibers pass through the dorsolateral tract of Lissauer (DLT), and their collaterals convey excitatory influences to marginal and gelatinosa cells in several spinal levels. (2) A low threshold nociceptive A delta afferent from the dorsal root passes through the medial bundle and, through collaterals, conveys excitatory influences to the gelatinosa and relay spinothalamic neurons. (3) A marginal cell of lamina I receives excitatory input from C fibers and inhibitory input from gelatinosa cells of many spinal levels and projects output via the anterior white commissure to the lateral spinothalamic tract. (4) A gelatinosa cell is incorporated into a glomerulus (circled in lamina II; see text). These cells receive excitatory input from A delta and C fibers and project inhibitory influences via the posterolateral (PLT) and dorsolateral (DLT) tracts for about five and six spinal levels up and down to synapse with marginal and relay cells of the spinothalamic tract. (5) The relay cells of the spinothalamic tract receive excitatory input from the A delta afferents and inhibitory input from the gelatinosa cells and project output via the spinothalamic tract. The numerals I through IV indicate Rexed laminae.

the complexity of the processing that occurs. The axons of a few relay cells project via the spinothalamic tracts to the thalamus (see Fig. 5-17).

Evidence indicates that some of the small neurons within the substantia gelatinosa contain somatostatin, a polypeptide with potent depressant activity. Possibly this substance is an inhibitory transmitter within the sensory path-

ways. Another peptide, substance P, is found in other small cells and their processes, passing through Lissauer's tract before terminating in laminae I, II, and III; this substance may be an excitatory transmitter. Opiate receptors (associated with chemical substances that alleviate pain, Chap. 8) have been identified as being located on neurons in laminae I, II, and III.

Lamina III This lamina consists primarily of a matrix of small neurons with small and medium-sized axons. It is clearly separate from lamina II (Ralston and Ralston).

Laminae IV, V, and VI (nucleus proprius) The large relay neurons of these laminae with their apical dendrites extending into the substantia gelatinosa are radially oriented. The basilar dendrites extend within the lamina containing the cell body. The projections to these neurons are derived from several sources: (1) terminals of apical dendrites receive input from gelatinosa glomeruli, (2) basilar dendrites receive input from descending fibers from brain including the corticospinal tract, and (3) neurons in general receive input from the collaterals of dorsal root afferents in the medial bundle and from intersegmental and intrasegmental local circuit neurons. Some of the neurons have axons which project via the anterior white commissure to join the lateral spinothalamic tract and other fibers which project to the spinospinalis tract. Progressing from laminae IV, V, and VI, the neurons are stimulated by larger receptive fields and receive input from a larger variety of modalities. This is apparently the result of convergence associated with neural processing.

Direct spinothalamic pathway (neospinothalamic pathway, lateral pain system, or spinal lemniscus) (Figs. 5-15 and 5-16)

Fine naked free nerve endings are the pain receptors. They are the only endings in such pain-producing sites as the pulp cavity of a tooth and the cornea of the eye.

It is thought that the *thermal senses are conveyed by one pathway system and that pain is conveyed by two or more pathway systems*. The thermal pathway and one of the pain pathways form the *direct* or *lateral spinothalamic* (spinal cord to thalamus) *tract*, which consists of a sequence of at least three neurons with long axonal processes. The other pain pathway is the *indirect spinoreticular thalamic pathway*, which consists of a sequence of many neurons. Fibers of the spinotectal tract may also be involved. Of the first order are largely the lightly myelinated A delta fibers. As a consequence, this direct pathway has been called the *A delta pathway* to the ventral posterolateral nucleus of the thalamus (also called ventrobasal complex). All fibers of the direct spinothalamic pathway are lightly myelinated.

Second-order cells (spinothalamic cells), distributed unevenly in laminae I through VIII of the spinal gray matter, have axons that decussate transversely or in a slightly upward oblique course through the anterior commissure to the contralateral anterolateral lateral funiculus (see Figs. 5-11 and 5-13 to 5-15). Each fiber traverses the equivalent of one spinal segment during its crossing. The nociceptive (pain) spinothalamic cells are mainly located in laminae I, IV, V, and VI. Cells responding to gentle mechanical stimuli (movement of hairs and light touch) are primarily located in laminae IV, V, and VI (refer to "Anterior Spinothalamic Tract," later on). Some lamina I cells are excited by thermoreceptors. A few spinothalamic cells located in laminae IV and VIII respond to stimulation from receptors in the deep tissues. Much convergence of inputs from both nociceptive and innocuous sources is directed upon spinothalamic cells, especially those in the deep laminae of the spinal gray matter. Some spinothalamic cells receive convergent input from receptors in both the viscera and the skin and other spinothalamic cells receive such input from both cutaneous and muscle receptors. Other spinothalamic cells are sensitive to light mechanical stimuli; these cells with relatively large receptive fields are probably involved with the perception of crudely localized touch. Many of these posterior horn cells, including those responsive to light mechanical stimuli, can be excited by thermal stimuli.

After decussating, the axons of the second-order neurons bend and ascend rostrally through the lateral funiculus and brainstem tegmentum (and hence are called the lateral pain system or spinal lemniscus) to terminate in the ventral posterolateral nucleus of the thalamus (ventrobasal complex), the posterior thalamic nucleus or region (magnocellular portion of the medial geniculate body or posteromedial nucleus), and the intralaminar thalamic nuclei (see Fig. 5-16). The ventrobasal complex (VB) and the posteromedial nucleus (PO_m) are physiologically defined nuclear groups. The VB complex is the equivalent of the posterior ventral thalamic nucleus. The PO_m is the equivalent of the posterior thalamic nucleus (region), and portions of the pulvinar and the suprageniculate nuclei (Chap. 13).

The posterior thalamic nucleus and the intralaminar nuclei receive bilateral sensory input of both noxious and nonnoxious qualities. From cell bodies within these nuclei, axons course through the posterior limb of the internal capsule and corona radiata to the postcentral gyrus (somatosensory area I) and somatic sensory area II. The precise significance of the cortex in pain perception is not known. Lesions of the postcentral gyrus may be accompanied by hypalgesia, rarely by analgesia, and possibly by a minor loss of pain sensibility in the appropriate body part on the contralateral side. Stimulation of the postcentral gyrus may produce the sensations of numbness and tingling but rarely that of pain. The thalamus and the somatic sensory area II may contain the critical substrates underlying conscious pain appreciation. It is unlikely that the somatosensory areas I and II (Chap. 16) are essential for the appreciation of pain because ablation of these areas is said to leave chronic clinical pain undiminished.

Each second-order neuron has collateral branches which extend from its ascending axon to the gray matter of the spinal cord at higher levels, into the brainstem reticular formation, and into the periventricular and periaqueductal gray matter and superior colliculi of the midbrain. In fact, some of the fibers of the tract terminate as spinoreticular fibers in the brainstem reticular formation. Probably only about one-third of the 2000 or so fibers of the lateral spinothalamic tract actually reach the thalamus. Within the brainstem the lateral spinothalamic tract is called the spinothalamic tract. This phylogenetically new pathway in mammals, called the neospinothalamic tract, conveys sensory influences perceived as sharp, localized pain sensations. The lateral spinothalamic tract exhibits both anatomic and physiologic lamination. Fibers from the lower segments of the spinal cord tend to be located posterolateral to those that are added to the tract at higher levels (see Fig. 5-14). This anatomic somatotopic lamination results because the fibers decussating through the anterior white commissure are added from each successive higher level on the medial aspect of the tract. Within the brainstem

this tract is less precisely somatotopically organized. Claims are made that the fibers conveying pain impulses tend to be located more anteriorly in the tract and that those conveying thermal impulses tend to be located posteriorly in the tract.

Indirect spinothalamic pathway (spinoreticulothalamic pathway, paleospinothalamic pathway, or medial pain polyneuronal system; visceral sensory pathway) (Figs. 5-15 and 5-16)

The spinoreticulothalamic pathway is a multineuronal, multisynaptic pathway that courses from the spinal cord through the brainstem reticular formation before terminating in the intralaminar nuclei of the thalamus, especially the paracentral and central lateral nuclei. The main input to this pathway presumably comes from C pain fibers. As a consequence, this indirect pathway has been called the C fiber pathway to the thalamus.

From cell bodies in the posterior horn and intermediate zone, fine axons ascend as both crossed and uncrossed fibers in the white matter of the anterolateral regions of the spinal cord; some of these fibers are interspersed among the fibers of the lateral spinothalamic tract. These fibers course through the reticular formation of the medulla posterior to the inferior olivary nuclear complex and anteromedial to the spinal trigeminal tract. These fibers (sometimes called spinoreticular or spinobulbar fibers) terminate in nuclei of the medial reticular formation of the medulla, pons, and midbrain. This pathway, composed of sequences of neurons within the brainstem reticular formation, terminates in the periaqueductal gray matter (midbrain), the thalamic intralaminar nuclei, the posterior thalamic nucleus, and the hypothalamus. Influences are also projected to general somatic area II (see Fig. 16-16). This fine fibered medially located pain pathway is the phylogenetically old system concerned with the disagreeable, diffuse, poorly localizable, and burning aspects of pain; it is likely that visceral sensations are conveyed by this system.

Electrical stimulation of the periaqueductal gray induces analgesia in experimental animals (Chap. 8). This so-called stimulus-produced analgesia suggests that both somatic and visceral pain can be modulated from this region. The pathway to the hypothalamus and the limbic system (Chaps. 11 and 15) presumably conveys some pain influences which may evoke responses associated with the autonomic nervous system activity (e.g., gastrointestinal activity) and with aggressive and aversive behavioral patterns (e.g., facial grimaces).

An *anterolateral chorodotomy* (cutting of the spinal cord) is a neurosurgical procedure designed for the relief of intractable pain in the body. *Intractable pain* is an obstinate form of pain which persists for weeks or months and renders patients unable to sleep normally or carry out their usual daily duties. In the operation, each of the two anterior quadrants of the spinal cord is cut (anterior to the denticulate ligament, cortiocospinal tract, and rubrospinal tract) at a spinal level. Pain and temperature sensations are lost below the transected level because the fibers of the lateral spinothalamic tract and spinoreticulothalamic pathway have been severed. After an elapse of some time, some pain and temperature sense may return in some patients. Two explanations have been suggested: (1) some persisting spinoreticular fibers may reconstitute a functional pathway and (2) a new functional pain pathway may develop through the posterolateral tract of Lissauer and bridge the sectioned region. A unilateral section through the spinal cord does not abolish visceral pain, because such influences are projected rostrally in both crossed and uncrossed ascending fibers.

Strong analgesic drugs have no effect on the peripheral receptors. They act by modifying either the perception of pain or the emotional reaction to pain.

Spinotectal tract

The *spinotectal tract* is composed of fibers which originate in the intermediate gray zone, decussate in the anterior white commissure, and ascend as a small bundle located adjacent to the spinothalamic tract (see Fig. 5-19). Its fibers terminate in the deep layers of the superior colliculus and in the periaqueductal gray matter. This pathway may have a role in the transmission of somatic and visceral, pain, and other noxious stimuli. In a sense, the spinotectal fibers may be considered as one expression of the spinoreticular and spinoreticulothalamic pathways.

Neural mechanisms associated with pain

What is pain? The answer depends on the respondent. With some reservations, pain is viewed by psychologists as a basic sensory modality; by neurophysiologists, neurologists, and neurosurgeons as a pattern of neurophysiologic activity in certain neural centers; by biologists as an activity of significance to survival; by psychiatrists as an affect or emotion; and by the analyst as the product of internal psychic conflict. Objectively, pain is an expression of the interpretation by some centers in the brain of the input to these centers.

Several clinical conditions indicate that the influences conveyed from the free nerve endings via the A fibers and the C fibers have different critical roles in the appreciation of pain. Some persons are congenitally insensitive to pain. In certain such subjects with markedly elevated pain thresholds the small-diameter C fibers are said to be absent, whereas the A fibers are relatively intact. In contrast, patients afflicted with *herpes zoster*—a skin eruption due to a virus infection—experience excruciating pain when the involved skin area is exposed to normally innocuous stimuli such as light touch. In this condition there is said to be a reduction in the number of A fibers relative to C fibers in the peripheral nerve. This abnormal sensitivity to pain may be a consequence, in part, of the inability of the fewer lightly myelinated A fibers to exert suppressor effects on the fine-fiber activity. As explained below, the intense delayed pain may be a response to repetitive stimulation of C fibers. No one, as yet, has advanced a proven explanation of why so-called painless people (those who do not usually feel any pain reaction to everyday stimuli that produce pain in normal people) do not feel pain.

Supraspinal influences from higer levels, which can modify the effect associated with pain, may be conveyed from the cerebral cortex and subcortical centers to the posterior horn.

These descending pathways include the cortico-spinal tract (especially from the parietal lobe) and other reflected fibers to the brainstem reticular nuclei within the reticulospinal tracts. Many of our subjective experiences of pain are modified through higher centers in the brain. Anxiety and depression may magnify the intensity of pain; hypnosis and intense emotional involvement or cognitive activity can suppress it. After prefrontal lobotomy (Chap. 16), the affective component of intractable pain may be markedly reduced, with the retention of the discriminative component.

Gate theory of pain

One concept utilizing the pattern theory of pain is the *gate-control theory* in which the neural substrates are supposed to be organized into a gating mechanism for the control of pain input. Utilizing the known neuronal organization of the dorsal horn, the following formulation is a possible explanation of how the rapidly conducting large-fiber pathway suppresses or modulates activity of the slowly conducting small (A delta and C) fiber pathway that conveys noxious information. The large fibers excite the gelatinosa cells of laminae II and III and the transmission cells of laminae IV and V. The latter are the source of some lateral spinothalamic tract fibers. The small afferent fibers inhibit the gelatinosa cells and excite the transmission cells. In turn, the gelatinosa cells can tonically inhibit the input from both large and small fibers by presynaptic inhibition. When the C fiber activity is great, the gelatinosa cells are inhibited from exerting their presynaptic inhibitory influences on the transmission cells. In this way the excitatory effects of the A delta and C fibers "open the gates" so the transmission cells can fire. When the large-fiber activity is elevated, the gelatinosa cells are excited to exert more presynaptic inhibitory influences on the transmission cells, thereby "closing the gates" to suppress and to modulate the activity of the transmission cells. This is consistent with the concept noted above, that subjects with A fibers but few C fibers have elevated pain thresholds. Their A fibers tend "to close the gates." The phenomenon of gating refers to the synaptic responses to degrees of facilitation and inhibition.

Spinoreticular tract

The *spinoreticular* (*spinobulbar*) *tract* is composed of fibers originating from cells in laminae V, VI, VII, and VIII of the spinal cord. The fibers ascend in the anterior and anterolateral funiculi and brainstem reticular formation; they terminate in the medial two-thirds of the medullary and pontine reticular formation. The spinoreticular tract is not somatotopically organized. The fibers of this tract which terminate in the nucleus reticularis gigantocellularis and lateral reticular nucleus are primarily uncrossed axons, whereas those which terminate in the nucleus reticularis pontis oralis and caudalis are both crossed and uncrossed axons. These pathways are integrated into the "ascending reticular system" and the spinoreticulothalamic *pain* pathway, and, in addition, probably convey visceral sensory impulses from the thoracic, abdominal, and pelvic viscera.

Touch and deep-sensibility pathways

The nerve endings associated with the conscious pathways for touch and deep sensibility include Merkel's disks, Meissner's corpuscles, terminals surrounding the hair follicles (peritrichial arborization), and Pacinian corpuscles. These modalities are conveyed by two pathways: light (tickle or crude) touch (stroking without deforming skin or moving hair) via the *anterior spinothalamic tract* (see Fig. 5-19); and tactile discrimination, stereognosis, pressure (deep touch), and associated discrimination senses via the *posterior column* (*spinal cord*)-*medial lemniscal* (*brainstem*) *pathway* (see Fig. 5-18).

Anterior (ventral) spinothalamic pathway (Figs. 5-11, 5-13, 5-14, and 5-19) The concept of an anterior spinothalamic tract has its basis in clinical observations that a lesion in the anterolateral region of the lateral funiculus may result in patients' having deficits of pain and temperature perception while retaining light touch perception (even after impairment of the posterior columns). However, this dichotomy of the spinothalamic tracts into a lateral and an anterior spinothalamic tract may be arbitrary. Anatomic evidence supports the concept that the two tracts are, in fact, one tract because the fibers of "both" tracts have similar terminations in the thalamus. In addition, physiologic evidence indicates that no anatomic segregation of the functional categories exists among the spinothalamic fibers; hence gross segregation of functional components is not likely. Many authorities refer to these tracts and the spinotectal tract collectively as the *anterolateral system*.

The following is the standard course usually described for the anterior spinothalamic tract (see Fig. 5-19). The first-order neurons consist of lightly myelinated fibers that pass through the dorsal root into the posterolateral tract of Lissauer and terminate in the posterior horn. The short ascending and descending collateral branches in the posterolateral tract extend up and down through about three spinal segments and terminate in the posterior horn. The second-order neurons project their axons obliquely from cells in laminae VI and VII through the anterior white commissure to the anterior funiculus, where they bend and ascend rostrally through the spinal cord and brainstem to terminate in the periventricular gray matter, ventral posterolateral nucleus of the thalamus, the posterior thalamic nucelus, and the intralaminar thalamic nuclei. The third-order neurons project from the thalamus through the posterior limb of the internal capsule to the postcentral gyrus of the cerebral cortex.

Posterior column — medial lemniscal pathway (Figs. 5-18 and 5-19)

Modalities This major system conveys information from mechanoreceptors in the skin, muscles tendons, and joints. Their activity is subjectively perceived in basically three forms of sensibility: touch-pressure, kinesthesia (position sense), and vibratory sense. Touch-pressure is the sense resulting from deformation of the skin; kinesthesia includes the sense of position and movement of joints (angle-movement detectors). Vibrations sensed from Meissner's corpuscles are called flutter-vibrations (30 to 40 Hz), while recognition of those from deep structures such as joints and bone is called the vibratory sense. Vibratory sense (roughly 400 Hz from Pacinian corpuscles) is actually a sensing of rapid, successive stimuli of tactile sense. In general, the fibers of first order of this posterior column-lemniscal system are modality specific. In turn, this modality

specificity is preserved throughout this system, commencing with first-order neurons and including the processing nuclei (nuclei gracilis and cuneatus and ventral posterolateral nucleus of the thalamus), second- and third-order neurons, and in the neurons of the postcentral gyrus (primary somesthetic cortex).

Touch-pressure and the flutter component of flutter-vibration are monitored by the fast-adapting fibers innervating hair follicles (movement detectors) and Meissner's corpuscles (flutter vibrations) in the skin. Touch-pressure is also sensed by slowly adapting fibers innervating Merkel corpuscles in the epidermis and Ruffini-like endings in the dermis of the skin, fascia, and periosteum. Vibratory sensibility (high-frequency sense) is picked up by Pacinian corpuscles of the dermis and deep tissues, while kinesthesia is sensed by receptors in the joint capsules and joint ligaments. Its free nerve endings monitor position sense, pains, and movement in the joints. The receptors in the joint "know" where the limb is (angle of joint). This information, signaling positive active movement and resistance to movement to the nervous system, is essential for the regulation of normal movements.

Pathway The first-order neurons of this system with their cell bodies located in the spinal ganglia consist generally of heavily myelinated modality-specific fibers which pass the spinal cord through the medial bundle of the dorsal root. Upon entering the cord of the medial aspect of the posterior horn, the fibers divide into ascending and descending branches which are located within the *posterior column (fasciculi gracilis* and *cuneatus)* on the same side of the spinal cord. About one-fourth of the ascending fibers extend rostrally and terminate in the nuclei gracilis and cuneatus, which are located in the lower medulla. Collateral fibers branch off the main axon within the segment of entrance and also from the ascending and descending branches into other segments; these collaterals terminate in the spinal gray matter. Approximately one-fifth of the ascending fibers terminate in the immediate gray matter within two or three spinal segments above their segment of entry. Many of these intraspinal collaterals are involved with intersegmental spinal reflexes.

The ascending fibers are somatotopically organized within the posterior columns. Those conveying input from the lower body caudal to T6 (including the lower extremity) are located more medially, in the *fasciculus gracilis*, and those from the upper body rostral to T6 (including the upper extremity) are located more laterally, in the *fasciculus cuneatus*. Fibers from each spinal segment are added successively on the lateral aspect of the posterior column; this maintains the somatotopic organization within the posterior columns. Thus at the cervical levels, the lamination from posteromedial to lateral consists, in order, of fibers from the sacral, lumbar, thoracic, and cervical segments of the body (see Fig. 5-14). Thus, the fibers from the sacral, lumbar, and lower six thoracic segments form the fasciculus gracilis, and those from the upper six thoracic levels and all cervical levels (including the back of the head) form the fasciculus cuneatus. The longest neurons in the body are those of the fasciculus gracilis; they extend without interruption from the foot to the nucleus gracilis in the medulla. These neurons in a 7-ft-tall giant are over 6 ft long. Each posterior column fiber terminates after dividing into two or three branches which, through collaterals, synapse directly with several neurons of the second order. The somatotopic organization is maintained in the nuclei gracilis and cuneatus.

Cells in the nucleus gracilis and nucleus cuneatus receive input from peripheral receptors by both convergence and divergence. Those cells with large receptive fields derive their input from many similar peripheral receptors via convergence. On the other hand, several similar peripheral receptors may project their influences via convergent routes to a cell in these nuclei. The relay cells in these nuclei exhibit center-surround physiological responses (excitatory center surrounded by an inhibitory zone), which are the basis of sharpening to maintain labeled lines.

Neural processing within these nuclei occurs through synaptic interactions among the nerve terminals of the ascending fibers, intrinsic interneurons, descending (reflected fibers, Chap. 3) corticofugal fibers from the cerebral cortex, and the neurons of the second order. The corticofugal fibers originate in the somatosensory (postcentral gyrus) cortex and course through the corona radiata, internal capsule, and basilar portion of the brainstem (among the fibers of the corticospinal tract) before terminating with the posterior column nuclei (nuclei gracilis and cuneatus). Each descending fiber divides before spreading over wide areas within these nuclei. The interneurons are not intercalated between the first- and second-order neurons, but rather are integrated into recurrent circuits (recurrent collateral fibers from second-order neurons) and are interposed between the reflected fibers and second-order neurons. These neuronal connections with these nuclei are organized into center-surround units (Chap. 12). Within this organization the discriminative nature of the sensations (e.g., two-point discrimination) maintains individuality within the processing nuclei by the excitatory center and inhibitory-surround organization. The information from each distinct point on the body is preserved and prevented from being dispersed from the center by the inhibitory activity of the surround (Chap. 12).

The second-order neurons, with their cell bodies in the nucleus gracilis and nucleus cuneatus, have axons which course transversely in an arc as the decussating *internal arcuate fibers* of the medulla into the contralateral *medial lemniscus* (see Fig. A-2) and ascend through the brainstem to the *ventral posterolateral nucleus* (ventrobasal complex) of the thalamus. Apparently all fibers of this pathway decussate in the low medulla and terminate in cone-shaped bushy endings in the ventral posterolateral nucleus. In the medulla, the medial lemniscus is located in the anterior portion just posterior to the pyramid between the midline raphe and the inferior olive. In the pontine region, the medial lemniscus shifts laterally along the anterior margin of the tegmentum of the pons. In the midbrain it shifts posterolaterally as a crescent-shaped bundle lateral to the nucleus ruber and medial to the medial geniculate body before terminating in the ventral posterolateral nucleus (see Figs. 8-6 through 8-13).

Although the lamination is not precise, the somatotopical organization is maintained within the medial lemniscus. In general, the second-order fibers from the nucleus gracilis ascend in the anterior portion of the medial lemniscus within the medulla and the lateral portion of the medial lemniscus within the pons and synapse in the lateral portion of the ventral postero-

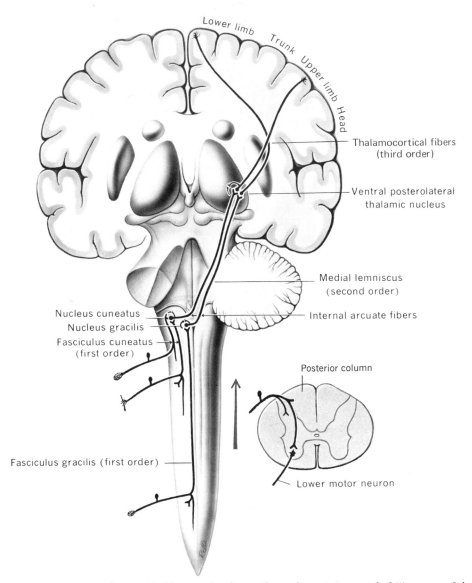

Lower limb   Trunk   Upper limb   Head

Thalamocortical fibers
(third order)

Ventral posterolateral
thalamic nucleus

Medial lemniscus
(second order)

Internal arcuate fibers

Nucleus cuneatus

Nucleus gracilis

Fasciculus cuneatus
(first order)

Posterior column

Fasciculus gracilis (first order)

Lower motor neuron

FIGURE 5-18 Posterior column-medial lemniscal pathway. This pathway is composed of (1) neurons of the first order with cell bodies in the spinal ganglia and with axons that ascend in the posterior column to the nuclei gracilis and cuneatus; (2) neurons of the second order with cell bodies in the nuclei gracilis and cuneatus and with axons that decussate as the internal arcuate fibers in the lower medulla and ascend in the medial lemniscus to the thalamus; and (3) neurons of the third order with cell bodies in the thalamus and with axons that project to the cerebral cortex (postcentral gyrus). Collateral branches of the neuron of the first order pass to the posterior horn, the anterior horn (see Fig. 5-13), and the posterior column; the last are descending association fibers.

lateral nucleus of the thalamus. Those fibers from the nucleus cuneatus ascend in the posterior portion of the medial lemniscus within the medulla and the medial portion of the lemniscus within the pons and synapse in the medial portion of the ventral posterolateral nucleus.

Axons of neurons of the third order with their cell bodies in the ventral posterolateral nucleus of the thalamus pass through the posterior limb of the internal capsule and corona radiata before terminating in the general somatic area I (primary somatic area, postcentral gyrus) and somatic sensory area II (general somatic area II, secondary somatic area; see Figs. 5-15 and 16-16).

The relay cells from the posterior ventrolateral nucleus project to cerebral cortical lamina IV, where they make excitatory synapses with the dendritic spines of stellate cells and the spines of basilar dendrites of pyramidal cells (Chap. 16). The processing within the somesthetic cortex is expressed in the functional vertical columns (Chap. 16). Group I afferents project to area 3A, cutaneous afferents to area 3, and the joint and periosteal afferents from bone to areas 1 and 2 (see Figs. 16-7 and 16-8).

According to a recent view, the posterior column–medial lemniscal pathway belongs to a

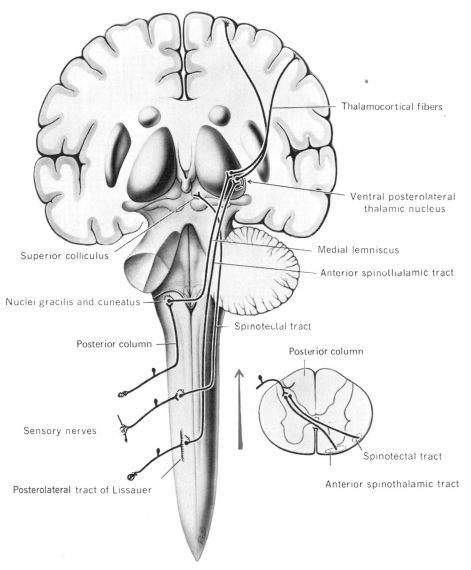

Thalamocortical fibers

Ventral posterolateral thalamic nucleus

Medial lemniscus

Anterior spinothalamic tract

Superior colliculus

Spinotectal tract

Nuclei gracilis and cuneatus

Posterior column

Posterior column

Sensory nerves

Spinotectal tract

Anterior spinothalamic tract

Posterolateral tract of Lissauer

FIGURE 5-19 Touch pathways and spinotectal tract. The touch pathways include (1) the posterior column–medial lemniscus-thalamocortical pathway, and (2) the anterior spinothalamic tract–thalamocortical pathway. The spinotectal pathway is composed of (1) neurons of the first order with cell bodies in the spinal ganglia, and (2) neurons of the second order with cell bodies in the posterior horn and with axons that decussate and ascend as the spinotectal tract to the superior colliculus.

system involved with so-called active touch. This is the touch associated with the capacity for learning tactile discrimination. This capacity is said to be lost following lesions of the posterior columns. On the other hand, the anterolateral pathways belong to a system involved with so-called passive touch. This is the touch associated with tactile discriminations upon which correct performance is dependent. The modalities include roughness, texture, form, and localization discriminations. Passive touch is said to persist following posterior column lesions.

In summary, the modalities associated with the posterior column–medial lemniscus system include discriminative touch, two-point discrimination, stereognosis, awareness of shape, size, and texture, awareness of passive movement, position sense, flutter vibration, vibratory sense (as in use of a tuning fork), and weight perception.

The view that muscle sense is "unconscious" has prevailed because it has been thought that muscle afferents do not have access to the cerebral cortex. Studies on monkeys indicate that this is *not* so. Stimulation of Group I muscle afferents utilizing the posterior column–medial lemniscal pathway and the spinocervicothalamic route (through nucleus Z, Fig. 8-6) elicit activity in the contralateral ventral posterolateral thalamic nucleus and a cortical area just rostral to area 3 called area 3A. The as yet to be answered question is to what extent muscle afferent activity is perceived as a discriminable cue.

Spinocervicothalamic pathway (spinocervicolemniscal pathway, spinodorsolateral-paralemniscal system)

This spinocervicothalamic pathway receives its afferent input from a variety of mechanoreceptors, including endings on hair follicles, tactile, touch-pressure, vibratory sensors in the skin receptors in muscles and joints, and some visceroceptors (see Fig. 5-20). The first-order lightly myelinated afferents pass through the medial bundle to laminae IV and V. Second-order fibers ascend from cells in these laminae and the thoracic nucleus of Clarke in lamina VII within the ipsilateral posterolateral tract. These ascending fibers are mainly of the posterior spinocerebellar tract; they and probably others send collateral branches to the lateral cervical nucleus (a small nucleus in humans located in the lower medulla and upper three cervical spinal levels on the lateral border of the dorsal horn) and the following nuclei in the medulla: cuneatus, gracilis, lateral reticular, accessory cuneate, and X and Z of Brodal and Pompeiano. The latter three nuclei project to the cerebellum. Nuclei X and Z are located just dorsal of the nucleus cuneatus (see Fig. 8-6). The axons of the lateral cervical nucleus decussate in the anterior white commissure of the upper cervical levels and in the lower medulla, ascend just lateral to the medial lemniscus within the brainstem, and terminate in ventral posterolateral and posterior thalamic nuclei. The pathway projects from the thalamus to both the primary and secondary somatic areas of the cerebral cortex (somatic sensory areas I and area II). This pathway has been demonstrated in the rhesus monkey and is thus assumed to be a functioning pathway in humans. Apparently this pathway does not convey nociceptive information (Kerr and Wilson).

SPINOCEREBELLAR PATHWAYS

General characteristics (Fig. 5-21)

Receptors in the extremities and body wall, especially those in the muscles and tendons, are continually monitoring the immediate status of muscle contraction and the momentary degree of tension within the tendons. The resulting "unconscious" proprioceptive information from the muscles, tendons, and joints is projected to the cerebellum via four pathways whose fibers terminate as mossy fibers in the cerebellar cortex (Chap. 9).

Some input to the cerebellum comes from exteroceptive receptors in the skin. The *posterior and anterior spinocerebellar tracts* convey these influences from the lower extremities and the caudal half of the body, while the *cuneocerebellar tract* and the *rostral spinocerebellar tract* (the latter as yet unidentified in humans) convey influences from the upper extremities and upper half of the body. In general, the posterior spinocerebellar and cuneocerebellar pathways receive their input from the muscle spindles, tendon organs, touch receptors, and pressure receptors,

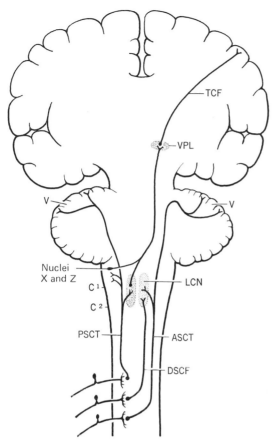

FIGURE 5-20 Spinocervicothalamic pathway. This tactile and kinesthetic system relays influences via the lateral cervical nucleus (LCN) to the ventral posterolateral (VPL) nucleus of the thalamus. This pathway projects to both the primary and secondary somatosensory areas of the cortex. ASCT, Anterior spinocerebellar tract; DSCF, Direct spinocervical fibers; PSCT, Posterior spinocerebellar tract; TCF, Thalamocortical fibers; V, Vermis; VPL, Ventral posterolateral nucleus. (*From Noback and Harting, Spinal Cord, S. Karger, Publisher, Basel.*)

both contralaterally and ipsilaterally in the rhesus monkey and presumably also in human beings.

It is not possible to determine the clinical effects of a lesion to the spinocerebellar tracts, because other tracts, such as the corticospinal tract, are usually included in the lesion. Loss of a conscious modality is not a consequence of the interruption of a pathway because the cerebellum has no role in the appreciation of conscious sensations (Chap. 9).

Posterior spinocerebellar tract (Fig. 5-20)

The neurons of the first order with cell bodies in the spinal ganglia convey coded information from the stretch receptors (muscle spindles and Golgi tendon organs) and some exteroceptive receptors (touch and pressure) directly to the neurons of the second order in the dorsal nucleus of Clarke (Clarke's column) of lamina VII. The neurons of this nucleus receive monosynaptic excitatory influences mainly from group Ia and Ib fibers with some from exteroceptive group II afferents. The axons of the dorsal nucleus of Clarke (located at levels T1 through L3) ascend ipsilaterally as the somatotopically organized uncrossed spinocerebellar tract (see Fig. 5-20). The fibers of this tract are among the fastest conducting fibers—120 m/s. Its large fibers ascend successively through the posterolateral aspect of the lateral funiculus of the spinal cord, the inferior cerebellar peduncle, and the white matter of the cerebellum before terminating as mossy fibers (Chap. 9) in the ipsilateral anterior (lobules I to IV) and caudal (pyramis and paramedian lobule) portions of the cerebellar vermis. Within the spinal cord the tract is superficial to the lateral corticospinal tract.

Because the dorsal nucleus of Clarke does not extend caudal to L3, (1) the fibers entering the spinal cord via the dorsal spinal roots of lumbar and sacral levels ascend in the posterior columns before synapsing with the neurons of the dorsal nucleus of Clarke, and (2) the posterior spinocerebellar tract, as such, is not found within the spinal cord caudal to the L3 level. In summary, the somatotopically organized posterior spinocerebellar tract relays unconscious proprioceptive information from the caudal half

while the anterior spinocerebellar and rostral cerebellar pathways receive input via neurons with large receptor fields of Golgi tendon organs and flexor reflex afferents. These flexor reflex afferents are those receptors in skin and joints conveying information via neurons of groups II and III; they are involved with the general flexor reflex, with two or more neurons intercalated within the reflex.

Projections from the spinal cord to the cerebellum arise from cells in nuclei located in the gray matter of each segmental level of the spinal cord (Petras). The axons from these cells ascend

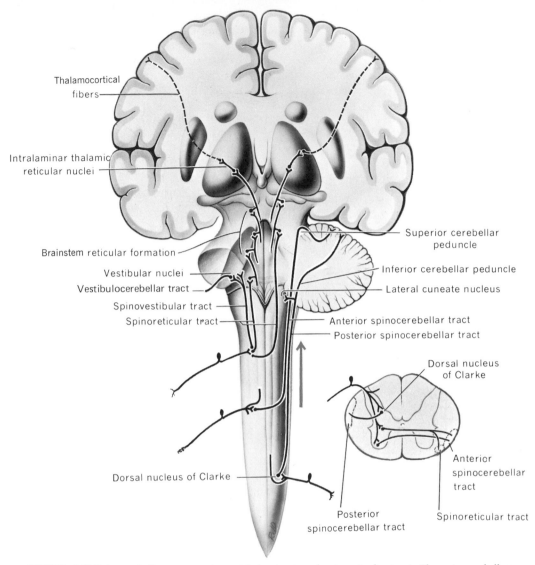

FIGURE 5-21 Spinocerebellar tracts, spinovestibular tract, and spinoreticular tract. The spinocerebellar tracts include (1) the uncrossed posterior spinocerebellar tract that passes through the inferior cerebellar peduncle and terminates in the paleocerebellum, and (2) the crossed anterior spinocerebellar tract that passes through the superior cerebellar peduncle and terminates in the paleocerebellum. The spinovestibular tract includes fibers that terminate in the vestibular nuclei. The spinoreticular tract is composed of crossed and uncrossed fibers that terminate in some brainstem reticular nuclei.

of the body and lower extremities to the cerebellar cortex via a two-neuron linkage with synaptic connections in the dorsal nucleus. This pathway has a role in the fine coordination of individual muscles during postural adjustments and movements of individual limb muscles.

Anterior spinocerebellar tract (see Fig. 5-21)

Fibers of neurons of the first order from the Golgi tendon organs, high-threshold muscle and joint receptors, and other receptors located in the lower extremity and lower half of the body enter the spinal cord via the dorsal roots and terminate with neurons in laminae V, VI, and VII in the lumbosacral levels. Each second-order neuron receives monosynaptic excitatory influences derived primarily from Ib afferents of Golgi tendon organs located in widely separated muscle tendons. The flexor reflex afferent fibers include those of groups II and III which evoke flexor reflexes via polysynaptic circuits mediated via two or more interneurons. These neurons also receive inhibitory and excitatory stimuli from the cutaneous afferent fibers. The axons of the neurons of the second order decussate in the anterior white commissure and ascend as the somatotopically organized anterior spinocerebellar tract located in the anterolateral aspect of the lateral funiculus. Some fibers of this tract are uncrossed. The tract can be identified as low as the lower lumbar levels. The tract courses through the lateral brainstem and along the posterior surface of the superior cerebellar peduncle before terminating in the vermis of the anterior lobe (lobules I to IV). This pathway has a role in the general coordination of posture and movement of the entire limb.

Cuneocerebellar tract

Groups Ia and Ib (muscle spindles and Golgi tendon organs) and some cutaneous (touch and pressure receptors) afferent fibers of first-order neurons innervating the upper extremities and rostral half of the body pass through the dorsal roots, ascend in the ipsilateral fasciculus cuneatus, and terminate in the somatotopically organized accessory cuneate nucleus. The accessory cuneate nucleus, located in the lower medulla just lateral to the cuneate nucleus, is the rostral equivalent to the dorsal nucleus of Clarke (see Fig. 8-6). Axons of the accessory cuneate nucleus course via the uncrossed cuneocerebellar tract through the inferior cerebellar peduncle and terminate in the ipsilateral lobule V of the cerebellar cortex. This pathway is the upper limb counterpart of the posterior spinocerebellar tract.

Rostral spinocerebellar tract

This pathway serves the same role for the rostral half of the body and upper extremity as the ante-
rior spinocerebellar tract for the lower extremity. Although its presence has been established so far only in the cat, it is presumed to exist in humans. This rostral spinocerebellar pathway relays influences from the group I muscle afferents and flexor reflex afferents (movement patterns of the whole extremity) from the ipsilateral upper extremity via uncrossed fibers. These course through both superior and inferior cerebellar peduncles and terminate in lobules I to V of the anterior cerebellar lobe.

Other ascending pathways

Fibers have been described that project directly to the cerebral cortex (*spinocortical tract*), to the (inferior) vestibular nuclei (*spinovestibular tract*, see Fig. 5-21), and to the pons (*spinopontine tract*). The nuclei of orgin of these tracts are in the gray matter. The general visceral afferent influences conveyed to the spinal cord are probably relayed rostrally via the *spinoreticular tract* (see Fig. 5-21).

The spinoolivary fibers originate from neurons in laminae V, VI, VII, and VIII and ascend mainly as uncrossed projections with some crossed projections in the anterior white columns to the inferior olivary nucleus.

The clinical effects of lesions of the spinocerebellar tracts in the spinal cord are not apparent, probably because they are masked by signs produced by lesions to other tracts.

SPINAL REFLEXES

The descending motor pathways from the brain to the spinal cord exert their influences on the intrinsic neural circuits of the spinal cord. These intrinsic neurons are important because they form the basic circuitry that eventually interacts with the lower motor neurons which innervate the voluntary muscles.

The *neuromuscular spindles* are arranged in parallel with the voluntary muscle fibers; they monitor *muscle length* (*length detectors*). The *Golgi tendon organs* are arranged in series with the voluntary muscles; they are *tension detectors*. When the muscle is stretched (lengthened), the spindle and the bag region of its intrafusal fibers are passively stretched and "loaded." The "loaded" spindle stimulates the Ia fibers to increase their firing rate. When the muscle is contracted, the spindle and its bag region are shortened and "unloaded." The "unloaded" spindle fires less actively. The Golgi tendon organs are not activated by passive stretch. Rather they respond to increases in tension during the contraction of a muscle by increasing their rate of discharge (see Fig. 2-12). The roles of the spindle and Golgi tendon organs are discussed further on in this chapter under "Monosynaptic Extensor Reflex." These sensory receptors are integral elements of negative feedback or servo loops; the feedback information is utilized by the various reflex circuits.

Neurons of spinal reflex arcs and the lower motor neurons

The neurons that comprise the intrinsic circuits within the spinal cord are classified into three categories (see Figs. 5-12 and 5-23 through 5-25).

1. The afferent neurons, those that enter the spinal cord via the dorsal roots and terminate in the gray matter. These neurons commence distally as endings in receptors within muscles, joints, and tendons, and in cutaneous receptors in the skin. The deep receptors include the primary (annulospiral) and secondary (flower spray) endings in the neuromuscular spindles, Golgi tendon organs, Ruffini and Pacinian corpuscles, and free nerve endings. The cutaneous (superficial) receptors comprise the Merkel, Meissner, Pacinian, and Ruffini corpuscles; hair endings; and free nerve endings (see Figs. 2-19, 2-20).
2. The interneurons, those that lie wholly within the spinal cord and interact with other interneurons or with lower motor neurons. These interneurons are classifed as (a) intrasegmental interneurons, those located entirely within a spinal cord segment on one side; (b) commissural interneurons, those projecting their axons to the same segment on the opposite side; and (c) intersegmental interneurons, those projecting their axons to other segments of the same side and of the opposite side (see "Intrinsic Spinal Interneurons and Fasciculi Proprii," later on).
3. The lower motor neurons. Each has its cell

body in the anterior horn; it projects its axon through a peripheral nerve to a voluntary muscle. The lower motor neurons are of two types, alpha and gamma (Figs. 2-1, 2-20). The *alpha motor (skeletomotor) neuron* is a heavily myelinated, fast-conducting neuron that terminates in the motor end plate of a voluntary muscle (extrafusal) fiber. The *gamma efferent (fusimotor) neuron* is a lightly myelinated neuron that innervates the small muscle (intrafusal) fibers within the neuromuscular spindle receptor. The lower motor neurons have their cell bodies located within the central nervous system (anterior horn of the spinal cord for spinal nerves; motor nuclei of cranial nerves III, IV, V, VI, VII, and XII and nucleus ambiguus, see Fig. 7-4). They have axons coursing within the peripheral nerves before terminating as motor end plates with extrafusal muscle fibers or intrafusal muscle fibers of the neuromuscular spindles. In summary, lower motor neurons include all alpha and gamma motor neurons associated with the cranial and spinal motor nerves. Movements of the body are produced by the contractions of skeletal muscles; muscle contractions result from the discharge of lower motor neurons. When adequately stimulated, each lower motor neuron conveys excitatory influences which evoke the contraction of all voluntary muscle fibers of the motor unit. This results because all motor end plates are obligatory excitatory synapses. All inhibitory synaptic influences upon the somatic motor circuits occur within the central nervous system.

Monosynaptic extensor reflex (Fig. 5-22)

The *simple knee jerk* results from the tapping of the tendon of the relaxed quadriceps femoris muscle—the muscle that extends the knee joint. This reflex is also known as the *patellar reflex, myotatic reflex, deep tendon reflex,* or *stretch extensor reflex.* It may be characterized as two-neuron (i.e., it involves a sequence of a set of afferent neurons and a set of efferent neurons), ipsilateral (it is restricted to the side tapped), and intrasegmental (each receptor stimulates an afferent neuron which excites alpha motor neurons in the

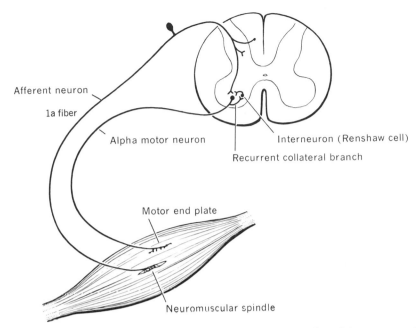

Afferent neuron

1a fiber

Alpha motor neuron

Interneuron (Renshaw cell)

Recurrent collateral branch

Motor end plate

Neuromuscular spindle

FIGURE 5-22 Extensor reflex (knee jerk). This two-neuron, monosynaptic, ipsilateral, intrasegmental reflex is composed of a "primary secondary ending" (annulospinal ending) of the neuromuscular spindle, afferent neuron, alpha motor neuron, and voluntary muscle.

same spinal segment). The sudden tap stretches the muscle and the neuromuscular spindles within the muscle. The stretched spindles (bag region) excite the sensitive low-threshold annulospiral endings to set up generator potentials that initiate a volley of impulses in the group Ia afferent fibers. The resulting action potentials are conveyed via these fibers through the dorsal roots of the L2 or L3 levels to the ipsilateral alpha motor neurons. In turn, these bombarded alpha neurons convey excitatory influences via the axons, which course through the ventral roots, spinal nerves, and peripheral nerves, to excite the motor end plates of muscle fibers of the quadriceps femoris to contract, thereby producing the knee jerk. During contraction, the spindles are passively shortened. The *brisk knee jerk* is a *phasic motion* (as in kicking a football); it is initiated by the synchronous discharges of many spindles. The *slow knee jerk* (as in contractions during stance) is a *tonic or postural jerk;* it is initiated by the asynchronous discharges from many spindles. The spindle acts as a *strain gauge monitor* (*length detector*) for these extensor reflexes. It is not a receptor associated with con-

scious sensations. Because the spindles are oriented "in parallel" to the extrafusal muscle fibers, the contraction of the extrafusal fibers results in the shortened spindles; this "unloads" the spindle so that it may cease to discharge momentarily ("*silent*" *period of spindle discharge*). As soon as the muscle relaxes, the spindle is stretched and firing resumes. Thus the spindles are involved in the autogenic excitation of the extrafusal fibers.

This two-neuron reflex, consisting of the afferent neuron innervating the spindle and the alpha motor neuron to a muscle, is known as the alpha (reflex) loop. Actually this monosynaptic reflex does not exist in isolation; collateral branches from the Ia afferent fibers (see Fig. 5-21) are integrated into a polysnaptic flexor reflex (reciprocal innervation).

Gamma motor (fusimotor, efferent neurons)

The gamma motor neurons are the lower motor neurons innervating the intrafusal muscle fibers of the neuromuscular spindles (see Fig. 2-20).

Their two roles are (1) to regulate the excitability of the spindles and (2) to contribute to the initiation of a movement. To appreciate the functional interactions of the gamma motor neurons and the activity of the spindle, it may be helpful to consider the following:

1. In the elongated spindle of a stretched muscle, the intrafusal muscle fibers of the spindle may be likened to a taut rope. In this state the firing rate of the gamma motor neurons is low to absent, while the firing rate of the Ia and II afferents from the spindle to the central nervous system is high.
2. In the shortened spindle of the contracted muscle, the intrasfusal fibers of the spindle may be likened to a slack rope. In this state the firing rate of the gamma motor neurons is low to absent and the firing rate in the Ia and II afferents is also low.
3. In the contracted muscle, the (slack) intrafusal fibers of a spindle can be stimulated to contract and become taut by increasing the firing rate of the gamma motor fibers. During the interval, the firing rate of the Ia and II afferents will change from a low rate (intrafusal fibers slack) to a high rate (intrafusal fibers taut).

There are two types of gamma efferent fibers: (1) dynamic gamma or gamma I fusimotor efferents and (2) static gamma or gamma II fusimotor efferents. The dynamic gamma fibers mainly innervate the bag fibers (with collaterals to the chain fibers). The static gamma fibers mainly innervate the chain fibers and to a lesser extent the bag fibers. The static outnumber the dynamic gamma fibers. The increased activity of the static gamma efferents results in an increased level of discharge of both group Ia and group II afferents for a given muscle length (static phase of stretch). The group Ia afferents are said to be velocity- and length-sensitive; during the dynamic phase they fire rapidly (determined by rate of muscle stretch) and then fire at a steady but reduced rate during the static phase (determined by muscle length). In brief, the group Ia afferents respond to both velocity and steady state. The group II afferents are only length-sensitive; they have a low dynamic sensi-

tivity. These are the fibers that mainly innervate the chain fibers of the spindle. The response of these fibers mainly to steady state is consistent with their sensitivity to muscle length.

Gamma reflex loop (Fig. 5-23)

As a muscle contracts, the neuromuscular spindles within the muscle become passively shorter (rope is slack); with this shortening there is a concomitant reduction in the rate of spindle firing via the Ia afferent neurons to the alpha motor pool. With this rate reduction, the system is not able to maintain the continuous contraction of any muscle mass. Continuous contraction of a muscle mass results when the muscle fibers are in various degrees of contraction (rope is slack) in response to asynchronous volleys of alpha motor neurons (a volley is the firing of a group of neurons). This continuous contraction is dependent upon the gamma reflex loop, which comprises (1) *gamma motor neuron*, (2) *neuromuscular spindle*, (3) *afferent neuron*, (4) *alpha motor neuron*, and (5) *voluntary muscle*. Note that the gamma loop commences with the gamma efferent neuron.

The *gamma control of spindle sensitivity to stretch* by the contraction of the intrafusal muscle fibers is important because the gamma neurons influence the quality of the sensory input from the spindle to the spinal cord. Gamma activation has a critical role in alpha motor neuron output. This process of sensitization of the spindle through the gamma efferents is known as *"gamma bias"*; it modulates the activity of the spindle. When intrafusal fibers contract, the equatorial region (bag) is stretched (rope is restretched), just as if the main muscle had been extended; the ensuing deformation pulls the coils of the annulospiral part and increases the rate of firing in the Ia fibers. Through gamma efferent stimulation, the slack in the muscle spindle (a consequence of the shortened muscle) is taken up by the pull exerted on the bag by the intrafusal muscle fibers. This acts to maintain spindle firing, which, through excitatory influences conveyed via Ia fibers to the alpha motor neurons, acts to smooth out the muscle contraction. The "biasing mechanism" of the gamma system is readily altered by changes in muscle tension. In general, increasing the load on the

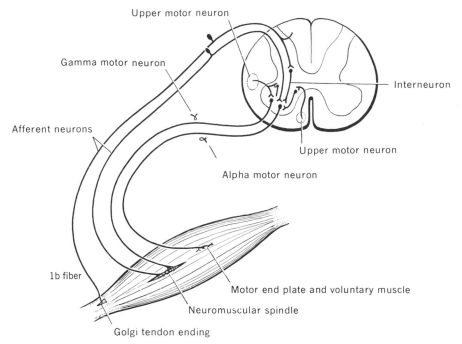

FIGURE 5-23 Gamma reflex loop and the Golgi tendon endings. The gamma loop comprises gamma motor neuron, neuromuscular spindle, afferent neuron (Ia fiber), alpha motor neuron, and voluntary muscle. The upper motor neurons can facilitate the gamma motor neurons. The Golgi tendon endings are involved in the loop composed of Golgi tendon endings, afferent neuron, spinal intrasegmental neuron, and alpha motor neuron.

muscle will increase the gamma efferent activity. When the slack occurs in the initial phase of the extrafusal muscle contraction, the spindle bags are unloaded and their firing ceases. This cessation is known as the *silent period*. Thus one role of the gamma efferents is to wipe out the silent period by stimulating the intrafusal fibers to contract; thus the bag assumes its normal tension status and the firing rate of its Ia fibers is resumed. In effect, this activity sustains the smooth ongoing muscular contraction. To summarize, the gamma motor neurons have two roles: they can change the sensitivity of the spindle—with the gain in the sensitivity of the bag region the firing rate of the Ia fibers increases; and they can obliterate the silent period.

The gamma neurons can be stimulated (1) by Ia fibers from the muscle spindle, (2) actively from the periphery through cutaneous stimulation by direct connections through interneurons synapsing with the gamma neurons, or (3) actively by upper motor neurons, especially those originating in the brainstem reticular formation. The cutaneous input acts rapidly; the reticular input via the upper motor neurons acts more slowly. Facilitatory and inhibitory influences from the brainstem reticular formation are conveyed via the medial and lateral reticulospinal tracts to laminae VII and VIII. Other descending tracts also contribute. The upper motor neurons stimulate the gamma motor neurons to excite the intrafusal muscle fibers slightly before stimulating the alpha motor neurons. This prior excitation of the gamma loop slightly before the alpha motor neuron discharge acts, in a sense, to condition the muscle. In effect, the gamma motor neurons act to load the spindle at the same rate as it is unloaded through the muscle contraction; this results in a smooth, coordinated muscle activity. Stated otherwise, to get a smooth contraction, the tension remains constant when the length shortens. The normal gamma motor neuron activity acts to prevent jerky, clonic movements.

Role of Golgi tendon organ

The *Golgi tendon organs* (*GTOs*) have a critical role in the maintenance of muscle tension through an inhibitory three-neuron reflex arc of afferent neuron, interneuron, and alpha motor neuron (see Fig. 5-23). In contrast to the spindles, which are muscle length detectors, the GTOs are muscle *tension detectors*. Because the GTOs within the tendons are *in series* with the extrafusal muscle fibers, they respond to an increase in tension within the tendon as the collagen fibers within the GTO squeeze the nerve endings (see Fig. 2-21). The GTOs act as biological force transducers that convert tension forces into a frequency code transmitted by the Ib afferent fibers. These tension forces are generated during the contraction or excessive stretch of the muscle. The threshold to stretch is slightly higher in the GTOs than in the neuromuscular spindles. As the tension within the tendon mounts, these endings are stimulated to increase the rate of discharge in the Ib fibers conveying influences from the GTOs to interneurons, which, in turn, increase their rate of discharge of inhibitory stimuli into the alpha motor neuron pool of the muscle undergoing contraction. In this way, the GTOs tend to counteract the excitatory effects of the gamma loop on the alpha motor neurons. The GTOs, through the Ib fibers, are thought to provide a steady inhibitory feedback so that the stretch reflex develops consistently less tension than it would in the absence of GTO influences. The exquisite balance of the excitatory effects of the gamma loop and the inhibitory effects of the Golgi tendon arcs are basic to the precise integration and timing of reflex activity. Through reciprocal innervation the GTO in a tendon inhibits the agonist but excites the antagonist. In this arrangement, the antagonists are said to be protected against excessive stretch by the Ib on the agonists.

The inhibition of the motor neuron in reflex pathway by means of a GTO in the tendon of the muscle being inhibited is called *autogenic inhibition*. This type of reflex inhibition resulting from a stimulated GTO of a stretched or overly contracted muscle is important because it can serve a protective function. The principal function of the GTOs is in autogenic inhibition. Unlike the sensitivity of neuromuscular spindles, that of the GTOs cannot be adjusted by the central nervous system because no efferent fibers from the central nervous system innervate the GTOs. Another important expression of GTO activity is in the inverse myotatic reflex (later on in chapter).

Tonus

When muscles are "at rest" some muscle fibers in any muscle are always contracted. This results in a residual tautness known as *muscle tone*. It is due to the continuous asynchronous discharge of a few motor units. Tonus is related primarily to the functional activity of the muscle spindles. Because muscles inserted to bones are in a continuous state of stretch, some of their muscle spindles must also be partially stretched. As a consequence some muscle spindles are always firing asynchronously. This is sufficient to produce the activity essential to maintain muscle tonus.

Flexor reflex responses (protective or withdrawal reflexes) (Fig. 5-24)

The flexor responses are initiated by a heterogeneous group of afferents called *flexor reflex afferents* (*FRAs*) with receptor endings in the skin, muscles, joints, and viscera. They include A delta and C pain fibers, group II (secondary spindle afferents) fibers, and groups III and IV (free nerve endings of myelinated afferents) fibers (see Fig. 2-20). These FRAs activate interneuronal circuits with widespread polysynaptic connections within the spinal cord. The eventual effects of this spinal activity are (1) excitation of the alpha motor neurons to flexor muscles and (2) inhibition of the alpha motor neurons to the antagonistic extensor muscles.

If the level of reflex excitability within the cord is highly elevated and the stimulus is intense, the flexor reflex activity may spread to evoke responses in the circuits influencing the contralateral extremity. This spread excites the neurons involved with the crossed extensor response (reflex) with the synchronous excitation of the extensor motor neurons and inhibition of the flexor motor neurons. The functional value of

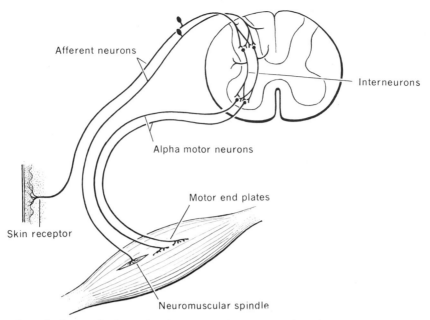

FIGURE 5-24 The flexor reflex loop. This three-neuron, disynaptic, ipsilateral, intersegmental reflex is composed of a sensory receptor in the skin, afferent neuron, spinal intersegmental neurons, alpha motor neurons, and voluntary muscles. This reflex can be facilitated by the "secondary sensory ending" (flower spray ending) of neuromuscular spindle, afferent neuron, spinal interneurons, alpha motor neurons, and voluntary muscles.

this added crossed extensor response is in supporting the body; when the right lower extremity withdraws from an intense stimulus by flexion, the extension of the contralateral extremity acts to support the body.

Principle of reciprocal innervation (Fig. 5-25)

In a movement of a joint, the contraction of the agonist (prime mover) muscles is coordinated with the synchronous relaxation of the antagonist muscles, as in walking or running. For example, to obtain the smooth flexion movement, the flexor muscle groups (agonist muscles) contract while the extensor muscle groups (antagonist muscles) relax synergistically during the movement. In the reflex circuits, interneurons integrate the excitatory and inhibitory stimuli (*reciprocal inhibition of an antagonist*) upon the lower motor neurons; this ensures the coordinated reciprocal innervation of the agonist and the antagonist. In the monosynaptic extensor reflex (knee jerk), the Ia fibers from the stretched neuromuscular spindles of the quadriceps muscles monosynaptically facilitate the alpha motor neurons innervating the extensor quadriceps muscles to contract. In addition, a collateral branch of the Ia fibers facilitates the "inhibitory" interneurons which inhibit the alpha motor neurons innervating the antagonistic flexor muscles. The Ib afferent fibers may also be integrated into this circuitry. The influences conveyed via the Ib fibers from the stimulated Golgi tendon organs (1) may excite the inhibitory interneuron, which, in turn, inhibits the alpha motor neurons innervating the agonist and (2) may facilitate an excitatory interneuron, which, in turn, excites the alpha motor neuron innervating the antagonist muscles. In *crossed extensor reflexes*, the coordination of the ipsilateral limb with the contralateral limb reflex activity is possible because of a double reciprocal innervation via commissural neurons.

In a static situation such as quiet standing, the Ia inhibitory interneurons are partially inhibited by other interneurons; as a consequence flexion and extension are simultaneously active.

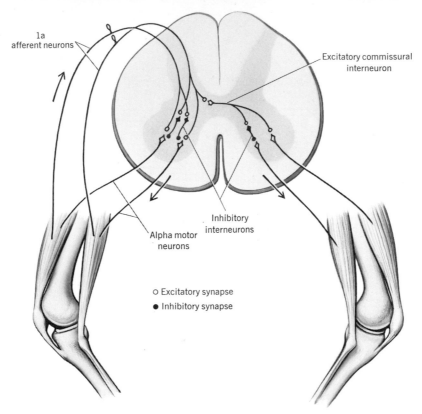

FIGURE 5-25 Reciprocal innervation of the agonist and antagonist muscles in an ipsilateral reflex (left side) and in a contralateral "crossed" reflex (right side).

Monosynaptic flexor reflex

The *jaw jerk* or *pluck reflex* is a powerful antigravity action which results in clenching the teeth. A tap on the jaw evokes a set of synchronous volleys from the annulospiral endings of the spindles in the flexor muscles of mastication. The Ia neurons of the trigeminal nerve (cell body in trigeminal ganglion) monosynaptically excite the alpha motor neurons in the motor nucleus of the trigeminal nerve; hence a monosynaptic reflex.

Intrinsic spinal interneurons and fasciculi proprii (Fig. 5-12)

The spinal interneurons whose axons course and terminate within the spinal cord are organized into complex circuits which have not, as yet, been described in detail. Some spinal interneurons have axons which are distributed ipsila-

terally within their own spinal segment on one side. These interneurons are actually intercalated within the circuits of ipsilateral intrasegmental multineuronal reflexes. Other spinal interneurons, called *commissural interneurons*, have axons which cross to the contralateral side and terminate in the same and other spinal segments. Most interneurons have collateral branches which extend up and down for a number of segments. Some of these fibers course within the gray matter. Others pass into the white matter adjacent to the gray matter as intersegmental fibers and ascend or descend for various distances before entering and synapsing within the gray matter. These fibers form the *fasciculi proprii* (*propriospinal or spinospinalis tracts*). These fasciculi are present in all three funiculi (see Fig. 5-12). The posterolateral fasciculus (or tract) is a portion of the spinospinalis tract in the lateral funiculus adjacent to the posterior horn (see Fig. 5-17).

The *commissural interneurons* and the *intersegmental interneurons* of the fasciculi proprii have significant roles in the more complex reflexes. The *crossed extensor reflex* utilizes commissural neurons to relay neural information across the midline (see Fig. 5-25). A painful stimulus on the foot may result in the reflex flexor withdrawal of the ipsilateral extremity and especially the enhancement of extensor musculature contractions of the contralateral limb to enable this contralateral extended limb to support the body when the flexed ipsilateral limb is off the ground. This interplay is utilized in the alternate rhythms of the extremities during walking and running, as one extremity is in active flexion while the contralateral extremity is in active extension.

A reflex utilizing ipsilateral intersegmental interneurons is the scratch reflex in a dog. This reflex is elicited when an irritation of the chest wall evokes a scratching response by the ipsilateral lower limb. This reflex utilizes intersegmental neurons with axons coursing through the ipsilateral fasciculi proprii.

Descending fibers in the posterior columns (Fig. 5-14)

Most of the descending branches of the dorsal root fibers within the posterior columns extend caudally only a few segments, although some may project for as many as 10 spinal segments. These descending fibers cluster into small bundles which tend to locate medially and posteriorly to the ascending pathways. In the sacral region, the descending fibers, called the *triangle of Gombault-Philippe*, are located in the dorsal part of the posterior column near the midline. In the lumbar region, the descending fibers, called the *septomarginal fasciculus*, are located deep adjacent to the posterior septum. In the cervical and most thoracic segments, the descending bundle of fibers, called *fasciculus interfascicularis*, is located in the middle of the posterior column, between the fasciculus gracilis and fasciculus cuneatus.

Renshaw cell

An interneuron, called the *Renshaw cell*, is intercalated between the recurrent collateral branches of the axon of the alpha motor neuron and the dendrites of the same alpha motor neuron (see Fig. 3-12). This negative feedback circuit (Chap. 3) acts as an autoinhibitor which dampens the alpha motor neuron (Chap. 13). This circuit probably serves to inhibit momentarily (recurrent inhibition) the discharge of the alpha motor neuron. The fiber of the Renshaw cell that synapses with the alpha motor neuron is probably a collateral branch of a neuron with connections with other neurons. The alpha motor neurons originating in the medial anterior horn (lamina IX) do not have recurrent collateral branches; this suggests that the neurons innervating the axial musculature do not require this form of antidromic feedback to the Renshaw and other neurons. The alpha motor neurons originating in the lateral anterior horn (lamina IX) do have recurrent collateral branches, suggesting that the neurons innervating the appendicular musculature require feedback inhibition.

Each alpha motor neuron receives input through its 2000 to 10,000 excitatory and inhibitory synapses with other neurons. This neuron is the final integrative battleground for excitation (EPSPs), inhibition (IPSPs), spatial summation, temporal summation, occlusion, and other neural processes. The integration of these activities by this neuron can result in the generation of an action potential in the axon capable of stimulating muscle contraction.

Central control of sensory input (reflected feedback pathways, descending pathways, and sensory input)

The central nervous system has a significant role in regulating the sensitivity by which the sensory receptors respond to both external and internal environmental stimuli. Through these centrally derived influences, the sensitivity of receptors may be enhanced or suppressed. This is one means by which the organism selects, biases, or rejects the influences of certain environmental stimuli.

The descending pathways from higher centers to relay nuclei of ascending pathways are called *reflected feedback pathways*. It is through these pathways that the cerebral cortex and brain stem exert their influences. Among these are pathways originating in the cerebral cortex, periaqueductal gray of the midbrain, some reticular nuclei of the brainstem, and the nucleus raphae magnus of the medulla (see Figs. 8-6 and 8-7). The descending influences from the cerebral cortex originate in the postcentral gyrus (somatosensory cortex, areas 1, 2, 3) and adjacent portions of the precentral gyrus and parietal cortex (area 5). They are conveyed by slow-conducting fine fibers of the corticospinal tract to laminae IV, V, and VI of the posterior horn. Some projections also terminate in Clarke's nucleus, the lateral cervical nucleus, and the nuclei gracilis and cuneatus. These spinal cord and lower medullary nuclei are processing stations of the major ascending pathways from the spinal cord.

Descending fibers from the periaqueductal gray (midbrain), nucleus raphae magnum (serotinergic nucleus in the medulla), and the medullary reticular formation (lateral reticulospinal tract) are mutually interconnected and project influences to the posterior horn (see Fig. 8-21). These influences can produce selective inhibitory effects on nociceptive transmission at the spinal level without any apparent change in the level of consciousness and other modalities. Endogenous substances such as endorphins may also modulate nociceptive input (Chap. 8). Electric stimulation in mammals of the periaqueductal gray and nucleus raphae magnus may produce analgesia. This effect following such stimulation is called *stimulus-produced analgesia* (Chap. 8).

After an animal is stressed, the sensitivity of the corpuscles of Meissner is enhanced so that these receptors are more responsive to tactile stimulation. Apparently the activity of the sympathetic nervous system is responsible, because the hypersensitivity is due, at least in part, to the increased concentrations of norepinephrine within the receptors. The central control of the responsiveness of the neuromuscular spindle by the gamma efferent neurons is an example of the influences exerted by the central nervous system in biasing the activity of a peripheral receptor. The sensitivity of the hair cells of the spiral organ of Corti is suppressed by the activity of the efferent cochlear bundle (olivocochlear bundle, Chap. 10). The fibers of this bundle arise in the superior olivary complex of the brainstem and terminate by synapsing on the hair cells. Influences conveyed by these fibers are inhibitory, making the hair cells less responsive to auditory stimuli.

Substrates for coordination of muscle activity — motor programs

The circuitry within the infratentorial brainstem and spinal cord contains the neural substrates for the basic patterns of motor activities including locomotion (walking, running, and flying), eye and head movements, respiration, chewing, and swallowing. These patterns of activity have been demonstrated to be centrally generated and are not dependent for their existence upon inputs from the peripheral sensors or the higher centers in the brain. Such central patterns are known as *motor programs*. The existence of the central rhythm generation within the spinal cord is demonstrable in the hind-leg movements in a decerebrate animal (transected through upper brainstem) in the absence of sensory input from the periphery (dorsal roots to hind limbs severed). Under appropriate conditions, these animals can walk on a moving treadmill, and the temporal sequences of flexion and extension of the limb movements are rhythmic. To obtain this rhythm the animal must be supported. The decerebrate animal cannot stand because of its inability to regulate muscle tone.

In the execution of fine movements, feedback influences from the periphery are essential, especially continuous feedback inputs from neuromuscular spindles, Golgi tendon organs, and joint receptors. The angle at which a joint is held is a major source of information for position sense and the detection of movement. These inputs are critical in making the continuous compensatory actions essential in carrying out any movement. For example, the information generated in the sensors modifies the motor program in making continuous adjustments in the activity of the muscles (1) in the lower extremities while walking on a rough terrain and (2) in the upper extremities in manipulating, handling, and gripping objects of different shapes, sizes, and weights. The sensory input functions to modify the motor program and to integrate actions responsive to the environmental demands. The responses may be phasic as in walking or static as in assuring balance and stability. The modulation of motor programs are additionally responses to inputs from the visual system and the vestibular system.

The volitional expressions of activity are influences by such higher levels as the cerebral cortex (Chap. 16) and basal ganglia (Chap. 14). The cerebral cortex is involved with the initiation, maintenance, and change of motor activities. The motor programs are not preformed in these higher levels; rather, these levels act to set activities in other centers in the brainstem into motion. In turn, these centers activate, modulate, and bias the motor programs intrinsic within the brainstem (for motor activity in the head) and within the spinal cord (for motor activity in the body).

Descending pathways from the brain (upper motor neurons)

The neurons that form the descending motor pathways from the brain to the spinal cord (and from the cerebrum to the brainstem) are known as upper motor neurons (see Figs. 5-26 through 5-31). In contrast to the lower motor neurons, which commence in the central nervous system and terminate in the muscles of the body, the upper motor neurons are wholly within the central nervous system. The pathways of these neurons are listed and outlined below according to the locations of their nuclei of origin. Opinions differ concerning many of the detailed features of the pathways. Those descending fibers that terminate in the cervical spinal segments are largely involved with the motor activities of the neck (position of the head) and of the upper extremity, and those that terminate in the lumbosacral spinal segments are largely involved with the motor activities of the lower extremity. All spinal cord segments have a role in axial (trunk) muscle integration.

The upper motor neurons exert their influences primarily upon the spinal reflex loops and circuits by modifying and biasing their activities. Other descending fibers exert influences to the preganglionic fibers of the autonomic nervous system (Chap. 6) and to nuclei of the ascending pathways (Chap. 8). In general, the upper motor neurons synapse with interneurons which, in turn, terminate on either the alpha motor neurons or the gamma motor neurons. Some upper motor neurons terminate directly on alpha and gamma motor neurons. Through these connections, the higher centers of the nervous system can control the alpha motor neurons independently of the gamma motor neurons.

Cerebral cortex

The *corticospinal tracts* (*pyramidal tracts*) originate from widespread areas of the cerebral neocortex and descend through the corona radiata, the internal capsule, and the basilar portion of the brainstem (including the pyramids of medulla and hence the pyramidal tracts) to the caudal end of the medulla, where the pathways diverge before entering the spinal cord (see Figs. 5-11 and 5-26). The pyramidal tract is topographically organized in its course from the cortex to the medulla (pyramids); this organization is obscured during the decussation and is not regained. About 60 percent of the corticospinal fibers originate from areas 4 and 6 of the frontal lobe (see Fig. 5-26; see also Fig. 16-7); the remaining 40 percent arise from areas 1, 2, 3, and 5 of the parietal lobe. Of the pyramidal fibers, about 90 percent are small fibers ranging in diameter from 1 to 4 μm. Fewer than 9 percent range from 5 to 10 μm in diameter, and fewer than 2 percent are large fibers, ranging from 10 to 22 μm in diameter.

Approximately 85 to 90 percent of the 1 million or more fibers cross over as the pyramidal decussation to form the lateral corticospinal tract of the spinal cord (see Fig. 8-5). Most of the remaining fibers continue as the anterior (ventral) corticospinal tract, as uncrossed fibers. A few uncrossed fibers are present in the lateral corticospinal tract. The lateral corticospinal tract extends throughout the spinal cord, with roughly 50 percent of its fibers terminating in the cervical segments, 20 percent in the thoracic segments, and 30 percent in the lumbosacral segments. The uncrossed anterior corticospinal tract crosses within the cervical spinal cord through the anterior white commissure and terminates largely in laminae VII and VIII of the

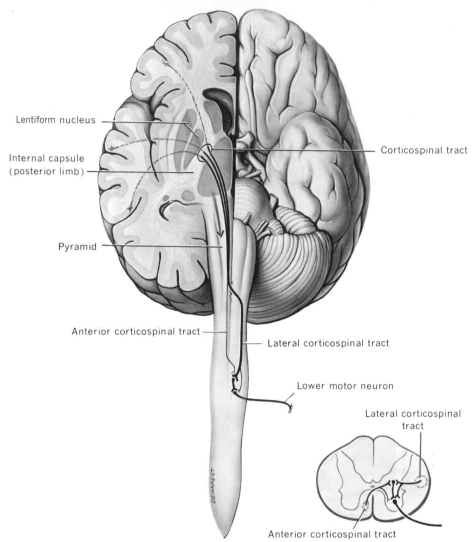

Lentiform nucleus

Internal capsule
(posterior limb)

Pyramid

Anterior corticospinal tract

Corticospinal tract

Lateral corticospinal tract

Lower motor neuron

Lateral corticospinal
tract

Anterior corticospinal tract

DEMAREST

FIGURE 5-26 Corticospinal pathways. These pathways are composed of descending fibers that originate from wide areas of the cerebral cortex, pass through the posterior limb of the internal capsule, crus cerebri, pons, pyramid, and spinal cord. Many of these fibers terminate upon spinal interneurons that, in turn, synapse with the lower motor neurons. Some fibers terminate directly upon lower motor neurons. The lateral corticospinal tract crosses over at the lower medulla as the pyramidal decussation, and the anterior corticospinal tract crosses over in upper spinal cord levels.

cervical segments. In humans, an estimated 90 percent of the corticospinal fibers from area 4 synapse with interneurons in laminae IV, V, VI, and VII, and a few synapse directly with the dendrites of the alpha lower motor neurons (lamina IX, see Figs. 5-11, 5-14, and 5-26).

It is through these monosynaptic connections with the alpha motor neurons that the cerebral cortex can exert a rapid and direct control of fine and delicate muscular activity. Depending upon the muscle group, the "motor cortex" of a given cerebral hemisphere may influence a muscle group of the contralateral side only or the same muscle group on both sides. The muscles of an extremity receive input from the contralateral cerebral cortex while those of the larynx, pharynx, and trunk (axial) muscles of one side receive their input from cortices of both hemispheres.

The corticospinal tract plays a significant role in precise and dexterous voluntary movements, mainly by facilitating flexion in the extremities. When this tract is damaged, there is marked impairment of volitional activity, especially of the finer movements in the distal segments of the extremities. The movements of the proximal joints and the grosser actions are less severely and less permanently affected. The descending fibers originating from the postcentral gyrus and adjacent parietal cortex (areas 1, 2, 3, and 5 of the "sensory" cortex) terminate within laminae IV, V, and VI of the posterior horn of the spinal cord; it is through these connections that the cortex can regulate, in part, sensory input largely by presynaptic inhibition.

Apparently the corticospinal tract exerts facilitatory influences on both the alpha and gamma motor neurons to the flexor muscles and inhibitory influences on the alpha and gamma motor neurons to the extensor muscles during flexion. These excitatory and inhibitory activities are primarily mediated through interneurons of the intrinsic circuits in the spinal cord.

Midbrain

Three tracts originate in the midbrain and terminate in the gray matter of the spinal cord: the rubrospinal, tectospinal, and interstitiospinal tracts (see Figs. 5-14, 5-27, 5-30).

The *rubrospinal tract* originates in the magnocellular portion of the nucleus ruber of the midbrain tegmentum (see Fig. 8-21). Its fibers cross immediately to the opposite side as the ventral tegmental decussation, and many descend through the entire length of the spinal cord to terminate in the posterior and intermediate spinal gray matter in a somatotopic pattern.

The rubrospinal tract seems to have a similar pattern of termination in the spinal laminae, and it produces effects on the flexor and extensor muscles similar to those of the corticospinal tract. In a way the corticorubrospinal tract is the indirect route from the cerebral cortex to the spinal cord (tract also receives cerebellar influences in the nucleus ruber). In contrast, the corticospinal tract is the direct route from cortex to spinal cord. The nucleus ruber and the rubrospinal tract are topographically organized.

The nucleus ruber receives its major input from the motor cortex (precentral gyrus) of the same side (*corticorubral tract*) and from the emboliform nucleus of the contralateral cerebellar hemisphere (*cerebellorubral fibers*). Within the spinal cord, the fibers of the rubrospinal tract are located anterior to and overlap with the fibers of the lateral corticospinal tract. They terminate upon interneurons in the lateral aspect of laminae V and VI and in the central portions of lamina VII. The excitatory influences on extension and inhibitory influences on flexion are exerted upon both the alpha and gamma motor neurons.

The combination of corticorubral tract and rubrospinal suggest the functional system as corticorubrospinal tract (see Fig. 8-21). The origin of this tract in the motor cortex and its termination in the spinal cord overlaps that of the corticospinal tract.

The *tectospinal tract* originates from cells in the intermediate and deep layers of the superior colliculus of the midbrain tectum (Figs. 5-27 and 5-30). After crossing through the region around the periaqueductal gray of the upper midbrain as the dorsal tegmental decussation (see Fig. A-10), its fibers descend through the brainstem as a bundle located anterior to the medial longitudinal fasciculus (MLF). These fibers join the MLF in the anterior funiculus of the spinal cord. They terminate upon interneurons in laminae medial VI and VII and VIII of all cervical levels, but mainly those of the upper four cervical segments (see Fig. 5-30). Because the superior colliculus is a major subcortical center of the visual system, it is probable that the tectospinal tract mediates visually directed reflex movements of the head through the musculature of the neck.

The small *interstitiospinal tract* originates from the *interstitial nucleus of Cajal* and nucleus of Darkschewitsch located in the midbrain dorsolateral to the oculomotor nuclei. Its fibers descend bilaterally within the MLF and terminate in parts of lamina VIII of all spinal levels (see Fig. 8-12).

Descending fibers originate from (1) ante-

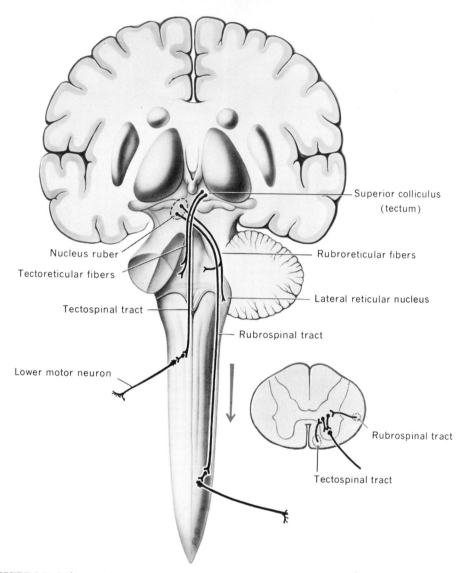

FIGURE 5-27 Rubrospinal tract and tectospinal tract. The rubrospinal tract originates in the nucleus ruber, decussates as the ventral tegmental decussation in the midbrain, and descends into the spinal cord. The tecto-spinal tract originates in the superior colliculus, decussates as the anterior tegmental decussation in the mid-brain, and descends into the spinal cord. The descending fibers of these tracts terminate largely upon inter-neurons, which, in turn, synapse with the lower motor neurons. The rubroreticular and tectoreticular (tectobulbar) fibers terminate in the brainstem reticular nuclei, which, in turn, are integrated into other path-ways (Chap. 8).

rior and lateral periaqueductal gray matter, (2) lateral tegmentum (nucleus cuneiformis; see Fig. 8-10), and (3) central tegmentum. This ipsila-terally projecting pathway may have an important role in the anterolateral pathways. Fibers of the lateral spinothalamic tract do ter-minate in the nucleus cuneiform. The periaque-ductal gray is involved with stimulus-produced analgesia and endorphins (Chap. 8).

Pons and medulla

Two significant pathway complexes originate in the lower brainstem and terminate in the spinal

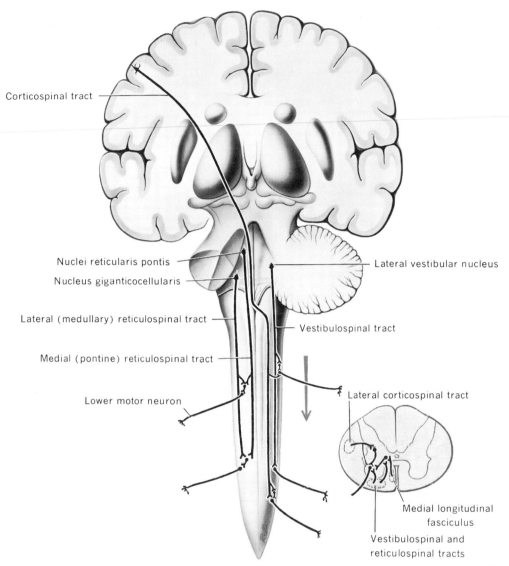

Corticospinal tract

Nuclei reticularis pontis

Nucleus giganticocellularis

Lateral (medullary) reticulospinal tract

Medial (pontine) reticulospinal tract

Lower motor neuron

Lateral vestibular nucleus

Vestibulospinal tract

Lateral corticospinal tract

Medial longitudinal fasciculus

Vestibulospinal and reticulospinal tracts

FIGURE 5-28 Reticulospinal tracts, vestibulospinal tract, and corticospinal tract. The pontine reticulospinal tract originates in the nuclei reticularis pontis oralis and caudalis of the tegmentum of the pons. The medullary reticulospinal tract originates in the nucleus gigantocellularis of the medulla. The vestibulospinal tract originates in the lateral vestibular nucleus. The medial longitudinal fasciculus is illustrated in Fig. 10-11.

cord: the vestibulospinal and the reticulospinal tracts.

The *vestibulospinal tracts* arise from cells located in the vestibular nuclei of the upper dorsolateral medulla (see Figs. 5-11, 5-14, 5-28, and 5-31). The vestibular nuclei receive their input from receptors in the vestibular labyrinth and from the cerebellum. The main input to the lateral vestibular nucleus is from the vestibular labyrinth of the utricle. The (*lateral*) *vestibulospinal tract* originates from the lateral vestibular nucleus and descends as uncrossed fibers within the lateral tegmentum of the medulla and throughout the entire length of the spinal cord within the anterolateral funiculus. The fibers of this somatotopically organized tract originating in the rostroventral lateral vestibular nucleus terminate in the cervical levels; those originating in the dorsocaudal part of the nucleus terminate in the lumbosacral levels; and those originating in the intermediate part terminate in the thoracic levels. The fibers synapse primarily with interneurons of lamina VIII and the medial part of lamina VII, although a few terminate directly on dendrites of the lower motor neurons in lamina IX. The descending influences of this tract act by facilitating spinal reflex activity and extensor muscle tone in the ipsilateral extremities. Some inhibitory activity on flexor neurons is exerted. The role of vestibular influences upon equilibrium and posture is expressed by the numerous fibers which terminate in the cervical levels (musculature of the neck and upper extremities) and in the lumbosacral levels (musculature of the lower extremities).

The *medial vestibular nucleus* gives rise to fibers (sometimes called the *medial vestibulospinal tract*) which descend ipsilaterally within the MLF primarily to cervical levels. These fibers terminate as do those of the vestibulospinal tract, in lamina VII and adjacent portions of lamina VII. These fibers exert inhibitory influences upon extensor muscle tone. There may be a reciprocal innervation by both vestibulospinal pathways upon the same alpha motor neurons to the neck musculature. In one respect these fibers from the medial vestibular nucleus are unusual; they are the only supraspinal descending fibers known to exert inhibitory effects directly upon alpha motor neurons.

The *reticulospinal pathways* include the descending fibers whose nuclei of origin are tegmental nuclei of the brainstem reticular formation (see Figs. 5-11, 5-14, 5-29, and 5-31; see also Figs. 8-9 and 8-10). The *pontine (medial) reticulospinal tract* originates in the medial pontine tegmentum from the *nucleus reticularis pontis oralis* (located in the rostral pons) and the *nucleus reticularis pontis caudalis* (located in the caudal pons). It descends primarily as an uncrossed tract in the vicinity of the MLF in the brainstem and within the anterior funiculus throughout the entire spinal cord. The fibers terminate upon interneurons in lamina VIII and adjacent portions of laminae VII and IX. Some of its fibers decussate in the anterior white commissure. The *medullary (lateral) reticulospinal tract* originates from the *nucleus reticularis gigantocellularis*, located in the medial reticular formation of the rostral

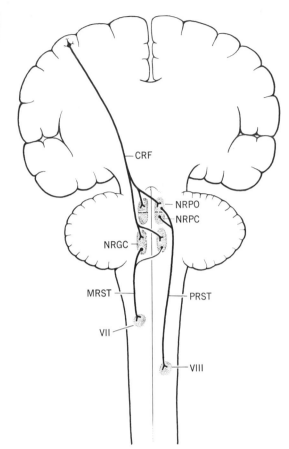

FIGURE 5-29 The reticulospinal tracts and the corticoreticulospinal system. CRF, corticoreticular fibers; MRST, medullary reticulospinal tract; NRGC, nucleus reticularis gigantocellularis; NRPC, nucleus reticularis pontis caudalis; NRPO, nucleus reticularis pontis oralis; PRST, pontine reticulospinal tract. (*From Noback and Harting, Spinal Cord, S. Karger, Basel.*)

medulla (see Fig. 8-8). It descends as an uncrossed tract, with some crossed fibers, within the anterior aspect of the lateral funiculus throughout the entire spinal cord. The fibers terminate upon interneurons in lateral lamina VIII and adjacent parts of laminae VI and IX. This tract contains some of the fastest axons in the CNS (conducting up to 138 m/s).

The input to these pontine and medullary reticular nuclei is largely derived from (1) descending corticoreticular fibers from the pre- and postcentral gyri (motor, premotor, and somesthetic cortex), (2) *spinoreticular fibers*, and (3) cerebellum (Chap. 9). The descending fibers are distributed bilaterally, but most of them termi-

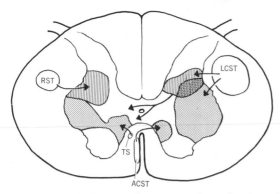

FIGURE 5-30 The location of some major descending (motor) tracts within the white matter and their sites of termination within the gray matter. ACST, anterior corticospinal tract; LCST, lateral corticospinal tract; RST, rubrospinal tract; and TS, tectospinal tract. (*From Noback and Harting, Spinal Cord, S. Karger, Publisher, Basel.*)

nate contralaterally in the lower brainstem tegmentum. These *corticoreticulospinal tracts* are not somatotopically organized; they apparently exert their influences through interneurons upon the gamma motor neurons. The medial reticulospinal fibers terminate in the same neuronal pool as the vestibulospinal fibers, while the lateral reticulospinal fibers terminate in some of the neuronal pools as the corticospinal and rubrospinal fibers (see Figs. 5-27, 5-30, and 5-31).

In general, the reticulospinal tracts convey influences which regulate motor activities related to posture and muscle tone through alpha and gamma motor neurons. The medial reticulospinal tract facilitates the extensor reflex and inhibits the flexor reflex (reciprocal innervation); the lateral reticulospinal tract inhibits the extensor reflex and facilitates the flexor reflex. Stimulation of the medullary reticular formation generally inhibits reflexes and muscle tone and movements evoked by cerebral cortical stimulation (*cortically induced movements*). Stimulation of the pontine reticular formation generally produces opposite effects.

Medial longitudinal fasciculus (MLF)

The *medial longitudinal fasciculus* (MLF) is a composite bundle of fibers extending from the upper midbrain (level of the nucleus of the oculomotor nerve) through the spinal cord (Fig. 10-11). It is located in the posteromedial part of the

anterior funiculus (see Figs. 5-11 and 5-14). The MLF of the lower brainstem and spinal cord is composed of the descending fibers of the tectospinal, interstitiospinal, pontine reticulospinal, and "medial" vestibulospinal fibers (Chap. 10).

Descending autonomic fibers

Within the lower brainstem reticular formation are neuronal pools of the autonomic nervous system which receive inputs from the hypothalamus (via the midbrain reticular formation), other levels of the brain, and cranial nerves (Chaps. 6 and 11). From these pontine and medullary pools, influences are relayed via "reticulospinal" fibers to interneurons within the spinal gray matter. These interneurons are in synaptic contact with the preganglionic neurons of the sympathetic system located in levels T1 through L2, and with preganglionic neurons of the parasympathetic system located in levels S2 through S4. The descending spinal autonomic (reticulospinal) fibers are apparently located in the anterior and anterolateral funiculi in close proximity to the spinal gray matter.

Descending somatic influences

The descending pathways from the higher centers in the brain probably produce movements (1) by sending "direct" influences to the alpha motor neurons and (2) by sending "indirect" in-

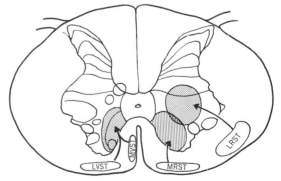

FIGURE 5-31 The location of some major descending (motor) tracts within the white matter and their sites of termination within the gray matter. MRST, pontine (medial) reticulospinal tract; MVST, "medial" vestibulospinal tract; LRST, medullary (lateral) reticulospinal tract; LVST, "lateral" vestibulospinal tract. (*From Noback and Harting, Spinal Cord, S. Karger, Publisher, Basel.*)

fluences to the gamma motor neurons and thereby acting through a feedback loop from the spindle to produce the desired contraction. Upon stimulation, the central nuclei in the brain have been shown to produce or to inhibit movement; hence the basic generalization that each central nucleus probably is able to excite (or to inhibit) the alpha and gamma motor neurons involved in the same basic contraction in much the same manner. In brief, both alpha and gamma motor nuclei are normally coinfluenced by descending pathways (this is called *"servo-assistance" of movement*). Thus in finger movements and respiratory movements, for example, the essential contraction of a muscle group through the alpha motor neurons commences just prior to the rise in the spindle firing from gamma stimulation. The latter has facilitated the essential contraction. Stated simply, the descending tracts from the brain convey influences which essentially bias the intrinsic activity of the spinal reflex circuitry.

In general usage, spinal reflexes are basically responses to neural influences conveyed as action potentials from the peripheral receptors. In contrast, voluntary activities are responses to neural influences conveyed as action potentials from the brain to the spinal cord. Voluntary activities need not be initiated by volitional drives. Under natural conditions neurons function in groups; thus a natural stimulus evokes many action potentials, called a volley, which influence the functional activity of a group of physiologically characterized neurons—called a neuronal pool. The inputs to a neuronal pool are expressed as excitatory and inhibitory postsynaptic potentials (EPSPs and IPSPs), whereas the output of reflex and voluntary activity via the lower motor neurons is expressed as obligatory excitatory responses of muscle contractions.

Coactivation The state of contraction of the infrafusal muscles of the neuromuscular spindles and that of the extrafusal muscles are synchronized by the integrated stimulation from the alpha and gamma motor neurons. This coordination is accomplished by the stimultaneous activation of these motor neurons (called *coactivation*) by influences from each of the following: Ia fibers from the spindles, Ib fibers from the Golgi

tendon organs, and some fibers of descending tracts from the brain. The functional role of this alpha-gamma coactivation system in a voluntary movement can be illustrated by the activity initiated by the influences through the corticospinal tract.

The descending pathways from the cortex and brainstem centers have a significant role in the coactivation of the alpha and gamma motor neurons. The net result of this normal flow is to sustain a steady "tonic" background input to the alpha motor neuron during the maintenance of a joint angle. In this regard the static gamma efferents are critical.

In a voluntary movement such as pointing a finger, the impulses in the pyramidal system activate the alpha and gamma motor neuronal complex controlling the finger movements in an approximately synchronous pattern. The alpha motor neurons are stimulated to produce an obligatory contraction of extrafusal muscle fibers. At the same time the gamma motor neurons are stimulated to convey impulses which excite the intrafusal fibers of the spindles to contract. In this way the appropriate gamma loop is activated. The slight time it takes for the influences to travel over the gamma loop means that the resulting alpha motor neuron discharge, generated by the Ia fibers from the spindle, occurs just after the extrafusal fibers had commenced to contract following the direct stimulation of the alpha motor neurons by the pyramidal system. Thus the voluntary stimulation of the extrafusal fibers by the corticospinal fibers occurs at the precisely right moment just prior to the onset of the servomechanism control via the gamma loop from the spindle to the extrafusal muscle fibers. In a voluntary movement, therefore, the pyramidal influences excite the initial contraction of the extrafusal fibers just prior to a close follow-up from the excitatory stimulation from the gamma loop. The automatic adjustments at the spinal level associated with voluntary movements are further regulated by influences conveyed from the spindles and Golgi tendon organs via the Ia and Ib fibers. In turn these fibers can coactivate both the alpha and gamma motor neurons.

The influences of the descending tracts are upon the reflex arcs of the spinal cord. The spinal reflex arcs contain the basic substrates for trunk and extremity movements essential to walking and running. In addition to their function of modifying and coordinating the spinal reflexes, the descending pathways are crucial to the ability to stand; a *"spinal human"* is unable to stand (see "Paraplegia," further on in this chapter). This is the basis of the statement that spinal humans (or animals) could walk or run, if they could stand unsupported.

Peripheral control theory and central control theory

Motor activities involve the participation of both the peripheral and central nervous systems. *Peripheral control theory* states that coordinated movements are products of linking reflex movements into the overall movement from smaller, discrete phases of motor parameters. According to this concept, the feedback involving the peripheral nervous system from each phase of the motor activity results in the excitation (or inhibition) of each subsequent phase. In contrast, the *central control theory* states that the feedback from the periphery is not essential for the elaboration of coordinated motor activities because the central nervous system contains all the circuitry and information required for the control of organized movements (refer to "Substrates for Coordination of Motor Activity" earlier in the chapter). The experimental evidence indicates that the central control of movements is the more critical and that the peripheral system exerts its role by modulating the intrinsic motor program of the central nervous system.

Some of the evidence favoring the central control theory is derived from observations of experimental studies on monkeys (Taub et al.). With all of its dorsal roots innervating either one or both upper extremities, a monkey can make purposeful movements, including those used in climbing and in gathering and eating food. Visual clues are not needed, for these movements can be made in the absence of visual stimuli. The ventral root afferents are probably not involved because these fibers are not associated with reflex and feedback mechanisms. Those monkeys with deafferented limbs do demonstrate that the central motor programs are capable of initiating and sustaining the basic movements. However,

the animals do not have the fluency of control, timing, and rapidity possessed by normal animals; the finer coordination requires the participation of peripheral influences.

In the monkey, these central motor programs develop within the central nervous system endogenously during fetal life. This is indicated in young monkeys that have had an entire limb deafferented by dorsal root section as early as just prior to the middle of pregnancy. After birth, these young monkeys can learn to make purposeful movements with the deafferented limb. The basic conclusion is that the central circuits involved with motor programs develop during the fetal period and that the somatosensory peripheral system is required for precision, accuracy, and smoothness of movements. In addition, the primate central nervous system can generate movements of almost all types autonomously in the absence of guidance from sensory cues from the organism's own body.

BLOOD SUPPLY OF THE SPINAL CORD (Figs. 5-32 and 5-33)

The adult spinal cord derives its arterial supply from a variable number of small spinal arteries which are branches of larger arteries just outside the vertebral column. These larger arteries include the *vertebral, ascending cervical, deep cervical, intercostal,* and *lumbar* and *sacral arteries.* The small spinal arteries travel along with the spinal nerves, pass through the intervertebral foramina, penetrate through the dura mater, and divide into the *dorsal* and *ventral radicular (spinal) arteries,* which accompany the corresponding nerve roots. There is much variation in the number of large and small radicular arteries. Generally the anterior radicular arteries are larger than the posterior radicular arteries. The number of larger radicular arteries on both sides ranges from 15 to 34 in humans (average 24).

These arteries form three main longitudinal channels along the entire spinal cord: an *anterior spinal artery (anterior longitudinal arterial channel)* at the anterior median fissure, and a pair of *posterior spinal arteries (posterior longitudinal arterial channels)* adjacent to the entering dorsal spinal rootlets. An anastomotic network of

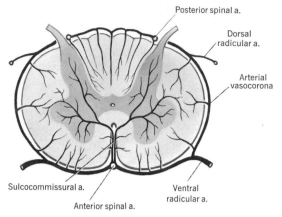

FIGURE 5-32 The arterial supply of the spinal cord.

branches from the anterior and posterior spinal arteries, called the *arterial vasocorona*, is located on the anterior and lateral surface of the spinal cord. Branches from the vertebral arteries supply most of the cervical spinal segments; these include the anterior spinal, posterior spinal, and inferior cerebellar arteries (Chap. 1). The *ascending and deep cervical arteries* give rise to the radicular arteries to spinal segments C7 to T2. The spinal cord levels caudal to T2 derive their blood supply from branches of the *aorta* and *internal iliac arteries*. The *anterior* and *posterior spinal arteries* arise from the intracranial portion of the vertebral arteries. These arteries supply part of the lower medulla and upper cervical spinal segments. The posterior spinal arteries descend and join the posterior longitudinal arterial channels. The anterior spinal arteries join on the anterior median surface of the medulla (see Fig. 5-32) to form the unpaired spinal artery, which descends to join the anterior longitudinal arterial channel of the spinal cord.

Certain levels of the spinal cord, especially those in a zone between two regions deriving their blood supply from different major arteries, have sparse collateral circulatory anastomoses. These levels are vulnerable to vascular injury, i.e., *ischemic necrosis*, which may result in a transection of the cord. C2 to C3, T1 to T4, and L1 are considered to be such vulnerable levels (see Fig. 5-33).

The distribution of the veins of the spinal cord is similar to that of the spinal arteries. They course along with the arteries and drain out-

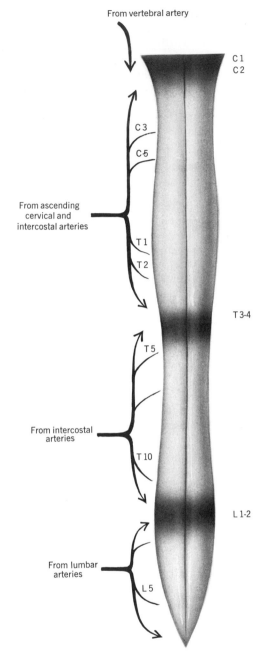

FIGURE 5-33 The sources of the arterial supply of the spinal cord. The upper cervical, upper thoracic, and upper lumbar spinal segments are zones located between two regions deriving their blood supply from different major arteries.

ward via the dorsal and ventral roots into the massive *internal vertebral venous plexus (spino-vertebral venous plexus, epidural venous plexus)* located between the dura mater and the periosteum of the vertebral column. There are about 6 to 11 large anterior radicular veins and roughly an equal number of posterior radicular veins. This valve-free venous plexus has rich and ample connections with the azygous vein and other veins of the thoracic, abdominal, and pelvic cavities.

FUNCTIONAL AND APPLIED CONSIDERATIONS

Some functional aspects of the spinal cord are emphasized in the following illustrations (see Fig. 5-34).

Afferent correlations

Dorsal roots and posterior columns The irritation of the fibers of one *dorsal root (radix)* by mechanical compression (by a slipped disk or extra-

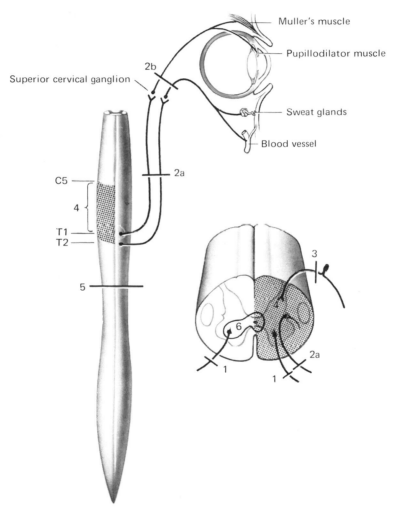

FIGURE 5-34 Some lesions of the spinal nerves and spinal cord. Lesions discussed are at (1) ventral roots of spinal nerves; (2a) preganglionic sympathetic fibers from T1 and T2 levels; (2b) postganglionic sympathetic fibers from the superior cervical ganglion; (3) posterior roots of spinal nerves; (4) hemisection of the spinal cord (Brown-Séquard syndrome) extending through the cervical enlargement; (5) transection of the spinal cord at a midthoracic level; and (6) region surrounding central canal throughout the cervical enlargement and extending into the anterior horn at the C8 and T1 level on one side. C5 to T1 is the cervical enlargement.

THE SPINAL CORD

medullary tumor) or a local inflammation may produce pain with a *radicular distribution* over the entire *dermatome* (Fig. 5-34). In herpes zoster (shingles) there is either a spontaneous, severe, intense pain, or a pain readily evoked by touch or pressure on one or more dermatomes. This pain is a consequence of the varicella zoster virus, which primarily affects one or more spinal ganglia. Because adjacent dermatomes overlap, the destruction of but one dorsal root (e.g., by transection, called rhizotomy) results in diminution of all sensations (hypesthesia) in that part of the dermatome innervated by the dorsal root. Destruction of several consecutive dorsal roots results in the complete absence of all sensations (anesthesia) in all but the rostral and caudal dermatomes of the roots sectioned. Irritation to the dorsal root fibers may result in paresthesia (abnormal spontaneous sensations such as numbness and prickling) or hyperesthesia (excessive sensibility to sensory stimuli in pain). The stimulation of a dorsal root may result in a dermatomal vasodilatation (due to the reflex arc involving the autonomic nervous system).

If a limb is completely deafferented, it is generally not used. For example, if all the dorsal roots innervating the upper extremity are sectioned (C5 through T1), the upper extremity is completely anesthetic (i.e., there is a complete absence of all forms of sensibility because of the lack of input). Because the afferent limbs of the reflex arcs are interrupted, reflex activity is absent (areflexia) and the muscles lack tone (i.e., they are hypotonic or atonic). Although the limb muscles are not paralyzed (lower motor neurons are intact), motor activity is impaired. The deafferented limb hangs by the side and is generally not used. The loss of muscle tone illustrates the significance to motor activity of peripheral sensory input from the neuromuscular spindles and Golgi tendon endings. Contraction of muscle is obtained when the volleys from the brain conveyed via upper motor neurons are sufficient to stimulate alpha motor neurons. On the other hand, a limb with only one dorsal root intact may be useful, as, for example, if dorsal root C8 is present but dorsal roots C5 to C6 and C7 and T1 are interrupted. Dorsal root C8 innervates the skin of the hand and palm. This indicates the importance of the skin sensations from this sensitive region in influencing movements.

A monkey with a completely deafferented limb does not use the limb; in the free situation no purposive movements occur. If the normal limb is restrained, the deafferented limb will make crude movements (e.g., grasp food). A monkey with both upper limbs completely deafferented will use both limbs for climbing the sides of the cage or one limb to grasp food. These actions are due to motivation, attention to body parts, and reinforcement.

Lesions and irritation of the dorsal roots or posterior horn result in segmental (dermatomal) sensory disturbances. In dorsal root lesions all general senses are involved, whereas in posterior horn lesions a *dissociated sensory loss* may occur in the dermatome, with pain and temperature sensibilities lost or reduced but with touch and other associated general senses intact and normal. Dissociated sensory loss (loss of one sensation and preservation of others) of pain and temperature also occurs with lesions in the vicinity of the central canal (see "Syringomyelia," farther on in this chapter).

The degeneration of the dorsal column neurons of the lumbosacral nerves in the disease *tabes dorsalis* impairs the proprioceptive and discriminative touch pathways. Tabes dorsalis is a consequence of a syphilitic infection of the dorsal roots with secondary degeneration of the posterior columns. General tactile sensibility is retained, but two-point tactile discrimination is lost. A stumbling, staggering gait known as *locomotor ataxia* is characteristic. The motor impairment is a result of a deficiency in proprioceptive input, not in the motor pathways per se. Because patients have difficulty in translating information about position and joint sense, they are only vaguely aware or "don't know where their legs are." To compensate, they walk with a broad base. Their feet slap sharply on the ground with each step. The use of visual cues by looking at the feet helps to compensate for the proprioceptive deficit.

Referred pain Pain of visceral origin is usually vaguely localized on the body surface. The pain may be interpreted as being located on the surface of the body somewhat removed from the primary source. This phenomenon, when visceral pain is subjectively felt in a somatic area, is known as "referred pain." The pain of coronary heart disease (angina pectoris) is referred to the left axilla, where the pain is subjectively felt. Irritation of the gallbladder may actually be felt under the shoulder blade. A stone in the ureter (duct from the kidney) results in an intense pain in the loin and groin.

Several explanations have been advanced to account for the subjective misinterpretation of the source of pain. The stimulation of the nerve endings within a viscus can evoke activity that may be referred from the viscus (such as the appendix, ureter, and heart, structures that are vaguely or not consciously perceived) to the skin or muscles (structures within our sphere of consciousness or expression action). Because the visceral source-location of the pain and the somatic area where the pain is felt are innervated by neurons utilizing a common dorsal root, the visceral sensory fibers and the somatic sensory fibers are presumed to discharge into a small common pool of neurons in some region of the central nervous system. Discharges from this pool to the cerebrum result in the referral of the pain. It has been documented that some cells in the posterior horn respond to both somatic and visceral stimulation. In essence, visceral afferent fibers are able to tap into the circuits normally used by the somatic afferent fibers from the skin. Thus, the brain can misinterpret the source of the pain and refer information from a viscus as coming from the skin. The response of the organism can be pain and tenderness of the skin and spasm by some muscles.

Muscle pain

Deep muscle pain, as in a "charley horse," occurs when the high-threshold muscle Group III and IV afferents are stimulated. These afferents correspond to the A delta and C fibers in other regions of the body. The stimulus for such pain is likely to be local anoxia or the stimulation of nociceptors by chemicals released in the connective tissues of the muscle.

Phantom limb An amputee is normally aware of his amputated extremity. This phantom limb moves easily, even through objects or the normal limb. The ring and wristwatch that were formerly worn can be felt on the finger and wrist, respectively. The phantom sensations of pain, pins and needles, arches, and thermal sense are felt by some amputees for many months, even years, following the amputation. Usually the phantom limb seems short, telescoped, embedded in the stump of the limb, or even separated from the stump; the distal segments of the phantom are felt to the exclusion of the proximal segments. The joints are felt more than the interjoint segments. With a limb amputated at the knee, the amputee is more aware of his foot than of his leg; with a limb amputated at the ankle, the amputee is more aware of his toes than of the rest of his foot. The phantom perceptions disappear last in those regions with the largest representation in the cerebral cortex (i.e., the thumb, hand, and foot). Pain may be considerable. Patients often feel that if they could only open their hands, the pain would leave.

The neural mechanisms involved in the phantom limb have not been conclusively explained; some of the pain may be psychologically based. By some means, pools of neurons associated with sensory perception of the missing segments are activated. These pools, perhaps in the thalamus and cortex, are hypersensitive (see "Denervation Hypersensitivity," in Chap. 6) and in an abnormally disturbed state. Irritation of the proximal stump of the peripheral nerve may initiate a series of impulses that trigger these pools of neurons in the central nervous system.

Pain in the phantom limb may be abolished by nerve blocks in the stump. Sectioning of the spinothalamic tract can relieve the pain in the phantom but not the sensation of the phantom. A lesion of the parietal lobe in an amputee has been noted to abolish both the pain and the phantom.

Efferent correlations

Lower motor neuron paralysis When the lower motor neurons to the voluntary muscles are severed physically or impaired metabolically (poliomyelitis is caused by a neurotropic virus which has a predilection for impairing the function of the lower motor neurons), the voluntary muscles become denervated. A lower motor neuron (flaccid) paralysis results. This paralysis is characterized by muscle weakness and loss of reflexes (areflexia), loss of muscle tone (atony), wasting away of muscle tissues because of the loss of the trophic influences of the nerve (atrophy) and lack of resistance to passive movement (movement produced by another source, another person). Fasciculations (muscle spasms) are exhibited by the denervated muscles. These spasms are probably due to denervation sensitivity (see Chap. 6) to trace amounts of acetylcholine or some unknown chemical substance. If only a percentage of the muscle fibers of a muscle mass is denervated, the reflexes are weaker (hyporeflexia), the tone is reduced (hypotonia), and the atrophy is less pronounced.

Upper motor neuron paralysis When the descending motor tracts on one side of a segment of the spinal cord are interrupted, a paralysis known as an *upper motor neuron (spastic) paralysis* results in the body segments innervated by spinal segments below the level of the lesion. Many clinicians equate the upper motor neuron with the corticospinal pathway; hence the common conception that the signs exhibited in an upper motor neuron paralysis are due to the lesion of the corticospinal tract. This is not correct, because confirmed lesions limited to the corticospinal tract do not produce all the upper motor neuron signs. Thus the interruption of the fibers of the corticospinal system and portions of other descending systems are necessary to produce the classical upper motor neuron paralysis.

Immediately after the occurrence of the lesion, the deep tendon reflexes are temporarily depressed (*areflexia*), and the paralyzed muscles are flaccid. In time, weeks and months later, the muscles become *spastic*, i.e., *increased muscle tone* (*hypertonus*), *increased deep tendon reflexes* (*hyperreflexia*), and other signs are present. In upper motor neuron paralysis, *spasticity* is associated with hypertonicity of the antigravity muscles. Hence an upper motor neuron paralysis is called a *spastic paralysis.* Hypertonus and muscle weakness are significant features of a spastic paralysis. Such a paralysis of the upper and lower extremities on one side is called a *hemiplegia.*

Several weeks or months after the lesion occurs, an upper motor neuron paralysis is characterized by a *paresis* (the impairment of motor function, partial paralysis with incomplete loss of muscle power) or *paralysis* (loss of motor function), hyperactive deep tendon reflexes (hyperreflexia), increase in muscle tone (hypertonus), clonus, increased resistance to passive movement and clasp-knife (jackknife) response, loss or diminution of cutaneous or superficial reflexes, positive Babinski reflex, and disuse atrophy. The *brisk knee jerk* (*hyperactive myotatic reflexes*) following the tapping of the quadriceps tendon is an example of hyperreflexia. *Hypertonus* is expressed in the firmness and stiffness primarily, but not exclusively, of the flexors in the upper extremity and in the extensors in the lower extremity. Apparently the stronger groups of muscles in each limb predominate. The more powerful muscle groups are the antigravity muscles, because they help the body oppose gravity—the extended lower extremity supports the body during standing, and the flexed upper extremity elevates the limb. The spasticity is primarily due to an increase in gamma motor neuron activity, and the increased sensitivity of the neuromuscular spindles to the stretch of the antigravity muscles. Gravitational forces act as a trigger to sustain hypertonus or spasticity. Apparently the loss of certain inhibitory upper motor neuron influences sets the stage.

Clonus is the rhythmic oscillation of a joint (e.g., ankle or knee) which occurs when a second party suddenly dorsiflexes the foot (pressure on the sole of the foot pushes toes toward the knee) and maintains the dorsiflexion under elastic pressure. The dorsiflexion actually puts the gastrocnemius muscle and its Achilles' tendon under moderate stretch. The stretched neuromuscular spindles fire, and the activated myotatic reflex results in contraction of the gastrocnemius and plantar flexion of the ankle. The plantar flexion produces a stretch of its antagonist, the anterior tibialis muscle; its sensitive neuromuscular spindles activate a myotatic reflex which produces a contraction of the anterior tibialis muscle and dorsiflexion of the ankle. The dorsiflexion of the ankle produced by the contraction of the anterior tibialis muscle and the elastic pressure produced by the second party maintain the cycle of the rhythmic oscillation. Clonus is actually a self-perpetuating rhythmic series of myotatic reflexes. It persists as long as a muscle agonist is kept under a moderate state of stretch. Clonus ceases as soon as the state of stretch ceases.

The *increased resistance to passive movement*

and the *"clasp-knife response"* are expressed as follows: When a second party attempts to extend the elbow by applying pressure on the palmar side of the hand, the spastic flexors of the elbow resist stretch. At the beginning of the action the resistance is strong; if the pressure on the hand is maintained, the resistance yields suddenly, in a clasp-knife (jackknife) fashion. When the tension stretches the biceps muscle to a certain point, the Golgi tendon endings suddenly commence to fire; their inhibitory influences act upon the unstable positive-feedback situation, maintaining the spasticity by inhibiting the hyperreflexia; hence the marked sudden shift in the passive resistance of the clasp-knife reflex. This so-called *inverse myotatic reflex* is a consequence of the activity of the Golgi tendon endings triggered by the lengthening of certain muscles involved in the movement (*lengthening reaction, autogenic inhibition*). The characteristic of Golgi tendon endings to fire inhibitory influences into neuronal pools has been regarded as a safety device to prevent a muscle from being damaged by excessive externally applied forces.

The *loss or diminution of the cutaneous reflexes* is difficult to explain on a neuronal basis. Stimulation of the skin of the thorax, abdomen, or extremities evokes weak or no reflex response—these are all disynaptic and multisynaptic reflexes. The *Babinski reflex (sign)* accompanies an upper motor neuron paralysis. When the lateral aspect of the sole of the foot is stroked with a blunt point, the big toe dorsiflexes (hyperextension), the tip of the toe points to the knee, and the other toes spread (fan). This reflex can be elicited in the newborn infant and baby during the first months after birth. Atrophy of these innervated muscles occurs because of disuse, hence it is called *disuse atrophy*. Passive exercise of the muscle is helpful in delaying disuse atrophy.

Several additional explanations have been suggested to account for some of the signs associated with upper motor neuron paralysis. All may be contributory. The spinal cord below the lesions retains its basic intrinsic neural circuits. These circuits have been deprived of many of the excitatory and inhibitory influences from the brain. In one interpretation, the basic intrinsic circuits are released more from the inhibitory influences than from the excitatory influences derived from supraspinal levels. Greater release from inhibition than from excitation may account for the hyperactivity. Denervation sensitivity (Chap. 6) and collateral sprouting (Chap. 2) of more nerve fibers have been proposed as explanations. In fact, the central mechanisms accounting for spasticity are not fully known.

HEMISECTION OF THE SPINAL CORD (BROWN-SÉQUARD SYNDROME)

A hemisection (unilateral transverse lesion) of the spinal cord damages structures, which results in a number of changes in the body at, and below, the levels caudal to the lesion (see Fig. 5-34). For instructional purposes, assume that the lesion is a hemisection extending from spinal levels C5 through T1; the peripheral nerves associated with these spinal levels innervate the upper extremities.

In relating the side of a lesion (right or left) in the nervous system to the side of the body where signs are expressed, one must relate the site of the pathway's crossing over to the location of the lesion. Symptoms occur on the same side (ipsilateral) and below the level of the lesion when the damaged neurons are those which normally convey influences from the same side of the body (ascending sensory tract) or to the same side of the body (descending motor tracts). In the spinal cord, structures involved with ipsilateral functional roles include the posterior columns, dorsal roots, lateral corticospinal tract (and other upper motor neurons), and ventral roots. Symptoms occur on the opposite (contralateral) side below the level of the lesion when the damaged neurons convey information from or to the opposite side of the body. In the spinal cord, this includes the decussated fibers of the lateral and anterior spinothalamic tract. In the brain, this includes the spinothalamic tract, medial lemniscus, and corticospinal tract. The fiber tracts injured and resultant symptoms and signs include:

1. Posterior column (fasciculi gracilis and cuneatus). Loss of position sense, appreciation of passive movement, vibratory sense, weight discrimination, and two-point discrimination

on the same side at and below the spinal levels of the lesion. The modalities from the neck are unaffected because the fibers conveying them are located wholly above the level of the lesion.

2. Lateral spinothalamic tract. Loss of pain and temperature on the opposite side at and below the spinal levels of the lesion. This includes the contralateral upper extremity, because lateral spinothalamic fibers decussate within one or two levels of the spinal root origin.

3. Anterior spinothalamic tract. Tactile sensibility is probably little affected on the opposite side below the spinal level of the lesion because this modality is also conveyed in the uncrossed fasciculi gracilis and cuneatus.

4. Corticospinal tracts and other descending supraspinal tracts. The spastic syndrome following the interruption of these fibers results in an upper motor neuron paralysis including spasticity, hyperactive deep tendon reflexes (*DTRs, hyperreflexia*), diminution or loss of superficial reflexes. Babinski sign, and muscle clonus below (but not at the level of) the site of lesion on the ipsilateral side. The hyperactive DTRs are illustrated by a brisk knee jerk.

5. At the spinal levels of the transection (C5 through T1), the entering fibers of the dorsal roots and the emerging fibers of the lower motor neurons and preganglionic sympathetic fibers (C8 and T1) are interrupted. The result is the complete absence of all sensations in the upper extremity on the lesion side and loss of pain and temperature on the contralateral upper extremity. Paresthesias and radicular pain may be sensed over the ipsilateral C5 and T1 dermatomes from the irritation of some intact dorsal root fibers; because of dermatome overlap from C4 and T2, the C5 and T1 dermatomes have a hypesthesia. The upper ipsilateral limb is flaccid; it exhibits all the signs of a lower motor neuron paralysis. Horner's syndrome on the ipsilateral side of the face and trophic changes in the ipsilateral upper extremity are due to the interruption of the preganglionic sympathetic neurons (see the discussion of Horner's syndrome later on).

AMYOTROPHIC LATERAL SCLEROSIS

Amyotrophic lateral sclerosis is a degenerative motor tract disease with bilateral involvement of the pyramidal tracts and anterior horns; there is degeneration of both upper and lower motor neurons. Most of the affected muscles show evidence of the degeneration of lower motor neurons, including paralysis, atrophy, fasciculations, and weakness; these signs are initially expressed by the muscles of the hands and arms. Some muscles exhibit signs of upper motor neuron paralysis, hyperreflexia, and, at times, Babinski signs. The lower motor neurons of cranial nerves may also exhibit signs of degeneration.

COMBINED SYSTEM DISEASE

Combined system disease is a complication of pernicious anemia—lack of intrinsic factor for the absorption of vitamin B_{12}—in which there is a bilateral subacute degeneration of the fibers of the posterior columns and lateral columns, especially those involved with the lumbosacral cord. The clinical symptoms include (1) loss of position and vibratory senses, numbness and dysesthesias in the lower extremities, and (2) such upper motor neuron signs as spasticity, muscle weakness, hyperactive deep tendon reflexes, and Babinski reflexes.

TRANSECTION OF SYMPATHETIC FIBERS TO THE HEAD (HORNER'S SYNDROME)

Lesions of preganglionic sympathetic fibers in the ventral roots of T1 and T2, the cervical sympathetic trunk, or of the postganglionic sympathetic neurons of the superior cervical ganglion (see Chap. 6) will result in *Horner's syndrome* on the ipsilateral side of the face (see Fig. 5-34). The affected pupil is smaller than the pupil of the opposite eye; it does not dilate when the pupil is shaded (pupillodilator muscle unit is not stimulated to contract). The affected eyelid droops a bit (ptosis) because the superior palpebral smooth muscle (Muller's muscle) is denervated. The face is dry (denervated sweat glands), red, and warm (vasodilatation of cutaneous blood vessels). In humans, Horner's syndrome regresses because of denervation hypersensitivity (Chap. 6).

SYRINGOMYELIA

A syrinx (cavity) may develop in the region of the central canal as, for example, in the cervical enlargement; from these the gliosis and cavitation may extend to other sites (see Fig. 5-34). The initial clinical signs are the loss of pain and temperature sensibility with a bilateral segmental distribution in both upper extremities. This dissociated sensory loss is due to the interruption of the decussating lateral spinothalamic fibers in the anterior white commissure. There is no sensory loss in the body and lower extremities because the spinothalamic tracts and posterior columns are intact. The extension of the degeneration into the anterior horn (lower motor neurons) results in a lower motor neuron paralysis.

PARAPLEGIA

Paraplegia is the condition in which both lower extremities are paralyzed; *quadriplegia (tetraplegia)* is the paralysis of all four extremities. The paralysis of the upper and lower extremity on one side is called *hemiplegia*.

Paraplegia is a direct consequence of a complete transection of the spinal cord. Several aspects of this condition in a person who has had a midthoracic transection are outlined. Immediately after the complete transection of the spinal cord, the body innervated by spinal segments caudal to the lesion site is devoid of detectable neural activity. All voluntary movements and somatic and visceral reflex activities are abolished. During the first month or so following the trauma, several symptoms are noted below the level of the lesion: loss of all sensations, loss of all reflex activities, bilateral flaccid paralysis of the lower extremities, visceral deficits such as loss of thermoregulatory control (dry, cool skin with no sweating), loss of voluntary control of a spastic urinary bladder, and loss in sexual potency in the male. Tidal drainage of the urinary

bladder must be maintained to prevent retention of urine. This extremely depressed neural activity, called *spinal shock*, usually lasts about 2 to 3 weeks in humans, though the period varies from 4 days to 6 weeks. Experimentally, spinal shock occurs at the moment of complete transection.

It is a transient state of decreased synaptic activity below the transection, and is related to the acute interruption of normally active descending supraspinal influences that maintain the excitability of the spinal neurons. Spinal shock is not due to the irritation of the cut surface. In time, the intrinsic spinal cord circuits become active. In general, the reappearance of any reflex is a sign of recovery from spinal shock.

The isolated spinal cord and its spinal nerves below the level of the transection gradually exhibit autonomous neural activity, which is divided into a sequence of phases of variable lengths: (1) minimal reflex activity, (2) flexor spasm activity (superficial reflexes), (3) alternation between flexor and extensor spasm activities, and (4) predominant extensor spasm activity (deep reflexes). Some symptoms are retained, while others are altered, until a stabilized condition is reached within a year or so. No sensations, no voluntary control of motor activities, and no thermoregulatory mechanisms can ever be elicited below the transection site. The muscular reflex activities are modified with the return of muscle tone and flexor reflex activities. A slight pinprick on the foot, for example, may initiate a mass withdrawal of the entire lower extremity by the *triple reflex*—flexion at the hip, knee, and ankle. This response is considered to be an expression of the protective primitive withdrawal of the limb from noxious stimuli, even though no sensation is felt. Later, extensor activities become more marked, until some spasticity may occur. At times the body weight may be supported in a transitory manner by the extended lower extremity, but patients cannot stand on their own without support. Later changes may be associated with collateral sprouting. After a year or two, the paraplegic patient will be in one of several conditions: (1) *paraplegia-in-extension*, in which extensor spasms predominate over flexor spasms (observed in about two-thirds of paraplegics); (2) *paraplegia-in-flexion*, in which flexor spasms predominate; (3) flaccid paralysis (occurring in fewer than 20 percent). The basic reason why the paraplegic subject cannot stand or walk is that the extensor monosynaptic reflexes are depressed; adequate extensor reflex activity is essential to maintaining the upright posture for standing or walking. The excitatory influences from the upper motor neurons are apparently necessary to facilitate the subliminal excitatory influences from the neuromuscular spindles; otherwise our lower extremities cannot support our weight. In theory, the brain projects neural influences which bias and facilitate the basic activity of the intrinsic circuits of the spinal cord.

The urinary bladder may be evacuated by reflex activity (reflex bladder) but is not under voluntary control. The absence of influences from the higher centers of the autonomic nervous system in the brain results in a variety of disturbances in the control of the autonomic activity in the urinary, genital, and anorectal systems. A spinal tap may induce *spinal reflex sweating*—this may be a phenomenon related to denervation sensitivity. Similarly, sweating may be associated with anxiety (e.g., as a consequence of the insertion of a hypodermic needle).

BIBLIOGRAPHY

Beal, J. A., and M. H. Cooper: The neurons in the gelatinosal complex (laminae II and III) of the monkey (*Macaca mulatta*): a Golgi study. J Comp Neurol, 179:89–122, 1978.

Burton, H., and A. D. Loewy: Projections to the spinal cord from medullary somatosensory relay nuclei. J Comp Neurol, 173:773–792, 1977.

Brodal, A.: *Neurological Anatomy in Relation to Clinical Medicine*, Oxford University Press, New York and London, 1969.

Castiglioni, A. J., M. C. Gallaway, and J. D. Coulter: Spinal projections from the midbrain in monkey. J Comp Neurol, 178:329–346, 1978.

Chouchkov, C.: Cutaneous receptors. Adv Anat Embryol Cell Biol, 54:1–62, 1978.

Coggeshall, R. E., D. G. Emery, H. Ito, and C. W. Maynard: Unmyelinated and small myelinated axons in rat ventral roots. J Comp Neurol, 173:175–184, 1977.

Dubner, R.: Neurophysiology of pain. Dent Clin Am, 22:11–30, 1978.

Gobel, S., and S. Hockfield: "An Anatomical Analysis of the Synaptic Circuitry of Layers I, II and III of Tri-geminal Nucleus Caudalis in the Cat," in D. J. Anderson and B. M. Matthews (eds.), *Pain in the Trigeminal Area*, Elsevier Publishing Company, Amsterdam, 1977, pp. 203–211.

Gilman, S., and L. A. Marco: Effects of medullary pyramidotomy in the monkey. Brain, 94:495–514, 1971.

Ha, H., and C. N. Liu: Organization of the spinocervico-thalamic system. J Comp Neurol, 127:445–470, 1966.

Henneman, E.: Peripheral mechanisms involved in the control of muscle, in V. B. Mountcastle (ed.), *Medical Physiology*, The C. V. Mosby Company, St. Louis, 1968, vol. 2, pp. 1697–1716.

Iggo, A. (ed.): Somatosensory system, in *Handbook of Sensory Physiology*, vol. II, pp. 1–851, Springer-Verlag New York Inc., New York, 1973.

Kerr, F. W. L., and P. R. Wilson: Pain. Ann Rev Neurosci, 1:83–102, 1978.

Langford, L., and R. Coggeshall: Branching of sensory axons in the dorsal root and evidence for the absence of dorsal root efferent fibers. J Comp Neurol, 184:193–204, 1979.

Matthews, P. B. C.: *Mammalian Muscle Receptors and Their Central Actions*, The Williams and Wilkins Company, Baltimore, 1972.

Melzack, R., and P. D. Wall: Pain mechanisms, a new theory. Science, 150:971–979, 1965.

Nyberg-Hansen, R.: Functional organization of descending supraspinal fibre systems to the spinal cord. Ergeb Anat Entwicklungsgesch, 39:1–48, 1966.

Oscarsson, O.: "Functional Organization of Spinocerebellar Paths," in A. Iggo (ed.), *Handbook of Sensory Physiology, vol. 2, Somatosensory System*, Springer-Verlag OHG, Berlin, 1973, chap. 2, pp. 339–380.

Petras, J. M.: Spinocerebellar neurons in the rhesus monkey. J Comp Neurol, 130:146–151, 1977.

Petras, J. M.: Spinocerebellar neurons in the rhesus monkey. Brain Res, 130:146–151, 1977.

Pubols, B. H., and L. M. Pubols: Forelimb, hindlimb and tail dermatomes in the spider monkey (*Ateles*). Brain Behav Evol, 2:132–159, 1968.

Ralston, H. J., and D. D. Ralston: The distribution of dorsal root axons in laminae I, II and III of the macaque spinal cord: a quantitative electron microscope study. J Comp Neurol, 184:643–684, 1979.

Rexed, B.: A cytoarchitectonic atlas of the spinal cord in the cat. J Comp Neurol, 100:297–380, 1954.

Scheibel, M. E., and A. B. Scheibel: Spinal motorneurons, interneurons and Renshaw cells: A Golgi study. Arch Ital Biol, 104:328–353, 1966.

Schmidt, R. F. (ed): *Fundamentals of Sensory Physiology*, Springer-Verlag New York Inc., New York, 1978.

Shriver, J. E., B. M. Stein, and M. B. Carpenter: Central projections of spinal dorsal roots in the monkey. Am J Anat, 123:27–74, 1968.

Sinclair, D. C.: *Cutaneous Sensation*, Oxford University Press, London, 1967.

Swanson, A. G., G. C. Buchan, and E. C. Alvord: Anatomic changes in congenital insensitivity to pain. Arch Neurol, 12:12–18, 1965.

Taub, E.: "Movement in Nonhuman Primates Deprived of Somatosensory Feedback," in J. F. Keough (ed.), *Exercise and Sport Science Reviews*, Journal Publishing Company, Santa Barbara, 1977, vol. 4, pp. 335–374.

Taub, E., G. Barro, R. Heitmann, H. C. Grier, and D. P. Martin: "Effect of Forelimb Deafferentation During the Mid-prenatal Period on Motor Development in Monkeys," in E. Asmussen and K. Jorgenson (eds.), *Biomechanics VI-A*, University Park Press, Baltimore, 1978, pp. 125–129.

CHAPTER SIX

THE AUTONOMIC NERVOUS SYSTEM

REGULATION OF THE INTERNAL ENVIRONMENT

The autonomic nervous system is the regulator, adjuster, and coordinator of vital visceral activities, including digestion, body temperature control, blood pressure, and many expressive facets of emotional behavior. Many of the activities are mediated below the conscious level or are recognized by the mind in a vague way. Synonyms for this system reflect these functional expressions: *involuntary nervous system*, *vegetative nervous system*, and *general visceral efferent system*.

The primary function of the autonomic nervous system is to help maintain a stable internal environment, or *milieu interne*, in the body against those forces that tend to alter it. The concept expressing the maintenance of the steady state of the internal environment is that of *homeostasis*. It is a form of negative feedback (Chap. 3) and represents the equilibrium level of activity. For example, a relatively constant body temperature is critical for the survival of warm-blooded animals. Compensatory thermostatic mechanisms are constantly operating to adjust and to prevent excessive fluctuations of this temperature. Heat is produced by such metabolic activities as the oxidation of glucose, active muscular movements, and shivering; it is conserved by the constriction of the skin blood vessels (to reduce loss by radiation); and it is dissipated by perspiration and dilatation of skin blood vessels.

Blushing, pallor, palpitations of the heart, clammy hands, and dry mouth are several emotional expressions mediated through the autonomic nervous system.

This system is not necessarily "involuntary," for it is known that humans and animals can be conditioned to be able to lower their blood pressure and rate of heartbeat volitionally. This is the basis of the modern use of biofeedback in therapy.

THE CONCEPT OF THE AUTONOMIC NERVOUS SYSTEM

The autonomic nervous system is represented in both the central nervous system and the peripheral nervous system. Classically the autonomic nervous system is defined as the motor (efferent) system innervating visceral organs; hence it is called the "general visceral efferent system." In this traditional view, both the somatic and visceral afferent (sensory) system act as the input arm of the reflex arcs, utilizing the general visceral efferent system as an output channel.

A more inclusive view broadens the widely used definition so that the autonomic nervous system includes both the general visceral afferent and the general visceral efferent systems. Both definitions are used and are valid.

The following account stresses some generalizations concerning the autonomic nervous system. However, it must be understood that many exceptions and paradoxes to these generalizations exist. Thus, many morphologic and functional aspects of the autonomic nervous system with respect to each organ system must be approached individually. For example, the autonomic nervous system by tradition (1) is divided into a parasympathetic system and a sympathetic system, (2) consists of preganglionic and postganglionic neurons, and (3) contains cholinergic neurons (neurotransmitter is acetylcholine) and adrenergic neurons (neurotransmitter is norepinephrine). Some aspects of this conceptualization are being modified at present by the discovery of a complex system of cell types each elaborating different neurohumeral and neurotransmitters such as serotonin, somatostatin, substance P, and enkephalin.

THE VISCERAL NERVOUS SYSTEM AND THE SOMATIC NERVOUS SYSTEM – SOME INTERACTIONS, DIFFERENCES, AND SIMILARITIES

Although the nervous system is conceptually divided into the visceral nervous system and the somatic nervous system, the two divisions are not mutually exclusive. Many neural activities are the product of interactions between these two divisions. For example, the somatic sensory input from "light," conveyed via the optic pathways, may be expressed via the visceral motor system by the dilation or constriction of the pupil of the eye, and via the somatic motor system by the movements of the eye or of the head

and body. The sensory input from visceral receptors within the body may be expressed (1) via the somatic motor system, as the respiratory rhythms of voluntary muscles and (2) via the visceral motor system, as adjustments in the rate and force of the heartbeat. The response to cold may be reflected by the visceral motor system, which stimulates the contraction of involuntary skin muscles (goose pimples), and by the somatic motor system, which stimulates the activity of voluntary muscles (shivering). In addition, a variety of influences acts upon the autonomic nervous system, including pain from both somatic and visceral sources, memory, and worry; these may be expressed in the form of blushing, pallor, sweating, and heart palpitations.

Fundamental differences and similarities between the two systems are expressed in the anatomy (Fig. 6-1) and the physiology of their peripheral motor neurons (Table 6-1).

Anatomy Each effector cell influenced by the autonomic nervous system is innervated by a sequence of two neurons called, respectively, the *preganglionic neuron* and the *postganglionic neuron* (see Figs. 6-1 through 6-4). Each preganglionic neuron has a cell body (and dendrites) that is located within the central nervous system; it

Table 6-1
Comparison of somatic motor system with the autonomic nervous system

Structure or function	Somatic motor system	Autonomic nervous system
I. Morphologic		
A. Structures innervated	Voluntary (skeletal) muscle	Cardiac and smooth (involuntary) muscles and glands
B. Ganglia outside central nervous system	None	Paravertebral (chain), prevertebral (collateral), and terminal ganglia
C. Neurons from central nervous system to effector	One	Two
D. Fibers	Myelinated lower motor neuron alpha and gamma fibers	Preganglionic fibers, myelinated; B fibers; postganglionic fibers, usually unmyelinated; C fibers.
E. Peripheral plexus	None	Numerous (e.g., aortic, hypogastric plexuses)
II. Functional		
A. Role in periphery	Excitatory	Either excitatory or inhibitory
B. Effect of denervation on effectors	Paralysis and atrophy	Remains functional, little change in automaticity
C. General role	Adjustments with external environment	Adjustments with the internal environment (homeostasis)
III. Neurotransmitter	Acetylcholine	Acetylcholine and norepinephrine

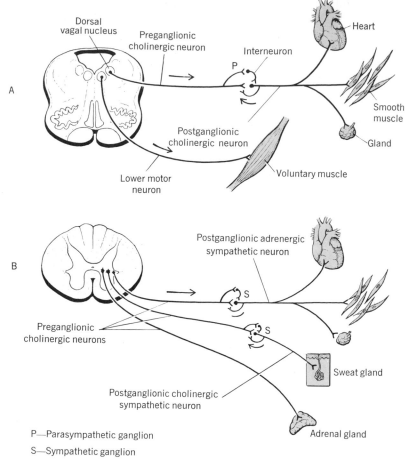

FIGURE 6-1 Motor innervation to the peripheral effectors. *A.* The parasympathetic outflow from the medulla innervates the heart, smooth muscle, and glands. The lower motor neuron innervates a voluntary muscle. *B.* Sympathetic outflow from the spinal cord innervates the heart, smooth muscle, and glands. See text for discussion of the various types of neurons.

has a lightly myelinated axon that courses through the peripheral nerves and terminates by synapsing with postganglionic neurons. Each postganglionic neuron has a cell body which is found in a peripherally located ganglion (i.e., outside the central nervous system) and an unmyelinated axon that terminates at or near an effector cell.

The autonomic nervous system innervates, either directly or indirectly, three types of effector cells: involuntary (smooth) muscle cells, cardiac (heart) muscle cells, and glandular (secretory) cells. In contrast, each effector cell influenced by the somatic motor system is innervated by a neuron with a cell body (and dendrites) located within the central nervous system and with an axon that courses through the peripheral nerves and directly synapses at a motor end plate with a voluntary muscle cell. The somatic motor system innervates only one type of effector cell: a voluntary (striated) muscle cell (including the intrafusal muscle of the neuromuscular spindle). The anatomic relationship of the autonomic nerve terminals with the smooth muscles, cardiac muscles, and glandular cells is unresolved; the terminations do not form identifiable end plates on these target cells. Neurotransmitter chemicals are released from the axon terminal.

The spinal nerves of the somatic system form interjoining branches of relatively simple, proximally located *plexuses* (e.g., cervical, brachial, or lumbosacral plexuses). In contrast, the nerves of the autonomic nervous system form peripherally located plexuses, which are complex networks along blood vessels and associated organs. These *terminal plexuses* include among others the cardiac, pulmonary, mesenteric, and pelvic plexuses.

Physiology The autonomic nervous system acts more slowly than the somatic system. The more slowly conducting fine fibers (B and C fibers) and the synaptic delay in the autonomic nervous system contrast with the faster-conducting, more heavily myelinated fibers (alpha neurons and gamma neurons, Chap. 5) of the somatic motor nerves. The nature of the neurotransmitter substances associated with these two sytems is significant. The neurotransmitter substance *acetylcholine* is released at the synaptic junctions between each preganglionic neuron and each postganglionic neuron. *Acetylcholine* is released at each parasympathetic synaptic junction between a postganglionic neuron and an effector cell, while *norepinephrine* is released at each sympathetic synaptic junction between a postganglionic neuron and an effector cell (see below). *Acetylcholine* is the chemical mediator released at the myoneural junction (motor end plate) between a somatic motor nerve and a voluntary muscle. A neurotransmitter released by the autonomic nervous system may evoke either an excitatory response or an inhibitory response from an effector (e.g., it may stimulate or inhibit muscle contraction). In the somatic nervous system the neurotransmitter (acetylcholine) always evokes an excitatory response (e.g., obligatory contraction of the muscle).

An effector is not completely dependent on its innervation by the autonomic nervous system. Smooth muscles and glands express their "functional independence" by not atrophying if deprived of their innervation (see "Denervation Hypersensitivity," at the end of this chapter); they remain functional. In contrast a voluntary muscle is dependent on its somatic motor innervation; in time it atrophies and becomes functionless if deprived of its innervation.

Visceral afferent system

Visceral afferent input constitutes a substantial portion of the total input to the spinal cord and brainstem. Influences from the viscera are conveyed via *visceral afferent fibers* to the central nervous system. These fibers are located in the somatic nerves (e.g., the sciatic nerve) and the visceral plexuses (e.g., cardiac and mesenteric) and nerves (e.g., the vagus and splanchnic). Although some of these afferents are lightly myelinated fibers, most of them are unmyelinated. Those afferent fibers terminating in the spinal cord have their cell bodies in the spinal ganglia, while those coursing in the glossopharyngeal and vagus nerves to the medulla have their cell bodies in the inferior ganglia of these nerves (Chap. 7). One estimate indicates that about four-fifths of the fibers in the vagus nerve are visceral afferent fibers. Influences from the peripheral blood vessels, especially those of voluntary muscles, and from glandular structures in the skin pass via afferent fibers in the somatic nerves.

Apparently these fibers of the afferent limb of a reflex arc of the autonomic nervous system terminate and synapse upon interneurons in the spinal cord. In turn, these interneurons have connections with the preganglionic sympathetic neurons. The visceral afferent fibers do not synapse directly with the preganglionic fibers of the autonomic nervous system.

The visceral afferent fibers are involved with the mediation of (1) visceral sensations, including pain, referred pain, cramps, fullness, and others; (2) vasomotor, respiratory, and viscerosomatic reflexes; and (3) interrelated visceral activities (e.g., digestion and peristalsis). The glossopharyngeal and vagus nerves convey the afferent influences from the chemoreceptors in the carotid and aortic bodies (they monitor O_2 and CO_2 levels of the blood) and the pressoreceptors in the carotid sinus and the aortic arch (mechanoreceptors) to the medulla. These are involved in the reflex control of heart rate, blood pressure, and respiration.

The carotid body and sinus have quite similar morphologic features; each contains glomerular aggregations of large globular cells (the probable receptors) upon which the afferent fibers terminate. The pressoreceptors of the carotid sinus are associated with a rich arteriovenous anastomotic network. The chemoreceptor cells are filled with catecholamine dense-core vesicles.

THE SYMPATHETIC NERVOUS SYSTEM AND THE PARASYMPATHETIC NERVOUS SYSTEM

The autonomic nervous system is subdivided into two parts, the sympathetic (orthosympathetic) and the parasympathetic (see Figs. 6-2 and 6-3). In general, the *sympathetic system* stimulates those activities which are most dramatically expressed and *mobilized* during emergency and stress situations—otherwise called the "fight, fright, and flight activities." These reactions are accompanied by the expenditure of energy stores: the acceleration of the rate and force of the heartbeat, increase in the blood pressure, increase in the concentration of blood sugar, and an emphasis on directing the blood flow largely to the voluntary muscles at the expense of flow to the viscera and the skin. Although this system operates at all times in the moment-to-moment adjustments throughout life, it is during stress that it acts with its stops removed.

In contrast, the *parasympathetic system* stimulates those activities that are associated with the conservation and restoration of the energy stores of the organism. The reactions to accomplish these functions are associated with decrease in the rate and force of the heartbeat, with decrease in the blood pressure, and with stimulation of the digestive system to encourage the digestion, movement, and ultimate elimination of ingested food and water.

The two systems integrate their actions and are not antagonistic. In the economy of the body they usually act synergistically, although at times some actions are executed independently. They function in concert to maintain the internal activities of the organism at a level commensurate with the intensity of the stress situation and with the emotional state of the individual (Table 6-2).

The *enteric nervous system* comprises the intrinsic neural network of the gastrointestinal tract (gut). This system can operate independently and possesses sensory neurons, coordinating interneurons, and motor neurons. In effect, it is a self-contained unitary functional unit which can be modulated by the sympathetic and parasympathetic systems (see later on in chapter).

Sympathetic (orthosympathetic) nervous system

Anatomy The *sympathetic nervous system* (Fig. 6-1) is also called the *thoracolumbar system* (*thoracolumbar outflow*), because all preganglionic neurons of this system emerge from the spinal cord via the motor roots of all thoracic and the upper two lumbar spinal nerves (T1 through L2). The preganglionic neurons terminate and synapse with postganglionic neurons located either in the paravertebral ganglia (ganglionic chain) or in the prevertebral ganglia. The bilateral paravertebral ganglionic chains (sympathetic chains) are series of ganglia located on and along the entire length of the bony vertebral column, extending from the upper cervical to the coccygeal regions (see Fig. 6-2). There are usually 3 pairs of cervical (upper, intermediate, and lower), 10 to 12 of thoracic, 4 of lumbar, and 4 or 5 of sacral ganglia. The two chains meet in front of the coccyx as the *median unpaired terminal* (*coccygeal*) *ganglion* (*ganglion impar*). The lower cervical and first thoracic ganglia are often fused into the stellate ganglion. Some variability exists in the number of ganglia. Some of the synaptic linkages between the preganglionic neuron and the postganglionic neurons are displaced from the paravertebral ganglion toward the spinal nerve. This displaced linkage is called an intermediate ganglion. When present, these ganglia may escape removal in a paravertebral sympathectomy. They are not reached in a "complete sympathectomy."

The cell bodies for the preganglionic sympathetic fibers are located in lamina VII (primarily in the intermediolateral cell column and some in a line extending medially to the vicinity of the central canal, where they join the medial compo-

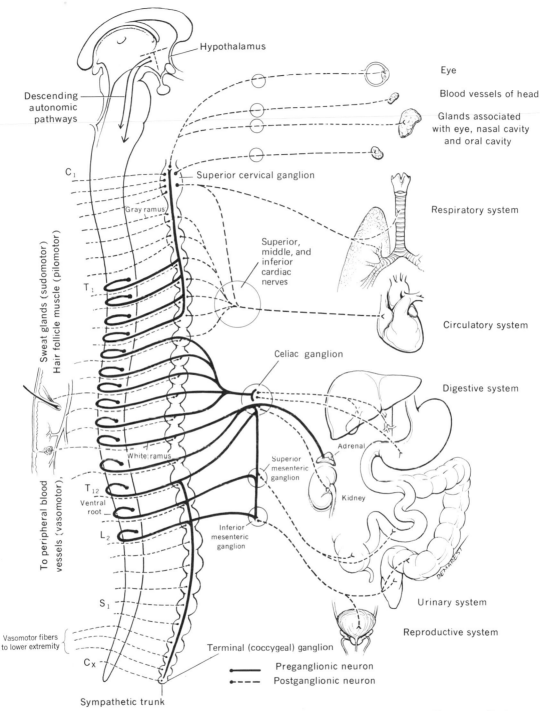

Hypothalamus

Descending autonomic pathways

Eye

Blood vessels of head

Glands associated with eye, nasal cavity and oral cavity

C_1

Gray ramus

Superior cervical ganglion

Respiratory system

Superior, middle, and inferior cardiac nerves

T_1

Sweat glands (sudomotor) Hair follicle muscle (pilomotor)

Circulatory system

Celiac ganglion

Digestive system

White ramus

Adrenal

Superior mesenteric ganglion

Kidney

T_{12}

Ventral root

To peripheral blood vessels (vasomotor),

L_2

Inferior mesenteric ganglion

Urinary system

S_1

Reproductive system

Vasomotor fibers to lower extremity

Terminal (coccygeal) ganglion

C_x

Preganglionic neuron

Postganglionic neuron

Sympathetic trunk

FIGURE 6-2 The sympathetic (thoracolumbar) division of the autonomic nervous system. The preganglionic neurons are cholinergic. The postganglionic neurons are adrenergic (see Table 6-3 for cholinergic sympathetic neurons). A preganglionic cholinergic neuron innervates the adrenal medulla. The posterior portion of the hypothalamus is involved with sympathetic activities (Chap. 11). The white rami with their preganglionic fibers are located at spinal levels T1 through L2. The gray rami with their postganglionic fibers are located at all spinal levels.

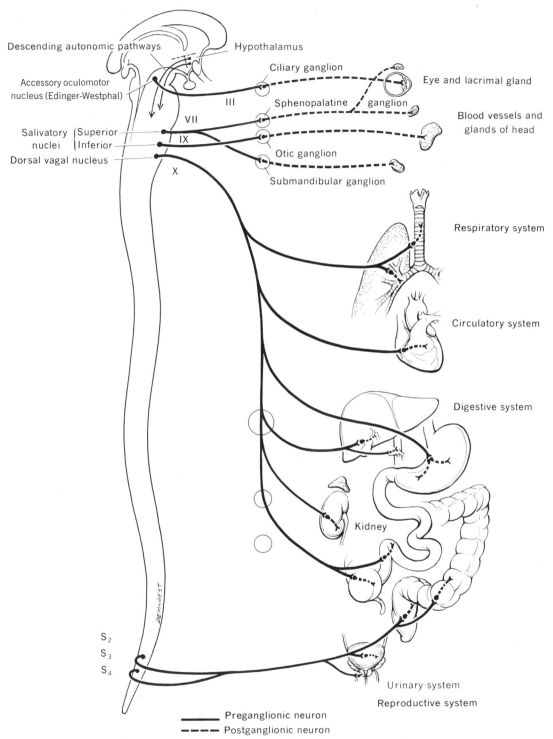

FIGURE 6-3 Diagram of the parasympathetic (craniosacral) division of the autonomic nervous system. The preganglionic and postganglionic neurons are cholinergic. The superior and inferior salivatory nuclei are actually diffuse and diffuse groups of cells located within the parvicellular reticular nucleus (Chap. 8, Fig. 8-9). The rostral portion of the hypothalamus is involved with parasympathtic activities (Chap. 11).

nent, the mucleus intercalatus). The fibers from the cell bodies of these nuclei enter the fasciculus proprius, then divide into ascending and descending branches that extend for many spinal levels before emerging at a number of spinal levels into ventral roots before reaching sympathetic ganglia (Petras and Faden). Classically, many preganglionic fibers are said to pass successively through the ventral roots, spinal nerves, and white rami communicantes (see Figs. 6-1 and 6-4) to the paravertebral ganglia (sympathetic chain) either at the same spinal level or by branches; these branches ascend and descend in the sympathetic chain so that each fiber has branches that terminate in many postganglionic neurons in many ganglia of the chain. These rami are called white rami because the preganglionic fibers are myelinated.

In humans, the distal or white rami appear white on gross inspection and contain an abundance of myelinated fibers, whereas the proximal or gray rami usually appear gray (but may appear white) and contain a variable number of myelinated fibers. Unmyelinated fibers are numerous in both rami, which include visceral afferent fibers on their way to the dorsal roots. Evidence indicates that (1) the gray rami contain both myelinated and unmyelinated afferent fibers and both myelinated and unmyelinated postganglionic sympathetic fibers, and (2) the white rami contain unmyelinated afferent, preganglionic, and postganglionic fibers and myelinated preganglionic and afferent fibers.

The visceral afferent input often merges with the somatic afferent input and may become indistinguishable. This is because the inputs from both sources can be fed to the same relay cells in the central nervous system as well as to both somatic and visceral motor outflow to the body. Thus, visceral sensory input from a portion of the gastrointestinal tract can evoke a somatic muscle spasm on the body wall.

The preganglionic neurons are outnumbered by the postganglionic neurons. Each preganglionic fiber may synapse with as many as 30 or more postganglionic neurons (the postganglionic neurons innervated by one preganglionic neuron may be located in several ganglia—an expression of divergence). In turn, each postganglionic neuron receives synaptic stimulation from many preganglionic neurons—an expression of convergence. The axons of the preganglionic neurons of the sympathetic system are relatively short, while those of the postganglionic neurons are relatively long, with many terminal branches (see "Parasympathetic Nervous System," farther on).

The postganglionic neurons of the paravertebral ganglia reach their effector cells via several routes. Some fibers return to the spinal nerves via the gray rami (appear gray because the postganglionic fibers are largely unmyelinated) and are then distributed to smooth muscles (blood vessels, hair follicles) and sweat glands of the skin, extremities, and body wall (see Fig. 6-4). Other fibers form small nerves and plexuses around major blood vessels and reach the smaller blood vessels and organs in the head, neck, and thorax (see Fig. 6-2).

Some preganglionic fibers reach the prevertebral ganglia (located in the abdomen) by passing successively through the ventral root, spinal nerve, white rami, and small nerves terminating in the ganglia (see Figs. 6-2 and 6-4). The postganglionic fibers reach their effector cell via perivascular plexuses and are distributed to the blood vessels and organs of the abdomen and pelvis. In general, the sympathetic outflow is distributed as follows: T1 to T4, to the head and neck; T2 to T9, to the upper extremity; T9 to L2, to the lower extremity; C8 and T1, to the eye; T1 to T5, to the heart and lungs; T4 to T9, to the upper abdominal viscera; T10 to T11, to the adrenal gland; and T12 to L2, to the urinary, genital, and lower digestive systems, including the kidney, ovary, testis, and pelvic organs (Table 6-3).

Note that the origin and outflow of the preganglionic neurons is restricted to the thoracic and upper two lumbar levels, but that the chain extends the entire length of the vertebral column. The postganglionic neurons projecting from these chain ganglia provide the sympathetic innervation to the visceral muscles and glands of the eye, lungs, heart, and skin and the muscles of the blood vessels of the head, neck, body, wall, and extremities.

The *prevertebral (collateral) ganglia* are located in the abdomen in close proximity to the aorta and its major branches, after which the

Table 6-2
Some comparisons between the sympathetic and parasympathetic nervous systems

	Sympathetic nervous system	Parasympathetic nervous system
GENERAL		
Outflow from CNS	Thoracolumbar levels	Craniosacral levels
Location of ganglia	Paravertebral and prevertebral ganglia close to CNS	Terminal ganglia near effectors
Ratio of preganglionic to postganglionic neurons	Each preganglionic neuron synapses with many postganglionic neurons	Each preganglionic neuron synapses with a few postganglionic neurons
Distribution in body	Throughout the body	Limited primarily to viscera of head, thorax, abdomen, and pelvis
Metabolism	Energy mobilization during emergency	Conservation and restoration of energy resources
General homeostasis	Central mechanism to obtain mass discharge of system	No central mechanism to obtain mass discharge of system
SPECIFIC STRUCTURES		
Eye		
Radial muscle of iris	Dilation of pupil (mydriasis)	
Sphincter muscle of iris		Contraction of pupil (miosis)
Ciliary muscle (accommodation)	Relaxation for far vision	Contraction for near vision
Glands of head		
Lacrimal gland		Stimulates secretion
Salivary glands	Scanty thick, viscous secretion	Profuse, watery secretion
Heart		
Rate	Increases	Decreases
Force of ventricular contraction	Increases	No direct effect
Blood vessels	Generally constricts*	Slight effect
Lungs		
Bronchial tubes	Dilates lumen	Stimulates constriction of lumen
Bronchial glands	Inhibits secretion	Stimulates secretion
Gastrointestinal tract		
Motility and tone	Inhibits	Stimulates
Sphincters	Stimulates	Inhibits (relax)
Secretion	May inhibit	Stimulates
Gallbladder and ducts	Inhibits	Stimulates
Liver	Glycogenolysis increase (blood sugar)	
Spleen (capsule)	Contracts	
Adrenal medulla	Secretion of epinephrine* and norepinephrine	
Sex organs	Vasoconstriction, constriction of vas deferens, seminal vesicle, and prostatic musculature (ejaculation)	Vasodilatation and erection
Skin		
Sweat glands	Stimulates*	None
Blood vessels	Constricts	Slight effect
Pilomotor	Contracts	
Urinary tract		
Ureter (motility and tone)	Increases	
Bladder detrusor	Relaxation (usually)	Contraction
Trigone and extension into urethra	Relaxation (see text)	Contraction

	Sympathetic nervous system	Parasympathetic nervous system
Metabolism		
Liver	Glycogenolysis	
Adipose tissue	Free fatty acid release	
NEUROCHEMICAL BASIS		
Neurotransmitter at neuro-effector junction	Usually norepinephrine* Adrenergic	Acetylcholine Cholinergic
Inactivation of transmitter	Slow and re-uptake	Rapid
Reinforcement in body	Secretion of norepinephrine and epinephrine by adrenal medulla	

* *Exceptions: Some postganglionic neurons of the sympathetic nervous system are cholinergic neurons. Sympathetic neuroeffector transmission mediated by acetylcholine includes (1) some blood vessels in skeletal muscles and (2) most sweat glands. The sweat glands of the palms are innervated by adrenergic fibers. The adrenal medulla is innervated by preganglionic cholinergic sympathetic neurons.*

ganglia are named (celiac ganglia, superior mesenteric ganglia, inferior mesenteric ganglion, and others; the celiac ganglia and their associated nerves are known as the solar plexus). These *prevertebral ganglia* receive their innervation from neurons whose cell bodies are located in the lower six thoracic and first two lumbar levels. The postganglionic neurons in these ganglia have axons that terminate distally in association with the smooth muscles and glands of the abdominal and pelvic viscera and their blood vessels, including those of the digestive, urinary, and genital systems. The medulla of the adrenal gland is innervated by preganglionic neurons.

Sympathetic reflex (see Fig. 6-4) The *autonomic visceral reflex arc* comprises a sequence of (1) afferent neuron (general visceral afferent neuron), (2) interneurons within the gray matter, and (3) a sequence of two efferent neurons (a preganglionic general visceral and a postganglionic general visceral neuron). The postganglionic neurons innervate involuntary muscle, cardiac muscle, and glandular cells. The afferent neurons convey influences from visceral structures via somatic and visceral nerves and the dorsal roots to interneurons in the base of the posterior horn. These interneurons interconnect with preganglionic neurons in the intermediolateral nucleus (sympathetic nervous system). The preganglionic neurons course through the ventral root and terminate in sympathetic ganglia with both

intraganglionic interneurons and postganglionic neurons. The interneurons are involved with processing within the ganglia (Fig. 6-4).

Interneurons within sympathetic ganglia These ganglia contain some interneurons which contain dopamine. Being small and fluorescent, they have been called *SIF cells* (*small intensely fluorescent*). These dopaminergic neurons are presynaptic to the postsynaptic neuron. They have inhibitory endings which are responsible for the IPSP on the postsynaptic neuron.

Table 6-3
Efferent segmental distribution
of sympathetic outflow

Head: eye, lacrimal gland and salivary glands	T1–3
Heart	T1–5
Bronchi and lungs	T1–5
Esophagus (near stomach)	T5–6
Stomach	T6–10
Small intestine	T9–10
Proximal large intestine	T12–L1
Distal large intestine and rectum	L1–2
Spleen and pancreas	T6–10
Kidney	T10–L1
Ureter	T11–L1
Urinary bladder	T11–L2
Testis and ovary	T10–T11
Prostate	T11–L1
Uterus	T12–L1
Upper extremity	T2–T6
Lower extremity	T10–L2

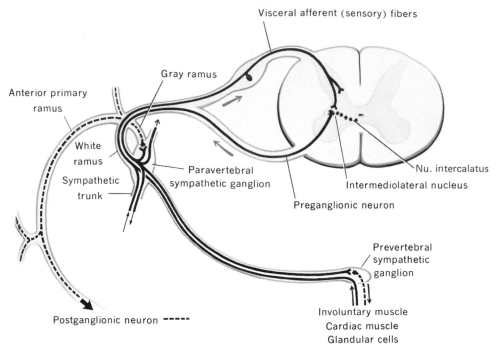

Visceral afferent (sensory) fibers

Gray ramus

Anterior primary
ramus

White
ramus

Sympathetic
trunk

Paravertebral
sympathetic ganglion

Nu. intercalatus

Intermediolateral nucleus

Preganglionic neuron

Prevertebral
sympathetic
ganglion

Postganglionic neuron ‑‑‑‑‑

Involuntary muscle
Cardiac muscle
Glandular cells

FIGURE 6-4 A visceral reflex arc of the sympathetic nervous system. An arc comprises an afferent neuron (general visceral afferent neuron), an interneuron (not illustrated), and a sequence of two efferent neurons (a preganglionic general visceral and a postganglionic general visceral).

Physiology The neurotransmitter mediator at the postganglionic effector junction is norepinephrine (noradrenaline), one of the catecholamines. Thus the sympathetic system is referred to as an *adrenergic system,* and its postganglionic fibers as *adrenergic fibers,* or *noradrenergic fibers.* Norepinephrine is slowly deactivated in the body. Some postganglionic neurons of the sympathetic nervous system are cholinergic neurons. Postganglionic sympathetic cholinergic fibers innervate (1) some blood vessels in voluntary muscles and (2) most sweat glands. The sweat glands of the palms are innervated by postganglionic adrenergic fibers.

The sympathetic nervous system is geared to act as a total unit throughout the body for sustained periods of time. Thus the catecholamine effect of the sympathetic nervous system can be widespread and lasting. Anatomic and biochemical factors contribute to this prolonged unit ac-

tion. Wide distribution and sustained activity result because (1) each preganglionic neuron with a short axon synapses with many postganglionic neurons, each having a long axon with many neuroeffector junctions, and (2) the blood-distributed epinephrine of the adrenal gland [see "Adrenal (Suprarenal) Gland," farther on] and the neurotransmitter norepinephrine are largely of adrenergic sympathetic nerve origin and are deactivated slowly.

The sympathetic nervous system is not essential to life, but it is critical for proper reactions to stress and strains. Animals without a sympathetic nervous system or an adrenal medulla can have a "normal" existence if kept in a sheltered environment. Their digestive, cardiovascular, and growth activities are essentially normal. They are sensitive to cold and have a slightly lowered basal metabolic rate. Under stress, such animals do not get excited, cannot adjust their body temperatures properly to heat or cold, and do not raise their blood pressure or their blood sugar levels.

Adrenergic neuron and synapse Several monamines are regarded as putative neurotransmitters in the nervous system (Table 6-4). Three of these are catecholamines—organic compounds that consist of a catechol nucleus and an amine group. They include dopamine (DA, dihydroxyphenylethylamine), norepinephrine (NE), and epinephrine (Adrenaline). Another is serotonin, which is an indoleamine called 5-hydroxytryptamine (5-HT). *Dopamine*, a precursor of norepinephrine, is also localized in the substantia nigra, nigrostriatal fibers, and striatum (Chap. 14). *Norepinephrine* is the catecholamine in the postganglionic sympathetic neurons of the autonomic nervous system; it is also found in the noradrenergic neurons of the brain (Chap. 8) and in the adrenal medulla (Chap. 6). *Epinephrine* is present in the adrenal medulla (absent in postganglionic sympathetic neurons). After its release into the circulation, epinephrine acts as a hormone. *Serotonin* is associated with the raphe nuclei of the brainstem (Chap. 8). Because these amines are synthesized in vivo, they are called biogenic amines.

Life cycle of the catecholamines (Table 6-4) Each neurotransmitter has a metabolic cycle which comprises synthesis, storage, combination with receptor sites, and, finally, degradation. The *metabolic cycle of NE*, as demonstrated in the postganglionic sympathetic neurons, is probably similar in the adrenergic neurons, of the central nervous system. Each postganglionic sympathetic neuron has axonal branches which terminate by arborizing into many branches with numerous varicosities; there may be as many as 25,000 varicosities per neuron (see Fig. 2-6).

The catecholamines are synthesized from the amino acid tyrosine in the following steps: tyrosine → dopa (dihydroxyphenylalanine) → dopamine → NE. Different enzymes are involved in each of these steps (Table 6-4). The synthesis of NE takes place within the postganglionic sympathetic neurons, in some neurons of the central nervous system (see Chap. 8 and Fig. 8-19) and in the cells of the adrenal medulla. The epinephrine of the adrenal medulla is formed by the *methylation of NE*. The metabolic cycle of the catecholamines in the cells of the central nervous system is thought to be similar to that described as occurring in postganglionic sympathetic neurons. All enzyme proteins involved in the biosynthesis of the neurotransmitter are formed by the action of the ribosomes of the endoplasmic reticulum in the cell bodies (not in the axons) of the neurons. The rate-limiting step in this biosynthesis is the conversion of tyrosine to dopa by the enzyme tyrosine hydroxylase. A feedback relation exists between NE and tyrosine hydroxylase: when the stores of NE are low, the tyrosine hydroxylase becomes active; when NE stores are high, the reverse occurs. After their formation, the enzymes are transported

Table 6-4
Biosynthetic pathways of some neurotransmitters

Precursor	Intermediates and enzymes		Neurotransmitter product
L-Tyrosine $\xrightarrow{\text{tyrosine hydroxylase}}$ L-dopa $\xrightarrow{\text{dopa decarboxylase}}$ dopamine $\xrightarrow{\text{dopamine } \beta\text{-hydroxylase}}$			
	L-norepinephrine $\xrightarrow{\text{phenylethanolamine } N\text{-methyltransferase}}$ epinephrine		
Choline + acetyl CoA $\xrightarrow{\text{choline acetylase}}$ acetylcholine			
L-Tryptophan $\xrightarrow{\text{tryptophan hydroxylase}}$ L-5-hydroxytryptophan $\xrightarrow{\text{5-HTP decarboxylase}}$ 5-hydroxytryptamine (5-HT, serotonin)			
L-Glutamate $\xrightarrow{\text{glutamate decarboxylase}}$ γ-aminobutyric acid (GABA)			

from the cell body via active transport and axoplasmic flow, or in conjunction with microtubules to the nerve terminals. Tyrosine is taken up from the bloodstream by active transport into the neurons. The synthesis of NE takes place within the cell body and in the varicosities of the axon terminal endings. The dopamine enters the dense-core vesicles, where it is converted to NE. From 90 to 95 percent of the NE is located in the dense-core vesicles (sometimes called storage granules). They are about 500 Å in diameter, with a 280-Å-diameter electron-dense core. These dense-core vesicles may possibly be derived from microtubules. Most vesicles are located in the varicosities. Estimates indicate that there are 1500 granules per varicosity. The NE is mainly bound with ATP (adenosine triphosphate), in the ratio of 4 NE to 1 ATP. The remaining 5 to 10 percent of NE is located in the axoplasm or on the plasma membrane; some is in a free form unbound to ATP. Some clear vesicles are present in the varicosities.

Some dense-core vesicles may be formed in the soma. Following their synthesis by the ribosomes of the endoplasmic reticulum, the enzymes and other components may be transferred to the Golgi apparatus, where they are enclosed in the membrane-limited vesicles. The NE may be synthesized within the soma or in the axon as the vesicle "flows" somatofugally. Most NE is elaborated in the nerve terminals. These sites of NE formation account for the observation that NE is found in varying amounts throughout the neuron.

Normally small amounts of free NE are released in quantal units into the synaptic cleft. The activity of these small amounts on the postsynaptic receptor sites accounts for the miniature graded postsynaptic membrane potentials (equivalent to miniature end plate potentials at the motor end plate of muscles). An action potential at the nerve terminal triggers the influx of some calcium ions into the neuron, which, in turn, triggers, within the nerve ending, the conversion of bound NE to free NE and the release of free NE into the synaptic cleft. The release of NE is dependent on calcium ions. Calcium is essential in the electrosecretory coupling process, i.e., the conversion of the action potential to the "secretion" of the neurotransmitter. One concept states that some synaptic vesicles aggregate near the presynaptic membrane and that, following the action potential, the entire contents of each vesicle is released by exocytosis through a formed opening in plasma membrane into the synaptic cleft. From these events, initiated by the action potential, the many quanta of NE in the synaptic cleft combine with enough receptor sites on the postsynaptic membrane to elicit the formation of an action potential on the postsynaptic neuron (central nervous system) or on the effector.

The released NE within the synaptic cleft has several fates (see Fig. 6-5). Some combines with receptor sites on the postsynaptic membrane. Most of the synaptically discharged catecholamines are inactivated by *re-uptake* through active transport into the nerve terminals that had released them. They end up in the synaptic vesicles or in the extragranular pool. Some NE in the cleft diffuses into tissue spaces or is absorbed on inert material.

Two enzymes—*monoamine oxidase (MAO)* and *catechol-O-methyl transferase (COMT)*—are primarily involved in the metabolic degradation of the catecholamines. Monoamine oxidase is considered to be the intraneuronal enzyme, located largely in the outer membrane of the mitochondria or in the axoplasm. It converts catecholamines by deamination to their corresponding aldehydes by acting on the amine group. The MAO probably acts on free NE and dopa and functions to regulate the amount of NE and dopa in the nerve ending; in effect MAO prevents the accumulation or release of an excess amount of NE from the nerve terminal. Catechol-O-methyl transferase is considered to catabolize the NE extracellulary by O-methylation; thus COMT terminates the action of NE liberated into the synaptic cleft. It converts catecholamines by transferring the methyl group from the catechol group. Neither MAO nor COMT is involved in the rapid inactivation of the neurotransmitter.

The catecholamine hypothesis of mood suggests that this group of chemicals has a role in our states of depression, euphoria, and well-being. A fall in the catecholamine level in the central nervous system results in a "catecholamine depression." A higher-than-normal central nervous system catecholamine level may result in euphoria. Some antidepressant drugs (e.g., nialamide) are MAO inhibitors which act by inhibiting the degradation of catecholamines. The resulting increase in the amount of catecholamines has an antidepressant role.

Amphetamine (pep pills) has an effect on the NE content in the brain. This drug blocks the re-uptake of NE into the neuron and, in addition, acts as an MAO inhibitor. This is presumed to be contributory to the euphoria and hallucinations which may follow administration of this drug. Amphetamine abuse from continued use may produce an "amphetamine psychosis," which is virtually indistinguishable from paranoid schizophrenia.

Chlorpromazine has been found to be useful in the treatment of schizophrenia. Chlorpromazine acts by preventing the re-uptake of NE by the nerve ending, and hence by producing more adrenergic activity. Prolonged intake of chlorpromazine may result in Parkinson-like symptoms (Chap. 14).

Parasympathetic nervous system

Anatomy The parasympathetic nervous system (see Fig. 6-3) is also called the *craniosacral system* (*craniosacral outflow*), because the preganglionic neurons of this system leave the brain via the cranial nerves from the brainstem and leave the spinal cord via the second through fourth sacral spinal nerves (S2 through S4). Each preganglionic neuron usually has a long axon that terminates and synapses with postganglionic neurons that are close to and located within the organ to be innervated. Each postganglionic neuron has a relatively short axon. This is in contrast to the neurons of the sympathetic nervous system.

The cranial portion of the parasympathetic system is associated with (1) four cranial nerves that supply the parasympathetic innervation to the head, thoracic viscera, and most of the abdominal viscera (some parasympathetic fibers are present in the eleventh cranial nerve) and (2) the sacral spinal cord that supplies the innervation to the lower abdominal and pelvic viscera (see Fig. 6-3).

The third (oculomotor) cranial nerve supplies the parasympathetic innervation to the eye; this nerve has its preganglionic neurons originating in the accessory oculomotor nucleus (of Edinger-Westphal) in the midbrain, and its postganglionic neurons originating in the ciliary ganglion behind the eye. The seventh (facial) cranial nerve and the ninth (glossopharyngeal) cranial nerve supply the parasympathetic innervation to the glands of the head, including the lacrimal (tear) glands of the eye, glands of the nasal cavities, and the salivary glands of the mouth; these nerves have their preganglionic neurons originating in the salivatory nuclei of the upper medulla and their postganglionic neurons originating in the sphenopalatine ganglion (seventh nerve), the submandibular ganglion (seventh nerve), and the otic ganglion (ninth nerve). The tenth (vagus) and the eleventh (cranial portion of spinal accessory nerve) cranial nerves supply the parasympathetic innervation to such organs as the heart, lungs, esophagus, stomach, liver, pancreas, small intestine, upper half of the large intestine, and numerous blood vessels; this nerve has its preganglionic neurons originating in the dorsal vagal nucleus and some cell bodies in the reticular formation near the nucleus ambiguus of the medulla and its postganglionic neurons located in or near the visceral organs innervated.

The sacral (pelvic) nerves supply the parasympathetic innervation to the lower half of the large intestine, rectum, urinary system, and genital system, including the uterus and erectile tissues. The preganglionic fibers from the sacral region pass successively through the ventral sacral roots, pelvic spinal nerves, and their plexuses to the effectors (see Fig. 6-3). These nerves have their preganglionic neurons originating in the sacral region and their postganglionic neurons located near or within the visceral organs innervated. The blood vessels and other visceral structures of the limbs and the body wall have no direct innervation from the craniosacral outflow.

Physiology The neurotransmitter substance at the parasympathetic postganglionic effector junction is acetylcholine. Thus the parasympathetic system is referred to as a "cholinergic system," and its postganglionic fibers are called "cholinergic fibers" (see Fig. 6-5). This chemical mediator is rapidly deactivated by hydrolysis by the enzyme cholinesterase in the synaptic area. Hence each parasympathetic discharge has an effect that is of short duration.

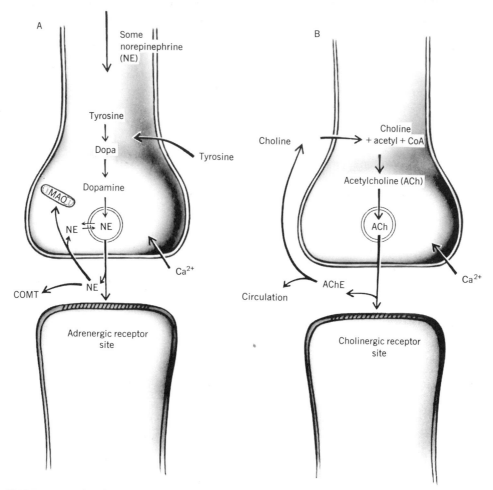

FIGURE 6-5 *A*. The adrenergic synapse. *B*. The cholinergic synapse. AChE, acetylcholinesterase; Ca²⁺, calcium ions; COMT, catechol-*O*-methyl transferase; MAO, monoamine oxidase. The postsynaptic receptor sites are cross-hatched.

Acetylcholine is synthesized primarily in the nerve terminal in two steps from acetate and choline. Acetate and coenzyme A (CoA) form acetyl CoA in the presence of ATP (energy source) in the presence of calcium ions. The acetyl CoA and choline form acetylcholine and CoA by the action of the enzyme choline acetylase (see Fig. 6-5).

The parasympathetic nervous system is geared to act in localized and discrete regions, rather than as a mass response throughout the body. Localized responses of short duration to a specific stimulus result because (1) each preganglionic neuron synapses with a limited number of postganglionic neurons; in turn, each of the latter exerts its effector action on a relatively limited number of neuroeffector (muscle and glandular cell) junctions; and (2) the neurotransmitter acetylcholine is rapidly deactivated by the enzyme cholinesterase. In contrast to the lasting, widespread catecholamine effect of the sympathetic nervous system, the acetylcholine effect of the parasympathetic system is discrete. There is no central nervous system mechanism to give a mass discharge of acetylcholine. For example, a drop in the blood pressure is not a response to the generalized action of acetylcholine activity on the cardiovascular system; actually the drop is due to the inhibition of the sympathetic nervous system.

The parasympathetic system is the conserver and the restorer of the energy stores of the body. The parasympathetic system is active when we are at rest and content. At these times there are a deceleration in the rate and force of the heartbeat, decrease in the blood pressure, and increase in the activity of the digestive system through glandular secretion and peristalsis. The protection of the eye from increased illumination (pupillary constriction) and the stimulation of urinary and bowel excretion are the result of parasympathetic activity. Because of the organs each innervates, the cranial parasympathetic portion is known as the "conserver of bodily resources," and the sacral portion as the "mechanism of emptying."

Massive discharges of the entire parasympathetic system do not usually occur. An excessively intense, massive discharge could even be detrimental to the organism; the heart could be decelerated to the point where beating would be reduced excessively.

ENTERIC NERVOUS SYSTEM

As previously noted, the enteric nervous system is the intrinsic neural system of the gastrointestinal tract; it is composed of sensory neurons, interneurons and motor neurons. This neuronal circuitry has the ability to mediate reflex activity even when completely separated from the central nervous system. The *sensory neurons* are the bipolar and pseudounipolar cells in the submucosal plexus. These afferent neurons have axons which are integrated into the intrinsic gut circuitry and also project to the prevertebral ganglia. The *interneurons* are serotonergic cells, i.e., serotonin acts as the transmitter. The *postganglionic motor neurons* are the motor neurons that can exert either excitatory effects (with acetylcholine as the transmitter) or inhibitory effects (with ATP as the putative transmitter). Serotonin, ATP, and such neuropeptides as somatostatin (Chap. 11) may be the transmitters not only of enteric neurons but also of neurons within such structures as the bronchial tubes and the blood vessels of the vascular system. These transmitters may account for many autonomic responses.

The enteric nervous system exhibits several features which resemble the central nervous system (Gershon and Bursztajn). Like the central nervous system, the myenteric plexus is characterized by a paucity of extracellular space and the absence of perineurial and endoneurial sheaths. The overall organization forms a blood-myenteric barrier similar to the blood-brain barrier in that the capillaries have tight junctions and are not fenestrated while the nonneural cells (neurolemmal cells) resemble astrocytes and not endoneurium in their fine structure.

The peripheral autonomic ganglia are more than just sites where simple neuron-to-neuron relays take place between the central nervous system (preganglionic neurons) and the neurons (postganglionic neurons), innervating the effectors. Rather they are neural processing centers exhibiting a number of chemical and structural features (Burnstock and Hökfelt). Two neurons illustrate morphologic modifications that alter simple relay sequences: (1) Intraganglionic processing is influenced by such interneurons as the SIF neurons (see earlier in chapter) located with sympathetic ganglia. (2) Input to the enteric plexus can be altered by sensory neurons with cell bodies located in the submucosal plexuses of the gut. Axons from these sensory neurons project to both the enteric nerve plexus and the prevertebral sympathetic ganglia (celiac, superior mesenteric, and inferior mesenteric ganglia). Through these afferent connections with the prevertebral ganglia, the gut is able to project neural influences which bypass the central nervous system and thereby modify its own neural input (Gershon).

THE AUTONOMIC NERVOUS SYSTEM AND THE ORGAN SYSTEMS

Dual innervation of the organs of the body by both the sympathetics and the parasympathetics is general but not universal.

1. The heart has a *true reciprocal* (*dual*) *innervation*, with the sympathetics acting to increase and the parasympathetics acting to decrease the force and rate of the heartbeat.
2. The salivary glands are stimulated *synergistically*, with sympathetic activity producing a thick, viscous secretion, and with parasym-

pathetic activity producing a profuse, watery secretion.

3. The constriction and dilation of the pupil offer an example of an activity resulting from the stimulation of different muscle groups. The pupil of the eye dilates when the dilator muscles (innervated only by sympathetic fibers) are stimulated by the sympathetics, and it constricts when the constrictor muscles (innervated only by parasympathetic fibers) are stimulated by the parasympathetics.

4. Some structures are innervated by only one system; the hair muscles (goose pimples) and the sweat glands are stimulated only by sympathetic fibers.

Not all the smooth muscle cells of a group or the cardiac muscles need be directly innervated by postganglionic fibers in order to respond to the influences conveyed by these fibers. This is so because smooth muscle cells of a group and the cardiac muscle cells are electrically coupled together by *gap junctions* (see "Nerve Impulse," Chap. 3). The junction between two smooth muscle cells is called a nexus, and that between two cardiac muscle cells is called an *intercalated disk* (see Figs. 2-6 and 2-9). A group of smooth muscles of the heart behaves like an *electrical syncytium*, because there is electrical continuity between these cells at their gap junctions. This method of propagation is essentially like that of a nerve. In effect, the neural influences sufficient to evoke a muscle action potential in some muscle cells of a group to contract can, via the gap junctions, stimulate all the muscle cells of the group to contract. The postganglionic autonomic fibers to the heart stimulate the conducting system (nodes, bundle of His, and Purkinje fibers) of the heart, which, in turn, stimulates the cardiac muscle cells through gap junctions.

Smooth muscle Depending upon their functional roles in various organs, smooth muscles exhibit a number of similarities and differences. Smooth muscle combines a slow prolonged contraction with a low metabolic demand. Their contractile elements are basically similar to those in voluntary muscle with some differences. Actin and myosin are present. The myofilaments are sparse and there is no neat arrangement of sarcomeres or T tubules. The small diameter of

smooth muscle cells apparently precludes the need for T tubules. It is likely that the sliding filament mechanism is operative. Many muscle cells exhibit electrotonic coupling through gap junctions (nexi). In some organs, smooth muscle cells pulse rhythmically; hence they act as pacemaker cells. The sympathetic and parasympathetic fibers within muscles have varicosities containing vesicles with neurotransmitters (see Fig. 2-6). These varicosities are found adjacent to troughs in the sarcolemma of the muscle cell. There are no specialized motor end plates.

Smooth muscle activities and their relation to their innervation vary. At one end of the spectrum are *multiunit smooth muscles* in which every muscle cell is innervated and is in synaptic contact with a varicosity (functionally a neuromuscular junction); these muscles have few gap junctions (electronic couplings) and only graded muscle potentials (no action potentials). Multiunit smooth muscles include muscles of the iris and ciliary body of the eye, the pilomotor system, the urinary bladder, and the blood vascular system.

At the other end of the spectrum are the *unitary smooth muscles* in which only a few cells are in synaptic contact with a few functional neuromuscular junctions. These muscles exhibit pacemaker potentials (similar to sinoatrial node cells on the heart), are electronically coupled through gap junctions, and propagate action potentials. Unitary smooth muscles are spontaneously active muscles which are intrinsically reactive to stretch. They are found in the gastrointestinal tract, ureter, and uterus.

Eye and lacrimal gland Parasympathetic stimulation results in the constriction (miosis) of the pupil, in the accommodation of the lens to near vision, and in the secretion of tears by the lacrimal gland. Pupillary constriction results from the contraction of the circular (constrictor) muscles of the iris. Accommodation requires a rounder (less flat) lens to effect the focusing on nearby objects.

Sympathetic stimulation results in the dilation of the pupil (mydriasis) by the contraction of the dilator muscles of the iris, slight elevation of the upper eyelid (there is some involuntary muscle in the eyelid), and possibly some accommodation to far vision.

Glands of the nose and mouth, including the salivary glands Parasympathetic stimulation conveyed via secretomotor fibers results in vasodilatation in the glands and in the secretion of a profuse watery secretion. Sympathetic stimulation results in vasoconstriction and in a diminution of blood flow through the glands and in a sparse, thick, viscous, mucinous secretion. The parotid glands lack adrenergic innervation.

Heart Parasympathetic stimulation results in a slower rate of the heartbeat (bradycardia), decrease in the blood volume expelled with each stroke, and probably the constriction of the coronary arteries (arteries supplying the heart muscle). The automatic rhythmic activity of the heart is basically maintained by the spontaneous depolarization of the automatic, or pacemaker, cells of the heart. In the order of the rate of rhythms (Chap. 3), the automatic cells are located in the sinoatrial node, specialized atrial fibers, atrioventricular node, bundle of His, and Purkinje fibers of the ventricle. Because the sinoatrial node has the fastest rate, it is *the pacemaker*. Acetylcholine slows the rate of depolarization and of the spontaneous depolarization; because the critical level is reached later than normally, the heart rate is slowed down. Of the automatic cells, acetylcholine acts only upon the sinoatrial node and the specialized atrial fibers.

Sympathetic stimulation results in a higher rate of the beat (tachycardia), increase in the blood volume expelled with each stroke, and dilation of the coronary arteries. By increasing the rate of depolarization, both NE and epinephrine raise the rate of the heartbeat. All the automatic cells of the heart are activated by both NE and epinephrine.

The upper three (or four) thoracic spinal levels are involved with the afferent and efferent innervation of the heart. The nerve fibers conveying this information are located in the spinal roots; rami communicantes of these thoracic levels; sympathetic chain (all cervical and upper thoracic ganglia); and the upper, middle, and inferior cervical and thoracic cardiac nerves. With the exception of the upper cervical cardiac nerve, which does not contain afferent fibers, all cardiac branches have both afferent and postganglionic sympathetic fibers (for functional relevance see "Angina Pectoris" at the end of this chapter).

The cardiac parasympathetic preganglionic fibers of the vagus nerve have their cell bodies in the reticular formation close to the nucleus ambiguus. Although most of these vagal fibers exert inhibitory influences (cardioinhibitory), some exert excitatory influences (cardioaccelleratory).

Lungs Parasympathetic stimulation results in the constriction of the bronchi and bronchioles of the lungs and in an increased secretion of the glandular cells of these tubes.

Sympathetic stimulation results in the dilatation of the bronchi and bronchioles. Respiration, or the inhalation and exhalation of air, is a function of the somatic nervous system, which innervates the respiratory voluntary muscles.

The free nerve endings in the respiratory tract are sensitive to irritant gases and particles —they can evoke the cough reflex.

Digestive system (see "Enteric System," described previously) Parasympathetic stimulation results in the increase in the contractility, motility, and tone of the digestive tract (peristalsis), in the relaxation of the muscle sphincters (between stomach and intestine, between small and large intestine, and at the anal orifice), and in the increase in the secretion of the digestive glands such as the pancreas. All these activities are directed to the digestion of food and its passage through and out of the digestive tract. The normal mechanical and secretory activities of the digestive tract are not wholly dependent on neural stimulation. Hormonal (humoral) agents are important. For example, contractions of the gallbladder are stimulated by the hormone cholecystokinin.

Sympathetic stimulation results in a decrease in the contractility, motility, and tone of the digestive tract, constriction in the sphincter muscles, inhibition of the secretion of the digestive glands, and an increase in the amount of glucose in the bloodstream. In times of excitement the organism does not readily digest food. Chewing and swallowing of food are essentially functions of the somatic motor system.

Genital system Parasympathetic stimulation results in the engorgement of the erectile tissues of the penis and clitoris and in the active secretion of the accessory glands of the reproductive system (glands of the cervix in the female, and prostate and seminal vesicles in the male).

Sympathetic stimulation results in the ejaculation of the semen by the involuntary muscles of the genital glands and ducts, accompanied by the somatic nervous stimulation of the voluntary muscles. Except for their blood vessels, the ovary, testis, and uterus do not respond to autonomic stimulation.

Urinary system Parasympathetic stimulation results in the increased tone and motility of the ureter and in urination as a consequence of the contraction of the urinary bladder (by the detrusor muscle).

Sympathetic stimulation inhibits urination by stimulating the relaxation of the detrusor muscle. Except for their blood vessels, the kidneys have no autonomic innervation. The voluntary sphincter of the bladder is innervated by the somatic motor system. A more complete discussion is presented below, under "The Autonomic Nervous System and the Urinary System."

Blood vessels The normal volume of blood is not sufficient to fill the blood vessels should all dilate (vasodilatation) simultaneously. The organism circumvents this consequence normally by dilating some vessels, especially arterioles, while contricting others, thereby maintaining a relatively constant blood vessel volume. In a fight, fright, or flight situation, the vasodilatation in the voluntary muscles is accompanied by vasoconstriction in the abdominal viscera and in the skin. In general, sympathetic stimulation results in dilatation of the coronary arteries of the heart and of the arteries of the voluntary muscles, and in the constriction of the blood vessels to the lungs, digestive system, and skin. Parasympathetic stimulation results in the dilatation of the blood vessels to the digestive system, as well as to the glands in the head, face (blushing), kidneys, and erectile tissues of the genital system.

The effect of the nervous system is largely over the tone of the arterioles. Vasoconstrictor fibers, by increasing the tone of the smooth muscles, decrease the size of these arterioles. Vasodilator fibers, by inhibiting the contractility of the smooth muscles, decrease the tone of the vessels and thereby allow the blood pressure to increase the diameters of these vessels. Humoral agents may influence that state of contractility of the blood vessels. For example, the cerebral vessels in humans react mainly to the circulating metabolic products, rather than to the autonomic nervous system. Carbon dioxide tends to enhance dilatation, and oxygen tends to stimulate constriction of the cerebral vessels. Many afferent fibers are present within the perivascular plexuses.

Sweat glands and pilomotor (hair) muscles of the skin Sympathetic stimulation results in the secretion of sweat glands (actually sympathetic fibers with cholinergic endings) and the contraction of the pilomotor muscles (goose pimples and hair standing on end). The cholinergic fibers to the sweat glands are usually called sympathetic because they are part of the thoracolumbar outflow. The sweat glands of the palms are innervated by sympathetic adrenergic fibers. These are involved in *"adrenergic" palm sweating,* which occurs during emotional stress.

Adrenal (suprarenal) gland The medulla of the adrenal gland secretes both epinephrine and NE into the bloodstream. In this respect, these catecholamines are hormones. The NE is produced by one type of cell. By the methylation of NE, epinephrine is formed in another type of cell. About 80 to 90 percent of the catecholamines secreted by the adrenal gland are epinephrine; the other 10 to 20 percent are NE. These catecholamines are released by *exocytosis* (see Fig. 3-6); in this process the vesicles discharge their contents directly through an opening in the plasma membrane into the extracellular space before it diffuses into the bloodstream. The adrenal medulla is controlled by the preganglionic cholinergic fibers of the sympathetic system.

The effect of the secretion of the adrenal medulla is similar to the action of the sympathetic system. This sympathetic activity of the adrenal medulla has a logical basis. The cells of the adrenal medulla, which are actually specialized postganglionic neurons, form the equivalent of a ganglion. These cells are embryologically derived, just as are many neurons, from neural crest cells (Chap. 4), and they are directly innervated by preganglionic cholinergic fibers (see

Fig. 6-1). The term *sympathoadrenal system* epitomizes this interrelationship. The widespread and sustained effects of the secretion of the adrenal medulla are the result of the distribution of epinephrine via the bloodstream and its slow deactivation. The adrenal medulla is not essential; its absence can be fully compensated for by the NE produced by the adrenergic fibers of the sympathetic system. Some differences do exist in the pharmacologic properties of NE and epinephrine. One difference, for example, is that epinephrine is more effective than NE in effecting a rapid increase of blood glucose from the glycogen stores in the liver.

THE AUTONOMIC NERVOUS SYSTEM AND THE URINARY SYSTEM

Innervation The peripheral innervation to the urogenital viscera is derived from three sets of nerves: *sympathetic nerves* from the lower thoracic and upper lumbar spinal levels; *parasympathetic nerves* from the midsacral spinal levels; and *pudendal nerves* (somatic nerves) from the second, third, and fourth sacral spinal levels. Within each of these sets are afferent as well as efferent fibers.

The sympathetic outflow passes from the spinal levels via the inferior mesenteric plexus (where synapses between the pre- and postganglionic neurons occur in the inferior mesenteric ganglion), hypogastric plexus (presacral nerve), and pelvic plexus to the pelvic viscera. The parasympathetic outflow passes from the S3 and S4 spinal levels via the pelvic splanchnic nerves (nervi erigentes) and hypogastric plexus to the pelvic viscera. The pudendal nerves convey the somatic motor influences via fibers (lower motor neuron) to the external sphincter of the bladder. Afferent fibers conveying the feeling of fullness and pain course via the pelvic splanchnic nerves to the midsacral levels. Other afferent fibers conveying pain may also pass via the hypogastric and inferior mesenteric plexuses to the lower thoracic and upper lumbar levels.

Urinary system Urine formed in the kidney drains into the renal calyces. When the pressure exerted by this urine reaches only 3 to 4 mmHg, the slightly stretched smooth muscles of the calyces are intrinsically stimulated into spontaneous contraction waves independently of innervation. This low-pressure response propels the urine along the ureter and protects the kidney from back pressure. The urine is forced along to the ureter by peristaltic waves. The sensory nerves in the ureter can, when stretched by a stone, evoke a most excruciating pain.

The emptying of the urinary bladder involves the following sequence of events. When the bladder fills (50 to 150 mL), influences from Pacinian receptors in the bladder wall are conveyed via afferent fibers in the pelvic nerves to the sacral cord, and from there pathways ascend to the cerebrum, where the conscious desire to urinate originates.

Voiding of urine is initiated primarily by the stretching of the smooth muscle of the bladder, called the detrusor muscle. This muscle is unusual in that it can be stretched to $2\frac{1}{2}$ times its normal resting length. As the bladder enlarges, the pressure upon the wall is elevated until it reaches the point that induces the smooth-muscle internal sphincter and the external sphincter (voluntary muscle innervated by the pudendal nerve) to relax. The stimulation of the spinal cord centers comes from stretch receptors in the bladder wall and external sphincter. Strong contractions by the detrusor muscle further elevate the pressure and tension. Thus voiding is initiated.

The sympathetics inhibit the detrusor muscle and excite the internal sphincter muscle, whereas the parasympathetics excite the detrusor muscle and the sympathetics inhibit the internal sphincter muscle.

Voluntary voiding can occur in the absence of spontaneous detrusor contractions. The intraabdominal pressure is increased with the contractions of the voluntary muscles of the abdominal wall (somatic fibers of the thoracic and lumbar nerves). The voluntary musculature of the perineum, urinary sphincter, and pelvic floor relaxes. The involuntary detrusor muscle is induced to contract; then voiding of urine takes place. Voiding quickly ceases as the voluntary muscles of the pelvic floor and external sphincter contract and the orifice of the bladder closes.

The initiation of voiding can be prevented

by strong contractions of both the external urinary sphincter and the pelvic floor musculature.

Disturbances in function of the bladder and rectum Lesions in various sites result in varying degrees of malfunction of these structures. A complete transection of the spinal cord above the sacral levels (supranuclear) results in an *automatic bladder*—also called a *reflex bladder* because its function depends upon the intact sacral spinal reflex arc. The retention of urine in the weeks immediately following the injury is due to the deranged reflex. Later, automaticity of the bladder occurs; it fills and empties, but never completely. Reflex voiding may be spontaneous or may follow the application of a stimulus to the skin of the perineum, abdomen, or lower extremity.

In lesions of the dorsal roots of sacral nerves or of posterior columns, as in tabes dorsalis, the afferent limb of the arc is interrupted. The result is a stretched and enlarged atonic bladder. Patients are unaware that their bladders are filled. Voluntary voiding is possible but is incomplete and is accompanied with dribbling and incontinence.

REPRESENTATION OF THE AUTONOMIC NERVOUS SYSTEM IN THE BRAIN AND SPINAL CORD

Structurally and functionally the autonomic nervous system is represented in the central nervous system as an intricate complex of centers and pathways whose details have been only partially unraveled.

The *segmental reflex arcs* are the fundamental anatomic and physiologic units of organization. In general, these arcs resemble the somatic reflex arcs. They are composed of (1) afferent neurons with their cell bodies in the spinal ganglia and in the geniculate ganglion of the facial nerve and inferior ganglia of the glossopharyngeal and vagus nerves, (2) interneurons in the central nervous system, (3) efferent neurons consisting of the sequence of preganglionic and postganglionic neurons, and (4) effector cells (smooth muscle, cardiac muscle, and glandular cell). Some reflex arcs involve other sequences of

neurons; e.g., the afferent neurons of the light reflex arc located in the retina, optic nerve, and optic tract (Chap. 12). The afferent neurons do not terminate in the nuclei containing cell bodies of the preganglionic neurons (dorsal vagal nucleus and intermediolateral nucleus); apparently at least one interneuron is intercalated between the afferent neuron and the preganglionic neuron of either the sympathetic or the parasympathetic system.

These reflex arcs respond to the everchanging and fluctuating demands of the internal environment. It is through these segmental arcs that the higher centers of the autonomic system in the brain ultimately exert their effects. The "centers" and the descending pathways of the system are identified essentially on the basis of physiologic criteria (e.g., the "respiratory center") and secondarily on the basis of anatomic criteria. Although some centers are relatively discrete morphologically (e.g., the hypothalamus and the dorsal vagal nucleus), many others are not (e.g., the cardiovascular centers in the brainstem tegmentum). The autonomic system in the brain and spinal cord may be thought of as a complexly organized, interacting network of pathways, with the centers as focal or nodal sites physiologically influencing a functional activity. The autonomic nervous system acts not alone but in concert with the somatic nervous system. Fight and flight reactions are expressions of both the somatic and the visceral systems. All autonomic activities are geared to function ultimately to maintain the homeostatic and homeokinetic balance of the organism.

The general visceral afferent input to the central nervous system is conveyed via the spinal nerves and the seventh, ninth, and tenth cranial nerves (Chap. 7). These visceral influences are (1) integrated into segmental visceral reflex arcs, whose motor nerves are the preganglionic and postganglionic neurons, and (2) relayed to higher centers via the spinoreticular tract and ascending tracts associated with the brainstem reticular system (Chap. 8).

Spinal cord The autonomic centers of the spinal cord are subject to the facilitatory and inhibitory stimuli from the centers in the brain. These stimuli are conveyed via descending pathways located mainly in the white matter in the anterior half of the spinal cord. Presumably the cord centers feed modulating influences back to the centers in the brain via ascending pathways. Ultimately this integrated activity is conveyed (1) via the preganglionic sympathetic neurons through the thoracolumbar outflow and (2) via the preganglionic parasympathetic neurons in the sacral gray matter through the sacral outflow.

Brainstem and cerebellum Many vital activities are mediated through the brainstem by "centers" definable largely by physiologic criteria. In the ventromedial tegmentum of the medulla is an inhibitory cardiovascular center; in the lateral tegmentum is an excitatory cardiovascular center. Stimulation of the lateral tegmentum may result in an acceleration of the heartbeat and an elevated blood pressure. Salivation may be a consequence of stimulation of the dorsolateral medullary tegmentum. Respiratory centers are located in the pons and medulla (Chap. 8). These centers and others project their influences via the reticulospinal tracts to the autonomic outflow in the spinal cord and through the reticular formation to the cranial nerve outflow in the brainstem.

The cerebellum may influence autonomic responses, probably acting through the brainstem reticular formation.

Hypothalamus The hypothalamus is a complex of visceral centers involved with the elemental visceral activities and behavioral patterns (Chap. 11). The visceromotor expressions of autonomic functions are transmitted from the hypothalamus by multineuronal pathways to visceral neuronal pools in the brainstem and spinal cord before being conveyed via the peripheral autonomic fibers to effectors.

The descending central visceromotor pathways from the hypothalamus to the brainstem and spinal cord are difficult to define precisely because direct descending hypothalamic efferents have not been demonstrated to project to the pons, medulla, or spinal cord. The caudally projecting fibers from the hypothalamus may be divided into two basic groups, both of which terminate in the midbrain.

1. The descending component of the medial forebrain bundle originates from cells in the lateral zone of the hypothalamus and descends (a) as the lateral division to the lateral midbrain tegmentum and (b) as the medial division to the paramedian midbrain tegmentum near the cerebral aqueduct of sylvius.
2. The descending component of the dorsal lateral fasciculus of Schütz originates from the more medial hypothalamus and descends to the anterior half of the periaqueductal gray substance. The nuclei of the paramedian tegmentum receiving input from these fibers include the superior central tegmental nucleus (raphe nucleus of Bechterew), dorsal tegmental nucleus, and ventral tegmental nucleus. This paramedian midbrain tegmentum, also known as the *limbic midbrain area* (Nauta), is the origin of ascending fibers which terminate in the hypothalamus (Chap. 13). They course in the dorsolateral fasciculus of Schütz and the mammillary peduncle. This "limbic midbrain area" is the caudal portion of the reciprocally organized hypothalamomesencephalic circuit (see Chap. 11).

Descending fibers from the midbrain tegmental nuclei terminate in the tegmental nuclei of the pons and medulla, including the nuclei reticularis pontis oralis and caudalis and the nucleus reticularis gigantocellularis. These descending reticulospinal pathways from the rhombencephalic tegmentum project through the white matter in the anterior half of the spinal cord to all spinal levels and terminate in the spinal gray matter. None terminates directly on the cells of the intermediolateral nucleus. Interneurons are the linkages between the fibers originating from the lower brainstem and the preganglionic sympathetic neurons. Interactions within these descending pathways from the hypothalamus occur through the rich interconnections and cross-linkages among the dendritic and axonal arborizations. In summary, the influences from the hypothalamus to the preganglionic neuronal outflow are conveyed via processing nuclear complexes in the midbrain, rhombencephalon, and spinal cord.

On the more elemental level, stimulation of the hypothalamus may result in the increase or decrease of the arterial pressure and the rate of the heartbeat, sweating, dilatation of the pupil, increase of the blood glucose concentration, stimulation or inhibition of activity in the gastrointestinal tract, and contraction of the urinary bladder.

On the behavioral level the hypothalamus affects (1) such behavioral patterns as savageness, rage, domestication, and wildness, (2) the sleep-wake mechanisms, (3) patterns of sexual behavior, (4) the overall metabolic activities related to such phenomena as food and water intake, obesity, and emaciation, and (5) the endocrine system through the pituitary gland.

Cerebrum and thalamus The neocortex, limbic lobe cortex, corpus striatum, and thalamus have their effects on autonomic activities. Details of the anatomy and physiology are scant. Cerebral structures are important to the emotional component of the total pattern of behavior. Animals live in a psychologic world with a support that is largely modulated through the autonomic nervous system. These higher centers have a role in such concepts as that excitable individuals are keyed to the sympathetic system and that placid individuals are keyed to the parasympathetic system. The basal ganglia influence the autonomic nervous system. For example, stimulation of the corpus striatum may produce changes in vascular tonus and in the state of contraction of pupillary, bladder, intestinal, and uterine muscles.

PHARMACOLOGY OF THE PERIPHERAL NERVOUS SYSTEM

Natural chemical mediators of the peripheral nervous system include (1) *acetylcholine*, at the cholinergic endings of (*a*) the preganglionic neurons of the autonomic nervous system, (*b*) the postganglionic neurons of the parasympathetic nervous system, and (*c*) the lower (somatic) motor neurons at the motor end plates; (2) *norepinephrine*, at the adrenergic endings of the postganglionic neurons of the sympathetic nervous system and released by the adrenal medulla; and (3) *epinephrine*, released by the adrenal medulla. These chemicals are the natural chemical mediators.

Pharmacologic agents and their mode of action

Many chemical substances have actions that may resemble some of the actions of the natural mediators. Those drugs which mimic the actions of acetylcholine are known as *parasympathomimetic drugs, cholinomimetic agents*, or *cholinergic drugs*. For example, carbachol mimics acetylcholine. Those drugs that mimic the actions of epinephrine and norepinephrine, e.g., ephedrine, are known as *sympathomimetic* or *adrenergic drugs.*

The general principles of neuropharmocology are based mainly on the action of chemical agents of the synaptic membranes or neurons. Some chemical substances modify the neural activity by acting at the synaptic sites to prevent the nerve impulse in the presynaptic neuron from stimulating the postsynaptic neuron (or effector structure). These drugs, known as blocking agents, do not prevent the release of the natural chemical mediators at the nerve endings but act just beyond the ending (probably in the synaptic cleft) to prevent the natural mediator from exerting its normal action.

Some blockers apparently stabilize the receptor site on the postganglionic neuron or effector cell so that the natural mediator cannot depolarize the postganglionic neuron or influence the effector cell. These blocking drugs are called *competitive blocking agents* (e.g., *d*-tubocurarine and tetraethylammonia) because they effectively compete at the synaptic site with the natural mediators.

Other blocking agents prevent the natural mediators from exerting their activity by depolarizing the postganglionic receptive sites, rendering these sites temporarily nonreceptive to further stimulation. These chemical substances are known as *depolarizing blocking agents* (e.g., nicotine). These blocking agents affect the receptor sites proper of the postganglionic cells, not their axons (the axon or the postganglionic neuron can still be directly stimulated to conduct).

Acetylcholine receptors

The acetylcholine receptors are classified as nicotinic receptors and muscarinic receptors. The nicotinic receptors are located predominantly at the neuromuscular junctions of voluntary muscles (motor end plates) and in the autonomic ganglia. These receptors are subject to stimulation by nicotine and to blockade by curare. Muscarinic receptors are located predominantly at effector cells (smooth muscle, cardiac muscle, and glands). They are subject to stimulation by muscarine and to blockage by atropine. In both types of receptors, acetylcholine is effective. The differences are thought to reside in the receptor sites; different parts of the acetylcholine molecule are involved at the different receptor sites. Stated otherwise, the differential action of muscarine and nicotine is explained by the concept that each of these chemicals reacts with a different kind of the many receptor proteins on the postsynaptic membrane.

Muscarine, a drug derived from a type of mushroom, is a parasympathomimetic agent that exhibits a cholinergic effect on such effectors as smooth muscle, heart muscle, and glands but has essentially no effect at the ganglionic synapses and at the motor end plates of voluntary muscles. These activities of muscarine are known as the *muscarinic effect*.

Nicotine has a dual effect (i.e., an effect with two phases) on the autonomic ganglia and on the voluntary muscles but has essentially no effect on smooth muscle, heart muscle, and glands. This agent initially stimulates and subsequently inhibits the excitation of the postsynaptic neuron or muscle. The initial effect of nicotine is to depolarize the postsynaptic membrane (depolarizing phase), which results in stimulation of the postganglionic neuron to fire. The subsequent effect is to maintain the depolarized state or phase so that the postsynaptic membrane cannot be stimulated. This dual action of nicotine is known as the *nicotinic effect*.

The so-called gamma receptors are stimulated by acetylcholine and yield an inhibitory response (cholinergic inhibitory). Some blood vessels have gamma receptors; vasodilatation is the response to stimulation. Such blood vessels are located in skeletal muscles, brain, and pia mater.

Cholinergic agents

The cholinergic endings of the autonomic neurons and of the somatic motor neurons at the motor end plates are the synaptic sites of action of a number of drugs. Carbachol is one such cholinergic drug that acts as a parasympathomimetic drug; its direct effect is similar to that of acetylcholine. Other pharmacologic agents have similar end effects but act by exerting an indirect mimetic action by inhibiting the enzyme cholinesterase; as a result, the concentration of acetylcholine increases in the synaptic clefts. These cholinesterase inhibitors or anticholinesterase agents include physostigmine and diisopropylfluorophosphate (DFP). DFP is a lethal nerve (war) gas. In short, similar cholinergic effects can be obtained either by the acetylcholine-like activity of such drugs as carbachol or by the inhibition of the enzyme cholinesterase (allowing acetylcholine to accumulate) by such drugs as physostigmine.

Blocking agents

Some drugs act as *blocking agents* at the synaptic sites. This blockage can be obtained by (1) such depolarizing agents as nicotine (depolarizing phase) and succinylcholine or (2) such competitive blocking agents as *d*-tubocurarine (derived from curare, the poison placed on arrow tips by certain South American Indians) and tetraethylammonia (TEA). Curare is an efficient blocker at the motor end plate (its paralytic action on the respiratory muscles can be fatal); TEA is a blocker that acts at the ganglionic synapses. Homatropine, a parasympathetic blocker at the postganglionic effector junction, is used by ophthalmologists in eye drops to dilate the pupil of the eye. This drug inhibits the pupillary constrictor muscle fibers from contracting by blocking the cholinergic endings. Dilatation results from the normal sympathetic activity of the unopposed dilator muscles of the pupil. *Atropine* and *homatropine* block the effect of acetylcholine at the neuroeffector receptive sites on the postsynaptic membrane; these agents do not interact chemically with acetylcholine.

Adrenergic receptors (adrenoceptive sites)

The effector cells innervated by the autonomic nervous system have two types of *chemically defined adrenoreceptive sites—namely alpha (α) and beta (β) receptors*. The alpha receptors have an affinity for both norepinephrine and epinephrine, while the beta receptors have a selectively stronger affinity for epinephrine.

The *alpha receptors* are generally excitatory, although some may be inhibitory in their response. Stimulation of most alpha receptors results in excitatory activity—contraction of smooth muscles or increased secretory activity of glandular cells. Excitatory responses are evoked in the following: (1) dilator (radial) muscles of the iris; (2) most blood vessels, including the coronary, skeletal muscle, salivary gland, cutaneous, pulmonary, and abdominal visceral vessels; (3) sphincters of the gastrointestinal tract; (4) muscle fibers of the trigone of the urinary bladder and of the vas deferens and uterus of the genital system; (5) sweat glands and pilomotor muscles in the skin; (6) smooth muscle in the capsule of the spleen; and (7) salivary glands (thick and viscous secretion). Inhibitory responses are obtained in some smooth muscle of the digestive system (relax intestine).

The *beta receptors* are generally inhibitory, with two significant exceptions. Inhibitory responses are evoked in the following: (1) ciliary muscles of the eye; (2) some blood vessels, including the coronary, skeletal muscle, pulmonary, and abdominal vessels (dilatation of arterioles); (3) musculature of the gastrointestinal tract (decrease in motility and tone); (4) bronchial muscles of the lung; and (5) detrusor muscle of the urinary bladder and smooth muscles of the uterus.

The two exceptions to the alpha-excitatory and beta-inhibitory responses are expressed by the heart and the gastrointestinal tract. Stimulation of the beta receptors in the sinoatrial node, atria, and ventricles produces excitatory cardiac effects; these include increase in the heart rate, increase in the force of the contraction, and increase in the excitability and automaticity. Stimulation of either the alpha or beta receptors produces inhibitory responses, and these responses are additive. Stimulation of both receptors acts to decrease gastrointestinal motility. Sympathetic responses can be eliminated by blocking both alpha and beta receptors. Some adrenergic blocking agents are *alpha receptor blockers* (e.g., dibenamines), while others are *beta receptor blockers* (e.g., dichloroisoproterenol).

Adrenergic agents

The *adrenergic mimetic drugs* that stimulate some of the actions of epinephrine and norepinephrine include ephedrine and amphetamine. These agents (as constituents of nose drops and nasal decongestants) act to constrict blood vessels and to inhibit mucous secretions.

CHEMOSENSITIVITY AND DENERVATION HYPERSENSITIVITY

When a muscle is deprived of its innervation, it becomes exquisitely sensitive to some chemical mediators (Chap. 4). Smooth muscles are most irritable when deprived of their postganglionic innervation and somewhat less hypersensitive if deprived only of their preganglionic innervation. The rate of beat of a totally denervated heart can be increased by a fractional amount of norepinephrine that normally stimulates the heart. This hypersensitivity is lost following the regeneration and functional recovery of these nerves. The *paradoxical pupillary reaction* is an example of denervation hypersensitivity to circulating epinephrine. The pupil of the eye without sympathetic innervation remains constricted because of the unopposed intact parasympathetic innervation of the pupillary constrictor muscles. When an individual without this sympathetic innervation is excited, the pupil may dilate. Presumably the minute amounts of circulating epinephrine secreted by the adrenal medulla are sufficient to excite the denervated dilator muscles to contract and dilate the pupil.

A denervated skeletal muscle is about 1000 times more sensitive to acetylcholine than is the normally innervated muscle. The muscle fibrillations associated with lower motor neuron damage probably result from the stimulation (depolarization) of the hypersensitive muscle fibers by the excitatory agents in the bloodstream (Chap. 5).

According to the *law of denervation*, denervation chemosensitivity, usually known as *denervation hypersensitivity*, is an expression of the response that is magnified as compared with that normally obtained by a neurotransmitter on a normally innervated effector. This heightened chemosensitivity resides in the number of active receptor sites on the plasma membrane of an effector—such as a voluntary muscle cell.

In the normal muscle cell the acetylcholine receptor sites are normally found to be restricted to the vicinity of the motor end plate (neuromuscular synapse).

In a denervated muscle changes occur with respect to the number and location of acetylcholine receptor sites on the muscle. Following the transection and subsequent degeneration of its motor neuron, the receptor sites increase in number, spread, and become distributed equally over the entire muscle fiber. This increase in the number of receptor sites and spread of chemosensitivity explains the phenomenon of denervation sensitivity. In this state, the muscle is capable of being reinnervated by one or more regenerating nerves which can form several motor end plates. Usually when reinnervation occurs (following denervation), one nerve terminal makes contact and several events are set in motion: (1) the motor end plate is formed, (2) widespread chemosensitivity is lost and, sensitivity becomes limited to the motor end plate, and (3) no other motor end plates are formed by any other motor nerve terminal with the muscle fiber.

The phenomenon of widespread chemosensitivity may be considered to be a retrogression of the muscle to a more undifferentiated embryonic state. It so happens that voluntary muscle fibers before they are innervated during their early development exhibit these features of the denervated muscle fiber. The spread of chemosensitivity is associated with an inactive muscle fiber. If a muscle is experimentally deprived of receiving stimulation (lack of action potentials), chemosensitivity appears throughout the muscle surface. If muscle is stimulated either by neural impulses or by mechanical means, there is no spread of the chemosensitivity.

Denervation of smooth muscle produces hyperresponsiveness to chemical mediators in addition to acetylcholine and norepinephrine, whereas this increased responsiveness in many neurons is limited to the transmitter removed. Thus, neurons and effectors can be either receptor-specific or receptor-nonspecific with regard to the spreading of chemosensitivity.

TROPHIC EFFECTS (NEUROTROPHISM)

The neurons may have other effects, independent of the influences exerted by the neurotransmitter activity, which are essential for the physiologic maintenance of other tissues. These so-called *trophic effects* (*trophic influences*) of neurons are directed to different types of target tissues, including epithelium and nerve endings (e.g., taste buds), muscle cells, and glandular cells. Even the maintenance of the nerve fiber itself may be dependent upon these influences. Chemical substances (macromolecular agents) elaborated in the cell bodies of neurons—called *neurotrophic factors or substances*—are thought to be involved in these *neurotrophic processes*. The precise nature and identity of these factors, or this factor, and the processes involved are not known at present. The concept of neurotrophism has been characterized as the nonimpulse transmitter neural function. It presumably involves some factor(s), which are conveyed by axoplasmic transport along the axon, are released and have a long-term interaction with the innervated tissues. Functionally this factor is essential for the maintenance of these tissues in their normal state. Specifically the trophic effects are "those interactions between nerves and other cells which initiate or control molecular modification in the other cell" (Guth).

Although trophic literally means nutrition, in neurobiology the term includes any relatively long-term influence that is passed from one cell to another or from one tissue to another. This may occur at any stage of the life cycle from early development through adulthood. Trophic interactions as they relate to the nervous system can occur in two ways: (1) the nervous system can be the source of the trophic influences upon nonneural or other tissues, or (2) the nervous system may be the recipient of trophic influences from nonneural tissues. In this sense, the nerve fiber and its neurolemma (Schwann) cells are presumed to interact trophically in these two ways.

The role of the gustatory nerve fibers with respect to the taste buds is illustrative of the effects of these "trophic influences" of the neuron. Not only do the gustatory nerve fibers convey coded "taste" information from the taste buds, but they also have an essential role in maintaining the morphology of the taste bud. Following the transection of the gustatory nerve fibers, the denervated taste buds degenerate. When the nerve regenerates and reinnervates the region, taste buds reappear. If nerve fibers other than gustatory fibers reinnervate the region, the taste buds do not reappear. Thus only gustatory nerves are capable of inducing the taste buds to appear. Motor fibers and nontaste fibers are not. The nature of the influences exerted by the nerve on the innervated structure to account for this phenomenon is not known. A plausible explanation is that certain substances—called trophic factors—in the nerves are conveyed via axoplasmic flow to the nerve terminals where they are released to the synaptic cleft. Then these "trophic" substances exert their roles of eliciting the formation of the taste buds and of maintaining their structural integrity.

Motor nerves are also implied to exert "trophic influences"; these include both somatic motor nerves (neuromuscular trophism) and nerves of the autonomic nervous system (neurovisceral trophism). "Trophic substances" may possibly have a role in some of the anatomic, biochemical, and physiologic differences between slow-red muscles and fast-white muscles. Red muscles are innervated slowly conducting axons (fire relatively slowly); white muscles are innervated primarily by rapidly conducting axons (fire relatively rapidly). Experimentally it is possible to sever the nerves innervating these muscles and have the slowly conducting axons regenerate to reinnervate the white muscles and have the fast conducting axons regenerate to reinnervate the red muscles. In such cross-innervation experiments, there is conversion of many but not all of the properties that are specific to each muscle type. These changes may be due, in part, to "trophic influences."

It is probable that the morphologic, physiologic, and biochemical parameters of a muscle cell are largely determined by the impulse pattern of the nerve innervating the muscle. The maintenance of white (or red) muscle and conversion of red to white muscle (or white to red muscle) is related to the rate of conduction of the nerve. Apparently the motor impulses are most critical for the differentiation of red (slow) and

white (fast) muscle because, through their activity, a rate of contraction is imposed on the muscle cell.

In effect, motor nerves with fast rates of conduction are associated with white muscles and those with slow rates with red muscles. Whether the control of the muscle type is mediated only by trophic factors or only by neuronal physiology or by both has not been resolved. In any case, the nerve innervating a muscle fiber has a significant role in influencing the muscle cells to express their genetic potential.

Clinically observed trophic changes include alterations that occur after lesions of the fibers of the autonomic nervous system. Among these disturbances are warm or cool, flushed or cyanotic skin (change in capillary circulation in skin), abnormal brittleness of the fingernails, loss of hair, dryness or ulcerations of the skin, and lysis of bones and joints, resulting, at times, in spontaneous fractures.

VISCERAL LEARNING

In the recent past it was said that the autonomic nervous system could not "learn" in the same sense as the somatic nervous system. This is true for humans and other mammals. By proper conditioned learning, the viscera can learn by *biofeedback*—a learned response to sensory input such that a specific thought complex or action can produce a desired response. For example, rats can be trained by the use of rewards to learn to control (1) their heart rate by making the heart beat faster or slower, (2) the rate of peristalsis, and (3) the rate of urine formation in the kidney.

Humans utilize visceral learning. Actors learn to regulate the flow of tears. Yogis can alter their heartbeat without resorting to physical exercise. We learn to control urination. Clinical applications are beginning to be found. For example, patients are being trained to control (1) the cardiovascular system, so that hypertensives can lower their blood pressure and hypotensives can raise their pressure; and (2) gut activity, so that mobility and peristalsis can be changed in certain gastrointestinal disturbances.

FUNCTIONAL CORRELATES

Angina pectoris

The frightening constricting pain of angina radiates from the left anterior chest wall and inner aspect of left arm. It is triggered by myocardial insufficiency as a consequence of reduced blood flow in the heart wall. The pain—referred from the heart to the chest and arm—is the result of the common afferent innervation of these structures to T1 and T3 segments of the left side of the spinal cord. Reduction or elimination of this referred pain can be obtained by (1) the application of a local anesthetic to skin over the sternum and left arm, (2) a neurosurgical operation in which the left sympathetic T1 to T4 ganglia are removed, or (3) transection of the dorsal roots of these same segments.

Megacolon (Hirschsprung's disease)

In this serious condition in young children, a portion of the large bowel is continuously constricted while the colon proximal to this obstructed segment is enormously dilated. The constricted segment contains the flaw responsible for the disease. Within this segment, there is an essential absence of intrinsic neurons of the intramural plexuses of the enteric nervous system. Because of the absence of the activity of these neurons, this aganglionic segment is unable to relax. This region does have an autonomic innervation consisting of both cholinergic and adrenergic axons. This disease illustrates the significance of the intrinsic neurons of the gut in peristalsis.

Painless childbirth

The normal activity of the uterus can be normally carried out, at least for a limited time, without its innervation. Because of this, the visceral afferent nerves from the uterus can be selectively anesthetized during childbirth to decrease the discomfort without abolishing the uterine contractions themselves.

BIBLIOGRAPHY

Appenzeller, O.: *The Autonomic Nervous System: An Introduction to Basic and Clinical Concepts*, American Elsevier Publishing Co., Inc., New York, 1970.

Botár, G.: *The Autonomic Nervous System*, Akadémiai Kiado, Budapest, 1966.

Burn, J. H.: *Autonomic Nervous System: For Students of Physiology and Pharmacology*, F. A. Davis Company, Philadelphia, 1971.

Burnstock, G., and T. Hökfelt (eds.): Non-adrenergic, non-cholinergic autonomic neurotransmission mechanisms. Neurosci Res Program Bull, 17:379–519, 1979.

Gershon, M. D., and S. Bursztajn: Properties of the enteric nervous system: limitation of access of intravascular macromolecules to the myenteric plexus and muscularis externa. J Comp Neurol, 180:467–487, 1978.

Guth, L.: "Trophic" influences of nerve on muscle. Physiol Rev, 48:645–687, 1968.

Koelle, G. B.: "Neurohumoral Transmission and the Autonomic Nervous System," in L. Goodman and A. Gilman (eds.), *The Pharmacological Basis of Therapeutics*, The Macmillan Company, New York, 1975, pp. 404–476.

Kuntz, A.: *The Autonomic Nervous System*, Lea & Febiger, Philadelphia, 1953.

Miller, A. E.: Biofeedback and visceral learning. Ann Rev Psychol, 29:373–404, 1978.

Mitchell, G. A.: *Anatomy of the Autonomic Nervous System*, Livingstone, Ltd., Edinburgh, 1953.

Neil, E. (ed.): "Enterceptors," in *Handbook of Sensory Physiology*, vol. III, sec. 1, Springer-Verlag, Berlin and New York, 1972, pp. 1–233.

Petras, J. M., and J. F. Cummins: Autonomic neurons in the spinal cord of the Rhesus monkey. A contribution of the findings of cytoarchitectonics and sympathectomy with fiber degeneration following dorsal rhizotomy. J Comp Neurol, 148:189–218, 1972.

Petras, J. M., and A. I. Faden: The origin of sympathetic preganglionic neurons in the dog. Brain Res 144:353–357, 1977.

Pick, J.: *Autonomic Nervous System: Morphological, Comparative, Clinical and Surgical Aspects*, J. B. Lippincott Company, Philadelphia, 1970.

Siegel, G. J., R. W. Albers, B. Katzman, and B. W. Agranoff: *Basic Neurochemistry*, Little, Brown and Company, Boston, 1976.

White, J. C., R. H. Smithwick, and F. A. Simeone: *The Autonomic Nervous System: Anatomy, Physiology and Surgical Application*, The Macmillan Company, New York, 1952.

CHAPTER SEVEN

THE CRANIAL NERVES

The cranial nerves are the peripheral nerves of the brain. They transmit input to the brain from the special sensors of smell, sight, hearing, and taste and from the same types of general sensors as do the peripheral spinal nerves. They convey output to the voluntary muscles involved with the movements of the eyes, mouth, face, tongue, pharynx, and larynx. They are the major outlet for the parasympathetic nervous system. Cranial nerves I and II are primarily associated with the cerebrum, whereas cranial nerves III through XII are nerves of the infratentorial brainstem.

The complexities of the 12 cranial nerves (see Table 7-1) will be outlined as follows:

1. Basic theory of the organization of the cranial nerves.
2. Cranial nerve nuclei within the brainstem.
3. Categories of cranial nerves based on their functional components.
4. General structural and functional aspects of the cranial nerves.
5. Peripheral ganglia associated with the cranial nerves.
6. Cranial nerve nuclei within the central nervous system.

BASIC THEORY OF THE ORGANIZATION OF THE CRANIAL NERVES

The cranial nerves can be better understood through an analysis of their functional components.

Components of the cranial nerves

The cranial nerves comprise the same four components of fibers present in the spinal nerves and three additional components (see Fig. 7-2). The four components found both in the spinal nerves and in the cranial nerves are the *general somatic afferent fibers* (GSA), the *general visceral afferent fibers* (GVA), the *general somatic efferent fibers* (GSE), and the *general visceral efferent fibers* (GVE). The three additional components found exclusively in the cranial nerves are the *special somatic afferent fibers* (SSA), the *special visceral afferent fibers* (SVA), and the *special visceral efferent fibers* (SVE). The special somatic afferent senses are vision, hearing, and equilibrium; the special visceral afferent senses are smell and taste. The special senses have their receptors located in restricted regions of the body. In contrast, the general senses have their receptors located over extensive regions of the body. The special visceral efferent fibers are the motor fibers innervating certain voluntary muscles of the head. They are the muscles of the branchial (visceral) arches, which in aquatic vertebrates (fish and amphibia) are the gill arches. Traditionally they are referred to as special visceral efferent musculature (branchiomeric or gill arch musculature). The term *visceral* is applied because these muscles are associated with the jaws, pharynx, and larynx, structures involved with such visceral functions as eating and breathing. No cranial nerve has all seven components.

The special visceral efferent fibers (SVE) are sometimes called special somatic efferent fibers

Nerve	Sensory peripheral ganglia
Olfactory nerve	Bipolar cells in nasal mucosa
Optic nerve	Bipolar cells located within the retina of eye
Trigeminal nerve	Trigeminal (Gasserian, semilunar) ganglion; mesencephalic nucleus of the midbrain
Facial nerve	Geniculate ganglion
Vestibulocochlear nerve	
Vestibular nerve	Vestibular ganglion (Scarpa's ganglion)
Cochlear nerve	Spiral ganglion
Glossopharyngeal nerve	Superior ganglion (somatic afferent)
	Inferior ganglion (visceral afferent)
Vagus nerve and spinal accessory nerve	Superior ganglion (somatic afferent)
	Inferior ganglion (visceral afferent)
Oculomotor nerve, trochlear nerve, abducent nerve, hypoglossal nerve	Cell bodies of proprioceptive neurons probably scattered along nerve, in trigeminal ganglion, or in mesencephalic nucleus of N. V

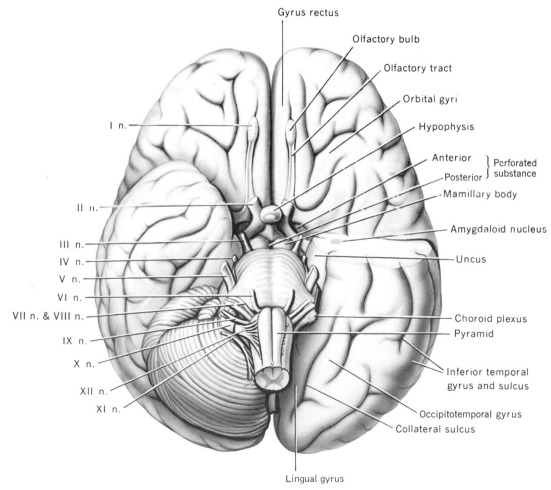

FIGURE 7-1 Basal surface of the brain and roots of the cranial nerves. Cerebellum and rostral portion of temporal lobe removed on right half of figure.

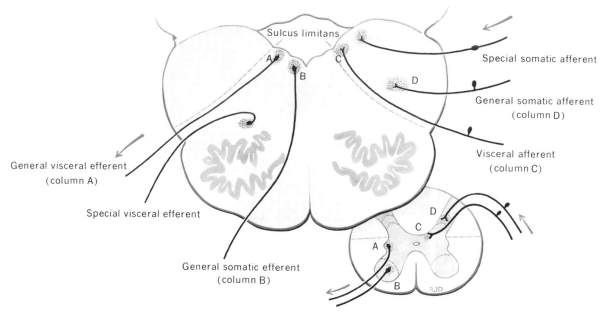

FIGURE 7-2 Functional components of the cranial nerve nuclei in the medulla and the spinal nerve nuclei in the spinal cord. In both regions, the afferent columns are located dorsal or dorsolateral to the dotted lines (derivatives of the alar plate, Chap. 4), and the efferent columns are located ventral or ventromedial to the dotted lines (derivatives of the basal plate; Chap. 4). In the medulla and the spinal cord, note the comparable locations of the general visceral efferent column (A), general somatic efferent column (B), general visceral afferent column (C), general somatic afferent column (D). Special somatic and special visceral nuclei are present only in the brain. The visceral afferent column in the brainstem is composed of special (such as taste) and general visceral afferent components.

(SSE) because the branchiomeric musculature innervated by these fibers are voluntary striated muscles.

CRANIAL NERVE NUCLEI WITHIN THE BRAINSTEM

The sensory nuclei of termination of the afferent fibers (see Fig. 7-3) and the nuclei of origin of the motor fibers of the cranial nerves (see Fig. 7-4) are organized in discontinuous nuclear "columns" within the brainstem. The olfactory nerve (N. I, SVA) and the optic nerve (N. II, SSA) are telencephalic and not brainstem cranial nerves.

Sensory nuclei of termination (Fig. 7-3)

There are three afferent columns of cranial nerve nuclei: (1) The *special somatic afferent column* includes the vestibular and cochlear nuclei (N.

VIII), which are located in the posterolateral tegmentum of the upper medulla and lower pons. (2) The *general somatic afferent column* includes the mesencephalic nucleus of N. V (proprioception), located in the posteromedial midbrain tegmentum; the principal (chief or main) sensory nucleus of N. V (touch), located in lateral midpontine tegmentum; and the spinal trigeminal nucleus (pain and temperature), located in the lateral tegmentum of the lower pons, medulla, and the upper two cervical spinal levels (fibers from nerves V, VII, IX, and X have fibers terminating in these nuclei). The mesencephalic nucleus of N. V is actually composed of cell bodies of neurons of the first order; it is a displaced portion of the trigeminal ganglion. (3) The *visceral afferent column* consists of the nucleus solitarius (and the commissural nucleus) located in the midposterior tegmentum of the medulla; its components include taste (SVA) and other visceral influences (GVA) which are conveyed via fibers in four cranial nerves, V, VII, IX, and X.

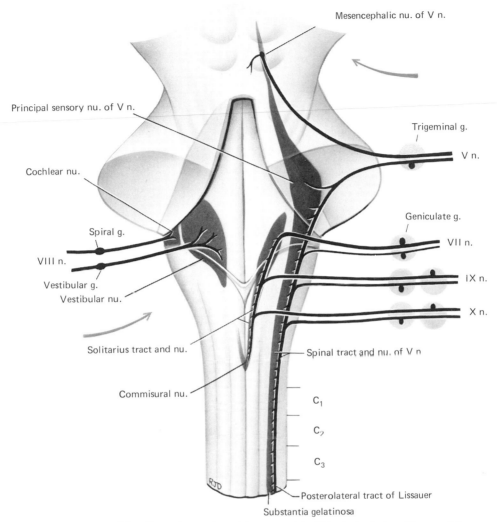

Mesencephalic nu. of V n.

Principal sensory nu. of V n.

Trigeminal g.

V n.

Cochlear nu.

Geniculate g.

VII n.

Spiral g.

VIII n.

Vestibular g.

Vestibular nu.

IX n.

X n.

Solitarius tract and nu.

Spinal tract and nu. of V n.

Commisural nu.

C₁

C₂

C₃

Posterolateral tract of Lissauer

Substantia gelatinosa

FIGURE 7-3 Location of the afferent (sensory) cranial nerve nuclei within the brainstem. These nuclei are organized into three nuclear columns. The general somatic afferent column includes the mesencephalic nucleus, the principal sensory nucleus, and the spinal nucleus of the fifth nerve. The general and special visceral afferent column includes the nucleus solitarius. The special somatic afferent column includes the cochlear and the vestibular nuclei. The sensory ganglia of the cranial nerves are indicated. The superior and inferior ganglia of both the ninth and tenth cranial nerves are illustrated but not labeled. g., ganglion; n., nerve; nu., nucleus.

Motor nuclei of origin

There are three efferent columns of cranial nerve nuclei: (1) The *general somatic efferent column* includes nuclei of the oculomotor nerve (midbrain), trochlear nerve (lower midbrain), abducent nerve (lower pons), and hypoglossal nerve (medulla). These nuclei, located in the posteromedial tegmentum, are composed of lower motor neurons innervating the voluntary muscles of the eye and tongue. (2) The *general visceral efferent column* includes the accessory oculomotor nucleus of Edinger-Westphal (midbrain N. III), the superior salivatory nucleus (posterior tegmentum of lower pons, N. VII), the inferior salivatory nucleus (posterior tegmentum of upper medulla, N. IX), and the dorsal motor nucleus of the vagus nerve (posterior tegmentum of

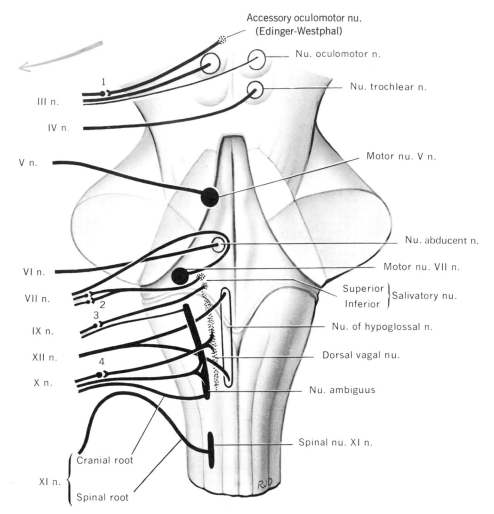

FIGURE 7-4 Location of the efferent (motor) cranial nerve nuclei within the brainstem. These nuclei are organized into three nuclear columns. The general somatic efferent column includes the nuclei of the third, fourth, sixth, and twelfth cranial nerves (outlined areas). The general visceral efferent (parasympathetic) column includes the accessory oculomotor nucleus (of Edinger-Westphal), salivary nuclei, and dorsal vagal nucleus (dotted areas). The special visceral efferent (gill arch) column includes the motor nucleus of the fifth nerve, facial nucleus, and nucleus ambiguus (solid areas). The numerals indicate the parasympathetic ganglia: (1) ciliary ganglion of the third cranial nerve, (2) pterygopalatine ganglion and submandibular ganglion of the seventh cranial nerve, (3) otic ganglion of the ninth cranial nerve, and (4) terminal parasympathetic ganglia (in the thoracic and abdominal viscera) of the tenth cranial nerve. The superior and inferior salivatory nuclei are actually diffuse and confluent groups of cells located within the parvicellular reticular nucleus (Chap. 8, Figs. 8-8, 8-9, 8-10).

medulla, N. X). These nuclei are composed of the cell bodies of preganglionic parasympathetic neurons of the autonomic nervous system. The salivatory nuclei are identifiable only by physiologic effects. (3) The *special visceral (branchial) efferent column* includes the motor nucleus of the fifth nerve (midpons, N. V), motor nucleus of the seventh nerve (lower pons, N. VII), and nucleus ambiguus (medulla, nerves IX, X, and XI). These nuclei of the lower motor neurons to the branchiomeric muscles are located in the middle of the tegmentum.

CATEGORIES OF CRANIAL NERVES BASED ON THEIR FUNCTIONAL COMPONENTS

The cranial nerves are tabulated according to their functional components in Table 7-2. Reference to this table indicates the rationale for the grouping of the cranial nerves into the following three categories.

Special afferent nerves The nerves primarily conveying special (somatic and visceral) afferent fibers from the special senses include the olfactory nerve (N. I), the optic nerve (N. II), and the vestibulocochlear nerve (N. VIII). The nerves with fibers transmitting the taste modality are located in the three visceral arch nerves noted further on.

General somatic efferent nerves The nerves conveying general somatic motor fibers to the voluntary muscles of the eye and the tongue include the oculomotor (N. III), trochlear (N. IV), abducent (N. VI), and hypoglossal (N. XII). The proprioceptive fibers (general somatic afferent component) innervating the extraocular muscles are located in the trigeminal nerve (see page 256). The oculomotor nerve has, in addition, general visceral efferent (parasympathetic) fibers to the eye.

Visceral arch nerves (branchiomeric, branchial, trematic, or gill arch nerves) The trigeminal (N. V), facial (N. VII), glossopharyngeal (N. IX), vagal (N. X), and the cranial root of the spinal accessory (N. XI) are nerves of the branchial arches. Each one of these nerves is associated with a specific gill arch in fish or with its evolutionary successor in higher vertebrates—the trigeminal nerve with the first arch (jaws), the facial nerve with the second arch, the glossopharyngeal nerve with the third arch, and the vagus nerve with the remaining arches. The basic similarities of the facial, glossopharyngeal, and vagus nerves are indicated by the fact that all have the same functional components (Table 7-2).

Each of these nerves has one or two sensory ganglia; significantly, these are the counterparts of the spinal ganglia of the spinal nerves (Table 7-1). In addition, parasympathetic ganglia are associated with the general visceral efferent component: the facial nerve is associated with the submandibular and pterygopalatine ganglia; the glossopharyngeal nerve with the otic ganglion; and the vagus nerve with small terminal ganglia within or on the viscera. In these ganglia are located the synapses between the preganglionic neurons and the postganglionic neurons (Chap. 6).

Each gill surrounds a gill slit, or *trema* (a hole from the pharynx to the outside for the passage of water in a fish or tadpole). Typically each of these nerves consists of three divisions: (1) The *pretrematic division*, which passes on the front margin of the trema, is an afferent nerve. It may contain parasympathetic fibers. (2) The *posttrematic division*, which passes on the hind margin of the trema, is a mixed nerve with afferent and efferent nerve fibers. The efferent fibers innervate the voluntary musculature of the gill. (3) The *pharyngeal division* is composed of afferent fibers to the pharynx. The relationship of the branchiomeric nerves to a gill slit is retained in a masked form in the land vertebrates, including humans. For example, in the trigeminal nerve, the pretrematic division is the maxillary nerve (a sensory nerve), the posttrematic division is composed of the mandibular and lingual nerves (collectively mixed sensory and motor nerves), and the pharyngeal division is the greater palatine nerve (a sensory nerve, Fig. 8-17).

The chorda tympani nerve of the seventh nerve and the tympanic nerve (nerve of Jacobson) of the ninth nerve are pretrematic nerves, whereas the main trunks of the seventh and ninth nerves are posttrematic nerves.

GENERAL STRUCTURAL AND FUNCTIONAL ASPECTS OF THE CRANIAL NERVES

Olfactory nerve (N. I)

The *olfactory*, or *first cranial*, *nerve* consists of from 15 to 20 small bundles of unmyelinated axons of neurons whose cell bodies are located in the olfactory mucosa of the nasal cavity. The olfactory neurons are bipolar neurons (SVA) which act as chemoreceptors, transducers of stimuli, and transmitters of nerve impulses to the olfactory bulb. The peripherally directed process of each cell (the "dendrite") commences on the sur-

Table 7-2
Components and functions of cranial nerves

Name	Components	Functions (major)
I. Olfactory nerve	Special visceral afferent (SVA)	Smell
II. Optic nerve	Special somatic afferent (SSA)	Vision and associated reflexes
III. Oculomotor nerve*	General somatic efferent (GSE)	Movements of eyes
	General visceral efferent (GVE) (parasympathetic)	Pupillary constriction and accommodation
IV. Trochlear nerve*	General somatic efferent (GSE)	Movements of eyes
V. Trigeminal nerve	Special visceral efferent (SVE)	Mastication Swallowing Movements of soft palate and auditory tube Movements of tympanic membrane and ear ossicles
	General somatic afferent (GSA)	General sensations from anterior half of head, including face, nose, mouth, and meninges
	General visceral afferent (GVA)	Visceral sensibility
VI. Abducent nerve†	General somatic efferent (GSE)	Movements of eyes
VII. Facial nerve	Special visceral efferent (SVE)	Facial expression Elevation of hyoid bone Movement of stapes
	General visceral efferent (GVE) (parasympathetic)	Lacrimation, salivation, and vasodilatation
	Special visceral afferent (SVA)	Taste
	General visceral afferent (GVA)	Visceral sensibility
VIII. Vestibulocochlear nerve	Special somatic afferent (SSA)	Hearing and equilibrium reception
IX. Glossopharyngeal nerve	Special visceral efferent (SVE)	Swallowing movements Raises pharynx and larynx
	General visceral efferent (GVE) (parasympathetic)	Salivation and vasodilatation
	Special visceral afferent (SVA)	Taste
	General afferent (GSA, GVA)	General senses in region of posterior third of tongue, tonsils, and upper pharynx Receptors of carotid sinus and carotid body
X. Vagus nerve and cranial root of N. XI	Special visceral efferent (SVE)	Swallowing movements and laryngeal control Movements of soft palate, pharynx, and larynx
	General visceral efferent (GVE) (parasympathetic)	Parasympathetic to thoracic and abdominal viscera
	Special visceral afferent (SVA)	Taste (epiglottis)
	General visceral afferent (GVA)	Sensory from viscera of neck (larynx, trachea, and esophagus), thorax, and abdomen
	General visceral afferent (GVA)	Visceral sensibility
XI. Accessory nerve (spinal root)	Special visceral efferent (SVE)	Movements of shoulder and head
XII. Hypoglossal nerve*	General somatic efferent (GSE)	Movements of tongue

* *General somatic afferent (GSA)–proprioception from the muscles of the eye and tongue.*
† *General somatic afferent (GSA)–cutaneous sense from small portion of and just behind external ear and external auditory meatus.*

face of the mucosa. The centrally directed process (the axon) joins one of the bundles, which passes through the cribriform plate of the ethmoid bone and the anterior cranial fossa before terminating in the olfactory bulb (Chap. 15).

These specialized special visceral afferent neurons are unusual among neurons for the following reasons:

1. They are the only sensory neurons in humans with cell bodies which are located distally in a peripheral structure (olfactory mucosa).
2. They are both receptors and neurons of the first order.
3. Each dendrite has specialized cilia, which extend into and are bathed in the secretion on the surface of the olfactory mucosa. In humans, these are the only nerve processes in direct contact with the external environment. In contrast, gustatory cells in the taste buds are neuroepithelial cells, rather than neurons (Chap. 8).
4. The axonal processes of a number of neurons collect into small groups of fibers. Each group is located within a trough ensheathed by neurolemma cells; the axons within each group are not separated from one another by processes of the neurolemma cell (see Fig. 2-15).

The total inability to perceive odors is called *anosmia*.

Optic nerve (N. II)

The *optic*, or *second cranial*, *nerve* is actually a tract of the central nervous system, not a true peripheral nerve (SSA); it consists of about 1 million fibers of the second order, which are invested by glial rather than neurolemma cells (Chap. 12). The optic nerve comprises the axons of the ganglion cells of the retina. Theoretically the bipolar cells of the retina are the equivalent of the peripheral nerves. These cells are located wholly within the retina and are intercalated between the photoreceptors (rods and cones, which may be considered to be neuroepithelial cells) and the ganglion cells.

The axons of ganglion cells of the retina converge to the optic disk and penetrate through the sclera of the eye (cribriform plate) to form the optic nerve, which is surrounded by all three meninges of the brain. The dura mater is continuous with the sclera of the eye. The subarachnoid and subdural spaces are continuous up to the region of the optic disk. The nerve passes successively through the orbit and the optic canal, including the common tendinous ring which is the origin of the four rectus muscles of the eye. The nerve is continuous with the optic chiasma, which is located in the middle cranial fossa, rostral to the hypophysis. The parasympathetic ciliary ganglion is found within the orbit lateral to the optic nerve. The *central retinal artery* (as well as the vein) enters the optic nerve from below about 10 to 20 mm behind the eye (see Fig. 1-32); it supplies the core of the nerve and the entire retina except for the pigment and rod and cone layers. An increase in the intracranial pressure is transmitted to the cerebrospinal fluid of the subarachnoid space surrounding the entire optic nerve, including the region of the optic disk. This increase may result in a condition called *papilledema*. In its early stages, it is characterized by engorgement of the retinal veins, pinkness of the optic disk, and blurring of the margins of the disk. In time, the indentation of the disk is obliterated and elevated.

The extraocular nerves — oculomotor (N. III), trochlear (N. IV), and abducent (N. VI) nerves (Fig. 7-5)

These three cranial nerves contain the lower motor neurons (GSE) which innervate the six extraocular and levator palpebral muscles. In addition, the oculomotor nerve has preganglionic and parasympathetic fibers (GVE), terminating in the ciliary ganglion with postganglionic neurons which innervate smooth muscles in the eye. Each nerve has proprioceptive fibers (from neuromuscular spindles, GSA), which may have their cell bodies along each nerve, in the trigeminal ganglion or in the mesencephalic nucleus of N. V. The coordinated activities of the extraocular muscles produce the normal conjugate movements of the eyes; the contraction of the levator palpebral muscles elevates the eyelids. The parasympathetic innervation, which is derived from the oculomotor nerve, has a role in accommodation (focusing) and constriction of the pupil. The sympathetic innervation to the eye is derived

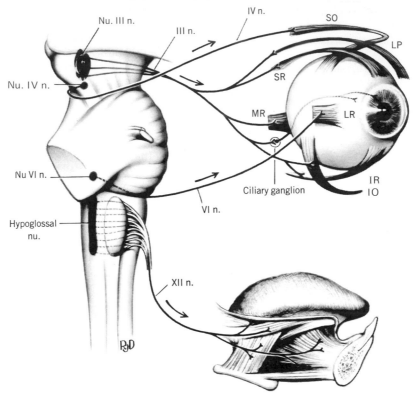

FIGURE 7-5 The cranial nerve nuclei and distribution of the oculomotor, trochlear, abducent, and hypoglossal nerves (III, IV, VI, and XII). The extraocular muscles are indicated as follows: IO, inferior oblique; IR, inferior rectus; LP, levator palpebral; LR, lateral rectus; MR, medial rectus; SO, superior oblique; SR, superior rectus.

from postganglionic sympathetic fibers from the superior cervical ganglion, which join the third, fourth, and sixth cranial nerves as they pass through the cavernous sinus (Fig. 5-32).

The *nuclear complex of the oculomotor nerve* is located in the anteromedial aspect of the periaqueductal gray at the level of the superior colliculus. The nucleus, which has a triangular shape in cross section, is flanked on its anterolateral sides by the medial longitudinal fasciculus (see Fig. 8-12). The root fibers of the oculomotor nerve from this nucleus sweep anteriorly through the medial longitudinal fasciculus and the medial tegmentum, including the red nucleus and substantia nigra, and enter the interpeduncular fossa as a number of rootlets, which join to form the oculomotor nerve within the interpeduncular cistern. The nerve passes between the posterior cerebral artery and the superior cerebellar artery and then successively through the cavernous sinus, inferior orbital fissure, and orbit, where it divides into a superior branch (innervating the superior rectus and levator palpebrae muscles) and an inferior branch (innervating the medial rectus, inferior rectus, and inferior oblique muscles).

The oculomotor nuclear complex is subdivided into several longitudinally oriented cell columns and nuclei. The extraocular muscles which are innervated by uncrossed nerve fibers from this complex include the inferior rectus muscle that is innervated by fibers from the posterior cell column, the inferior oblique muscle by the intermediate cell column, and the medial rectus muscle by the anterior cell column. The superior rectus muscle is innervated by crossed fibers from the medial cell column. Each levator palpebral muscle is innervated by both crossed and uncrossed fibers from the caudal central nucleus.

The parasympathetic nuclei (GVE) consist of a pair of narrow columns (accessory oculomotor nucleus of Edinger-Westphal) posterior to the rostral three-fifths of the oculomotor complex; these columns become continuous rostrally with the anterior median nucleus located in the raphe. The accessory oculomotor nucleus and anterior median nuclei give rise to uncrossed preganglionic parasympathetic fibers. They synapse in the ciliary ganglia with postganglionic parasympathetic fibers which innervate smooth muscle of the ciliary body and iris. Of the parasympathetic fibers to the eye, about 90 percent are said to innervate the ciliary musculature ("Accommodation," Chap. 12), while the remainder innervate the pupillary constrictor muscles of the iris diaphragm (miosis).

Functional roles   The precise roles of the extraocular muscles in eye movements are complex, with many actions depending upon the position of the eyeball within the orbit. The following is a summary (Fig. 12-3):

1. The medial and lateral recti muscles rotate the eyeball around its vertical axis. The medial rectus is an adductor, which deviates the pupil inward toward the nose; the lateral rectus is an abductor, which deviates the pupil outward toward the temple. These muscles are antagonists.
2. The superior and inferior recti muscles rotate the eyeball around its transverse axis. With the eye rotated outward, the superior rectus is a pure elevator (pupil directed upward), while the inferior rectus is a pure depressor (pupil directed downward). In other positions these muscles also have a role in adducting the eye.
3. The superior and inferior oblique muscles rotate the eyeball around its sagittal axis. With the eye directed inward, the superior oblique is a depressor and the inferior oblique is an elevator of the eye. With the eye directed outward, the superior oblique is an intorter of the eye (rotates on the sagittal axis), while the inferior oblique is an extorter of the eye. The superior rectus and inferior rectus act as intorter and extorter, respectively, when the eye is directed inward.

4. The levator palpebral muscles elevate the upper eyelids.

The movements of the eyes are precisely and delicately coordinated. *Conjugate movements* are those in which the eyes move in the same direction. On looking to the right, the lateral rectus of the right eye and the medial rectus of the left eye are the muscles involved in the movement. *Disjunctive movements* are those in which the eyes move in opposite directions. In close-up vision, the eyes converge. In this disjunctive movement the two medial recti contract and the two lateral recti relax. Conjugate and disjunctive movements are regulated and controlled by supranuclear (upper motor neuron) influences acting through circuits composed of interneurons (see "The Oculomotor System," p. 361).

The *trochlear nerve* originates from the small nucleus located in an indentation in the posterior margin of the medial longitudinal fasciculus at the level of the inferior colliculus (see Fig. 8-11). The nucleus is actually a caudal extension of the oculomotor nucleus. The fibers from the nucleus of the trochlear nerve curve posterolaterally and caudally along the edge of the periventricular gray; all fibers cross the midline and emerge on the dorsal surface of the brainstem just caudal to the inferior colliculus (see Fig. 1-15). The nerve courses through the sequence of rostral pons, along the under surface of the tentorium, lateral wall of the cavernous sinus, superior orbital fissure, and orbit before innervating the superior oblique muscle.

The *abducent (abducens) nerve* originates from the nucleus located in the floor of the fourth ventricle near the midline in the caudal pons (it forms the abducent or facial colliculus; see Fig. 1-16). All its fibers have an ipsilateral course. They pass from the abducent nucleus anteriorly through the tegmentum before emerging from the brainstem just lateral to the pyramid at the pons-medulla junction (see Figs. 1-13 and 8-9). The nerve then continues forward through the sequence of cisterna pontis, lateral wall of the cavernous sinus, superior orbital fissure, and orbit before innervating the lateral rectus muscle.

Lesions   The paralysis of one or more of the extraocular muscles results in diplopia (double vision) because of the faulty coordination of movements of the two eyes. A *complete lesion of an oculomotor nerve* results in the following: (1) *ptosis*, or drooping, of the eyelid and inability to elevate the eyelid because of unopposed action of the orbicularis oculi muscle which closes the eyelid (innervated by N. VII); (2) dilated pupil (*mydriasis*) which is unresponsive to the light reflex because of interruption of the parasympathetic fibers and the unopposed activity of the intact sympathetic fibers to the iris diaphragm (Chap. 12); (3) loss of accommodation due to interruption of parasympathetic fibers; lens may be permanently adjusted for distant vision; and (4) *external* (*divergent*) *strabismus*, with the pupil directed laterally and downward (*walleye*) because of unopposed action of the lateral rectus and superior oblique muscles, the inability to direct the affected eye inward, upward, and downward. Subjects with this lower motor neuron paralysis of the third nerve turn their heads away from the paralyzed side in an attempt to minimize the diplopia caused by the abnormal position of the involved eye.

A *complete lesion of the trochlear nerve* results in vertical diplopia, head tilt, and limitation of ocular movement on looking down and in. Diplopia occurs when subjects turn their eyes in any direction except upward; the double vision is maximal when the pupils are turned down; this makes walking difficult, especially when walking downstairs. To align the eyes in order to minimize or eliminate the diplopia, patients tilt their heads to the shoulder on the side opposite the paralyzed muscle. Because the trochlear fibers decussate within the dorsal brainstem, the nucleus of the trochlear nerve is on the opposite side from the trochlear nerve itself; hence a lesion of a nucleus of the trochlear nerve is expressed in the contralateral eye.

A *complete lesion of the abducent nerve* results in a horizontal diplopia, with the ipsilateral eye adducted (convergent strabismus) because of the unopposed action of the normal medial rectus muscle. Abduction is limited. The diplopia is maximal when the subject attempts to gaze to the side of the lesion (because the eye with the paralyzed lateral rectus cannot be adequately abducted). It is minimal with gaze to the normal side, because the visual axis of the normal eye can parallel that of the affected eye.

Trigeminal nerve (N. V)
(Figs. 7-6 and 8-17)

The *trigeminal*, or *fifth cranial*, *nerve* is the main general sensory nerve, composed of GSA fibers conveying the modalities of pain, temperature, touch, and proprioception from the superficial and deep regions of the face. The regions innervated include the skin of the anterior scalp and face; mucous membrane of the mouth (including gum and tongue), nasal cavities and paranasal sinuses, teeth, and meninges. In addition, its masticator (motor) nerve, with SVE fibers, innervates muscles involved with mastication, swallowing, movements of the soft palate and auditory tube, and movements of the tympanic membrane and ear ossicles.

The trigeminal nerve emerges from the anterolateral surface of the midpons as two adjacent roots: the large sensory root and the small motor root. These roots course anteriorly on the floor of the posterior fossa, across the tip of the petrous portion of the temporal bone into the middle cranial fossa, where it joins the massive trigeminal ganglia in the trigeminal cave. The latter is a cavity in the dura mater on the anterior surface of the petrosal bone. The internal carotid artery and the posterior aspect of the cavernous sinus are located medial to the trigeminal ganglion.

The unipolar neurons of the trigeminal ganglion (Gasserian ganglion, semilunar ganglion) give rise to the three large branches of the trigeminal nerve: the ophthalmic, maxillary, and mandibular nerves. The root fibers associated with these nerves are topographically represented within the sensory root. At the locale of emergence of the sensory root from the pons, the ophthalmic fibers are located caudally, the maxillary fibers in an intermediate position, and the mandibular fibers rostrally. In the region where the sensory root joins the trigeminal ganglion, the ophthalmic fibers are located medially, the maxillary in an intermediate position, and the mandibular fibers laterally. The motor root is generally located on the medial aspect of the sensory root; it courses laterally on the inferior aspect of the trigeminal ganglion before its fibers blend into the mandibular nerve.

Peripheral distribution The ophthalmic nerve passes forward in the dura mater on the lateral

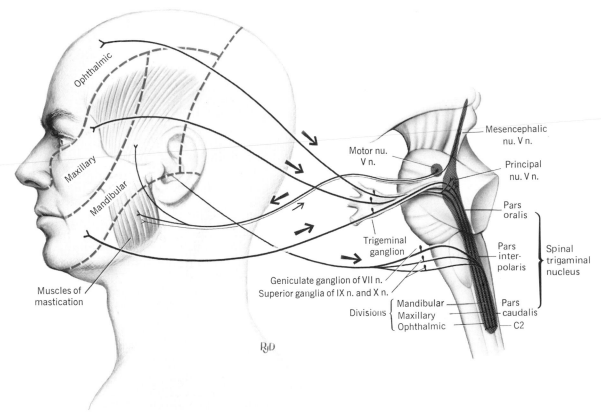

FIGURE 7-6 The cranial nerve nuclei and distribution of the trigeminal nerve (N. V). Fibers of nerves VII, IX, and X from the region of the outer ear to the spinal nucleus of N. V are illustrated.

wall of the cavernous sinus and through the superior orbital fissure before entering the orbit. Branches of this nerve innervate the dura mater, including the tentorium, orbit, eye [including the cornea (e.g., corneal reflex)], upper eyelid, skin of the nose, forehead, and scalp back to a line between the ears, and the mucosa of the frontal, sphenoid, and ethmoid paranasal sinuses.

The maxillary nerve passes out of the skull through the foramen rotundum into the pterygopalatine fossa, where it becomes associated with the pterygopalatine ganglion (parasympathetic ganglion which receives preganglionic fibers from the facial nerve). The branches of the maxillary nerve innervate the dura of the middle cranial fossa, lower eyelid, skin of the temple, upper cheek, adjacent area of the nose and upper lip, mucous membranes of the upper mouth, nose, roof of pharynx, and maxillary, ethmoid, and sphenoid paranasal sinuses, and the gums, teeth, and palate of the upper jaw.

The mandibular nerve passes from the middle cranial fossa through the foramen ovale into the infratemporal fossa. One of its branches, the lingual nerve, is associated with the submandibular ganglion (parasympathetic ganglion) which receives preganglionic fibers from the chorda tympani of the facial nerve. Branches of the mandibular nerve supply the sensory innervation to part of the dura mater of the middle and anterior cranial fossa; teeth and gums of the lower jaw; oral mucosa of the cheek, floor of the mouth, and anterior two-thirds of the tongue; skin of the auricular temporal region, lower lip, external auditory meatus, tympanic membrane, and lower jaw; and the temporomandibular joint. The pulp of the tooth contains only A delta and C (pain) fibers. The masticator nerve supplies the lower neuron innervation to (1) the four muscles of mastication (temporalis, masseter, and internal and external pterygoids), (2) the mylohyoid and anterior belly of the digastric muscles, and (3) the tensor tympani and tensor veli palatine muscles.

The jaw jerk is a two-neuron flexor reflex (similar to the extensor knee jerk), which involves the temporalis and masseter muscles. This reflex can be evoked by tapping the chin of the slightly opened mouth. The afferent limb of the reflex arc is composed of neurons of the mesencephalic nucleus of N. V, which convey influences from the neuromuscular spindles of these muscles to the motor nucleus of N. V. The lower motor neurons from the latter nucleus comprise the efferent limb, which innervates the muscles of mastication. The mylohyoid and anterior belly of the digastric muscles have a role in mastication and swallowing. During its contraction, the tensor tympani, through its pull on the malleus, tenses the tympanic membrane; this protects the tympanic membrane by dampening the amplitude of its vibration to loud noises. The tensor veli palatine muscle helps to prevent food from passing into the nasal pharynx by tensing the soft palate.

The branches of the trigeminal nerve are characterized by several special features.

1. Each of the three major branches—ophthalmic, maxillary, and mandibular—supplies a distinct dermatome of the head, face, and oral cavity (see Figs. 7-6 and 8-17). These three nerves show practically no dermatomal overlap, as do the nerves innervating the dermatomes formed by the spinal nerves.

2. Information from proprioceptive endings (e.g., neuromuscular spindles) in the extraocular muscles and muscles of facial expression are conveyed to the central nervous system by nerve fibers of the oculomotor, trochlear, abducent, and facial nerves, which join the trigeminal nerve. These fibers are presumed to have their cell bodies in the trigeminal ganglion and in the mesencephalic nucleus of the trigeminal nerve.

3. The lingual branch of the mandibular nerve contains gustatory fibers from the anterior two-thirds of the tongue. In fact, these fibers are facial rather than trigeminal nerve fibers. These taste fibers pass from the nucleus soli-

tarius through the nervus intermedius and one of its branches, the chorda tympani, which joins the lingual nerve.

4. Many fibers of the autonomic nervous system join the branches of the trigeminal nerve. Among these are the postganglionic sympathetic fibers from the superior cervical ganglion, which leave the external carotid artery plexus and join each of the major branches of the trigeminal nerve. These fibers supply the sympathetic innervation to the sweat glands of the skin, the mucosal glands (mucous and serous) of the nasal and oral cavities, and the blood vessels.

5. Each of the three major branches of the trigeminal nerve is associated with a parasympathetic ganglion. The ophthalmic nerve receives postganglionic fibers from the ciliary ganglion, the maxillary nerve from the pterygopalatine ganglion, and the mandibular nerve from the submandibular and otic ganglia. Recall that preganglionic fibers to these ganglia are derived from the oculomotor nerve (ciliary ganglion), from the facial nerve (pterygopalatine and submandibular ganglia), and from the glossopharyngeal nerve (otic ganglion). The trigeminal nerve is actually the vehicle for the distribution of the postganglionic parasympathetic fibers to the smooth muscles of the eye and to the glands of the head (including the lacrimal gland and those of the nasal and oral mucosa).

Central projections The sensory root (portio major) of the trigeminal nerve enters the pons and divides into an ascending limb (which terminates in the principal nucleus of the trigeminal nerve) and a descending limb (which forms the spinal tract of the trigeminal nerve, N. V). The fibers of the sensory root of the trigeminal nerve rotate so that the fibers from the caudally located mandibular nerve become located posteriorly in the spinal tract of N. V, those from the rostrally located ophthalmic nerve become located anteriorly in the spinal tract of N. V, and those from the maxillary nerve become located in an intermediate position between the other two nerves (see Fig. 7-6). The sensory root fibers consist of several types: (1) nonbifurcating ascending fibers to the *principal sensory nucleus*— these subserve touch, position sense, and two-point discrimination; (2) nonbifurcating A delta and C descending fibers of the spinal tract of N. V—these subserve pain and temperature; and (3) bifurcating fibers, each with an ascending branch to the principal sensory nucleus and a descending branch of the spinal tract of N. V—these subserve touch and two-point discrimination. The descending fibers of the ophthalmic, maxillary, and mandibular nerves have collateral branches, which terminate throughout the spinal nucleus of N. V., and terminal branches, which descend as far caudally as the first two cervical spinal levels. The spinal nucleus of N. V is a continuous structure which is subdivided into (1) the rostrally located *pars oralis,* which receives tactile input from the head, mouth, lips, and nose; (2) the intermediately located *pars interpolaris,* which receives input from cutaneous areas of the forehead, cheeks, and angle of the jaw, and from the tooth pulp; and (3) the caudally located *pars caudalis,* which receives the modalities of light touch, pain, and temperature from the entire anterior part of the head.

The pars oralis is located in the pons caudal to the principal sensory nucleus, which is in the midpons (see Fig. 7-6). The pars interpolaris extends in the upper medulla from the pars oralis to the level of the obex (see Fig. 7-6), while the pars caudalis extends from the obex level caudally through the second cervical spinal level. The pars oralis is composed of small, tightly packed cells, whereas the pars interpolaris is characterized by scattered, small cells. The pars caudalis is the posterior horn of the medulla because it is subdivided into a *marginal layer* equivalent to lamina I of the posterior horn, a *substantia gelatinosa,* equivalent to laminae II and III, and a *magnocellular layer* equivalent to lamina IV and V (see Fig. 7-6; see also Fig. 8-5). In fact, the spinal tract of N. V is the brainstem equivalent of the dorsolateral tract of Lissauer and the spinal nucleus of N. V is the continuation of the posterior horn of the spinal cord. The pars caudalis is often called the posterior horn of the medulla. Evidence indicates that a large proportion of the neurons in the pars oralis and pars interpolaris project to the cerebellum.

The motor root (portio minor) is composed primarily but not exclusively of motor fibers from the motor nucleus of the trigeminal nerve. In addition, the root contains a significant number of afferent fibers with their cell bodies in the trigeminal ganglion. As with the afferent fibers in the ventral roots of the spinal nerves (Chap. 5), the role and connections of the fibers is not known.

In general, the pain modality is conveyed from all trigeminal nerves via sensory root fibers which, after entering the pons, descend in the spinal tract N. V as far caudal as the C2 spinal level. These fibers terminate in the pars caudalis. The touch-pressure, position sense, and two-point discrimination modalities are conveyed via the sensory root fibers, which, after entering the pons, terminate in the principal nucleus and pars oralis of the spinal nucleus of the trigeminal nerve. Many collateral branches descend in the spinal tract before terminating in the spinal nucleus of N. V. Unconscious proprioceptive information (pressure and position sense) from the periodontal membrane of the teeth (tooth pressure receptors), palate, muscles, and temporomandibular joint is conveyed to the mesencephalic nucleus of the trigeminal nerve. This includes input from the neuromuscular spindles in the extraocular muscles, muscles of mastication, and probably all other facial muscles including those of the tongue. The motor nucleus of N. V is the nucleus of origin of the lower motor neurons which pass through the motor root and the mandibular nerve to the voluntary muscles innervated by N. V. Sensory root fibers conveying visceral afferents descend in the solitary tract and terminate in the caudal half of the solitary nucleus.

Lesions Interruption of all trigeminal fibers unilaterally results in anesthesia and loss of general senses in the region innervated by N. V and a lower motor neuron paralysis (weakness, fasciculations, loss of jaw jerk unilaterally, and atrophy) of the jaw muscles. The sensory changes include loss of smarting effect in one nostril from the insensitivity of the nasal mucosa to ammonia and other volatile chemicals and loss of corneal sensation. The complete interruption of the sensory fibers from the cornea results in loss of the ipsilateral and contralateral (consensual) corneal reflex. The afferent limb of the *corneal reflex* (N. V) stimulates through interneurons both facial motor nuclei, whose lower motor neurons innervate the orbicularis oculi muscles of both eyes. The loss of proprioceptive input may result in the relaxation of the ipsilateral muscles of facial expressions (innervated by N. VII). The loss of the *jaw jerk* results from the interruption of both the afferent and efferent limbs of the reflex arc. Because of the action of the contracting pterygoid muscles on the normal side, the jaw, when protruded, will deviate and point to the paralyzed side. The patient may experience partial deafness to low-pitched sounds because of the paralysis of the tensor tympani muscle. The floor of the mouth on the paralyzed side exhibits flaccidity because of the paralysis of the mylohyoid muscle and the anterior belly of the digastric.

Sharp, agonizing and excruciating pain localized and confined in the area of distribution of one or more branches of the trigeminal nerve is known as trigeminal neuralgia or *tic douloureux*. The slight stimulation of a region called a *trigger zone* may initiate an attack. The cause is unknown. One possibility is an abnormal, "epileptic-like" discharge triggered in neurons of the pars caudalis of the spinal nucleus of cranial nerve V. This is the rationale for the therapeutic use of anticonvulsant agents in this condition. Some success has been claimed in alleviating the pain by (1) *medullary tractotomy*—sectioning of the spinal tract of N. V; (2) sectioning roots of the trigeminal nerve proximal to the trigeminal ganglion (in this procedure the ophthalmic nerve is not severed in order to retain corneal reflex); and (3) electrocoagulation or alcohol block in the trigeminal ganglion.

The supranuclear (upper motor neuron) influences upon the motor nucleus of N. V are outlined in Chap. 8. Unilateral supranuclear lesions usually do not impair trigeminal motor activity. This is because (1) crossed and uncrossed corticobulbar fibers and (2) crossed and uncrossed corticoreticular fibers (through interneurons) project to the motor nucleus of N. V.

Facial nerve (N. VII) (Fig. 7-7)

The *facial*, or *seventh cranial*, *nerve* consists of the facial nerve proper with its lower motor neurons and the *nervus intermedius* with its sensory and parasympathetic components. The SVE fibers of the facial nerve proper convey motor impulses to the muscles of facial (*mimetic*) expression (i.e.,

those involved in closing the eyelids, frowning, smiling, whistling, wrinkling the forehead, puffing the cheek to blow up a balloon, and pursing the lips). Other muscles innervated by the facial nerve include the stapedius (controls the movements of the stapes) and the posterior belly of the digastric muscle (elevates the hyoid bone). All the sensory neurons of the first order in the *nervus intermedius* have their unipolar cell bodies in the geniculate ganglion. This includes taste (SVA) from the anterior two-thirds of the tongue, GSA information from the back of the external ear, and GVA input from the glands and other visceral structures of the face. The parasympathetic fibers (GVE) of the nervus intermedius, through their connections in the pterygopalatine and submandibular ganglia, exert influences on the lacrimal, nasal, oral, submaxillary, and sublingual glands and blood vessels.

The facial nerve emerges from the inferior lateral aspect of the brainstem at the pons-medulla junction just anterior to the vestibulocochlear nerve. The nervus intermedius is located between these two nerves. The three nerves pass successively through the cerebellopontine angle and the internal auditory meatus. The facial nerve proper continues through the facial canal, from which it emerges at the stylomastoid foramen; it then arborizes into branches which innervate the muscles of facial expression. Within the facial canal (distal to the geniculate ganglion), the facial nerve has three branches: the *nerve to the stapedius muscle;* the *chorda tympani* with its special (taste) and general visceral afferent fibers and preganglionic parasympathetic fibers to the submandibular ganglion (postganglionic fibers from this ganglion innervate the submandibular, sublingual, and other small salivary glands); and the *nerve to the external auditory meatus* and external ear (general somatic afferent).

The *greater petrosal nerve* is a branch of the nervus intermedius. It is composed of preganglionic parasympathetic fibers which synapse with postganglionic neurons in the pterygopalatine ganglion; the latter project influences to the lacrimal gland and the glands of the nasal cavity and palate. Some special (taste) and general visceral afferent fibers also pass through the greater petrosal nerve. Some postganglionic sympathetic fibers from the superior cervical ganglion

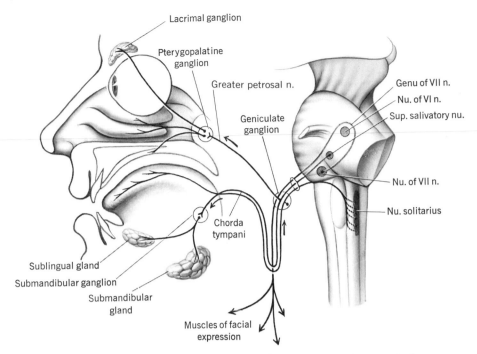

Lacrimal ganglion

Pterygopalatine ganglion

Greater petrosal n.

Geniculate ganglion

Genu of VII n.

Nu. of VI n.

Sup. salivatory nu.

Nu. of VII n.

Nu. solitarius

Chorda tympani

Sublingual gland

Submandibular ganglion

Submandibular gland

Muscles of facial expression

FIGURE 7-7 The cranial nerve nuclei and distribution of the facial nerve (cranial nerve VII). The superior and inferior salivatory nuclei are actually diffuse and confluent groups of cells located within the parvicellular reticular nucleus (Chap. 8, Figs. 8-8, 8-9, 8-10)

leave the carotid plexus to join some branches of the facial nerve.

Central projections and connections The special visceral efferent fibers to the muscles of facial expression arise from the motor nucleus of the seventh nerve. After leaving the nucleus, the fibers take a hairpin course through the lower pons as they recurve as the internal genu around the nucleus of the abducent nerve before passing into the cerebellopontine angle. The preganglionic parasympathetic fibers from the superior salivatory nucleus pass via the nervus intermedius and its two branches: the chorda tympani to the submandibular ganglion, and the greater petrosal nerve to the pterygopalatine ganglion.

All afferent fibers associated with the nervus intermedius have their cell bodies (unipolar neurons) in the *geniculate ganglion*. The gustatory fibers from the anterior two-thirds of the tongue course through the chorda tympani primarily and at times through the greater petrosal nerve to the lateral and rostral aspects of the nucleus solitarius (called the *gustatory nucleus*). The gen-

eral somatic afferent fibers from the external auditory meatus and back of the external ear course through the nervus intermedius and join the spinal tract of N. V before terminating in the spinal nucleus of N. V. General visceral afferent fibers from the visceral organs terminate in the nucleus solitarius.

Lesions A lesion interrupting the facial nerve (e.g., Bell's palsy) is primarily expressed as a lower motor neuron paralysis of the muscles of facial expression. There is an abolition of both voluntary and reflex movements of the facial muscles. The paresis of *Bell's palsy* may occur suddenly (it is believed to be due to an edema of the nerve following rheumatoid infection of the nerve in the facial canal of the petrosal bone) and may be followed within a few months by a spontaneous recovery. On the ipsilateral side, the face is masklike, the forehead is immobile, the corner of the muscle sags, the nasolabial folds of the face are flattened, facial lines are lost, and saliva may drip from the corner of the mouth. The patient is unable to whistle or puff the cheek because the buccinator muscle is paralyzed. When the patient is smiling, the normal muscles draw the contralateral corner of the mouth up while the paralzyed corner continues to sag. Corneal sensitivity remains (N. V), but the patient is unable to blink or close the eyelid (N. VII). To protect the cornea from damage (e.g., drying), the eyelids are closed therapeutically or other measures are taken (e.g., the patient wears an eye mask, or lids are closed by sutures). Lacrimation on the lesion side may be impaired (fibers which pass through the greater petrosal nerve). There may be a reduction in the secretion of saliva (fibers which pass through the chorda tympani). Taste will be lost on the ipsilateral anterior two-thirds of the tongue (fibers which pass through the chorda tympani). An increased acuity to sounds (*hyperacusis*), especially to low tones, results from the paralysis of the stapedius muscle, which normally dampens the amplitude of the vibrations of the ear ossicles.

A *unilateral supranuclear lesion* of the upper motor neurons (corticobulbar and corticoreticular fibers) to the facial nucleus (Fig. 8-22) results in a marked weakness of the muscles of expression of the lower part of the face on the side contralateral to the lesion. The frontalis muscle (which wrinkles the forehead) and the orbicularis oculi muscle (which closes the eyelid) are unaffected. The accepted explanation states that (1) bilateral upper motor neuron projections from the cerebral cortex influence the lower motor neurons innervating the frontalis muscle and orbicularis, and (2) only unilateral, crossed, upper motor neuron projections influence the lower motor neurons innervating the muscles of facial expression of the lower part of the face. Hence the contralateral muscles are deprived of upper motor neuron influences.

In some patients with unilateral supranuclear lesions, the contralateral weak lower facial muscles are paralyzed to volitional influences but will contract to emotional or mimetic influences (jokes, distress). In *voluntary facial palsy* the deficits of facial movements are accentuated when the patient is consciously trying to contract these muscles. This voluntary facial palsy is apparently due to the interruption of the cortical influences conveyed by the corticobulbar and corticoreticular fibers. The mimetic (involuntary) influences are presumed to originate from such subcortical nuclei as the globus pallidus and thalamus. When the seventh nerve is deprived of these influences, the patient will have a *mimetic facial paralysis*. This may or may not be accompanied by voluntary facial paralysis.

Note the distinction between a *lower motor (infranuclear) lesion* and an *upper motor (supranuclear) lesion* involving the muscles of facial expression. In a lower motor neuron paralysis these muscles on the entire half of the face have a marked weakness; in an upper motor neuron paralysis only those muscles on the lower half of the face have a marked weakness.

Vestibulocochlear nerve (N. VIII) (Fig. 7-3 and Chap. 10)

The *vestibulocochlear* (*auditory, acoustic, or statoacoustic*) or *eighth cranial nerve* is actually two nerves. The *cochlear nerve* is associated with hearing (exteroception) and the *vestibular nerve* is concerned with the state of equilibrium and orientation in three-dimensional space (proprioception). Both components are special somatic afferent. The bipolar cells of the cochlear nerve have their cell bodies in the spiral ganglion located within the spiral canal of the modiolus, and those of the vestibular nerve are in the vestibular ganglion located within the distal part of the internal auditory meatus.

After emerging from the lateral aspect of the pons-medulla junction, the vestibular root and the cochlear root join and pass laterally and slightly rostrally in the cerebellopontine angle and then through the internal acoustic meatus, accompanied, in part, by the facial nerve proper and the nervus intermedius. In the distal end of the meatus the nerve divides into cochlear and vestibular nerves. The cochlear nerve passes into the ganglion cells of the spiral ganglion lying within the spiral canal of the modiolus. The peripherally directed fibers of the bipolar spiral ganglion cells pass through small canals within the bony spiral laminae to form a spiral sheet of fibers, which innervates the hair cells of the spiral organ of Corti. Within the spiral organ, the nerve fibers are unmyelinated. The vestibular nerve divides into two parts, each with its own ganglion: the superior part and inferior part of the vestibular ganglion. The distally directed fibers ("dendrites") of the bipolar vestibular cells are distributed as follows: (1) the fibers of the superior part terminate in the receptor cells of the ampullae of the anterior and lateral semicircular canals, the macula of the utricle, and part of the macula of the saccule; (2) the fibers of the inferior part terminate in the receptor cells of the ampulla of the major part of the saccule and in the ampulla of the posterior semicircular canal; and (3) a small branch of the inferior part passes to the spiral ganglion of the cochlea; this branch is said to be composed of cochlear efferent fibers (Chap. 10). The vestibulocochlear nerve is the only nerve that terminates wholly within a bone (petrous portion of the temporal bone); all other cranial nerves emerge from the skull.

Glossopharyngeal nerve (N. IX) (Fig. 7-8)

The *glossopharyngeal,* or *ninth cranial, nerve* (from *glosso,* "tongue," and *pharynx,* "throat") is

a mixed branchiomeric nerve composed of (1) special visceral afferent fibers conveying taste sensations from the posterior third of the tongue; (2) general somatic afferent fibers from the back of external ear and external auditory meatus; (3) general visceral afferent fibers from the (*a*) mucous membranes of tympanic cavity, auditory tube, palatoglossal arches, tonsil, soft palate, posterior third of tongue, and upper pharynx, and (*b*) pressoreceptors in the carotid sinus and chemoreceptors in the carotid body; (4) general visceral efferent fibers (parasympathetic) conveying visceromotor influences to the parotid gland; and (5) special visceral efferent fibers to the stylopharyngeus muscle (elevates upper pharynx) and possibly to the muscles within the palatal arches and the upper pharyngeal constrictor muscle (involved with swallowing). The visceral afferent fibers have their unipolar cell bodies in the inferior (petrosal) ganglion, while the somatic afferent fibers have theirs in the superior ganglion.

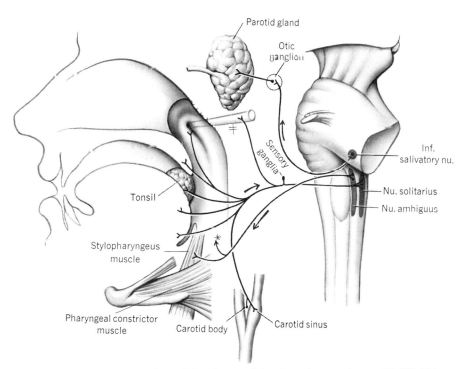

FIGURE 7-8 The cranial nerve nuclei and distribution of the glossopharyngeal nerve (N. IX). This cranial nerve supplies the motor innervation to the stylopharyngeus muscle, the muscles (*) of the anterior and posterior pillars of the fauces, and possibly some superior pharyngeal constrictor muscle fibers (involved in deglutition). The superior and inferior salivatory nuclei are actually diffuse and confluent groups of cells located within the parvicellular reticular nucleus (Chap. 8, Figs. 8-8, 8-9, 8-10). ‡Auditory tube.

The glossopharyngeal nerve emerges as five or six rootlets from the posterior lateral sulcus of the rostral medulla. These rootlets are located near the facial nerve and are in series to the caudally located rootlets of the vagus nerve. The rootlets of N. IX join to form the nerve, which passes, along with the vagus and accessory nerves, through the jugular foramen. It continues in an arc on the lateral aspect of the pharynx toward the region of the tonsils and soft palate.

Spinal and principal nucleus of the fifth nerve
The fibers conveying touch, pain, and temperature from the external ear, external auditory meatus, and tympanic cavity, and possibly from the region of the palatal arches and posterior third of the tongue, terminate in the spinal tract and nucleus of the fifth nerve, whereas those conveying tactile impulses terminate in the principal nucleus of the fifth nerve.

Nuclei solitarius and commissuralis (Fig. 7-3)
The primary visceral afferent fibers of nerves V, VII, IX, and X join the solitary tract and terminate in the *nuclei solitarius and commissuralis*. The latter (nucleus commissuralis) is the nuclear complex formed by the joining of the paired nuclei solitarius in the caudal medulla. The taste fibers in this solitary tract from nerves VII, IX, and X terminate in the rostral and lateral portions of the nucleus solitarius called the *gustatory nucleus* (see "Taste Pathways," Chap. 8). The fibers from N. VII descend and those from nerves IX and X ascend to the gustatory nucleus. The caudal portion of the solitary nucleus receives general visceral afferent input from nerves V, VII, IX, and X and afferent input involved with the respiratory and cardiovascular reflexes from nerves IX and X.

Many visceral reflexes are mediated via projections from the solitary nucleus to various regions of the midbrain, pons, and medulla involved with visceral activities (Chap. 8). A bilateral solitariospinal projection terminates (1) in the anterior horn pools of cervical levels 3 to 5 giving rise to the phrenic nerve (respiration) and (2) in pools giving rise to preganglionic autonomic fibers in the thoracolumbar region ("Intermediolateral Cell Column" and "Intercalated

Nucleus," Chap. 6) and the sacral region. The latter are involved with the cardiovascular and other visceral reflexes.

Specialized cords of epithelioid cells acting as sensors are located within the carotid body at the carotid bifurcation and the aortic bodies (associated with the major thoracic arteries). The carotid body consists of two types of cells: (1) one type, called glomus type I, contains dense-core vesicles rich in catecholamines and serotonin; these cells monitor the blood in the surrounding bed of fenestrated and sinusoidal capillaries, and they respond to changes in the oxygen and carbon dioxide tension and in the blood pH; and (2) another, called glomus type II, is free of granules. The function of these two types is not clear. These cells are arterial *chemoreceptors* which are stimulated by a decrease in the oxygen level, a rise in the carbon dioxide content, or a decrease in the hydrogen ion concentration in the arterial blood. General visceral afferent fibers convey influences from these chemosensitive cells via both the glossopharyngeal and vagus nerves. They terminate in the nucleus solitarius.

Stretch pressoreceptors are diffusely located within the adventitia of the carotid sinus at the carotid bifurcation, aortic arch, great veins near the heart, and in the atrium and ventricles of the heart. These *pressoreceptors* respond with changes in the intraarterial pressure. Nerve fibers commencing as rich networks of large nerve endings of cranial nerves IX and X convey influences from the pressoreceptors centrally to the nucleus solitarius. The input from these chemoreceptors and pressoreceptors is integrated into the activity of the cardiovascular and respiratory centers in the medulla (*carotid reflex*). In addition, collaterals of the glossopharyngeal fibers terminate in the parasympathetic dorsal motor nucleus of the vagus nerve. Concomitant with a rise in the blood pressure, there is an increase in the frequency of impulses in the fibers innervating these stretch receptors. These influences appear to inhibit sympathetic activity and to facilitate parasympathetic vagal activity (reduction in the heart rate and arterial pressure). Following a pronounced lowering of blood pressure, there is a decrease in the frequency of impulses. This results in an increase in sympathetic and a reduction in parasympathetic discharges (an increase in the heart rate and arterial pressure).

Inferior salivatory nucleus The preganglionic parasympathetic fibers originate in the so-called *inferior salivatory nucleus*—a physiologically defined nucleus located just rostral to the dorsal vagal nucleus. The fibers from these cells course via the lesser petrosal nerve to the otic ganglion. The postganglionic parasympathetic cells in this ganglion give rise to secretomotor fibers to the parotid gland. Sympathetic fibers do not appear to innervate the parotid gland.

Nucleus ambiguus The special visceral efferent fibers of the glossopharyngeal nerve originate from the rostral portions of the *nucleus ambiguus*. The stylopharyngeus muscle is often said to be the only muscle innervated by the glossopharyngeal nerve. However, the palatal arch and superior pharyngeal constrictors are probably innervated by the glossopharyngeal nerve as well as the vagus nerve. This is indicated because following the interruption of N. IX, there may be a deviation of the pharynx, lowering of the palatal arches, and difficulty in swallowing.

Lesions Interruption of all fibers of the glossopharyngeal nerve results in the following symptoms: (1) loss of sensation, including taste, in the posterior third of the tongue and adjacent area; (2) unilateral loss of the *pharyngeal* (or *gag*) *reflex;* (3) difficulty in swallowing (*dysphagia*); and (4) impairment of the *carotid reflex*. The *pharyngeal reflex* consists of the constriction of the pharyngeal musculature accompanied by the retraction of the tongue when the tonsillar region is stimulated; the afferent input to this reflex is conveyed via the glossopharyngeal nerve, while the efferent limb of the reflex arc is through the vagus and/or glossopharyngeal nerves. Thus the gag reflex may be accompanied by unilateral loss of the palatal and uvular reflexes with a deviation of the palate and uvula to the normal side (because they are unopposed by the paralyzed muscles). *Glossopharyngeal neuralgia* (similar to trigeminal neuralgia) may be triggered by chewing or swallowing.

The presence or absence of taste sensations in the posterior third of the tongue can be evaluated clinically by the topical application of galvanic current in the tonsillar region. Normally an acid taste sensation is induced.

Vagus nerve (N. X) (Fig. 7-9)

The *vagus* or *tenth cranial nerve* is a mixed nerve with functional components similar to those of the glossopharyngeal nerve. A few special visceral afferent fibers with their cell bodies in the inferior ganglion relay influences from the taste buds on the epiglottis to the "gustatory" nucleus of the nucleus solitarius. Sensory information is also conveyed via general visceral afferent fibers (cell bodies in the inferior ganglion) from many sources to the nucleus solitarius. These sources include (1) the pharynx, esophagus, stomach and intestinal tract (to the left colic flexure), larynx, bronchi and lungs, and such organs as the liver, pancreas, and their ducts; (2) pressoreceptors in the aortic arch, atrium, and ventricles of the heart and in the pulmonary tree; and (3) chemoreceptors in the aortic bodies and major thoracic arteries. The influences from these structures may be interpreted as hunger pangs, fullness and distention of the abdominal viscera, and nausea (this information may also be conveyed to the spinal cord and its sensory pathways). They are also utilized by the visceral centers (e.g., cardiovascular and respiratory centers) in the medulla.

The general somatic afferent fibers from the back of the external ear and external auditory meatus pass through the spinal tract of N. V before terminating in the spinal nucleus of N. V.

The general visceral efferent fibers from the cells of the dorsal vagal nucleus in the medulla relay the parasympathetic influences via the vagus nerve to the heart and the smooth muscles and glands of the thoracic and abdominal viscera. These include the larynx, trachea and lungs, esophagus, gastrointestinal tract (to the left colic flexure), and associated glands and their ducts. The vagus nerve contains some cardioacceleratory and many cardioinhibitory fibers. The functional aspects of this innervation are discussed in Chap. 6.

The special visceral efferent fibers from the nucleus ambiguus of the medulla supply the lower motor neuron innervation to all the mus-

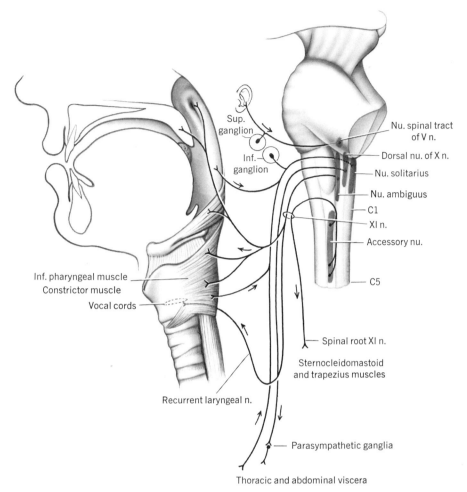

Sup. ganglion

Inf. ganglion

Nu. spinal tract of V n.

Dorsal nu. of X n.

Nu. solitarius

Nu. ambiguus

C1

XI n.

Accessory nu.

C5

Inf. pharyngeal muscle
Constrictor muscle

Vocal cords

Spinal root XI n.

Sternocleidomastoid and trapezius muscles

Recurrent laryngeal n.

Parasympathetic ganglia

Thoracic and abdominal viscera

FIGURE 7-9 The cranial nerve nuclei and distribution of the vagus and accessory nerves (X and XI).

cles of the soft palate (except the tensor veli pala-tini), pharynx (except the stylopharyngeus mus-cle), cricothyroid muscle, and all other intrinsic muscles of the larynx. Some of the palatal arch and pharyngeal constrictor musculature may be also innervated by fibers from the nucleus ambi-guus which course through the glossopharyngeal nerve. The intrinsic muscles of the larynx and possibly some pharyngeal constrictor muscles are innervated by fibers from the nucleus ambi-guus which pass through the cranial root of the accessory nerve before joining the vagus nerve. *In summary*, the special visceral efferent fibers of the vagus and cranial (bulbar) root of the ac-cessory nerves are functionally involved with the movements of the soft palate (velum), palatal

arches, pharynx, and larynx. These are asso-ciated with swallowing and regulating the laryn-geal apertures during respiration and phona-tion.

The vagus nerve emerges as rootlets from the posterior lateral sulcus. The rostral rootlets are primarily sensory, and the caudal rootlets are primarily motor. These rootlets join and, along with the glossopharyngeal and accessory nerves, pass through the jugular foramen into the neck. After this the vagus nerve and its branches are distributed to structures in the neck, thorax, and abdomen. The spinal portion of the accessory nerve joins the vagus within and just distal to the jugular foramen. Small branches leave the vagus in the vicinity of the superior ganglia: one branch innervates the dura mater of the posterior fossa of the skull, and the other branch (auricular) innervates the cutaneous area in the back of the external ear and the floor of the external auditory meatus.

Lesions A complete unilateral lesion of the vagus nerve results in the following: (1) the flaccid soft palate produces a voice with a twang, and (2) swallowing is difficult (*dysphagia*) because of the unilateral paralysis of the pharyngeal constrictors; the pharynx is shifted slightly to the normally innervated side. Because of the unilateral paralysis of the palatal, uvular, and palatine arch musculature, the soft palate is elevated and the uvula deviates to the normal side during vocalization. A transient *tachycardia* (increased heartbeat) is a consequence of the interruption of some parasympathetic stimulation. After a unilateral lesion of the bulbar root fibers (inferior laryngeal nerve) of the accessory nerve, the ipsilateral vocal fold becomes fixed and partially adducted to the midline; the voice is hoarse (*dysphonia*) and reduced to a whisper. Bilateral lesions of the vagus nerves are rapidly fatal because the adducted vocal cords obstruct the flow of adequate amounts of air to and from the lungs. Asphyxia follows unless a tracheostomy is performed. Paralysis following lesions of vagal neurons may occur in *bulbar poliomyelitis*.

Accessory (spinal accessory) nerve (N. XI) (Fig. 7-9)

The *accessory*, or *eleventh cranial*, *nerve* arises as two roots: spinal and bulbar (cranial). The fibers (SVE) of the *spinal root* originate from cells located in the lateral portion of lamina IX of spinal segments C1 through C5 (see Fig. 8-4). They course through the lateral funiculus and emerge as rootlets on the lateral side of the spinal cord between the dorsal and ventral roots. The rootlets join to form a common trunk which ascends within the vertebral canal on the posterior side of the denticulate ligament before passing through the foramen magnum. The rootlets of the *bulbar root* are actually composed of fibers (SVE) of the vagus nerve arising from the caudal portion of the nucleus ambiguus. The spinal and bulbar roots join and pass through the jugular foramen posterior to the jugular vein. The roots and nerve contain some parasympathetic fibers.

Just distal to the jugular foramen the bulbar root rejoins the vagus nerve; its special visceral efferent fibers form the inferior (recurrent) laryngeal nerve which innervates the intrinsic muscles of the larynx. The spinal root descends into the neck in a posterocaudal direction to innervate the ipsilateral sternocleidomastoid and upper portions of the trapezius muscles. Motor fibers of the cervical segments which course via the cervical nerves of the cervical plexus supply the lower portions of the trapezius muscle.

Lesions A lower motor neuron paralysis is a consequence of the interruption of the accessory nerve. A unilateral lesion of the spinal root fibers is indicated by a weakness in the ability to rotate the head so that the chin points to the side ipsilateral to the lesion (paralyzed sternocleidomastoid muscle) and in a downward and outward rotation of the scapula accompanied by the flaring of the vertebral border of the scapula, shoulder sag, and upper extremity droop (paralyzed upper portion of the trapezius muscle). The head is readily held in its normal position. Although the chin can be pointed satisfactorily to the paralyzed side, it can be turned away from the affected side only to a limited degree. The effects of a lesion of the fibers of the bulbar root are noted with the vagus nerve.

Hypoglossal nerve (N. XII) (Fig. 7-5)

The lower motor neuron fibers (GSE) of the *hypoglossal*, or *twelfth cranial*, *nerve* originate in the nucleus of the hypoglossal nerve, which is a 2-cm-long column of motor cells located underneath the floor of the fourth ventricle just lateral to the midline. It forms the bulge of the *hypoglossal trigone* (see Fig. 1-16). The uncrossed nerve fibers pass ventrally through the tegmentum of the medulla lateral to the MLF, lateral lemniscus, and pyramid and medial to the inferior olivary nuclear complex. They emerge as 10 to 15 rootlets in the anterolateral sulcus. The rootlets join in the hypoglossal canal to form the hypoglossal nerve, which passes in an arc lateral to the pharynx to the root of the tongue. The nerve divides into branches which innervate the ipsilateral intrinsic muscles of the tongue as well as the hypoglossus, styloglossus, and genioglossus muscles. Clinically, the chin to tongue muscle—

the genioglossus—is important because the contraction of this pair results in the protrusion of the tongue.

Lesions   Interruption of all the fibers of N. XII produces an ipsilateral lower motor neuron paralysis of the tongue. The fasciculations of the early stages are followed by atrophy of the muscles, which results in a wrinkled tongue surface on the side of the lesion. When protruded, the tip of the tongue deviates to the paralyzed side. This deviation is due to the unopposed contraction of the contralateral genioglossus, which pulls the base of the tongue forward. Otherwise functional disturbances are minimal because many intrinsic tongue muscle fibers cross the midline. Bilateral lesions of the hypoglossal nerves result in an immobile tongue which can be displaced into the throat, interfering with respiration. Tracheotomy may be required.

PERIPHERAL GANGLIA ASSOCIATED WITH THE CRANIAL NERVES

Two types of peripheral ganglia are associated with the cranial nerves: (1) *sensory ganglia,* which are the equivalent of the dorsal roots of the spinal nerves, and (2) *parasympathetic ganglia* of the autonomic nervous system.

Sensory ganglia   All the cell bodies of the sensory neurons of the spinal nerves are located in the spinal ganglia. In the case of each cranial nerve, the cell bodies of the sensory ganglia are usually located in one or more cranial ganglia (see Fig. 7-1). Table 7-1 lists the cranial nerves and the name and location of the cell bodies of the peripheral sensory neurons. All sensory ganglia of the cranial nerves (except for the mesencephalic nucleus of the fifth nerve and the bipolar cells of the retina) are located outside the central nervous system (as are the spinal ganglia of the spinal nerves). The retina is considered to be a distal extension of the central nervous system.

Parasympathetic ganglia   Within the head there are four parasympathetic ganglia where the preganglionic fibers (arising from cell bodies located within the brainstem) synapse with postganglionic neurons. These include the *ciliary ganglion* of the N. III, the *pterygopalative* and *submandibular ganglia* of N. VII, and the *otic ganglion* of N. IX. The parasympathetic ganglia associated with the vagus nerve are the terminal ganglia located near or within the visceral organs of the thorax and abdomen (Fig. 7-4).

CRANIAL NERVE NUCLEI WITHIN THE CENTRAL NERVOUS SYSTEM

The sensory neurons of the cranial nerves terminate and synapse within the brainstem in the sensory cranial nerve nuclei (see Fig. 7-3). The motor nuclei of the cranial nerves are the location of cell bodies whose axons course through the cranial nerves to voluntary muscles or to parasympathetic ganglia (see Figs. 7-4 and 7-9). These nuclei are arranged in six longitudinal columns in the brainstem: (1) *special somatic afferent,* (2) *general somatic afferent,* (3) *visceral afferent,* (4) *general somatic efferent,* (5) *general visceral efferent,* and (6) *special visceral efferent.* The nuclei are illustrated in Figs. 8-4 through 8-13 and A-1 through A-25.

Special somatic afferent column   This column includes the *four vestibular nuclei* and the *two cochlear nuclei* which are associated with the eighth cranial nerve. It is located in the dorsolateral tegmentum in the upper medulla and lower pons (see Fig. 7-3).

General somatic afferent column   This column is located throughout the brainstem from the upper midbrain into the upper cervical spinal cord levels (in the lateral tegmentum of the pons and medulla and the dorsomedial tegmentum of the midbrain). The nuclei of this column include the *mesencephalic nucleus of the fifth nerve* (proprioception), *principal sensory nucleus* (chief, superior, or main sensory nucleus) of the fifth nerve located in the midpons (touch), and the *spinal (descending) nucleus of the fifth nerve* located in the lower pons, medulla, and upper cervical spinal cord (pain and temperature). All general somatic afferent fibers of the fifth, seventh, ninth, and tenth cranial nerves terminate in these nuclei. The mesencephalic nucleus of the fifth nerve is unusual; it is actually composed of cell bodies of neurons of the first order. It may be considered as a portion of the trigeminal ganglion of the fifth cranial nerve displaced into the midbrain.

Visceral afferent column The visceral afferent column consists of the *nucleus solitarius*, located in the medulla just lateral to the dorsal vagal motor nucleus. The visceral senses conveyed by fibers of the seventh, ninth, and tenth cranial nerves terminate in this nucleus. This includes the impulses from taste endings (special visceral), pressoreceptors, and chemoreceptors (general visceral). All taste fibers are conveyed by three cranial nerves (N. VII, N. IX, and N. X), and they terminate in this nucleus. The rostral portion of the solitary nucleus, called the gustatory nucleus, is involved with taste; the intermediate portion is a link in the cardiovascular reflex; and the caudal portion has a role in respiration.

General somatic efferent column Consisting of the *nucleus of the oculomotor nerve* (midbrain), *nucleus of the trochlear nerve* (lower midbrain), *nucleus of the abducent nerve* (lower pons), and *nucleus of the hypoglossal nerve* (medulla), this column is located in the dorsomedial tegmentum adjacent to the medial raphe and ventral to the central canal. These nuclei consist of the lower motor neurons to the voluntary muscles of the eye and the tongue.

General visceral efferent column Also called the parasympathetic nuclear column, it includes the *accessory oculomotor nucleus* (*of Edinger-Westphal*) (midbrain), the *superior and inferior salivatory nuclei* (lower pons and upper medulla), and the *dorsal motor nucleus of the vagus nerve* (medulla). These nuclei tend to be located just lateral to the general somatic efferent column. The accessory oculomotor nucleus is the source of preganglionic neurons in the oculomotor nerve, the superior salivatory nucleus of preganglionic neurons in the facial nerve, the inferior salivatory nucleus of preganglionic neurons in the glossopharyngeal nerve, and the dorsal motor vagal nucleus of preganglionic neurons in the vagus nerve (Chap. 6). The salivatory nuclei are identifiable by their physiologic effects (stimulation evokes secretion), not by morphologic criteria. The superior and inferior salivatory nuclei are actually diffuse and confluent groups of cells located within the parvicellular reticular nucleus (Chap. 8, Figs. 8-8, 8-9, and 8-10).

Special visceral efferent column Consisting of the *motor nucleus of the fifth nerve* (midpons), *motor nucleus of the facial nerve* (lower pons), and the *nucleus ambiguus* (medulla), this column is located in the middle of the tegmentum. The nuclei consist of the lower motor neurons to the branchiomeric (gill) arch musculature. The motor nucleus of the fifth nerve innervates the muscles of mastication (first arch), the motor nucleus of the seventh nerve innervates the muscles of facial expression (second arch), and the nucleus ambiguus innervates the pharyngeal (swallowing) and laryngeal muscles (vocalization) via the glossopharyngeal, vagus, and cranial roots of accessory nerves (third and fourth arches). Several other muscles innervated by these nerves include the tensor tympani muscle (fifth nerve) and stapedius muscle (seventh nerve, Chap. 10).

BIBLIOGRAPHY

Anderson, J. E.: *Grant's Atlas of Anatomy*, sec. 8, The Williams & Wilkins Company, Baltimore, 1978.

Brodal, A.: *The Cranial Nerves: Anatomy and Anatomicoclinical Correlations*, Blackwell Scientific Publications, Ltd., Oxford, 1965.

Cogan, D. G.: *Neurology of the Ocular Muscles*, Charles C Thomas, Publisher, Springfield, Ill., 1978.

Romanes, G. J.: *Cunningham's Textbook of Anatomy*, Oxford University Press, New York, 1972.

Smith, R. Dale: The trematic interrelationships of the branchiomeric nerves. Acta Anat, 39:141–186, 1959.

Young, R. F., and R. Stevens: Unmyelinated axons in the trigeminal motor root of human and cat. J Comp Neurol, 183:205–214, 1979.

CHAPTER EIGHT

THE BRAINSTEM: MEDULLA, PONS, AND MIDBRAIN

The medulla, pons, and midbrain—the lower or infratentorial brainstem—are actually continuous structures (see Figs. 8-1 and 8-2). They will be analyzed as a unit rather than as distinct entities. The major ascending and descending pathways in the brainstem are linked rostrally with the cerebrum, dorsally with the cerebellum, and caudally with the spinal cord. In terms of this chapter, the brainstem comprises the medulla, pons, and midbrain. Descriptions of the surface anatomy and the sites of the emergence of the cranial nerves of the brainstem are to be found in Chap. 1. Illustrations of the gross anatomy of this region of the brain are found in a number of figures including Figs. 1-5 through 1-7, 1-9, 1-11, and 1-13 through 1-16.

BASIC ORGANIZATION OF THE BRAINSTEM

The schematic drawings of transverse sections through the medulla, pons, and midbrain (see Figs. 8-4 through 8-13) illustrate several salient features of the internal structure of the brainstem. The following account outlines basic relations and omits exceptions. Two fundamental similarities to the spinal cord should be noted.

1. *The major ascending and descending pathways are oriented parallel to the long axis of the brainstem.* Hence, they are illustrated in cross section in these figures. They include the spinothalamic tract (spinal lemniscus), medial lemniscus, lateral lemniscus, trigeminal lemniscus, medial longitudinal fasciculus, and corticospinal tract.

2. *The intrabrainstem course of each cranial nerve is usually oriented parallel to the transverse plane of the brainstem.* The cranial nerves illustrated comprise III and IV (midbrain), V (pons), VI, VII, and VIII (pons-medulla junction) and IX, X, XI, and XII (medulla) (see Figs. 1-11 through 1-14 and Figs. 8-1 and 8-4 through 8-12).

The brainstem consists of four regions called (1) *roof,* (2) *ventricular cavity,* (3) *tegmentum,* and (4) *basilar portion* (Fig. 8-3). The structures associated with these regions are different in the various levels of the brainstem. The central core of the tegmentum is known as the *reticular formation* (*reticular core*).

The relations of several structures of the brainstem can be understood by referring to Figs. 8-1 through 8-3. The basilar portion of the brainstem consists of the *crus cerebri* (midbrain), *basilar portion* of the pons, and *pyramid* (medulla), and within it is located the corticospinal tract (Figs. 1-11, 1-13, 8-3). In the lower medulla are indications of the pyramidal decussation. In these same figures note that the cranial nerves III (midbrain), VI (pons-medulla junction), and XII (medulla) emerge from the *basal (anterior) surface* as does the motor root of the first cervical nerve. These three cranial nerves of the brainstem are the functional equivalents of the motor roots of the spinal cord. Cranial nerve IV belongs with this group but is unusual because it emerges on the dorsal surface of lower midbrain (see Fig. 8-1; see also Figs. A-9 and A-20).

Five cranial nerves (V, VII, IX, X, and XI) emerge from the *lateral surface* of the pons and medulla. The equivalent spinal cord structures

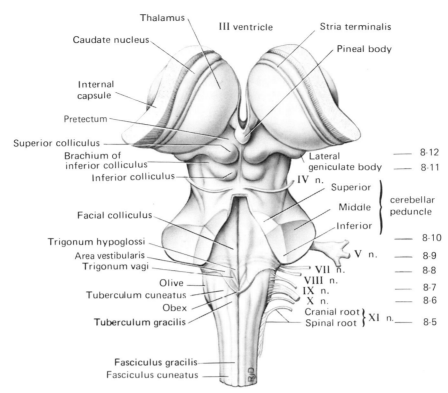

FIGURE 8-1 Posterior surface of the brainstem. The lines adjacent to the figure indicate the levels of the transverse sections illustrated in Figs 8-5 through 8 12. Roman numerals represent some cranial nerves (Chap. 7).

of these cranial nerves are (1) the dorsal roots and (2) the spinal root of N. XI (see Fig. 8-4; see also Fig. A-11). Cranial N. VIII emerges dorsal to N. VII (see Figs. 1-13 and 1-14). Cranial nerves VI, VII, and VIII emerge at the junction of the pons and medulla (see Fig. 1-13).

The cranial nerves have their sensory nuclei (sites of termination of fibers of sensory nerves) and their motor nuclei (sites of origin of motor nerves) located in the tegmentum (see Fig. 7-2). The sensory nuclei are always located lateral or dorsolateral to the motor nuclei (see Fig. 7-2). The latter are located in the medial tegmentum. As stated in Chap. 7, some cranial motor neurons are equivalent to the lower motor neurons in the anterior horn and others to autonomic neurons in laminae VII of the spinal cord.

Several major pathways pass through the tegmentum of the brainstem. They include the following:

1. The *medial lemniscus* is located in the posterior column-medial lemniscal pathway (Fig. 5-18). It is formed in the caudal medulla from internal arcuate fibers (see Figs. 5-18, A-2, and A-13) that arise from the contralateral nuclei gracilis and cuneatus (see Fig. A-2). The lemniscus ascends along the edge of the reticular formation to the ventral posterolateral nucleus of the thalamus (see Figs. 8-6 through 8-12; see also Fig. 5-18).

2. The *(neo)spinothalamic tract (spinal lemniscus)* is the continuation of the lateral spinothalamic tract in the spinal cord. It is located along the edge of the reticular formation always dorsolateral or dorsal to the medial lemniscus (see Figs. 8-5 through 8-12).

3. The *anterior trigeminothalamic tract (trigeminal lemniscus)* is the tract arising in trigeminal nuclei and terminating in the ventral posteromedial thalamic nucleus (see Figs. 8-11,

8-12, and 8-15). It is located on the edge of the reticular formation of pons and midbrain between the medial lemniscus and spinothalamic tract (spinal lemniscus).

4. The *lateral lemniscus* is a bundle of fibers arising from the cochlear nuclei (Figs. 8-9 through 8-11; see also Fig. 10-6). It is located on the edge of the reticular formation dorsal to the spinal lemniscus. It is a link in the auditory pathway of lateral lemniscus (pons), nuclei of inferior colliculus (lower midbrain, see Fig. 8-11), brachium of the inferior colliculus (midbrain, see Figs. 8-11 and 8-12), and medial geniculate body of the thalamus (see Figs. 8-12 and 8-13; see also Fig. 10-6).

5. The *paleospinothalamic tract and spinoreticular and reticulospinal pathways* (see Figs. 5-16 and 5-20) consist of fibers projecting to and from the spinal cord to the brainstem reticular formation (reticular core of telmentum).

Several other brainstem structures are excellent landmarks. *Ventricle IV* of the pons and medulla and the *cerebral aqueduct of Sylvius*

(midbrain) are the brainstem equivalents of the central canal of the spinal cord (see Figs. 8-3, 8-4, 8-11, and 8-12). In the midbrain the *periventricular gray matter* is called the periaquaductal gray; it surrounds these ventricular cavities. Within the raphe (midline) of the brainstem are the *raphe nuclei*. The prominent *medial longitudinal fasciculus (MLF)* is located ventral to the ventricular cavities and on either side of the raphe (see Figs. 8-5 through 8-13; see also Fig. 10-10); its fibers have a significant role in coordinating eye movements. Surrounding the corticospinal tracts in the pons are the pontine nuclei of the basilar portion.

ROOF, VENTRICULAR CAVITY, TEGMENTUM, AND BASILAR PORTION

The brainstem may be considered to be organized as four longitudinally oriented structures: roof, ventricular cavity, tegmentum, and basilar portion (see Figs. 8-3 through 8-13; see also Figs. 1-2 and 1-3).

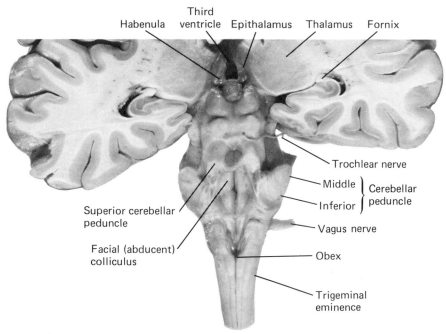

FIGURE 8-2 Photograph of the dorsal view of the brainstem and a section of the cerebrum. Surface structures can be identified by referring to Figs. 1-5, 1-6, and 8-1. Structures in the section can be identified by referring to Fig. 1-31. (*Courtesy of Dr. Howard A. Matzke, University of Kansas Medical Center.*)

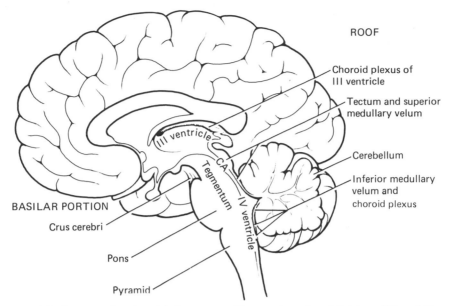

ROOF

Choroid plexus of
III ventricle

Tectum and superior
medullary velum

Cerebellum

Inferior medullary
velum and
choroid plexus

BASILAR PORTION

Crus cerebri

Pons

Pyramid

III ventricle

CA

Tegmentum

IV ventricle

FIGURE 8-3 Median sagittal section of the brainstem to illustrate the major subdivisions of (1) roof, (2) central canal, (3) tegmentum, and (4) basilar portion. The *roof* consists of the choroid plexus of the third ventricle, tectum (including superior and inferior colliculi), superior and inferior medullary velum, cerebellum, and choroid plexus of the fourth ventricle. The *central canal* comprises the cerebral aqueduct and the third (III) and fourth (IV) ventricles. The tegmentum is the diencephalon proper (thalamus, hypothalamus, subthalamus, and epithalamus, and the tegmentum of the infratentorial brainstem). The basilar portion comprises the internal capsule, crus cerebri, and the basilar portion of pons and pyramid. Refer to Figs. 1-1 and 1-7. CA, cerebral aqueduct.

Roof (Figs. 8-1 and 8-3)

The roof of the brainstem is located posterior to the ventricular cavity. The roof of the midbrain, called the *tectum* or *lamina quadrigemina*, is subdivided into the *pretectum* (rostral portion), paired *superior colliculi* of the optic system, and paired *inferior colliculi* of the auditory system. The colliculi are collectively called the *corpora quadrigemina*. The fourth cranial nerve emerges from the roof just caudal to the inferior colliculi. The cerebellum along with the thin superior and inferior medullary veli form the roof of the pons. The choroid plexus and the tela choroidea (layer of pia mater and ependyma) of the fourth ventricle form the roof of the medulla; the posterior columns and nuclei gracilis form the roof of the central canal of the caudal medulla, merging caudally with the central canal of the spinal cord.

Ventricular cavity (Figs. 1-10, 1-11, 8-3)

The *ventricular cavities* include the cerebral aqueduct of the midbrain, the fourth ventricle of

the pons and medulla, and the central canal of the caudal half of the medulla.

Tegmentum

The tegmentum, which comprises the bulk of the brainstem, is located anterior to the ventricular canal. It may be subdivided into several structural-functional units, including (1) the cranial nerves and their nuclei (2) the ascending lemniscal pathways, (3) the reticular formation with its reticular nuclei and pathways, (4) the "unconscious" proprioceptive systems, (5) the periventricular gray matter (called periaqueductal gray matter in the midbrain because it surrounds the cerebral aqueduct), and (6) the raphe.

The *cranial nerves and their nuclei* include sensory and motor nuclei (Chap. 7). The sensory nuclei receive input from the cranial nerves, and the motor nuclei project output via motor fibers of the cranial nerves.

The *ascending lemniscal pathways* include the long ascending pathways which commence in the nuclei of the spinal cord and lower brainstem, terminate in nuclei of the higher brainstem and thalamus, and convey one or more sensory modalities. These pathways project their influences rostrally to the higher centers of the diencephalon and the cerebral cortex. In this context, the tracts of the lemniscal systems in the brainstem include the medial lemniscus (touch and deep sensibility), the spinothalamic tract (spinal lemniscus for pain and temperature), the trigeminothalamic tracts (trigeminal lemnisci for touch, pain, and temperature), and the lateral lemniscus (audition) (see Figs. 8-4 through 8-13).

The *reticular formation* is the intricate neural network which forms most of the brainstem tegmentum. The *reticular system* is the functional system utilizing the reticular formation as its physical substrate. This widespread reticular system is not limited to the brainstem but is present throughout the central nervous system. The reticular formation is organized into reticular nuclei and into (1) ascending reticular pathways and (2) descending reticular pathways. The brainstem portion of the reticular system is integrated with (1) the ascending reticular pathways involved with the relative state of alertness of the organism (sleep-wake pattern) and with some pain, and (2) the descending reticular pathways associated with the somatic and visceral motor activities expressed largely via the reticulospinal tracts and pathways. The major intrinsic tract of the brainstem reticular formation is the central tegmental tract (Figs. 8-9 and 8-14).

The *"unconscious" proprioceptive systems* in the brainstem are the nuclei and tracts associated with the vestibular system (Chap. 10) and with the pathways to the cerebellum (Chap. 9). The medial longitudinal fasciculus and the vestibulospinal tract contain fibers of the vestibular system. The spinocerebellar tracts, inferior, middle, and superior cerebellar peduncles, inferior olivary nuclear complex, lateral reticular nucleus, reticulotegmental nucleus, paramedial reticular nuclei, and red nucleus are functionally integrated with the cerebellum.

The *periventricular gray matter* (see Figs. 8-7 through 8-12) is located in the immediate vicinity of the ventricular cavity. In the midbrain, it is called the periaqueductal gray matter. Within it is located the dorsal longitudinal fasciculus, a pathway of the autonomic nervous system and some small scattered groups of cells (Chaps. 6, 15).

Within the *raphe* are located the midline raphe nuclei (Figs. 8-6 through 8-13, 8-19, 8-20).

Basilar portion

The *basilar portion of the brainstem* is made up of the following: the *crura cerebri* (*crus cerebri*, singular) of the midbrain, the *ventral pons* of the metencephalon, and the *pyramids* of the medulla (Figs. 8-3 to 8-12 and 13-7). The corticospinal tracts, corticobulbar fibers, corticopontine tracts, and pontocerebellar tracts form the basilar portion (see Fig. 9-5). The corticospinal tracts descend through the entire basilar portion before decussating in the lower medulla. The corticobulbar and corticoreticular fibers descend in the basilar portion before entering the tegmentum (see Figs. 8-21 and 8-22). The corticopontine tracts descend in the crura cerebri and terminate in the pontine nuclei of the pons proper (see Fig. 9-5). Pontocerebellar fibers cross over in the pons proper, pass through the middle cerebellar peduncle, and terminate in the cerebellar cortex. The *substantia nigra* is a large nuclear complex which is often included in the basilar portion of the midbrain (see Figs. 8-12 and 8-13). The *cerebral peduncles* comprise the tegmentum, substantia nigra, and crus cerebri (the midbrain without the tectum; see Fig. 8-12).

TRANSVERSE SECTIONS THROUGH THE INFRATENTORIAL BRAINSTEM

In the following account, the anatomic relations of the intrinsic structures of the infratentorial brainstem are briefly described in a representative series of transverse sections. These comprise a sequence of successively higher levels from the upper cervical segment through the upper midbrain.

First cervical segment of the spinal cord (Figs. 8-4 and A-11)

The first cervical segment has several distinctive features. The fibers of the lateral corticospinal tract are located more medially than in the other spinal levels. Its location, abutting against the gray matter, indicates that the tract has not

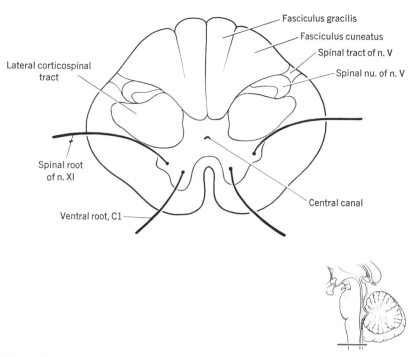

FIGURE 8-4 Transverse section of the upper portion of the first cervical segment. Refer to Fig. A-11.

completed its decussation. The myelinated fibers of the *spinal tract* and the large *spinal nucleus of the trigeminal nerve*, which extend to the C2 level, are the equivalents to the posterolateral tract and substantia gelatinosa of the spinal cord. The fibers of the *spinal root of cranial nerve XI* originate in the anterolateral aspect of the anterior horn and pass posteriorly and then laterally before emerging from the lateral side of the spinal cord. Although the dorsal root is absent at C1, the ventral root of the first cervical nerve is present.

Rearrangement of structures in the transition from the spinal cord to the medulla (Figs. 8-4 through 8-7, A-1 through A-3, and A-11 through A-14)

The junctional zone where the spinal cord merges into the medulla is usually defined as being located at the foramen magnum. It is also stated to be at a slightly different site either just rostral to the ventral root of C1 or at the level of the decussation of the corticospinal tract.

Although the external topography of the medulla differs from that of the spinal cord, many similarities are present (Figs. 8-4 through 8-7).

1. The fasciculus gracilis is continuous rostrally with the *tuberculum gracilis (clava)*, which is formed by the nucleus gracilis (Figs. 1-16, 8-1).
2. The fasciculus cuneatus is continuous with the *tuberculum cuneatus*, which is formed by the nucleus cuneatus (Figs. 1-16, 8-1).
3. The band of dorsal roots and posterolateral tract (zone of Lissauer) grades into the *trigeminal eminence (tuberculum cinereum)*; the longitudinal line of this band is directed to the trigeminal roots, which emerge from the middle cerebellar peduncle of the pons. The *trigeminal eminence* is formed by the spinal tract and nucleus of the trigeminal nerve (Fig. 1-16).
4. The longitudinal band of the ventral roots is represented in the medulla by the *rootlets of the hypoglossal nerve*, which emerge throughout the entire length of the anterior lateral sulcus of the medulla. The rostral continuation of this band comprises the sites of

emergence of cranial nerve VI at the ponto-medullary (preolivary) sulcus and of cranial nerve III into the interpeduncular fossa of the midbrain (see Fig. 1-13).

5. On the lateral aspect of the cervical spinal cord just posterior to the attachment on the denticulate ligament (halfway between the dorsal and ventral roots) is the longitudinal line formed by the sites of emergence of the rootlets and rostral course of the *spinal root of the accessory nerve* (*cranial nerve XI*). This is continuous rostrally along the lateral aspect of the medulla (posterior lateral sulcus) as the line formed by the emergence of the rootlets of the cranial part of N. XI and cranial nerves VII, IX, and X.

There are several other special topographic features of the medulla (Figs. 1-13 through 1-16).

6. Each *pyramid* on the anterior aspect is located between the rootlets of cranial nerve XII and the midline. The pyramids are formed exclusively by the fibers of the corticospinal tract. In the caudal medulla is a series of ridges which traverse across the anterior median fissure; they represent the pyramidal decussation.

7. The *olive* is located between the rootlets of nerve XII and those of nerves IX and X. Deep to the olive is the inferior olivary nuclear complex.

8. The central canal of the spinal cord continues rostrally into the diamond-shaped fourth ventricle of the medulla and pons; the medullary portion of the ventricle is covered posteriorly by the tela choroidea (choroid plexus). The obex is a posterior midline site at the caudal end of the fourth ventricle.

9. The floor of the fourth ventricle has several eminences. Adjacent to the midline is the *trigonum hypoglossus*, which is formed by the nucleus of the hypoglossal nerve. Just lateral to the trigonum hypoglossi is the *trigonum vagi* (*ala cinerea*), formed by the dorsal vagal nucleus (a parasympathetic nucleus) and the nucleus solitarius. On the caudolateral wall of the ventricle is a ridge called the *area postrema* (Chap. 11). The indentations on either side of the trigonum vagi constitute the inferior fovea, which represents the sulcus limi-

tans. The area vestibularis, an eminence formed by the vestibular nuclei, is located laterally.

Basic differences The differences in structure between the spinal cord and the medulla are primarily the consequence of several major features.

1. The large size and lateral spread of the fourth ventricle are associated with the topographic differences between the derivations of the alar plate and the basal plate of the embryo. The structures which develop from the alar plate and basal plate are located dorsally and ventral to the sulcus limitans, respectively, in the spinal cord. In contrast, the derivatives of the alar plate and basal plate are located lateral and medial to the sulcus limitans (fovea), respectively, in the medulla.

2. These differences in orientation have several consequences. In the spinal cord, the sensory nuclei (laminae) for the termination of the GSA and GVA fibers of the spinal nerves are located in the posterior horn dorsal to the sulcus limitans, while the motor nuclei or origin of GSE (alpha and gamma motor neurons) fibers of the spinal nerves are located in the gray matter ventral to the sulcus limitans. In contrast, the nuclei of the cranial nerves differ. The sensory cranial nerve nuclei (nucleus solitarius, spinal nucleus of N. V, and vestibular nuclei) are located lateral to the inferior fovea, while the motor nuclei of the cranial nerves (dorsal vagal nucleus, nucleus ambiguus, and hypoglossal nucleus) are located medial to a plane from the inferior fovea to the posterolateral sulcus (Fig. 7-4).

3. Lamina VII and the fasciculi proprii of the spinal cord are presumed to be the equivalent of the expansive reticular formation of the brainstem.

4. The posterior column–medial lemniscus pathway undergoes a major shift in its location in the lower medulla. The posterior columns and their nuclei of termination (nuclei gracilis and cuneatus) are present dorsally throughout the spinal cord and lower medulla. The axons of the neurons of the second order course from these two nuclei (located

dorsal to the central canal) in a curve, as the internal arcuate fibers, which cross the midline ventral to the central canal to form an ascending tract called the medial lemniscus. After passing through the brainstem, the medial lemniscus terminates in the ventral posterolateral nucleus of the thalamus (Fig. 5-18).

5. The descending corticospinal fibers of the pyramid, which is located ventrally in the medulla, cross in the lower medulla (just caudal to the crossing of the internal arcuate fibers) as the pyramidal decussation. In this decussation most of the fibers course dorsally and laterally to the dorsal aspect of the lateral funiculus of the spinal cord to form the lateral corticospinal tract. The uncrossed fibers of the pyramid just descend into the anterior funiculus as the anterior corticospinal tract.

Basic similarities With some slight modifications, several structures have the same basic morphologic relations of one to the other and to the spinal cord and medulla. The *medial longitudinal fasciculus (MLF)* is located (1) ventral to the central canal of the spinal cord or fourth ventricle and cerebral aqueduct of the brainstem and (2) medially on either side of the midline. The spinothalamic tract, posterior and anterior spinocerebellar tracts, spinotectal tract, and spinal nucleus and tract of the trigeminal nerve are located as a group laterally in the spinal cord and medulla. Within the brainstem, the lateral spinothalamic tract is called the spinothalamic tract; it may be joined by some fibers of the anterior spinothalamic tract.

Level of the pyramidal decussation
(Figs. 8-4, 8-5, A-1, A-11, and A-12)

The most distinguishing feature of this level is the crossing of 85 to 90 percent of the corticospinal fibers as the *pyramidal decussation*. It is

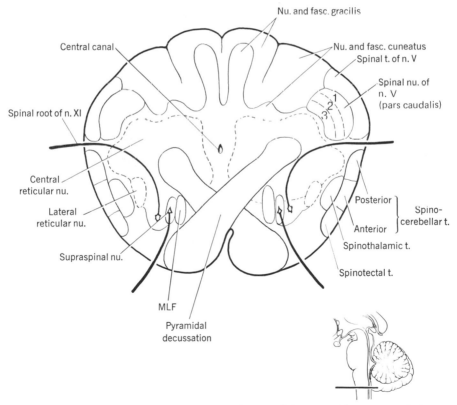

FIGURE 8-5 Transverse section of the lower medulla at the level of the pyramidal (corticospinal) decussation. The pars caudalis of the spinal trigeminal nucleus is called the posterior horn of the medulla because it is divisible into a (1) marginal lamina, (2) substantia gelatinosa, and (3) magnocellular layer (Chap. 7).

composed of interdigitating descending fibers which decussate and course in a caudal and posterior direction to the dorsal aspect of the lateral funiculus of the spinal cord. Dorsal and ventral spinal roots are absent. Fibers of the *spinal root of N. XI* arise in the anterior horn and pass dorsally and then laterally before emerging on the lateral aspect of the medulla. The spinal tract of N. V is composed of fibers from cranial nerves V, VII, IX, and X which descend as far as C2 (Fig. 7-6) to terminate in the spinal nucleus of N. V. The fasciculus gracilis is smaller than the fasciculus cuneatus; both fasciculi are in the same location as in the spinal cord. The *nucleus gracilis* is present; it is the nucleus of termination for the fibers of the fasciculus gracilis. The posterior and anterior spinocerebellar, spinothalamic, and spinotectal tracts have a relatively similar position as in the spinal cord. The medial longitudinal fasciculus and the anterior corticospinal tract pass on the ventrolateral side of the decussating pyramidal fibers. The *central reticular nucleus* of the medulla occupies the bulk of the reticular formation from the spinal cord-medulla

junction to the midolivary level. In the medial part of the ventral gray matter of the caudal medulla is a rostral extension of the anterior horn (lamina IX) of the spinal cord; this nucleus, which gives rise to ventral root fibers of the first cervical nerves, is called the *supraspinal nucleus.*

Level of decussation of the medial lemniscus (Figs. 8-6, A-2, and A-13)

The distinguishing feature of this level is the curve of the *internal arcuate fibers*, which, after arising from cells in the enlarged nuclei gracilis and cuneatus, sweep anteriorly in an arc and decussate across the midline to form the medial lemniscus of the opposite side. Upon entering the medial lemniscus, these fibers bend and ascend rostrally through the brainstem to the ventral posterolateral nucleus of the thalamus. The fasciculi gracilis and cuneatus are small because their ascending fibers terminate within the nuclei gracilis and cuneatus. The *spinal tract and nucleus of the trigeminal nerve* are displaced anteriorly. Some fibers arise from this nucleus and,

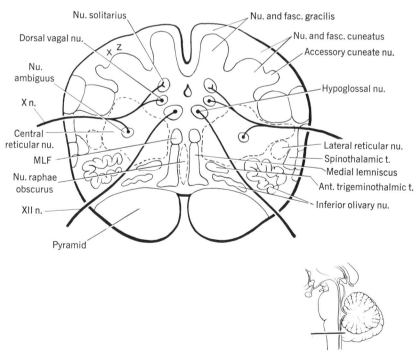

FIGURE 8-6 Transverse section of the lower medulla at the level of the medial lemniscus. Refer to Figs. A-2 and A-13.

with the internal arcuate fibers, cross to the opposite side, ascending as the anterior trigeminothalamic tract to the ventral posteromedial nucleus of the thalamus (Fig. 8-17). They are second-order neurons, conveying pain and temperature information derived from the trigeminal nerve, nervus intermedius (VII), and glossopharyngeal and vagus nerves.

In addition to the spinal nucleus of N. V, four other cranial nerve nuclei are present at this level. The sensory *nucleus solitarius* (GVA and SVA) and the parasympathetic motor *dorsal vagal nucleus* (GVE) and the motor *nucleus ambiguus* (SVE) are involved with the vagus nerve, which emerges through the dorsolateral sulcus of the medulla. The former two nuclei are located anterior to the nucleus gracilis and medial to the internal arcuate fibers; the latter (nucleus ambiguus) is located in the middle of the tegmentum just lateral to the internal arcuate fibers. Many of the fibers of the nucleus ambiguus from this level form the cranial root of the accessory nerve.

Anterior to the central canal on either side of the midline is the pair of *hypoglossal nuclei* (GSE); from each nucleus arises a hypoglossal nerve which passes through the medial tegmentum and emerges from the medulla between a pyramid and the olive (inferior olivary nuclear complex) at the preolivary sulcus.

The ascending tracts located in the lateral medulla—comprising the posterior and anterior spinocerebellar, spinothalamic, spinotectal tracts—occupy the same general location as in the more caudal levels.

Three prominent cerebellar relay nuclei are the source of fibers which pass through the inferior cerebellar peduncle before terminating in the cerebellum. The *accessory cuneate nucleus* of the lower medulla, located lateral to the cuneate nucleus, is the homologue to the dorsal nucleus of Clarke in the spinal cord; it receives proprioceptive input from the cervical and upper thoracic regions, especially the upper extremities, via uncrossed fibers ascending in the fasciculus cuneatus. The ipsilaterally projecting cuneocerebellar fibers from the accessory cuneate nucleus are the pathway from the upper extremity that is equivalent to the posterior spinocerebellar tract from the lower extremity. The *lateral reticular nucleus*, located anterolaterally in the vicinity of

the spinothalamic tract, extends rostrocaudally at the level of the caudal two-thirds of the inferior olivary complex. This nucleus receives afferent input from the spinal cord via spinoreticular and collateral branches of spinothalamic fibers and from rubrobulbar fibers from the red nucleus of the midbrain. The nuclei of the *inferior olivary nuclear complex* are discussed further on under "Level of the Middle Third of the Inferior Olivary Nucleus."

Of the descending tracts and fibers, the pyramids, composed of corticospinal fibers, are clearly demarcated. The anterior border of the medial longitudinal fasciculus (MLF) is not clearly defined because its fibers overlap with those of the medial lemniscus. At this level the MLF is composed of (1) the pontine reticulospinal tract from the pars oralis and pars caudalis of the pontine reticular nuclei, (2) the interstitiospinal tract from the interstitial nucleus of Cajal, (3) the tectospinal tract from the midbrain tectum, and (4) the vestibulospinal fibers from the medial vestibular nucleus.

Just posterior to the inferior olivary nuclear complex within the reticular formation are the fibers of the rubrospinal tract from the red nucleus in the midbrain, the medullary reticulospinal tract from the nucleus reticularis gigantocellularis of the medulla, and the vestibulospinal tract from the lateral vestibular nucleus. The fibers of these tracts are intermingled with other fibers; hence they are not clearly delineated.

Just rostral to this level are the *obex* and the caudal fourth ventricle (see Fig. 8-1). The *reticular nuclei* include the nucleus raphae magnus, central reticular nucleus, and lateral reticular nucleus; these belong to the raphae, central, and lateral nuclear groups, respectively.

Level of the middle third of the inferior olivary complex
(Figs. 8-7, A-3, and A-14)

The distinguishing features of this level are the nuclei of the inferior olivary complex, fourth ventricle, and cranial nerve nuclei. The *olivary complex* comprises the phylogenetically new *principal inferior olivary nucleus* and the phylogenetically old *dorsal and medial accessory olivary nuclei*. The fibers from the inferior olivary complex decussate and pass successively through the

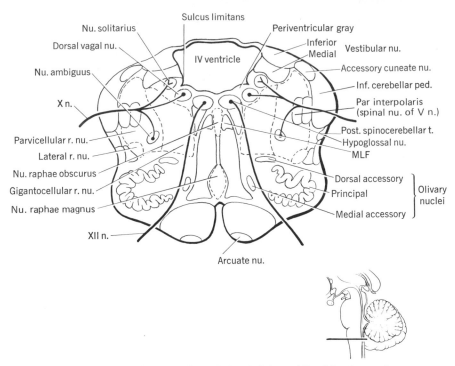

FIGURE 8-7 Transverse section of the medulla at the level of the middle of the olive. Refer to Figs. A-3 and A-14. The arcuate nuclei are minor nuclei projecting to the cerebellum.

medial lemnisci, the vicinity of the contralateral olivary complex, and the inferior cerebellar peduncle before terminating in the cerebellum. The accessory olivary nuclei and principal inferior olivary nucleus have fibers which project primarily to the vermis. The fibers from the principal olivary nucleus terminate in the contralateral cerebellar hemisphere. The olivo-cerebellar fibers convey excitatory influences to the deep cerebellar nuclei and to the entire cerebellar cortex. The input to the inferior olivary complex is derived from the spinal cord, cerebral cortex, deep cerebellar nuclei, red nucleus, and periaqueductal gray of the midbrain. The spinoolivary fibers ascend in the anterior funiculus and terminate in the accessory olivary nuclei; the existence of these fibers in humans has been questioned. All the descending fibers to the olivary complex terminate in the principal inferior olivary nucleus. Originating from the frontal, parietal, temporal, and occipital lobes, the corticoolivary fibers course with the corticospinal fibers before terminating bilaterally in the principal inferior olivary nuclei. The fibers from the

red nucleus and periaqueductal gray descend in the central tegmental tract. From the dentate and interpositus nuclei of the cerebellum, fibers pass through the superior cerebellar peduncle, cross in the lower midbrain, and descend to the olivary nucleus in the descending limb of the superior cerebellar peduncle.

In the tegmentum anterior to the floor of the fourth ventricle is a row of cranial nerve nuclei. Two motor nuclei, located medial to the fovea (sulcus limitans), are the hypoglossal (GSE) and dorsal vagal (GVE) nuclei. Two sensory nuclear groups, located laterally to the fovea, are the nucleus solitarius (GVA, SVA) and the medial and inferior vestibular (SSA) nuclei. The nucleus ambiguus (SVE) is a motor nucleus located in the middle of the tegmentum. The spinal nucleus of N. V is a sensory nucleus in the dorsolateral tegmentum. The vagus nerve is associated with the nucleus ambiguus, dorsal vagal nucleus, nucleus solitarius, and the spinal nucleus of N. V.

The *paramedian reticular nuclei* (nuclei lateral to medial lemniscus in vicinity of inferior olivary nucleus) and the nearby *arcuate* and *peri-*

hypoglossal nuclei relay influences via the inferior cerebellar peduncles to the ipsilateral and contralateral halves of the cerebellum. The cells of the *raphe nuclei* — the *nucleus raphe magnus* — contain serotinin (5-hydroxytryptamine). Fibers from these cells project to the spinal cord. The nucleus raphe magnus was formerly divided into a nucleus raphe obscurus and nucleus raphe pallidus.

The *central reticular nuclear group* in the upper medullary levels is the *gigantocellular reticular nucleus*, which is located posterior to the inferior olivary complex. This large-celled nucleus occupies the medial two-thirds of the reticular formation as far rostral as the medullary-pontine junction. Input to this nucleus is derived largely from (1) widespread areas of the cerebral cortex via crossed and uncrossed corticoreticular fibers, (2) higher brainstem levels via the central tegmental tract, (3) neurons from the parvicellular nucleus of the lateral nuclear group, and (4) spinoreticular fibers ascending in the anterolateral funiculus of the spinal cord. The output from this nucleus is projected (1) rostrally via the central tegmental tract to higher brainstem levels and the intralaminar nuclei of the thalamus and via the median forebrain bundle to the hypothalamus, and (2) caudally via the medullary (lateral) reticulospinal tract to the spinal cord. The reticular nucleus of the central group in the caudal medulla is called the ventral reticular nucleus.

The *lateral reticular group* comprises the *lateral reticular nucleus* and *parvicellular reticular nucleus* (see Fig. 8-14). Input to the parvicellular reticular nucleus is derived from (1) widespread areas of the cerebral cortex via crossed and uncrossed corticoreticular fibers, (2) collateral fibers conveying influences from the auditory, vestibular, trigeminal, and visceral pathways, and (3) spinoreticular fibers from the spinal cord. The output from the parvicellular reticular nuclei is directed medially to the gigantocellular reticular nucleus.

Except for possible minor changes, the locations of the ascending and descending tracts and pathways are similar to those described under "Level of Decussation of the Medial Lemniscus." The posterior spinocerebellar tract is close to the inferior cerebellar peduncle, which it is about to join.

Tangential section at the levels of the glossopharyngeal and vestibulocochlear nerves
(Figs. 8-8, A-4, and A-15)

This medullary level is in the vicinity of the medullopontine junction; it is basically different from the midolivary level in several respects. The hypoglossal and dorsal vagal nuclei are absent. The *inferior salivatory nucleus* is a physiologically defined nucleus (related to secretion of the parotid gland) located within the parvicellular reticular nucleus (see Fig. 8-8; see also Fig. 7-8). The cranial nerve nuclei associated with the glossopharyngeal nerve comprise the nucleus solitarius, spinal nucleus of the trigeminal nerve, inferior salivatory nucleus, and nucleus ambiguus. The large inferior cerebellar peduncle (left side of Fig. 8-8) is illustrated as it passes (right side of Fig. 8-8) into the cerebellum. The *inferior cerebellar peduncle* comprises the following fibers passing to the cerebellum: posterior spinocerebellar, cuneocerebellar, and olivocerebellar tracts, along with fibers from such nuclei as the lateral reticular and paramedian reticular nuclei. A portion of the inferior cerebellar peduncle, called the juxtarestiform body, is composed of fibers associated with the vestibular system conveying influences to and from the vestibulocerebellum and the fastigial nuclei of the cerebellum.

On the outer surface of the inferior cerebellar peduncle are the dorsal and ventral cochlear nuclei. The fibers of the cochlear nerve branch in an organized sequence so that each fiber is distributed in a precise pattern to both the dorsal and ventral cochlear nuclei. At a slightly higher level the fibers of the vestibular nerve pass at right angles among the fibers of the inferior cerebellar peduncle on their way to the four vestibular nuclei (the medial, inferior, and lateral vestibular nuclei are illustrated).

The *reticular nuclei* at this level include the *nucleus raphe obscurus* and *nucleus raphe magnus*, the *nucleus gigantocellularis* (a central reticular nucleus), and the *nucleus parvicellularis* (a lateral reticular group nucleus).

The four deep cerebellar nuclei, oriented in order from medial to lateral, are the fastigial, globose, emboliform, and dentate nuclei. The globose and emboliform nuclei are collectively

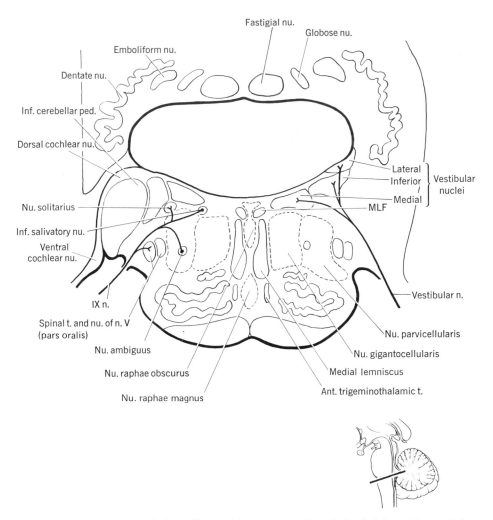

FIGURE 8-8 Transverse section (slightly oblique) of the upper medulla at the level of the cochlear and glosso-pharyngeal nerves (*left*) and the vestibular nerve (*right*). Refer to Figs. A-4 and A-15. Section includes the cerebellum through the deep cerebellar nuclei.

called the nucleus interpositum. The fibers of the inferior cerebellar peduncle pass lateral to the dentate nucleus. The juxtarestiform body is located between the deep cerebellar nuclei and the lateral border of the fourth ventricle.

Level of nuclei of sixth and seventh cranial nerves
(Figs. 8-9, A6, and A-17)

The general pattern of organization at this level differs from that of the levels of the medulla primarily because of the massive size of the *ventral* or *basilar pons* relative to the *dorsal* or *tegmental pons*. The *ventral pons* represents a modified, rostral continuation of the pyramids of the medulla. The *dorsal pons* represents the rostral continuation of the medulla exclusive of the pyramids. The boundary between the dorsal and ventral pons is a plane located just anterior to the medial lemniscus. The fourth ventricle is large.

The *ventral pons* is composed of (1) the longitudinally oriented corticospinal and corticobulbar tracts and (2) the terminal branches of the corticopontine fibers, the pontine nucleus, and the transversely oriented pontocerebellar fibers.

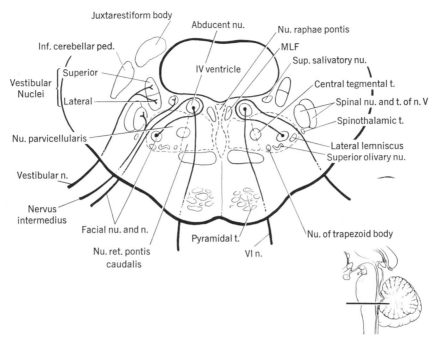

Labels in figure:
- Juxtarestiform body
- Abducent nu.
- Nu. raphae pontis
- Inf. cerebellar ped.
- MLF
- Sup. salivatory nu.
- Superior
- IV ventricle
- Central tegmental t.
- Vestibular Nuclei
- Lateral
- Spinal nu. and t. of n. V
- Spinothalamic t.
- Nu. parvicellularis
- Lateral lemniscus
- Superior olivary nu.
- Vestibular n.
- Nervus intermedius
- Facial nu. and n.
- Nu. of trapezoid body
- Pyramidal t.
- VI n.
- Nu. ret. pontis caudalis

FIGURE 8-9 Transverse section of the lower pons at the level of the sixth and seventh cranial nerves. Refer to Figs. A-16 and A-17.

The latter course laterally, decussate, and pass through the middle cerebellar peduncle before terminating in the contralateral half of the cerebellum (see Fig. 9-5).

Except for a few significant modifications, the dorsal pons resembles the medulla. The medial longitudinal fasciculus (MLF) is still located anterior to the fourth ventricle and just lateral to the midline, while the spinal tract and nucleus of the trigeminal nerve are in the dorsolateral tegmentum. The medial lemniscus has shifted from a ventromedial tegmental location in the medulla to a ventral tegmental location in the pons. The *central tegmental tract* is prominent in the middle of the reticular formation.

The cranial nerve nuclei present at this level have their equivalents in the medulla. The *abducent nucleus* (GSE), *motor nucleus of the facial nerve* (SVE), and the *superior salivatory nucleus* (GVE) are located within the tegmentum in sites similar to those occupied within the medulla by the hypoglossal nucleus (GSE), nucleus ambiguus (SVE), and dorsal vagal nucleus (GVE), respectively. The *superior vestibular nucleus* (SSA) is found in the posterolateral tegmentum. The course of the fibers of the abducent and facial

nerves is characteristic and significant. The lower motor neurons of the sixth nerve emerge from the abducent nucleus and pass ventrally through the medial tegmentum and basal pons lateral to the pyramidal tract before emerging medially at the pontomedullary junction. After leaving from the facial nucleus, the lower motor neurons form a bundle that follows a circuitous course. It passes posteromedially and ascends for a short distance medial to the abducent nucleus and posterior to the medial longitudinal fasciculus; at the rostral end of the abducent nucleus, the bundle turns laterally (as the internal genu of the facial nerve) and then continues anterolaterally through the lateral tegmentum and ventral pons before emerging at the cerebellopontine angle. The hillock in the floor of the fourth ventricle at the site of the abducent nucleus and the internal genu is called the facial or abducent dolliculus. Fibers of the nervus intermedius are in close association with the facial nerve; they originate in the physiologicaly defined superior salivatory nucleus (GVE) or terminate in the spinal nucleus of N. V (GSA) and nucleus solitarius (SVA, GVA). The superior and inferior salivatory nuclei are actually diffuse and confluent groups of cells located within the parvicellular reticular nucleus (see Figs. 8-8 through 8-10).

The upper motor neuron pattern of innervation is clinically significant. Bilateral upper motor neuron projections from the cerebral cortex via corticobulbar and corticoreticular fibers influence the lower motor neurons innervating the muscles in the upper part of the face and forehead (e.g., frontalis and orbicularis oculi). In contrast, unilateral upper motor neurons projecting from the contralateral cerebrum influence the lower motor neurons which innervate the muscles of the lower part of the face (i.e., buccinator and labial muscles). As a consequence, a unilateral lesion of the upper motor neurons to the facial nucleus results in paralysis of the muscles of facial expression in the contralateral part of the lower face; the other facial muscles are generally spared (see Fig. 8-22).

The trapezoid nucleus and superior olivary nuclei and fibers of the auditory pathways are located at this level. Dicussating fibers of the trapezoid body are present in the vicinity of the medial lemniscus; these fibers collect in the ventrolateral tegmentum as the lateral lemniscus, which is located roughly posterior to the spinothalamic tract. Nuclei of the auditory pathways include the superior olivary nuclei and nuclei of the trapezoid body.

The reticular nuclei at this level and those of the lower pons caudal to the principal nucleus of the trigeminal nerve are the *nucleus raphe pontis* (a raphe nucleus), the *nucleus reticularis pontis caudalis* (a central reticular group nucleus), and the *nucleus parvicellularis* (a lateral reticular nucleus).

Level of the trigeminal nerve
(Figs. 8-10, A-7, and A-18)

The characteristic features at this midpontine level are (1) the *principal sensory nucleus* and *motor nucleus of the trigeminal nerve* and (2) the *superior cerebellar peduncle* on the lateral aspect of the narrowing fourth ventricle.

The *principal nucleus of N. V* is a nucleus of termination of the sensory root of the trigeminal nerve; other fibers of this root have their cell bodies in the *mesencephalic nucleus of N. V*, which is located lateral to the ventricle. The *motor nucleus of N. V*, located medial to the principal nucleus, contains the cell bodies of origin of the lower motor neurons of the motor root of the trigeminal nerve.

The *superior cerebellar peduncle* is composed of primarily cerebellar efferent fibers originating in the dentate, emboliform, and globose nuclei; these fibers decussate in the lower midbrain tegmentum and (1) ascend to the nucleus ruber and to the rostral intralaminar and ventrolateral thalamic nuclei and (2) descend in the brainstem tegmentum to the reticulotegmental nucleus of the pons and the inferior olivary and paramedian nuclei of the medulla. The anterior spinocerebellar tract courses posteriorly in the superior cerebellar peduncle; its fibers terminate in the anterior vermal cortex. The roof of the fourth ventricle is covered by the superior medullary velum. Between the superior cerebellar peduncle and the fourth ventricle, extending from the rostral half of the principal nucleus of N. V to the level of the inferior colliculus, is a group of pigmented cells, the locus ceruleus (nucleus pigmentosus) (see Fig. 8-11). These cells are noradrenergic neurons and have axons which are distributed to (1) cerebellum, (2) cerebrum, (3) brainstem, and (4) spinal cord (see page 303 and Fig. 8-19). It appears cerulean blue in the gross specimen.

The medial lemniscus has shifted somewhat laterally, and the spinothalamic tract and lateral lemniscus have shifted slightly dorsolaterally along the outer margin of the reticular formation. The medial longitudinal fasciculus, central tegmental tract, rubrospinal tract, and the structures of the basilar pons have the same topographic relations to one another as those described earlier under "Level of Nuclei of the Sixth and Seventh Cranial Nerves." The lateral lemniscus contains a small synaptic collection called the nucleus of the lateral lemniscus.

The *reticular nuclei* extending rostrally from this level into the isthmus of the midbrain are (1) the *superior central nucleus* (a raphe nucleus), (2) the *nucleus reticularis pontis oralis* and *locus ceruleus* (a central reticular group nucleus), and (3) the *reticulotegmental nucleus*. The latter is actually an extension of the pontine nuclei of the ventral pons into the tegmentum; as do the pontine nuclei, the reticulotegmental nucleus projects its fibers to the cerebellum. The lateral

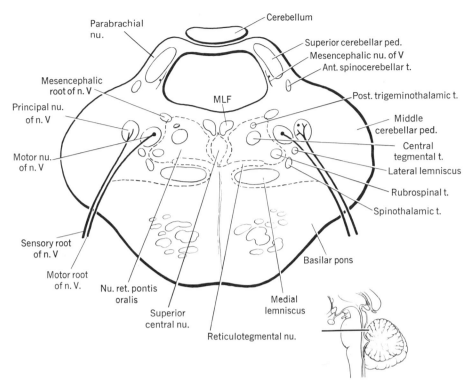

FIGURE 8-10 Transverse section of the midpons at the level of the entrance of the trigeminal nerve. Refer to Figs. A-7 and A-18.

reticular nuclear group is not represented in the midpontine level.

Level of the inferior colliculus
(Figs. 8-11, A-9, and A-20)

The distinguishing features at this level include the inferior colliculus, the decussation of the superior cerebellar peduncle, and the ventral pons. The ventricular system is represented by the narrow *cerebral aqueduct* (*iter*).

The large *nucleus of the inferior colliculus* is a major processing station in the auditory pathways. It receives input from ascending auditory fibers of the lateral lemniscus and descending fibers from the madial geniculate body; it projects influences (1) rostrally to the medial geniculate body via the brachium of the inferior colliculus and to the superior colliculus, and (2) caudally to auditory nuclei via the lateral lemniscus. The nuclei of the inferior colliculi are interconnected by fibers of the commissure of the

inferior colliculus. As a group, the medial lemniscus, spinothalamic tract, and lateral lemniscus have shifted laterally and dorsally along the outer margin of the reticular formation of the tegmentum. In this shift, the lateral lemniscus approaches the inferior colliculus; its fibers enter and terminate in the nucleus of the inferior colliculus. The rostrally projecting fibers from the nucleus form the brachium of the inferior colliculus, which is located in the dorsolateral tegmentum of the upper midbrain.

The posterior trigeminothalamic tract from the ipsilateral principal nucleus of N. V is located in the tegmentum posterior to the central tegmental tract (Fig. 8-17). The anterior trigeminothalamic tract from the contralateral spinal and principal nuclei of N. V is located between the medial lemniscus and spinothalamic tract. The medial longitudinal fasciculus (MLF) is notched posteriorly by the nucleus of the trochlear nerve (GSE). The fibers of the trochlear nerve pass as a dorsocaudally directed

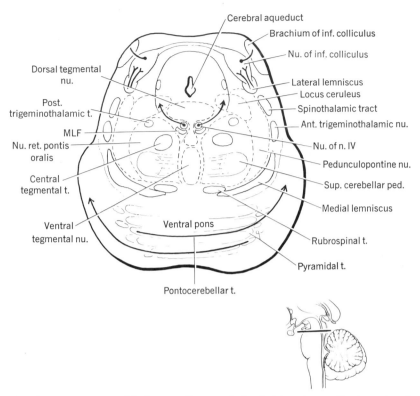

Cerebral aqueduct
Brachium of inf. colliculus
Nu. of inf. colliculus
Dorsal tegmental nu.
Post. trigeminothalamic t.
Lateral lemniscus
Locus ceruleus
Spinothalamic tract
Ant. trigeminothalamic nu.
MLF
Nu. ret. pontis oralis
Nu. of n. IV
Pedunculopontine nu.
Central tegmental t.
Sup. cerebellar ped.
Medial lemniscus
Ventral tegmental nu.
Ventral pons
Rubrospinal t.
Pyramidal t.
Pontocerebellar t.

FIGURE 8-11 Transverse section of the lower midbrain at the level of the inferior colliculus and nucleus of the fourth cranial nerve. Refer to Figs. A-8, A-9, and A-20.

arc from this nucleus along the outer edge of the periaqueductal gray matter; they decussate completely in the superior medullary velum and emerge from the posterior tectum caudal to the inferior colliculus. The locus ceruleus is located deep to the inferior colliculus. The reticulotegmental nucleus is present in the anteromedial tegmentum.

The *reticular nuclei* at this level include (1) the *dorsal and ventral raphe tegmental nuclei* (raphe nuclei), (2) the rostral portion of the *nucleus reticularis pontis oralis* and *locus ceruleus* (central reticular nuclei), and (3) *pendunculopontine and cuneiform nuclei* (lateral reticular group nuclei). The dorsal tegmental nucleus (supratrochlear nucleus) is located dorsal to the trochlear nucleus in the periaqueductal gray matter; it receives input from the mamillary body. The ventral tegmental nucleus is present ventral to the medial longitudinal fasciculus; it is apparently a rostral extension of the superior central nucleus. The locus ceruleus (nucleus pig-

mentosus pontis) is the ''blue place'' located in the upper pons to lower midbrain between the mesenchephalic nucleus of the trigeminal nerve and the medial longitudinal fasciculus. The pedunculopontine nucleus lies in the caudal midbrain lateral to the superior cerebellar peduncle and medial to the medial lemniscus. This nucleus receives input from the precentral gyrus and the ipsilateral globus pallidus. It is the only infratenorial brainstem reticular nucleus which receives direct input from the globus pallidus.

Section through midbrain at lower level of the superior colliculus
(Figs. 8-12, A-10, and A-21)

The major characteristic features at this level are the *superior colliculus, nucleus of the oculomotor nerve, red nucleus, substantia nigra,* and *crus cerebri* (see Fig. 8-13).

The *superior colliculi* are paired laminated hillocks of the tectum, which are complex pro-

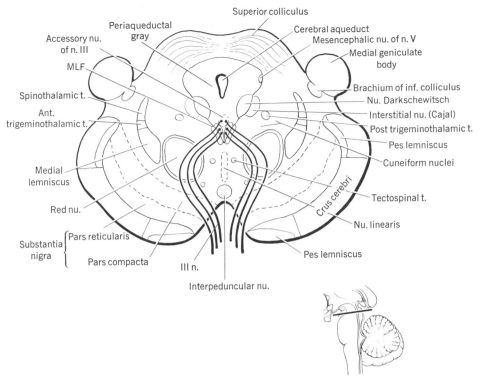

Accessory nu. of n. III
MLF
Spinothalamic t.
Ant. trigeminothalamic t.
Medial lemniscus
Red nu.
Substantia nigra { Pars reticularis
Pars compacta
III n.
Interpeduncular nu.
Periaqueductal gray
Superior colliculus
Cerebral aqueduct
Mesencephalic nu. of n. V
Medial geniculate body
Brachium of inf. colliculus
Nu. Darkschewitsch
Interstitial nu. (Cajal)
Post trigeminothalamic t.
Pes lemniscus
Cuneiform nuclei
Crus cerebri
Tectospinal t.
Nu. linearis
Pes lemniscus

FIGURE 8-12 Transverse section of the upper midbrain at the level of the superior colliculus and the third cranial nerve. Refer to Figs. A-10 and A-21.

cessing nuclei. Each superior colliculus should be referred to as cortex, because its neurons and their fibers are organized into laminae. Just rostral to the superior colliculus is a small area of nuclei called the pretectal area. The primary roles of the superior colliculi and pretectal area are in the light reflex, accommodation (focusing) reflex, and other responses to visual stimuli.

The *red nucleus* is a large oval nucleus in the medial tegmentum. It is composed of a caudal magnocellular part and a rostral parvocellular part. Some fibers of the superior cerebellar peduncle terminate within the nucleus, while others pass through and on its outer margins as a "capsule" on their way to the ventral lateral, ventral anterior, and some intralaminar thalamic nuclei. In the region between the two red nuclei is the dorsal and the ventral tegmental decussation. Cells in the deep layers of the superior colliculus give rise to the tectospinal tract; the fibers arc through the tegmentum and cross the midline as the dorsal tegmental decussation

before descending as the spinotectal tract located anterior to the medial longitudinal fasciculus. The rubrospinal tract originates from cells in the caudal three-fourths of the red nucleus; its fibers cross as the ventral tegmental decussation before descending as the rubrospinal tract in the anterior tegmentum.

The *oculomotor nuclear complex* is located in a V-shaped region formed by the paired medial longitudinal fasciculi. The fibers of the oculomotor nerve arise in this nucleus, course anterior through the medial tegmentum, including the red nucleus, on their way to emerge as rootlets into the interpeduncular fossa.

The *substantia nigra* is located between the tegmentum and the crus cerebri. It is divided into a pars compacta and a pars reticularis. The large cells of the compact or black part contain melanin pigment and primary catecholamines; these cells synthesize and convey dopamine via nigrostriatal fibers to the neostriatum (caudate nucleus and putamen). The cells of the reddish brown pars reticularis contain iron but no melanin pigment.

The *crus cerebri* is the basilar part of the midbrain. It is composed of descending corticofugal fibers which originate in the cerebral cortex. The corticospinal and corticobulbar fibers are located in the middle two-thirds (Fig. A-10). They are said to be somatotopically organized at this level with the head and upper- and lower-extremity musculature influenced by nerve fibers arranged from medial to lateral within the crus. Frontopontine fibers are located in the medial portion, and the corticopontine fibers from the parietal, temporal, and occipital cortical areas are located in the lateral portion of the crus. The most medial and lateral portions of the crus may contain some corticobulbar fibers; each of these regions is called a pes lemniscus.

The medial lemniscus, anterior trigeminothalamic tract, and spinothalamic tract have shifted to a slightly more dorsal location in the tegmentum. The brachium of the inferior colliculus (auditory tract) is located dorsolateral to the spinothalamic tract; it is heading to the medial geniculate body. The posterior trigeminothalamic tract is located in the dorsomedial tegmentum. The interpeduncular nucleus is located in the midline just dorsal to the interpeduncular fossa.

In the roof of the cerebral aqueduct at the level of the posterior commissure is a sheet of modified ciliated ependymal cells called the subcommissural organ (Chap. 11).

Reticular nuclei at this level include *nuclei linearis* (raphe nuclei); *nucleus ruber*, which is considered to be a specialized central reticular nucleus; and *cuneiform nuclei* (lateral reticular nuclear group). Other nuclei include the *interpeduncular nucleus, mesencephalic nucleus of the trigeminal nerve, interstitial nucleus of Cajal,* and the *nucleus of Darkschewitsch.*

Transverse section through junction of midbrain and thalamus (Figs. 8-13 and A-22)

The midbrain structures illustrated are similar to those depicted in the previous level. The fibers of the brachium of the inferior colliculus are terminating in the medial geniculate body of the thalamus. The medial lemniscus and the spino-

thalamic tracts will terminate just rostrally in the ventral posterolateral (VPL) nucleus of the thalamus. The optic tract is composed of fibers from the retinas of both eyes. Some fibers terminate in the lateral geniculate body of the thalamus. The other fibers pass through the brachium of the superior colliculus before terminating in the superior colliculus. The pulvinar of the thalamus is located above the lateral geniculate body.

RETICULAR SYSTEMS AND THE LEMNISCAL SYSTEMS

General concept

This classification is a means of conceptually dissecting the brainstem, as well as other parts of the central nervous system. However, the contrasting dichotomy implied in this characterization should not be considered absolute, for the structural and functional interrelations and interactions between the two systems are considerable and significant. They are functional systems based upon physiologic criteria.

The *lemniscal systems* are characterized as the specific, oligoneuronal, oligosynaptic, phylogenetically more recent, compactly grouped systems which convey the signals of most conscious sensory modalities.

The *reticular system* (*reticular core*) is characterized as the nonspecific, multineuronal, multisynaptic (polysynaptic), phylogenetically older system that integrates and conveys a great variety of ascending influences.

The lemniscal and reticular systems are composed of nuclei and tracts. The *lemniscal system* is called the specific system because its pathways convey those impulses of the specific conscious modalities ultimately recognized as pain, temperature, taste, audition, touch, discriminative touch, and appreciation of form, weight, and texture. The pathways associated with these senses are conceived of as having fewer sequences of neurons (oligoneuronal), fewer synapses (oligosynaptic), and somewhat more myelinated fibers (some fibers conduct faster) than are found in the reticular system. The specific systems are also characterized by point-to-point relays, by "secure" synaptic connections of the

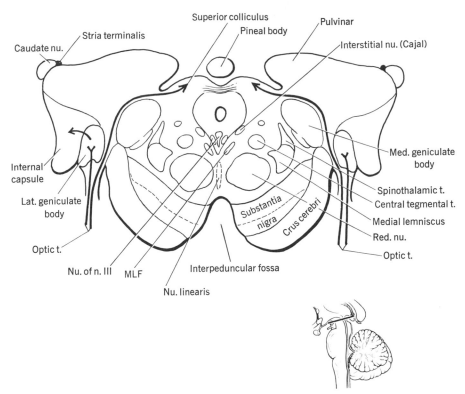

FIGURE 8-13 Transverse section at the junction of the upper midbrain diencephalon. Refer to Fig. A-22.

presynaptic neurons with the postsynaptic neurons, and by short latencies in the transmission times. These three characteristics are expressed by several observations. Stimuli from a spot (point) in the skin, mouth, joints, retina of the eye, or spiral organ of Corti of the ear project a limited number of neurons (points) in each of the relay nuclei of the pathway up to and including the primary sensory cortical area. This point-to-point relay from periphery to cerebral cortex is indicative of the secure connectivity within each pathway. In addition, the relay of a minimal sequence of neurons (many with long myelinated axons) results in the short latency it takes from the time a stimulus is applied in the periphery until the evoked activity is indicated in the sensory cortex. The activity of the lemniscal systems is only slightly affected by anesthetics; these pathways readily transmit impulses when the subject is unconscious from an anesthetic agent. Although the lemniscal system is defined as an ascending system, several descending

pathways may be considered to be "efferent lemniscal tracts." These are the corticobulbar, corticospinal and corticopontine tracts. These pathways are oligoneuronal, oligosynaptic, phylogenetically more recent, and organized in compact bundles (as compared with descending reticular pathways).

In addition to their role in the conveyance of information associated with appreciation of the specific senses, the lemniscal systems also make significant contributions to behavioral activities. An animal with a cerebrum deprived of lemniscal stimulation exhibits little affect and facial expression. Emotional and associated autonomic reactions require the specific stimuli of the lemniscal systems. The cerebral cortex, particularly the neocortex, requires the input from the lemniscal pathways for many expressions of affect.

The *reticular system* is present throughout the central nervous system in spinal cord, brainstem, cerebellum, diencephalon, and cerebral

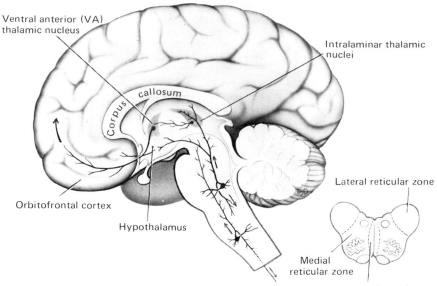

FIGURE 8-14 Ascending projections of the reticular pathway system associated with brainstem reticular formation. In general, the multineuronal, multisynaptic relays of the brainstem reticular formation extend rostrally into two telencephalic regions: (1) posteriorly into the intralaminar, ventral anterior and dorsomedial thalamic nuclear complexes; and (2) anteriorly into the subthalamic and hypothalamic complexes. The thalamic component projects, via the ventral anterior thalamic nucleus, to the orbitofrontal cortex. The cross section through the brainstem (medulla) illustrates the division of the brainstem reticular formation into (1) a midline raphe or paramedian zone, (2) a medial reticular or "motor" zone, and (3) a lateral reticular or "sensory" zone.

hemispheres (see Figs. 8-14 to 8-16). The *reticular formation* is the anatomic substrate of much of the reticular system. In the spinal cord the reticular formation comprises some of the gray matter, the fasciculi proprii (spinospinalis) tracts, and spinoreticular tracts. Estimates suggest that as many as half of the neurons of the spinal gray matter are neurons of the spinal reticular formation. The spinoreticular fibers are essentially fibers of the fasciculi proprii which extend into the brainstem. The fasciculi proprii and the reticuloreticular fibers (central tegmental tract) are the reticular pathways of the spinal cord and brainstem, respectively.

The reticular system is said to be nonspecific in the sense that it is not primarily associated with the specific modalities. The term *nonspecific* should be used judiciously; it must be clearly understood that the reticular system is *not* a diffusely projecting, functionally homogeneous, "nonspecific in the strict sense" neuronal system. The differentiated portions of this reticular formation (core), though operating

in a concerted manner, receive highly precise inputs and give rise to highly organized directed outputs. In fact, the brainstem reticular core is composed of heterogeneous subsystems that are highly differentiated in their morphology, the chemistry of their neurotransmitters, and their functional expressions. Morphologic diversity is illustrated in the differences between the neural organization of the paleospinothalamic tract from that of the locus ceruleus noted in Chap. 5 and in this chapter. Chemical diversity is observed in the organizations of the noradrenergic, serotinergic, and dopaminergic pathways (see Figs. 8-19 and 8-20). Functional diversities are expressed in a variety of physiologic centers and pathways associated with the autonomic nervous system (Chap. 6), oculomotor system for the control of eye movements, reticulospinal pathways for the control of posture through the alpha and gamma motor neurons, neospinothalamic pathways for "protopathic" pain, and the respiration (several respiratory centers).

In addition to the *reticuloreticular fibers*, the

central tegmental tract (see Figs. 8-9 to 8-11) also includes the rubrospinal fibers and ascending fibers from some brainstem reticular nuclei to certain thalamic nuclei (intralaminar nuclei and posterior thalamic region). The reticulospinal tracts are essentially reticuloreticular fibers which extend into the spinal cord (see Fig. 8-21). Many axons of the brainstem reticular neurons decussate before bifurcating into ascending and descending branches. This is a basis for the observations that some influences from the brainstem reticular formation are projected bilaterally. The reticular formation extends into the hypothalamus and into the thalamus as the intralaminar nuclei, reticular nucleus, and nuclei of the midline (refer to Fig. 8-14; see also Chap. 13). Some brainstem reticular nuclei project to the cerebellum. The axons of cells of the nonspecific thalamic nuclei probably do not project directly to the cerebral cortex. However, these nuclei generate activity which projects influences to widespread areas of the cerebral cortex. Through the neural networks of the reticular formation of the brainstem are conveyed those impulses associated with vaguely appreciated senses, such as poorly localized pain, neural activities associated with the arousal-sleep cycle, and affect behavior expressions. The effects of the reticular system are not actually random and indefinite but rather are organized and definite and hence, though mainly nonspecific, have some degree of specificity. These pathways have numerous neurons and many synaptic connections and consist essentially of unmyelinated and lightly myelinated fibers. The descending motor reticular pathways consist of the "extrapyramidal pathways" (Chap. 14) and the autonomic pathways that project their influences from the brainstem to the spinal cord as the reticulospinal tracts.

The nonspecific system is characterized by the lack of point-to-point relays, by the relative absence of "secure" synaptic connectivity of presynaptic neurons with postsynaptic neurons, and by long latencies in the transmission time. These three characteristics are expressed by several observations. Stimuli from many peripheral spots may exert their influences upon one neuron of the reticular system. This complex convergence does not permit point-to-point, secure relays. In addition, one peripheral spot may exert its influences upon many neurons. The multineuronal, multisynaptic connectivity results in the long latencies exhibited in the reticular pathways. The reticular system is extremely sensitive to even low levels of anesthesia.

Reticular formation

The *reticular formation* is a column of neurons which extends as a continuum with minimal histologic variation through the length of the spinal cord, brainstem, and basal regions of the diencephalon and telencephalon. The boundaries of the reticular formation cannot be precisely delineated, because its constituent neurons are not generally grouped into compact nuclei or tracts. The most constant structural substrate of the reticular formation is the presence of *generalized or isodendritic neurons* (see Fig. 2-7)—cells with long, sparsely branching dendrites (Ramón-Moliner and Nauta) (Chap. 2). Even the presence of this neuronal type is not always diagnostic, because it is also found in regions outside the classical reticular formation. The dendritic fields of one neuron overlap with those of other neurons; in addition, the fields are interlaced with the transit axons. The classical Golgi type II cells with axon arborization limited to the region of the dendritic field are absent in the reticular formation. The axons of the reticular neurons bifurcate into a long ascending branch and a long descending branch; these branches with their collaterals are transit axons (see Fig. 8-14). The long branches form the pathway systems which convey the output of these cells rostrally and caudally. These pathways are interrupted by numerous synaptic connections which are organized as orderly and precise linkages of neurons.

The following is a version of the extent of the reticular formation in the nervous system. In the spinal cord, the reticular formation is located in the intermediate zone (lamina VII), with extensions into parts of the anterior and posterior horns. The pathway of the spinal cord reticular formation is the fasciculus proprius. Rostrally it expands into the enlarged central region of the brainstem tegmentum, so that the brainstem reticular formation has been called the reticular core. The *nuclei of this reticular core of the medulla, pons, and midbrain* are arranged into three longitudinal columns (see Fig. 8-14): the *raphe nuclei* and *paramedian reticular nuclear group,* which are located within, and adjacent to, the midline raphe, the *central reticular nuclear group,* which occupies the medial subcolumn of the brainstem reticular core, and the *lateral reticular nuclear group,* located in the lateral subcolumn of the reticular core. The central tegmental tract (fasciculus) is the pathway of the brainstem reticular core.

The *raphe nuclei* include (1) the *nucleus raphe magnus* and *paramedian reticular nuclei* of the medulla; (2) the *nucleus raphe pontis, nucleus centralis superior, nucleus raphe dorsalis (dorsal tegmental nuclei* or *supratrochlear nucleus),* and *ventral tegmental nucleus of the pons* (the latter two nuclei extend into the midbrain) (see Fig 8-20); and (3) the *nuclei linearis of the midbrain* (see Figs. 8-5 through 8-13).

The *central reticular nuclear group* includes (1) the *nucleus reticularis centralis* and *nucleus reticularis gigantocellularis of the medulla,* (2) the *nuclei reticularis pontis caudalis oralis the reticulotegmental nucleus of the pons,* and (3) the *nucleus ruber of the midbrain.*

The *lateral reticular nuclear group* includes (1) the *nucleus reticularis parvicellularis* and *lateral reticular nucleus of the medulla,* (2) no nuclei in most of the pons, and (3) the *cuneiform nucleus, parabrachial nucleus,* and *pedunculopontine tegmental nucleus of the midbrain.*

The nucleus ruber, locus ceruleus, and interpeduncular nucleus of the midbrain and the inferior olivary nuclear complex may be considered as specialized nuclei which are not usually classified as reticular core nuclei.

The most rostral extension of the reticular formation into the diencephalon and telencephalon may include (1) the midline nuclei, intralaminar nuclei, reticular nucleus, and part of the ventral anterior nucleus of the thalamus; (2) hypothalamus; (3) zona incerta of the ventral thalamus; and (4) the septal nuclei and substantia innominata (located ventral to globus pallidus) of the telencephalon. Some investigators include the subthalamic nucleus and globus pallidus in the reticular formation. The reticular pathways link (1) the midbrain with the hypothalamus and septal nuclei and (2) the upper brainstem with the nuclei of the diencephalic reticular formation (see Chaps. 13, 14, and 15).

The brainstem reticular formation and its major rostral extension, the hypothalamus, have been called the *isodendritic core of the brain,* because they are composed primarily of isodendritic neurons. The dendritic fields of isodendritic neurons overlap extensively. Differential specificity of function among these neurons within the isodendritic core is presumed to occur. Apparently the dendrites of each isodendritic neuron receive specialized inputs; these differ from the inputs received by the other isodendritic neurons.

Reticular system

The brainstem reticular system is the phylogenetically ancient integrator, often called the "central core" (isodendritic core) (see Fig. 8-14) of the mammalian brainstem. The cell bodies of the neurons of the reticular system are organized into groups throughout the reticular formation as the relatively diffuse brainstem reticular nuclei. The very long dendrites of each neuron are generally oriented in the transverse plane at right angles to the longitudinal axis of the brainstem, while the axon bifurcates into one long ascending branch and one long descending branch oriented parallel to the long axis of the brainstem (see Fig. 8-14). Numerous collateral branches leave the main axonic branches. This organization permits a tremendous amount of interaction among the neurons of the system. Each neuron may receive synaptic input from over 4000 other neurons (convergence), and, in turn, each neuron may have synaptic connections with over 25,000 other neurons (divergence).

The *input to the brainstem reticular system* is derived from many sources (see Fig. 8-15). The ascending influences from the spinal cord include the spinoreticular tracts, the spinotectal tract, and the terminal and collateral branches of the spinothalamic tracts. The medial lemniscus does not have any branches which project into the reticular formation. All the sensory cranial nerves are sources of input. The brainstem reticular formation receives influences from visceral sources via the nucleus solitarius (facial, glossopharyngeal, and vagal nerves), from the vestibular and cochlear nuclei and their path-

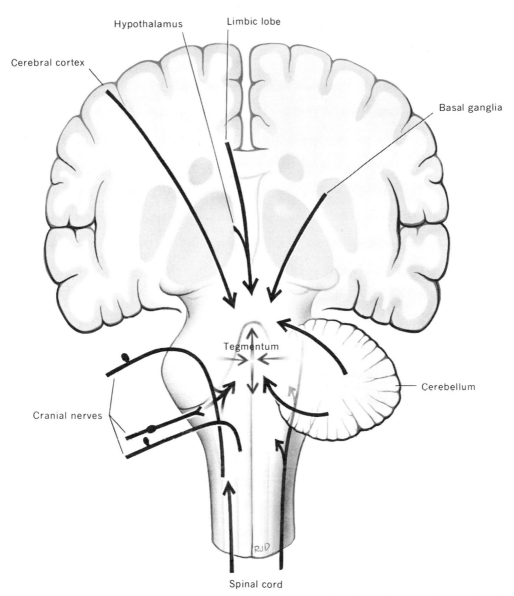

FIGURE 8-15 Input to the brainstem reticular formation. Projections from the cerebrum and the spinal cord are directed to the lateral reticular zone. From this zone influences are conveyed to the medial reticular zone, as indicated by the arrows pointing toward the midline. From this medial zone neural influences are conveyed rostrally toward the cerebrum and caudally toward the spinal cord via the central tegmental tract. Other influences are projected laterally to the cranial nerve nuclei and the cerebellum.

ways, from the olfactory system via the median forebrain bundle, and from the visual system via cells of the superior colliculus. The input from the trigeminal system—its nuclei and pathways—is important; influences from this system have a significant effect on arousal. Descending influences from the cerebrum are derived from the corticobulbar and corticoreticular tracts, from collateral branches of the corticospinal tracts, and from projections from the basal ganglia, limbic lobe, and hypothalamus. Fibers from the cerebellum are included. The intrinsic tract of the reticular formation, called the central tegmental tract, is essentially a reticuloreticular tract consisting of the axons of the brainstem neurons. This reticuloreticular tract in the brainstem is more prominent than the propriospinal tract, its counterpart in the spinal cord. The descending portion of the central tegmental tract is located largely in the medial tegmentum, and the ascending portion in the lateral tegmentum. The lateral brainstem reticular formation is essentially an "affector," "sensory," or associative zone, receiving input primarily from higher centers (descending pathways), from spinal levels, and from trigeminal sources. The parvicellular reticular nucleus of the medulla and pons is an important reticular nucleus of this zone. This affector region projects its output to the medial brainstem reticular formation, which acts as an effector or motor zone.

The *output from the brainstem reticular system* is extensive because its axonic projections have diffuse connections; the full extent of its physiologic influences is somewhat unsettled (see Fig. 8-16). Its ascending influences to the cerebral cortex and basal ganglia are largely directed to and through the thalamic intralaminar nuclei, hypothalamus, and septal region. The medial forebrain bundle (Chaps. 11 and 15) is the main ascending pathway from the midbrain to the hypothalamus and septal region. Its descending influences are expressed via reticulospinal tracts upon the gamma and alpha motor neurons of the spinal cord. Many actions are exerted via the cranial nerves and via the autonomic pathways upon the visceral output of the spinal cord and cranial nerves.

The *functional role of the brainstem reticular system* is the subject of considerable comment. The reticular formation is a most significant integrating structure; it is the region where impulses from the sensory modalities as well as from cerebral and cerebellar sources converge and interact. This region is able to modify the neural activity from these sources of stimulation and is capable of suppressing or enhancing the excitability of many neurons, thus inhibiting, facilitating, or modifying the transmission of neural information even through specific pathways. The stimulation of the brainstem reticu-

lar formation may heighten pain sensibility. Through its neural networks the reticular system may utilize slight shifts of the excitatory and inhibitory interplay to direct input into any of the numerous responses without in any way altering the neuroanatomic substrate. This implies a functional lability of paramount significance. The reticular system is probably crucial in evoking the myriad nuances that may result from a single stimulation such as a sound, including the range of responses from no reaction to an intense attraction or repulsion.

The reticular system is involved with the range of behavioral expressions, from animations of alertness and attention to the "passiveness" of sleep. Deprivation of the ascending reticular influences may produce sleep. Depending in part on the state of the animal, stimulation of the midbrain reticular formation may induce sleep or awakening. A *sleep center* may be present in the reticular formation of the lower pons–upper medulla. Thus it has been postulated that sleep is produced (1) actively by the stimulatory activity of this sleep center in the lower brainstem (*active reticular deactivation*) or (2) passively by the suppression of the influences of the ascending reticular system (*passive reticular deactivation*). A permanent coma, following a brain injury, is probably the result of damage to the reticular formation (deprivation of ascending influences) within the ascending reticular pathways. A lesion in the lower brainstem may result in a deep coma whereas a lesion in the upper brainstem reticular formation may result in a coma which is not deep.

The ascending reticular system has been implicated in the neural integrative mechanisms associated with many facets of behavioral activities, including emotion, perception, motivation, drive, wakefulness, sleep, and habituation. *Habituation* is the neural mechanism whereby the organism becomes inattentive to monotonously repeated stimuli, as when a student falls asleep during a dull lecture. It refers to decreased sensitivity to a repeated stimulus pattern. In contrast, *adaptation* is the decreased sensitivity to a continuing stimulus. The reticular system may have a role in reducing the impact of stimuli upon the cerebral cortex. An example would be the relative unawareness of a driver of traffic noises that persist.

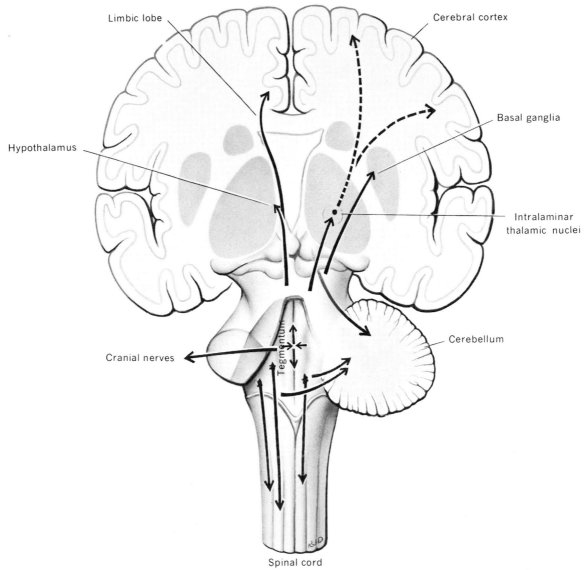

FIGURE 8-16 Output from the brainstem reticular formation. The output is directed from the medial reticular zone (1) rostrally to the hypothalamus and intralaminar and other nuclei of the thalamus (see Fig. 8-14) and from these structures to the limbic lobe and cerebral cortex, (2) laterally to the cerebellum and cranial nerve nuclei, and (3) caudally to the spinal cord via the reticulospinal tracts and descending autonomic pathways.

Pain and temperature pathways

The pain and temperature pathways are divided into two subsystems: (1) *neospinothalamic pathway* from the body and *neotrigeminothalamic pathway* from the head and (2) *paleospinothalamic pathway* from the body and *paleotrigemin-* *othalamic pathway* from the head (see Fig. 8-17; see also Figs. 5-11 and 5-15). The neopathways project directly to the ventral posterior (VP), intralaminar (mainly paracentral and centralis lateralis), and posterior (zone) nuclei of the thalamus. The paleopathways ascend in multineuronal sequences through the brainstem reticular formation to the periaqueductal gray, intra-laminar nuclei, and posterior nucleus of the thalamus.

Many neurons in these pathways show a high degree of modality specificity—nociceptors, thermoreceptors, and mechanoreceptors (light-touch). Many neurons can be activated by more than one stimulus modality. These latter cells may be a part of a generalized system for signaling overall afferent activity rather than conveying specific sensory information.

The neurons of these pathways generally have large receptive fields—larger than those of the posterior column–medial lemniscal pathway. The cells of the VP nucleus have small, discrete receptive fields, presumably associated with the rapidly felt sharp pain. In contrast the neurons of the posterior and intralaminar nuclei are activated by large receptive fields of bilateral origin, presumably subserving slow, diffuse pain that is poorly localized.

The neurons of the VP nucleus project to both somatosensory cortical areas SI and SII (see Fig. 16-16). It is possible that one cell in VP may project in both areas. The posterior nucleus projects to somatosensory area SII. Feed-forward inhibition does not apparently occur at any level in these pain and temperature pathways. Both inhibitory and facilitatory reflected feedback projection are present. For example, spinal posterior horn cells can be inhibited by reflected projections from the somatosensory cortex and be facilitated by reflected projections from the reticular formation.

Stimulus location is relatively less precise than in the medial lemniscal system. This is, in part, associated with the absence of afferent inhibition and large receptive fields in the paleo-system.

From the body (Chap. 5) The *lateral spinothalamic tract* conveying the pain and temperature modalities from regions innervated by the spinal cord (see Fig. 5-15) is located in the lateral column (spinal cord) and lateral tegmentum of the brainstem, where it is called the *spinothalamic tract* (*spinal lemniscus, lateral column–spinal lemniscal pathway*). This *spinal lemniscus tract* terminates in the ventral posterolateral nucleus posterior and intralaminar nuclei of the thalamus (Chap. 13). The spinothalamic tract atten-

uates as it ascends, for many of its fibers terminate in the brainstem reticular formation (including the lateral reticular nucleus of the medulla) and in the roof of the midbrain (spinotectal tract).

Other pain fibers ascend parallel to the spinothalamic tract near the medial lemniscus, in the brainstem reticular formation (*paleospinothalamic pathway, spinoreticulothalamic pathway*), and in the periventricular and periaqueductal gray to terminate bilaterally in the posterior and intralaminar thalamic nuclei (see Fig. 5-16). Deep pain and visceral pain are apparently associated with these diffuse pathways. The association of the primitive pain modality and the phylogenetically old ascending reticular system is geared to the basic self-preservation drive of the organism.

From the head The pain and temperature fibers from the head are conveyed chiefly via the fifth cranial nerve (with some contribution from the seventh, ninth, and tenth cranial nerves). Pathways from the head comprise two systems: (1) the neotrigeminothalamic pathway, also called the trigeminal lemniscus or the anterior trigeminothalamic tract (see Fig. 8-17); and (2) the paleotrigeminothalamic pathway, also called the trigeminoreticulothalamic pathway.

The A delta and C fibers of first-order neurons with the cell bodies in the trigeminal ganglion of the fifth nerve enter the midpons and descend without bifurcating as the ipsilateral spinal tract of the fifth nerve as far down as the second or third cervical spinal cord level (Fig. 8-17). They terminate in the caudal third of the spinal (descending) nucleus of the fifth nerve (*subnucleus caudalis*). The spinal tract and nucleus of the fifth nerve have as their functional and anatomic equivalents the posterolateral tract of Lissauer and the posterior horn of the spinal cord (Chap. 7). The fibers from the mandibular branch of the fifth nerve are located in the dorsal aspect of the spinal tract and terminate in the lower medulla level; those of the ophthalmic branch are located in the ventral aspect of the spinal tract and terminate in the second and third cervical levels; and those of the maxillary branch are located in the middle of the spinal tract and terminate largely in the first cervical level. The neurons of the spinal nucleus of the

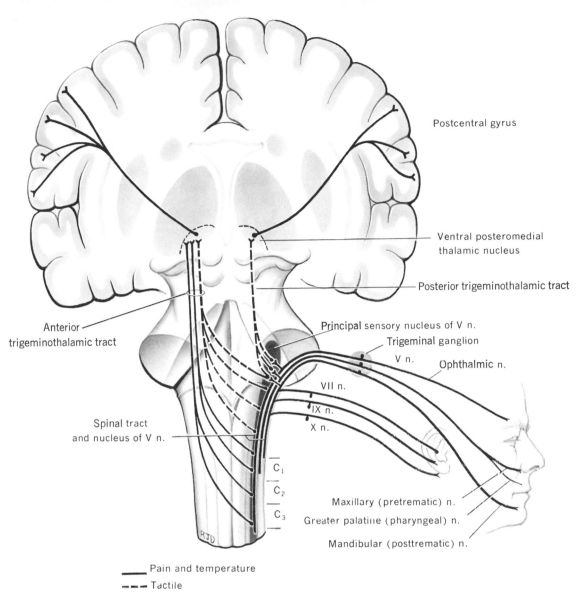

Postcentral gyrus

Ventral posteromedial thalamic nucleus

Posterior trigeminothalamic tract

Anterior trigeminothalamic tract

Principal sensory nucleus of V n.

Trigeminal ganglion

V n.

Ophthalmic n.

VII n.

IX n.

X n.

Spinal tract and nucleus of V n.

C₁

C₂

C₃

Maxillary (pretrematic) n.

Greater palatine (pharyngeal) n.

Mandibular (posttrematic) n.

RJD

―――― Pain and temperature

‑ ‑ ‑ Tactile

FIGURE 8-17 General somatic sensory pathways from the head in front of the ears. These pathways consist of (1) first-order neurons of cranial nerves V, VII, IX, and X, which pass through the spinal tract of the fifth nerve and terminate in the principal sensory nucleus and spinal nucleus of the fifth nerve; (2) second-order neurons, which either decussate and ascend as the contralateral anterior trigeminothalamic tract, or ascend as the ipsilateral posterior trigeminothalamic tract; and (3) third-order neurons, which project to the "head region" of the postcentral gyrus. This figure illustrates the older concept that the various components of the spinal tract of N. V descend to different levels: (1) fibers from the ophthalmic nerve descend as far as the third cervical level; (2) fibers from the maxillary division descend as far as the first cervical level; (3) fibers from the mandibular nerve and cranial nerves VII, IX, and X descend as far as the caudal medulla. The recent concept that fibers from all nerves descend as far as the second cervical level is illustrated in Fig. 7-6.

fifth nerve project fibers of the second order which decussate and ascend in the medial lemniscus or in the adjacent ventral tegmentum as the *anterior tract* or *neotrigeminothalamic tract* (quintothalamic tract, anterior trigeminothalamic tract, and trigeminal lemniscus) and terminate in the ventral posteromedial nucleus of the thalamus. This neotrigeminothalamic pathway is the cranial equivalent of the neospinothalamic tract. It conveys information associated with sensation of sharp pain.

The principal trigeminal nucleus and the subnucleus caudalis are the major sources of cells projecting to the thalamus (trigeminothalamic fibers, see Fig. 8-17). Evidence indicates that the subnuclei oralis and interpolaris are the source of a large cerebellar projection and a small trigeminothalamic projection (Burton and Craig). The primary afferent fibers of the trigeminal nerve extend (many via the spinal tract of the fifth nerve), either directly or via the spinal nucleus of N. V, to the brainstem reticular formation, nucleus solitarius, motor nucleus of the fifth nerve, and motor nucleus of the seventh nerve. The ascending projections in the reticular formation are incorporated into the multineuronal pathway known as the paleotrigeminothalamic pathway with bilateral terminations in the periaqueductal gray (midbrain) and in the posterior nucleus and intralaminar nuclei of the thalamus. They are integrated into the reflexes of the brainstem and into the ascending reticular system. As the trigeminoreticulothalamic pathway the input from the fifth nerve into the functional activity of the reticular system is crucial to the maintenance of the arousal state. The bilateral representation of the general senses of the head in the cerebral cortex may result from the presence of uncrossed ascending trigeminal fibers. This pathway is the cranial equivalent of the paleospinothalamic pathway. It conveys information associated with long-lasting, burning pain.

Functional analysis of pain Clinical observations indicate that lesions in VP produce a loss of cutaneous touch and sharp pain. However, chronic pain persists. In contrast, lesions in the intralaminar nuclei can relieve chronic deep pain but not cutaneous pain. These observations are consistent with the concept of the duality of pain at these sites. Lesions in the pulvinar are said to relieve intractable pain and are not accompanied by sensory loss. The somatosensory cortex has a role in the appreciation of localized and sharp pain—presumably conveyed via the neospinothalamic pathways. Extensive cortical ablation of somatosensory areas SI and SII does not relieve chronic dull pain. This indicates (1) that the thalamic nuclei are involved and (2) that the cortical projections from these nuclei are essential for the appreciation of pain.

Observations of patients indicate that a dissociation exists between the perception and the tolerance of pain. Patients with frontal lobotomies do report the perception of pain but are not bothered by the pain. Similar dissociation can occur in patients following lesions in the dorsomedial and anterior thalamic nuclei (Chap. 13).

Following the stimulation of the thalamus in human subjects, the sensory experience of pain, temperature, touch, or vibratory sense is not experienced. Electrical stimulation can evoke the feeling of "tingling" or "pins and needles." Stimulation of the intralaminar nuclei does not evoke the quality of pain; however, at low-frequency and low-amplitude stimulation, analgesic and relaxing effects are evoked. The patient can feel aroused and anxious and can feel the drive to escape when the frequency and amplitude are increased.

Opiate receptors and endorphins The cells in many regions of the brain and spinal cord have in their plasma membranes receptors with an affinity for opiates such as morphine. These opiate receptor or binding sites are in neural structures of or paralleling the paleospinothalamic and paleotrigeminothalamic pathways. These include laminae I, II, and III of the posterior horn, pars caudalis of spinal nucleus of N. V, periventricular gray (medulla and pons), periaqueductal gray (midbrain), raphe nucleus magnus (medulla), and intralaminar thalamic nuclei. This correlates with the well-known observation that dull, poorly localized, burning pain is effectively relieved by opiates. Other of the many structures with opiate receptors include nucleus solitarius, amygdaloid body, hypothalamus, medial thalamus, habenular nuclei, and corpus striatum.

The brain and the pituitary gland contain certain peptides called *endorphins*, the breakdown products of which are called *enkephalins*. The distribution of endorphins and enkephalin receptor sites closely parallels that of the opiate receptor sites. In addition, the endorphins and enkephalins are apparently acting as neurotransmitters in the pain-inhibitory pathways.

The functional significance of these peptides in pain may be summarized as follows. Endorphins and enkephalins are morphinelike substances that occur naturally in the nervous system. They are the brain's own opiates, which mimic the effects, including the analgesia, of opiates such as morphine. It is likely that all these substances produce their analgesic effects by combining with the specific receptor sites on neurons involved with the intrinsic pain pathways.

Another peptide called *substance P*, whose structural formula is known, is present in small-diameter pain fibers in the posterior horn of the spinal cord and in some regions of the brain. Substance P is thought to be a neurotransmitter in the pain pathways.

Stimulus-produced analgesia When certain regions of the brain are appropriately stimulated electrically, influences are conveyed to the dorsal horn of the spinal cord and the spinal nucleus of N. V. The effect is to inhibit actively somatic and visceral nociceptive afferent neurons with the result that the perception of pain is prevented but without any change in consciousness or in the perception of other sensory modalities. This *stimulus-produced analgesia* can be obtained in mammals, including humans. Following electrical stimulation of the periaqueductal gray, analgesic relief of chronic pain has lasted for more than one day.

Stimulation along the axis of hypothalamic periventricular gray, periaqueductal (midbrain), and periventricular gray (pons and medulla) matter produces a profound analgesia; abdominal surgery can be performed without use of an anesthetic upon rats so stimulated.

The most potent analgesia is obtained by stimulating the caudal periaqueductal gray, especially in regions of dorsal tegmental nucleus (Fig. 8-12) and medullary nucleus raphe magnus. Both nuclei are serotonin-rich. The descending inhibitory pain pathway apparently consists of descending fibers from the dorsal tegmental ra-

phae nucleus (midbrain; see Fig. 8-11) through the periventricular gray to the nucleus raphae magnus (nuclei pallidus and obscrus; see Figs. 8-6 through 8-8). From this nucleus magnus fibers project to the pars caudalis of N. V and via fibers in the spinal lateral funiculus (called dorsolateral tract) to the posterior horn. These are nuclei in the nociception pathways.

Thus, the projections from the nucleus raphe magnus to the pars caudalis of N. V and to the posterior horn have the significant role in inhibiting specific neurons in these regions. These are neurons that are excited by noxious stimuli. They contain the neurotransmitter *serotonin*. Additionally, neurons in the accessory oculomotor nucleus of Edinger-Westphal, located adjacent to the periventricular gray, are also involved. They project *directly* to the nucleus raphae magnus, laminae I and V of the spinal cord, pars caudalis of the spinal nucleus of N. V, and nuclei gracilis and cuneatus (Loewy and Saper). These projections may have roles in processing stimuli of many somatosensory modalities including pain.

Cortex and descending influences on pain The sensorimotor and limbic cortices are presumed to have a significant role in modulating the processing and transmission of nociceptive input at many levels. Influences from these areas to the hypothalamus, including its periventricular gray, are subsequently conveyed via the dorsal longitudinal fasciculus (Chap. 11) to the periaqueductal gray. These regions of the cerebrum are apparently critical in the integration of the emotional expressions associated with pain and in the modulation of pain input influences by the current emotional state of patient. Other projections from the hypothalamus terminate in the brainstem reticular formation. The reticulospinal pathways can, in turn, exert their influences on the nociceptive neurons in the posterior horn of the spinal cord.

In summary, within the brainstem are two systems: (1) one centered in midline structures including the periventricular gray substance from the hypothalamus to the medulla and the raphe nuclei and (2) another including the brainstem reticular formation and the reticulospinal pathways. The midline system is mutually interconnected and through its activity can exert powerful inhibitory effects on nociceptive transmission. Of significance is that this inhibition occurs without any apparent change in the level of consciousness and of other modalities. This complex descending system uses aminergic pathways (see Figs. 8-19 and 8-20) to exert its modulatory effects. In turn, this system is probably controlled to some degree by the endogenous transmitter endorphin.

The suggestion has been made that acupuncture analgesia may be associated with the release of endorphins from the hypophysis and some nerve endings. These substances then act through this intrinsic pain-inhibiting pathway. The jaw reflex resulting from tooth pulp pain can be selectively abolished by electrical stimulation of or by the injection of morphine into the periaqueductal gray.

Other regions of the brain can also be stimulated to obtain stimulus-produced analgesia. Furthermore, evidence suggests that stimulus-produced analgesia areas overlap extensively with those regions responsive to opiate analgesia. In addition, the serotoninergic raphe nuclei are also linked with both these methods of producing analgesia. For example, lesions of the raphe nuclei or depletion of serotonin blocks the ability of opiates or optimal stimulation to diminish pain.

Electrical stimulation of some portions of the tectum in humans has been reported to be painful. Apparently these are in the general region where spinotectal fibers terminate (deep layers of superior colliculus.). Of interest are the observations that electrical stimulation of the thalamus does not result in pain.

Touch-deep sensibility pathways
(Figs. 5-18, 5-21, 7-6, and 8-17)

The touch-deep sensibility pathways convey input from low-threshold mechanoreceptors responding to touch, joint movement, and position sense via large-diameter myelinated fibers. The receptive fields of the first-order neurons in the dorsal root ganglia and the trigeminal ganglia innervating regions of high discriminative sensations (e.g., fingertips and lips) are small, and those innervating regions of low discrimination (e.g., skin on back) are large. These pathways are somatotopically organized. The linkages within the relay nuclei are tightly coupled; this gives a great deal of security in the synaptic connections within the pathways. The integrity of the individual channels is also maintained by afferent inhibitory activity. These systems provide for rapid conveyance of information and preservation of each channel regarding the joint position of touch localization.

From the body The *medial lemniscus* is the brainstem tract of the *posterior column-medial lemniscus* pathway (see Figs. 5-18 and 5-19). The fibers (neurons of the first order) of the fasciculus gracilis and fasciculus cuneatus (posterior column) of the spinal cord terminate in the nuclei gracilis and cuneatus, respectively, in the lower dorsal medulla. Axons from the neurons in these nuclei cross over the midline of the medulla just dorsal to the pyramids as the internal acuate fibers and then ascend as the medial lemniscus. The medial lemniscus, found at all levels of the brainstem, gradually shifts laterally and then dorsally as the tract ascends, until it terminates in the ventral posterolateral nucleus of the thalamus. This tract does not contribute collateral fibers to the reticular formation.

From the head Tactile discrimination in the face and head in front of the ears, including the nasal and mouth cavities, is transmitted by sensory fibers in the fifth nerve to the principal sensory nucleus of the fifth nerve, located in the lateral tegmentum of the pons (see Fig. 8-17). This principal sensory nucleus is the cranial equivalent of the nuclei gracilis and cuneatus of the spinal pathways. Both nuclei contain neurons of the second order of the touch and deep sensibility pathways; the former nucleus receives input from the head and the latter two nuclei receive input from the body. Some neurons in this trigeminal nucleus project fibers that decussate in the pons and ascend in the medial lemniscus as the anterior trigeminal tract and terminate in the ventral posteromedial nucleus of the thalamus. Other neurons project uncrossed fibers that ascend in the dorsal tegmentum as the *posterior trigeminal tract* to the ventral posteromedial nucleus of the thalamus. These uncrossed ascending fibers convey influences from the mandibular nerve.

The proprioceptive input from the head, especially from the muscles of mastication, teeth, and gums and the voluntary extraocular eye and tongue muscles, is probably carried mainly by fibers of the ophthalmic and mandibular branches of the cranial nerve V with their cell bodies (neurons of the first order) in the mesencephalic nucleus of the fifth nerve. These fibers project their axons into the reticular formation and to the motor nucleus of the fifth nerve for the jaw reflexes, involving the muscles of mastication. This nucleus is unique, for it is the only nucleus within the brain that is actually composed of spinal (sensory) root ganglion neurons whose cell bodies interact through electronic (gap) junctions. The equivalence of the two-neuron extensor reflex in the arc of the spinal cord and of the flexor jaw reflex is apparent.

The ascending pathways from the spinal cord conveying *light touch* are incorporated in either the crossed *anterior spinothalamic tract* or the uncrossed *posterior columns* of the spinal cord (see Figs. 5-18 and 5-19). The anterior spinothalamic tract joins and ascends through the brainstem with the medial lemniscus and possibly with the lateral spinothalamic tract. The light-touch fibers in the posterior columns ascend in the posterior column-medial lemniscus pathway to the higher centers (thalamus and cerebral cortex). Light-touch impulses from the head may be conveyed after synapsing in the principal sensory nucleus of the fifth nerve as crossed fibers in the medial lemniscus or as the uncrossed fibers in the dorsal tegmentum (*posterior trigeminal tract*) (see Fig. 8-17). These ascending fibers terminate in the ventral posteromedial nucleus of the thalamus.

Taste pathways

"Taste," in its colloquial usage, is equated with flavor, and flavor is the complex subjective perceptive quality which is the composite of several sensations, including smell, texture, temperature, "common chemical sense," and even pain. Flavor is also influenced by sight, feel, and sounds. Receptors in the oral and nasal cavities are utilized in the "taste" perceptions involved in the evaluation and appreciation of the smells of aromatic spices, of the texture of liquids and solids, of the temperature of foods, of the astringency of a persimmon ("puckering" results from the competition for the moisture in the mouth),

of "chemical heat," of the buccal pain of hot Mexican chili, and of the tang of many cheeses. The sight or the sound of a frying steak can modify taste sensations. Even a "water sense" is indicated; distilled water applied to the taste buds may evoke discharges in "taste nerve fibers."

It is normally impossible to perceive pure taste without sensing an overlay of smell, because true taste is a much cruder and less sensitive sensation than smell; taste thresholds are significantly higher than smell thresholds. For example, estimates indicate that some 20,000 times more molecules are needed to induce a taste sensation than a smell sensation. This explains why it is that when we taste, we invariably also smell.

In humans, taste sensations can be obtained following appropriate stimulation of the taste receptors in the tongue, palate, and pharynx. To utilize all taste receptors, wine tasters swish the wine in their mouths and swallow slowly. Four taste modalities are generally recognized in humans: salt, sweet, sour, and bitter. Each of these modalities can be sensed in the following regions. Salt and sweet are perceived most acutely on the tongue, while bitter and sour are perceived most acutely on the palate. Bitter and sour are definitely but mildly tasted on the tongue and pharynx, while salt and sweet are mildly tasted on the palate and pharynx. Many taste sensations cannot even be described in terms of these four "elementary taste sensations." Among these are the taste qualities of numerous spices, fruits, and vegetables. In fact a truly objective classification of the tastes has not been developed; probably there are no primary taste qualities. All are chemically induced sensations. Salt taste is maximally perceived on the sides of the tongue, probably by the stimulation from chloride (Cl^-) and sulfate (SO_4^-) ions. Sour taste is maximally sensed part way back on the tongue by the stimulation of the hydrogen (H^+) ions of acids. Sweet is optimally perceived at the tip of the tongue, where sugars react with the fatty substances in the taste ending. Bitter is tasted mainly at the back of the tongue.

In addition to taste associated with the tongue and oral cavity, there is a form known as "intravascular taste." Certain nutrients such as sugar can be tasted when injected intravenously. The subjective sensation of taste can be readily modified by many factors including the state of health and hormone levels.

The true taste qualities in humans are derived from the stimulation of taste buds. Each brandy snifter-shaped taste bud contains upward of 25 *neuroepithelial taste cells.* In addition, other less-differentiated cells, called *"sustentacular cells,"* act as reserve cells to replenish the taste cells when they die out. The receptor taste cells are continuously turning over. Each mature taste cell is replaced every 200 to 300 h. A degenerated neuroepithelial cell can be replaced rapidly, usually within 10 h. If the nerve fibers to a taste bud are cut, the taste bud atrophies and disappears. After the nerve regenerates and reinnervates the tongue epithelium, the taste buds redifferentiate from undifferentiated basal cells of the taste bud. This control of the differentiation of taste cells by gustatory nerves is an expression of the role of neurotrophic factors.

The distal tip of each taste cell extends as a surface specialization of microvilli into the small taste pit, which is continuous with the oral cavity through the gustatory pore. The solutions containing sapid substances, either as ions or as dissolved molecules, enter the pore into the pit to interact with receptor sites on the taste cell. All substances must be in solution in order to be tasted. The proximal ends of the taste cells are in synaptic contact with nerve endings of the "taste" nerves.

The receptor sites are probably located on the surface of the microvilli. Not only does each taste cell have many different types of receptor sites, but the proportion of different types varies from taste cell to taste cell. Hence each gustatory cell can respond to several stimuli. No evidence indicates that a specific gustatory cell responds to but one group of stimuli (e.g., one cell for salts; another cell for hydrogen ion concentration). Another factor may regulate the types of stimuli that have access to the receptor sites. The proteins on the cell membrane surface may act to open or close gates of the membrane to different types of potential gustatory stimuli.

The exact mechanisms by which a taste cell is stimulated are now known, although many theories have been proposed. Each taste bud and each taste cell apparently responds to several "tastes." No structural differences in the 10,000 taste buds or in the taste cells of the young adult have been revealed. The taste cells stimulate the taste nerve fibers. Structurally each neuroepithelial cell in a taste bud is innervated by the nerve fibers of several nerve cells; and several neuroepithelial cells in a taste bud are innervated by the branches of one neuron. Functionally, each neuroepithelial cell apprently responds to several taste qualities; and each neuron from a taste bud also responds to several taste qualities. The taste buds of humans may well respond to as many as 10,000 different chemicals, of which many do not occur naturally. Discrimination by taste can be made between the dextro and levo forms of some amino acids. The numerous nuances of true taste are the result of transmission via many patterns of afferent impulses in the various nerve fibers and of processing in the nuclei of the taste pathways, the situation being comparable to the transmission of the qualities of sound (Chaps. 10 and 13). The variations in the intensity of taste are transmitted by the differences in the frequency of firing of nerve impulses. Adaptation is rapid, usually in seconds or minutes.

A decrease in the sensitivity of taste with age is paralleled by the decrease in the total number of taste buds after the age of 40. A human baby has more than 10,000 taste buds, including some even on the palate and pharynx. This large number explains, in part, why babies dislike spiced foods and prefer bland baby food. The latter is probably tasty to them. Elderly people use spices, sugar, and salt more liberally to make food more tasty for their jaded gustatory sense by stimulating the lesser number of taste buds present. For example, the young adult can taste sugar in concentration about one-third (0.4 percent sugar) that of elderly adults (1.2 percent sugar). The center of the tongue, with only a few taste buds, is relatively taste blind.

Taste impulses are conveyed from the anterior two-thirds of the tongue by the fibers of the chorda tympani branch of the facial nerve and from the posterior third of the tongue, palate, and pharynx by fibers in the branches of the glossopharyngeal and vagus nerves. The sensory nerves in this region terminate either in the taste buds or as free nerve endings in the connective tissues and epithelium other than taste buds. Many of the free nerve endings are of terminals of general sensory fibers of the trigeminal nerve.

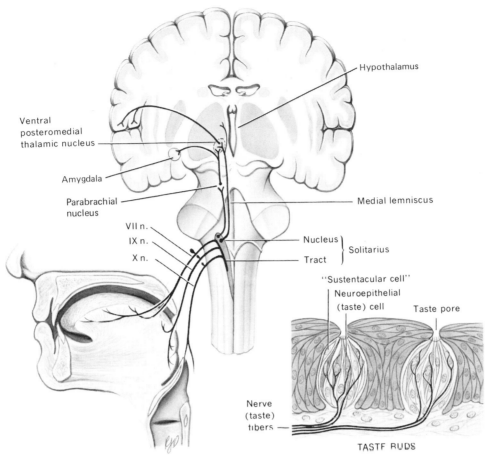

FIGURE 8-18 The taste (gustatory) pathway The taste pathway is composed of (1) first-order neurons of cranial nerves VII, IX, and X which pass through the solitary fasciculus and terminate in the solitary nucleus; (2) second-order neurons which ascend ipsilaterally in the medial lemniscus, and terminate in the ventral posteromedial nucleus of the thalamus; and (3) third-order neurons (thalamocortical fibers) which project to the inferior aspect of the postcentral gyrus (see text).

The taste buds on the anterior two-thirds of the tongue are located on the free surface of the fungiform papillae, with each papilla containing from one to eight taste buds (Fig. 8-18). These *fungiform papillae*, which are scattered singly, are especially numerous near the tip of the tongue. In the region of the V-shaped sulcus terminalis is a linear series of 10 to 12 large *circumvallate papillae;* they cover a portion of the posterior third of the tongue. The numerous taste buds on each papilla are generally located along the sides of the papilla facing the moat surrounding the structure. In humans, taste buds are also present on the surface of the hard and soft palate, pharynx, and larynx.

Taste buds are in synaptic contact with afferent taste fibers and sympathetic terminals. Each taste papilla usually receives branches from several different trunk axons. In turn, each axon divides and sends branches to several papillae. The sympathetic fibers may exert a neurotrophic role; they are said to have cell bodies in the nucleus solitarius.

The taste fibers of the facial, glossopharyngeal, and vagus nerves pass into the medulla and terminate in the rostral and lateral portions of the nucleus solitarius; this portion is called the *nucleus gustatorius.*

The axons from the gustatory nucleus ascend ipsilaterally in the tegmentum and terminate directly in the medial portion of the ventral posteromedial nucleus of the thalamus in the monkey and presumably in humans (Becksted and Norgren). Axons from the caudal nucleus solitarius (general visceral afferent input) ascend to the ipsilateral parabrachial nucleus, which is a brainstem reticular nucleus located in the lower midbrain on either side of and within the superior cerebellar peduncle (see Figs. 8-11 and 8-18). The parabrachial nucleus projects rostrally to the ipsilateral substantia innominata, lateral hypothalamus, central nucleus of the amygdaloid body, and bed nucleus of the stria terminalis (see Figs. 15-3 and A-43). Fibers from the amygdaloid body feed back to the parabrachial nucleus. Some of these nuclei are integrated into the activities of the hypothalamus (Chap. 11) and the limbic system (Chap. 15).

Fibers from neurons in the VPM nucleus pass through the posterior limb of the internal capsule and terminate in the lower end of the postcentral gyrus (opercular region of the parietal lobe) and possibly in the cortex of the insula and superior temporal gyrus.

The ability to taste certain chemicals has a hereditary basis. Some individuals have a taste blindness to certain substances that other individuals can taste. One such compound is phenylthiourea (PTC), which is tasteless to some and bitter to others. Two-thirds of males are tasters and one-third are nontasters. Some taste abnormalities are known to be associated with the alteration of the body metabolism as a consequence of the action of certain chemical substances. Miracle fruit, a tropical fruit found in southeastern United States, will, after being eaten, modify taste perception drastically. Foods which formerly tasted sour and bitter will then taste sweet.

Taste may have a role in the preservation of life itself. A rat without its parathyroid glands will die unless it ingests quantities of calcium salts. A parathyroidectomized rat selects calcium or calcium-containing foods from a mixed diet. By increasing its intake of calcium, the rat maintains its blood calcium at a level essential to life. This same animal with its "taste nerves" severed does not select sufficient quantities of calcium out of the same mixed diet. As a result, its blood calcium level drops, tetany results, and death follows. A rat without its adrenal glands will die within a few days unless it ingests extra sodium chloride. An adrenalectomized rat will drink a solution of sodium chloride in preference to plain water, and in such quantities as to maintain good health for months. This same rat with its "taste nerves" severed loses its ability to discriminate between a saline solution and plain water. As a consequence it does not selectively drink the saline solution in sufficient quantities to maintain life. The animal soon dies. An adrenalectomized rat with taste perception intact is so specific in its salts preferences that it will select a sodium chloride solution and neglect available potassium chloride solutions or calcium chloride solutions. This predilection for salt is related to the seeking out of salt licks by wild herbivorous animals living on salt-deprived vegetation.

Altered taste sensations have been reported in some patients. This condition is thought to be associated with lesions of the limbic system or with seizure discharges of the insular cortex. The similarity to "uncinate fits" associated with the olfactory system (Chap. 15) is probable.

Auditory pathway (lateral lemniscus) and vestibular pathways

The nuclei and other structures contributing to the lateral lemniscal pathways of the auditory system and those contributing to the medial longitudinal fasciculus, vestibulospinal tract, and the cerebellar connections of the vestibular system are discussed elsewhere (Chap. 10).

Monoaminergic and cholinergic pathways of the central nervous system

Several pathway systems have been identified and described by biochemical and pharmacologic criteria as well as in anatomic terms. These pathway systems originate in the nuclei of the brainstem reticular formation and raphe and they project rostrally to the forebrain, laterally to the cerebellum, and caudally to the spinal cord. A number of monoaminergic pathways and a cholinergic pathway system are recognized.

The neurons of monoaminergic pathways contain one of the following monoamines: norepinephrine, 5-hydroxytryptamine (serotonin, 5-HT), and dopamine. These monoamines are present in the cell bodies, axons, and endings of these neurons. Hence, they are collectively called *monoamine (aminergic, monoaminergic) neuronal pathways* (see Figs. 8-19 and 8-20). Evidence indicates that these monoamines and their precursors and associated enzymes are presumably synthesized in the cell bodies of neurons and distributed in monoamine vesicles via axoplasmic flow to to the nerve terminals. These putative neurotransmitters are also synthesized in axon terminals. Neurons with norepinephrine comprise the *noradrenergic pathways* (see Fig. 8-19), those with serotonin, the *serotoninergic pathways* (see Fig. 8-20), and those with dopamine, the *dopaminergic pathways* (see Fig. 8-20).

The cholinergic pathway, characterized by neurons containing acetylcholine, is an ascending pathway projecting from the midbrain to the many structures of the cerebrum.

The cell bodies of the neurons comprising the aminergic pathways have been identified in limited regions of the infratentorial brainstem and hypothalamus. With respect to the brainstem, the cell bodies of the *noradrenergic neurons* are localized in the tegmentum of the pons and medulla (apparently they are absent in the midbrain tegmentum), those of the *serotoninergic neurons* are found in the raphe nuclei; and those of the *dopaminergic neurons* are restricted to the substantia nigra and to regions surrounding the interpeduncular nucleus of the midbrain. The aminergic pathways within the central nervous system may be classified into several groups: (1) descending noradrenergic (NA) pathway, (2) descending serotoninergic (5-HT) pathway, (3) ascending noradrenergic (NA) pathway, (4) NA pathways from the locus ceruleus, (5) ascending serotoninergic (5-HT) pathway, and (6) dopaminergic (DA) pathway.

Descending noradrenergic (NA) pathway (system) and descending serotoninergic (5-HT) pathway (system) (Figs. 8-19 and 8-20)

The descending aminergic pathways originating in the medulla and terminating in the spinal cord include the *NA and the 5-HT pathways.* The NA fibers originate from cells in the ventrolateral part of the reticular formation of the caudal medulla; the 5-HT fibers originate from cells of the raphe nuclei of the medulla. Many of the NA fibers and 5-HT fibers descend in the anterior funiculus and ventral part of the lateral funiculus and then terminate in the anterior horn of the spinal gray matter. Other NA and 5-HT fibers descend in dorsal part of the lateral funiculus and then terminate in the posterior horn and the intermediolateral nucleus of the spinal cord.

Ascending noradrenergic (NA) pathway (system) (Fig. 8-19)

Ascending NA fibers originate from cells of the brainstem reticular nuclei located in (1) the ventrolateral medulla, (2) the lower pons dorsal and lateral to the superior olivary nuclei, and (3) the upper pons ventral to the superior cerebellar peduncle. These fibers ascend as *the ventral NA pathway* within the medial and ventromedial brainstem reticular formation and medial forebrain bundle of the hypothalamus. The fibers of this pathway terminate as nerve endings in the lower brainstem, mesencephalon, and cerebrum. Some of the structures in which these fibers terminate include the dorsal vagal nucleus and nucleus solitarius of the medulla, some reticular nuclei and periaqueductal gray matter of the midbrain.

Many fibers of the medial forebrain bundle (Chaps. 11 and 15) terminate in virtually all regions of the hypothalamus including (1) the paraventricular, supraoptic, and arcuate nuclei and (2) the bed nucleus of the stria terminalis and septal nuclei and the preoptic region. Some fibers continue to the amygdaloid body (primarily the central nucleus). None of the fibers of the ventral noradrenergic pathway terminate in the hippocampus and neocortex. These sites of termination are structures associated with the limbic system (Chap. 15). This pathway is said to be involved in the mediation of feeding behavior and reward processes (Chap. 15).

Locus ceruleus (NA pathways from the locus coeruleus) (Figs. 8-11 and 8-19)

The *locus coeruleus* is a brainstem nucleus whose entire complement of several thousand cell bodies contains norepinephrine. This nucleus re-

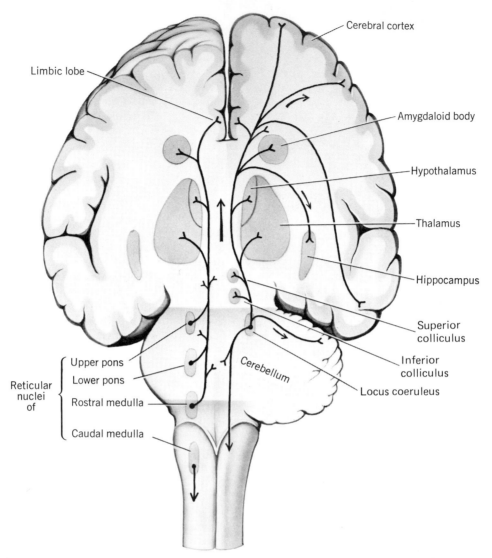

FIGURE 8-19 Noradrenergic pathways. The ascending pathway on the left originates from the medullary and pontine reticular nuclei and terminates in the cerebrum. The descending pathway on the left originates from medullary reticular nuclei and terminates in the spinal cord. The projections from the locus ceruleus on the right course (1) via the lateral pathway to the cerebellum, (2) via the ascending pathway to the midbrain and cerebrum, and (3) via the descending pathway to the spinal cord.

ceives its input from and projects its output monosynaptically to many widespread regions located in each of the major subdivisions of the central nervous system—cerebrum, cerebellum, brainstem, and spinal cord. The widespread and diffuse projections of the locus ceruleus are unique among the nuclei in the brain. It is likely that some cell bodies have several main axonal

branches, one of which terminates in the cerebellar cortex and another in the cerebral cortex. In addition, many collaterals from these two main branches may terminate in many nuclei along their course. This unusual distribution spectrum has suggested such general overriding roles as expressed in (1) modulating the electrophysiology of the cerebral and cerebellar cortices, (2) regulating the autonomic nervous system, (3) paradoxial sleep, (4) regulating vigilant states and behavior arousal, and (5) the involvement with learning ("forebrain information processing").

Afferent influences are derived from such neuronal complexes as the insular cortex; central nucleus of amygdaloid body; parafascicular thalamic nucleus; hypothalamus; reticular formation (including noradrenergic neurons) and raphe nuclei of the medulla, pons, and midbrain; contralateral locus ceruleus; deep cerebellar nuclei and spinal nucleus of N. V, solitary nucleus and marginal nucleus of posterior horn of spinal cord (Cedarbaum and Aghajanian).

These direct projections comprise an extensively ramifying plexus of fine axons innervating the entire cerebral, hippocampal and cerebellar cortices, amygdaloid body, septal nuclei, thalamus, bed nucleus of stria terminalis, habenular nucleus, lower brainstem, and spinal cord. The terminal of the noradrenergic fibers forms a geometrically orderly distribution in all laminae of the cerebral cortex. With this distribution, the locus ceruleus can presumably modulate neural activity over a vast expanse of cortex.

The coeruleospinal pathway extends through the entire length of the spinal cord, its noradrenergic terminals innervating laminae IV through IX of the spinal gray matter. The adrenergic reticular neurons in the caudal medulla (see Figs. 8-5, 8-16, and 8-21) project axons that terminate in laminae I, II, and III and in the intermediolateral cell column of the spinal cord.

Ascending serotoninergic (5-HT) pathway (system) (Fig. 8-20)

The cell bodies of the raphe nuclei of the pons and lower midbrain (nucleus raphe pontis, superior central nucleus, and dorsal and ventral tegmental nuclei) have high concentrations of serotonin. Axons originating from these cell bodies form the ascending serotonin (5-HT) pathway. It ascends through the brainstem and cerebrum and terminates in the hypothalamus, amygdaloid body, septal nuclei, and cerebral cortex.

These raphe nuclei are, in some way, related to various aspects of behavior and to the sleep-wake cycle. Total insomnia occurs when these raphe nuclei are destroyed or when the serotonin stores are depleted by the drug reserpine. In contrast, an increase in the brain serotonin level decreases the sensitivity to pain.

Dopaminergic (DA) pathway (system) (Fig. 8-20)

The cell bodies of the compact zone of the substantia nigra and of the region dorsal to the interpeduncular nucleus have high concentrations of dopamine (DA). The axons originating in the compact zone ascend to the neostriatum (caudate nucleus and putamen). This *nigrostriatal DA system* is integrated in the basal ganglia circuits (Chap. 14). Some DA fibers from the substantia nigra terminate in the amygdala. The fibers originating from the cells dorsal to the interpeduncular nucleus ascend within the medial forebrain bundle and terminate in the hypothalamus, amygdaloid body and other portions of the limbic lobe. Some dopaminergic neurons project to the hypophysis.

Ascending cholinergic pathway (system)

The ascending cholinergic pathway system arises from cells located in the midbrain tegmentum and substantia nigra. The cuneiform nucleus (see Fig. 8-12) is the principal site where cholinergic cells in the tegmentum are located.

Anatomically, this ascending pathway projects both directly and indirectly to virtually all nuclear complexes of the limbic system and to the archicortex, paleocortex, and neocortex. Functionally, this pathway system is presumed to be a substrate of the important *ascending reticular activating* system (Chap. 8).

Like the ascending monoaminergic pathways, the cholinergic system projects influences widely to virtually all limbic system structures (Chap. 15), the neocortex, and some subcortical nuclei. Unlike the monoaminergic pathways that project from the brainstem nuclei directly, without synaptic interruption, to numerous forebrain centers, the cholinergic pathways from the midbrain synapse with other cholinergic neurons located more rostrally and, in turn, some of these cholinergic neurons synapse with still other cholinergic neurons. This complex of se-

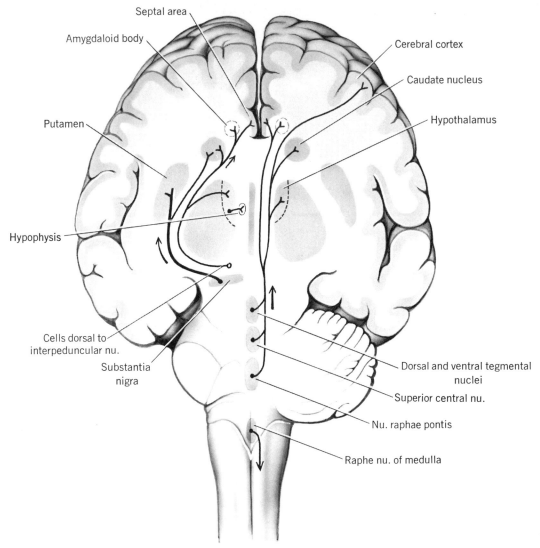

Septal area

Amygdaloid body

Putamen

Hypophysis

Cells dorsal to
interpeduncular nu.

Substantia
nigra

Cerebral cortex

Caudate nucleus

Hypothalamus

Dorsal and ventral tegmental
nuclei

Superior central nu.

Nu. raphae pontis

Raphe nu. of medulla

FIGURE 8-20 The dopaminergic pathways (*left*) and the serotoninergic (5-HT) pathway (*right*). These pathways are described in the text. The raphe nucleus of medulla is called the *nucleus magnus*.

quences comprises the *ascending cholinergic system.*

Direct projections from the midbrain nuclei that terminate on noncholinergic neurons in the tectum, thalamus, and subthalamic region may constitute the so-called thalamic division of the reticular activating pathway. The other direct projections that form the so-called hypothalamic division comprise fibers that terminate in several forebrain regions including the posterior

and lateral hypothalamus, the preoptic region, the bed nucleus of stria terminalis, and the globus pallidus.

The cells of the preoptic region are the sources of a number of neuronal sequences: (1) to the anterior perforated substance and associated nuclei; (2) to the bed nucleus of the stria terminalis, from there via the stria terminalis to the amygdaloid body, and from there to the entorhinal and pyriform cortices; (3) to the septal nuclei and from there to the hippocampus and dentate gyrus; and (4) to the cingulate gyrus and adjacent neocortex. These sequences of neurons are primarily composed of cholinergic neurons (Chap. 15, Figs. 1-10 and 15-3).

Many cholinergic projections from the midbrain tegmentum terminate on noncholinergic neurons in such nuclei as the paraventricular and supraoptic nuclei of the hypothalamus (Chap. 11).

STRUCTURES ASSOCIATED WITH THE CEREBELLUM

Tegmental connections

A number of major structures in the brainstem tegmentum are involved with the input and output of the cerebellum (Chap. 9). The nuclei and tracts associated with the inferior cerebellar peduncle include (1) vestibular pathways to and from the archicerebellum (see Figs. 9-6 and 10-12), (2) the posterior spinocerebellar tract from the spinal cord, and (3) nerve fibers from the inferior olivary nuclei (olivocerebellar tract), accessory cuneate nucleus, and the paramedian reticular nuclei in the medulla (reticulocerebellar tract) to the cerebellar cortex (see Fig. 9-4). The cerebellum receives influences from the lower extremity via the posterior spinocerebellar tract and from the upper extremity via fibers from the accessory (lateral) cuneate nucleus (see Figs. 5-20 and 8-6). Fibers from the reticulotegmental nucleus of the pons pass through the middle cerebellar peduncle to the entire vermis except for the nodulus. The nuclei and tracts associated with the superior cerebellar peduncle include: input via the anterior spinocerebellar tract from the spinal cord; and outflow via (1) ascending fibers to the nucleus ruber (a reticular nucleus) and the ventrolateral and intralaminar nuclei of the thalamus, and (2) descending fibers of the descending division of the superior cerebellar peduncle to the reticulotegmental nucleus of the pons (see Fig. 8-10), paramedian reticular nuclei of the medulla (see Fig. 8-14 and 9-4), and the inferior olivary nuclear complex (see Fig. 8-7).

Corticoreticular fibers from the cerebral cortex project to the paramedian reticular nuclei and lateral reticular nucleus of the medulla and the reticulotegmental nucleus of the pons.

Basilar connections

The *corticopontine tracts* arise from all lobes of the cerebral cortex and descend through the internal capsule and the crus cerebri before terminating by synapsing with the ipsilateral pontine nuclei (see Fig. 9-5). The frontopontine fibers from the frontal lobe are located in the anterior limb of the internal capsule and the medial part of the crus cerebri. The parietooccipitopontine fibers are located in the posterior limb of the internal capsule and in the lateral part of the crus cerebri. The corticopontine tracts are a link in the corticopontocerebellar pathways (Chap. 9). The pontine nuclei give rise to axons which decussate (a few fibers are uncrossed) as the pontocerebellar tract that passes through the middle cerebellar peduncle before terminating in the neocerebellum.

DECENDING PATHWAYS: INPUT TO BRAINSTEM RETICULAR FORMATION (FIGS. 8-16 AND 8-19)

The descending pathways of the brainstem reticular system receive input from many sources. Its motor activities are expressed via influences exerted upon the somatic and visceral (autonomic) effectors. The sources of neural input to this system include the ascending reticular system, collateral fibers from some ascending lemniscal pathways (except the medial lemniscus), and descending direct and indirect pathways from higher centers (hypothalamus, globus pallidus, thalamus, and cerebral cortex). Many influences from subcortical cerebral centers are conveyed to the cerebral cortex, from which they are projected via corticoreticular fibers to the brainstem reticular formation. The *reticuloreticular fibers* (*central tegmental fasciculus*) constitute the brainstem intrareticular integrating pathway.

DESCENDING SOMATIC TRACTS FROM BRAINSTEM RETICULAR FORMATION

Reticulospinal tracts (Fig. 8-21)   The two descending pathways from the brainstem reticular formation to the spinal cord comprise the pontine (medial) reticulospinal tract and the medullary (lateral) reticulospinal tract. The *pontine re-*

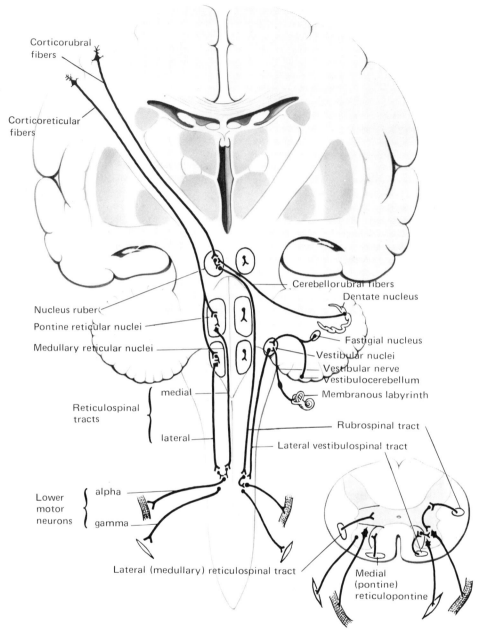

FIGURE 8-21 Descending motor pathways to the spinal cord, including the reticulospinal tracts (corticoreticulospinal pathways), rubrospinal tracts (corticorubrospinal pathways), and vestibulospinal tracts.

ticulospinal tract arises in the nuclei reticularis oralis and caudalis and descends as an uncrossed tract adjacent to and within the medial longitudinal fasciculus through the entire length of the spinal cord. Its fibers terminate in the me-dial part of the anterior horn (lamina VIII and adjacent parts of lamina VII). The *medullary reticulospinal tract* originates in the nucleus gigantocellularis of the medulla. Its fibers are primarily uncrossed; they descend in the anterolateral funiculus and terminate primarily in lamina VII of all levels of the spinal cord. A major input to these tracts is derived from the motor (area 4), premotor (area 6), and somesthetic (areas 3, 1 and 2) areas of the cerebral cortex.

These *corticoreticular fibers* descend in the vicinity of the corticospinal tracts and terminate bilaterally (with slightly more crossed than uncrossed fibers) in the nucleus reticularis pontis oralis and nucleus reticularis gigantocellularis. As a total unit, these pathways should be called corticoreticulospinal pathways. The fibers of the reticulospinal tracts are presumed to terminate upon interneurons of laminae VII and VIII, which, in turn, influence gamma (and also alpha) motor neuron activity, especially that related to posture and muscle tone.

Stimulation of the medullary reticular formation generally inhibits the myostatic reflexes and extensor muscle tone (a rigid limb in the decerebrate animal becomes flaccid) and movements evoked by cerebral cortical stimulation (cortically induced movements). In the normal animal, this medullary component tends to inhibit antigravity muscle tone and facilitate flexor muscle tone. Inhibitory effects are largely evoked from the medullary reticular formation and are mediated via the medullary reticulospinal fibers. Facilitatory effects are largely evoked by stimulation of the pontine reticular formation (increased muscle tone); these are mediated via pontine reticulospinal tracts. The response evoked by these stimulations is produced by the activity of antagonistic muscle groups (e.g., flexors and extensors) through reciprocally organized interneuronal intrinsic circuits within the spinal cord. In the normal animal, the pontine component has the opposite effect from the medullary component. Reticulospinal tracts convey influences involved with respiratory movements and with activities of the autonomic nervous system. Those fibers which terminate upon neurons of the ascending pathways have a role in the processing and biasing of sensory input.

Vestibulospinal tracts and medial longitudinal fasciculus The (*lateral*) *vestibulospinal tract* from the lateral vestibular nucleus passes from the lateral vestibular nucleus through the lateral medullary tegmentum and anterolateral funi-

culus of the spinal cord. This uncrossed tract exerts facilitatory influences upon muscle tone, especially the extensor musculature, associated with posture and maintenance of equilibrium. The *medial longitudinal fasciculus* (*MLF*) is a bundle of fibers, mainly involved with reflexes of the vestibular system (see Figs. 8-6 through 8-13; see also Fig. 10-11). These reflexes include movements of the eyes (vestibulomesencephalic and associated fibers) and neck movements for maintaining position of the head in space (medial vestibulospinal tract, Fig. 10-11). The MLF contains some descending interstitiospinal descending fibers of unknown function from the interstitial nucleus of Cajal of the midbrain (Fig. 8-13).

Rubrospinal and tectospinal tracts The *rubrospinal tract* originates in both large and small neurons of the nucleus ruber, decussates in the midbrain as the ventral tegmental decussation, and extends through the entire length of the spinal cord (see Figs. 8-12 and 8-21; see also Figs. 5-27, 5-30, A-3, A-6, A-8, and A-10). The nucleus ruber, actually a nucleus of the reticular formation, receives input from the cerebellum (dentatorubral tract) and cerebral motor cortex (uncrossed corticorubral tract). As a total unit, this pathway is called the corticorubrospinal tract. The rubrospinal tract exerts facilitatory influences on the tone of flexor musculature. This is presumed to be important to posture and locomotion as well as in skilled voluntary movements of the extremities.

The nucleus ruber has some descending projections which terminate in the inferior olivary nuclear complex and in some pontine and medullary reticular nuclei.

The *tectospinal tract* originates in the deep layer of the superior colliculus, decussates in the midbrain as the dorsal tegmental decussation, and extends through the spinal cervical region (see Figs. 5-27, 5-30, and A-10). This tract, a component of the medial longitudinal fasciculus, is presumed to be involved with postural movements initiated by visual stimuli.

Descending autonomic pathways

The autonomic pathways in the brainstem may be thought of as a complexly organized interacting, multineuronal network with certain tegmental regions acting as focal or nodal sites. The autonomic nervous system acts not alone but in concert with the somatic nervous system, also represented in the reticular formation.

The descending influences of the autonomic nervous system are derived primarily from diffuse pathways from the hypothalamus. Other cerebral structures, including the cerebral cortex, basal ganglia, and the thalamus, direct their effects essentially through connections in the hypothalamus (Chap. 11). The hypothalamic output to the brainstem is conveyed via (1) the dorsal longitudinal fasciculus and diffuse fibers located in the periventricular gray, terminating primarily in the dorsal tegmental nucleus of the lower midbrain, and (2) the median forebrain bundle and mamillotegmental tract, terminating largely in the midbrain tegmentum (Chap. 15). The multineuronal nets of the reticular formation (reticuloreticular tract) convey the influences to the rest of the brainstem. The dorsal longitudinal fasciculus has indirect connections with the parasympathetic dorsal vagal nucleus of the medulla.

The descending autonomic pathways from the hypothalamus and the cerebellum also interact in the brainstem reticular formation with the input from the peripheral viscera (via the cranial nerves, especially the vagus nerve) and with the various ascending influences and modulating feedbacks from the spinal cord. These complex patterns in the reticular formation are organized for the regulation of many visceral functions.

Many vital activities are mediated through the brainstem by "centers" definable largely by physiologic criteria. These "centers" project their influences (1) to the spinal cord via reticulospinal fibers and (2) to the body, largely, but not exclusively, through the parasympathetic and sympathetic outflows (Chap. 6). The ventromedial tegmentum of the medulla contains an *inhibitory cardiovascular center* and an *inspiratory respiratory center;* the lateral tegmentum of the medulla and lower pons contains an *excitatory cardiovascular center;* and the dorsolateral tegmentum contains the *salivatory centers* and an *expiratory respiratory center.*

These medullary respiratory centers are responsible for the rhythmic discharges which result in the spontaneous respiratory cycle. Anatomically, the two respiratory centers overlap. A neuronal group in the rostral pontine tegmentum is called the *pneumotaxic center.* This area is presumed to exert inhibitory influences on neurons of the medullary inspiratory center and lower pontine apneustic center. The pontine pneumotaxic center acts to prevent sustained inspiration. The arrest of respiration in the inspiratory phase is called apneusis. In the caudal pontine tegmentum is a neuronal group called the *apneustic center.* When released from the influences of the pneumotaxic center, the activity of the cells of the apneustic centers produces *apneusis.* This apneustic center is presumed to be facilitatory to respiration, when uninhibited; normally it receives inhibitory influences from the vagal nerves and the pneumotaxic centers.

Each of these bilateral centers is composed of scattered neuronal groups, which are not delineated as morphologically discrete nuclei. These centers are involved in the following phenomena. Stimulation of the ventromedial tegmentum may result in deceleration of the heartbeat, lower blood pressure, and an inspiratory (inhalation) phase of the respiratory cycle. Stimulation of the lateral tegmentum may result in an acceleration of the heartbeat and a higher blood pressure, and stimulation of the dorsolateral tegmentum may evoke salivation, vomiting (*vomiting center*), and the expiratory phase (exhalation) of the respiratory cycle. The area postrema of the medulla (see Figs. 11-6 and A-15) may have a role in certain vomiting (emetic) reflexes; the area may be a chemoreceptor which acts upon the vomiting center (Chap. 11).

Input from peripheral receptors to the respiratory and cardiovascular centers of the brainstem is derived from (1) the *pressoreceptors* located in the lung (stretch receptors), in the atrium and ventricle of the heart, in the carotid sinus in the vicinity of the carotid bifurcation, and in the walls of the aorta and its major branches (monitors of the blood pressure); and (2) the *chemoreceptors* in arterial receptors located in the carotid body (innervated by the glossopharyngeal nerve), the aortic bodies, the roots of the main thoracic arteries (innervated by the vagus nerve), and the medulla (called *central receptors*). The stretch (Hering-Breuer) reflex is an activity initiated by pulmonary pressoreceptors; it is protective to the lungs. When the lung is inflated, these receptors are stimulated to convey influences which act to inhibit inspiration. In contrast the pressoreceptors of the deflating lungs initiate activity which results in stimulating inspiration. Pain, heat, or cold may excite an increase in respiration (e.g., spanking a newborn infant). The pressoreceptors in the heart, aorta, and carotid sinus can influence vasomotor (cardiovascular) centers in the medulla, which have a role in regulating cardiovascular activity.

The chemoreceptors of the carotid and aortic bodies are stimulated to increase their rate of discharge by a lowered P_{O_2}, elevated P_{CO_2}, and increased hydrogen ion concentrations (H^+) in their arterial blood supply. These bodies have a high rate of blood flow passing through them. They are rugged receptors, which drive respiration. They remain active even when the chemoreceptors within the central nervous system are depressed by anesthetics or shock. Some neurons within the ventrolateral tegmentum of the medulla act as central chemoreceptors. They respond to an increase in P_{CO_2} primarily through the hydrogen ions of the carbonic acid. Carbon dioxide is known as a most sensitive and potent stimulant to respiration; this activity is mediated largely through these central chemoreceptors. The CO_2 in cerebrospinal fluid, which readily diffuses through the pia-glial membrane, is another source of carbonic acid. Pulmonary chemoreceptors are either nonexistent or not important.

The parasympathetic nuclei include the accessory oculomotor nucleus of Edinger-Westphal of the oculomotor nerve, the salivatory nuclei of the facial and glossopharyngeal nerves, and the dorsal vagal nucleus of the vagus nerve.

Corticobulbar and corticoreticular pathways to cranial nerve motor nuclei

The corticobulbar fibers transmit impulses from the cerebral cortex to the motor nuclei of the cranial nerves. The precise course of these upper motor neuron fibers has not been fully documented. The pathway commences in the lower aspect of the precentral gyrus (area 4) and other cerebral cortical areas such as 8 and 44. Direct

stimulation of these cortical areas produces movements of cranial nerve–innervated muscles. A topographic representation of the head is present in area 4 (Chap. 16). The corticobulbar fibers descend in order through the genu of the internal capsule, the middle of the crus cerebri of the midbrain, and the pons proper (see Fig. 8-22). These fibers enter into the brainstem tegmentum to interact with interneurons that innervate the lower motor neurons of the cranial nerves. Because practically all the corticobulbar fibers terminate on interneurons in the reticular formation, they are often called corticoreticular pathways. The "aberrant" corticobulbar fibers have a similar course until they reach the upper midbrain. In the brainstem these fibers take variable paths through the tegmentum, which may account for the margin of safety from limited injury of these pathways.

The corticobulbar pathways consist of both crossed and uncrossed fibers, so that many cranial nerve nuclei receive both crossed and uncrossed upper neuron innervation. In general, all the cranial nerve motor nuclei are innervated by crossed corticobulbar fibers. In addition, many nuclei are innervated by a significant number of uncrossed corticobulbar fibers.

In this account, *direct corticobulbar fibers* are those projecting from the cerebral cortex directly, without interruption, to the lower motor neurons of the cranial nerves (see Fig. 8-22). The *indirect corticobulbar (corticoreticular) fibers* are those projecting from the cerebral cortex to brainstem interneurons, which, in turn, innervate the lower motor neurons of the cranial nerves (see Fig. 8-22). This is comparable to the process in which some *corticospinal fibers* terminate and synapse directly with lower motor neurons, while others terminate and synapse with spinal interneurons that, in turn, synapse with lower motor neurons (Chap. 5). In effect, direct corticobulbar projections are associated with those nerves which innervate muscles which contract somewhat independently from the others of the group (e.g., control of a few of the muscles of facial expression).

The cranial nerves which innervate the extraocular muscles of the eye (cranial nerves III, IV, and VI), the pharynx and soft palate (swallowing), and larynx (cranial nerves IX and X and

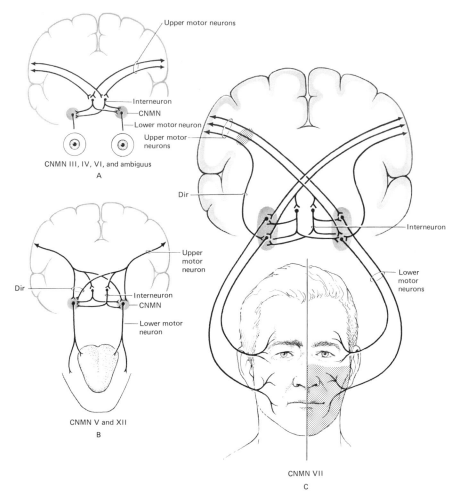

FIGURE 8-22 The three groups of cranial nerve motor nuclei (CNMN) according to their upper motor neuron (UMN) innervation. *A*. CNMN III, IV, VI, and ambiguus. The UMNs exert influences through direct bilateral projections to interneurons, which, in turn, innervate the lower motor neurons (LMN) of these motor nuclei. *B*. CNMN V and XII. The UMNs exert influences both through (1) indirect bilateral projections to interneurons and (2) direct (Dir) bilateral projections to the LMNs of these motor nuclei. *C*. CNMN VII. The UMNs exert influences through indirect bilateral projections to LMNs. Of importance: (1) the LMNs innervating muscles of upper face and forehead receive direct (Dir) bilateral UMN projections and (2) the LMNs innervating muscles of lower face receive predominantly direct crossed UMN projections. The UMN lesion (shaded) results in a paralysis limited to muscles of contralateral lower face (shaded).

cranial root of XI) are innervated by both un-crossed and crossed indirect corticobulbar fibers (see Fig. 8-22). Apparently the lower motor neu-rons of these cranial nerves do not receive direct corticobulbar innervation.

The cranial nerve nuclei that innervate the muscles of mastication (cranial nerve V), the muscles of facial expression (cranial nerve VII), and the muscles of the tongue (cranial nerve XII) are innervated by both uncrossed and crossed direct and indirect corticobulbar fibers (see Fig. 8-22). These nuclei receive bilateral upper motor neuron influences. The spinal nucleus of cranial nerve XI (mainly to the sternocleidomastoid muscle) is presumably innervated by uncrossed (not crossed) direct corticobulbar fibers. The rel-ative number of crossed and uncrossed direct corticobulbar fibers may vary from individual to individual.

The direct corticobulbar innervation of the

motor nucleus of the seventh nerve differs from the above in a way that is clinically significant. The neurons of the facial nucleus innervating the muscles of the upper part of the face (forehead, eyelids) receive a substantial number of crossed and uncrossed fibers. Those neurons of the facial nucleus innervating the muscles of the lower part of the face (lips, nose, and cheek) receive crossed direct corticobulbar fibers almost exclusively (i.e., they receive few, if any, uncrossed fibers).

Paralysis of the voluntary muscles of the head may result from the interruption of cranial nerve fibers (lower motor neurons) or of the corticobulbar tracts (upper motor neurons). A lower motor neuron paralysis results when the cranial nerve fibers to a muscle group are transected. An upper motor neuron paralysis is not necessarily a consequence of the unilateral interruption of a significant number of upper motor neurons. Muscles innervated by the cranial nerves that have bilateral cortical representation generally do not show any signs of paralysis, while those with only a crossed unilateral representation show signs of upper motor neuron paralysis on the contralateral side. The consequences of damage to the corticobulbar pathways to the facial nucleus may be expressed with several variations. A unilateral lesion of the corticobulbar tracts to the facial nucleus may result in an upper motor neuron paralysis of the lower facial muscles of the contralateral side and a complete sparing of the upper facial muscles. The affected muscles may not respond to voluntary stimulation (*central facial palsy*) but may respond to an emotional stimulus (*mimetic palsy*); e.g., the patient cannot smile when asked to smile but can smile when told a joke. The facial muscles may respond to voluntary stimulation but not to emotional stimulation, or vice versa. The precise neural mechanisms involved in these diverse expressions are unknown.

Descending corticobulbar (reflected feedback) fibers from cortex to nuclei of ascending pathways

Influences from the cortex on the nuclei of the ascending pathways are important in neural processing (Chap. 16). These descending reflected feedback pathways (Chap. 3) terminate in the nuclei gracilis and cuneatus of the posterior column–medial lemniscus pathway, in the trigeminal nuclei of the brainstem, in the nuclei of the auditory pathways, and in the nucleus solitarius (Chap. 5). The descending influences are mainly inhibitory; they have a role in the sharpening effect by enhancing the signal and reducing the noise accompanying the signal (Chap. 10).

Cells in the nucleus gracilis and nucleus cuneatus give rise to axons that descend to laminae I, IV, and V of the spinal cord.

Corticospinal tract

The *corticospinal* (*pyramidal*) tract is composed of motor fibers from the cerebral cortex passing through the basilar portion of the brainstem on their way to the spinal cord (see Fig. 5-26). Throughout the brainstem course numerous collateral branches which leave the main axon and terminate in the reticular formation. The corticospinal tract is located in the middle two-thirds of the crus cerebri of the midbrain, in fascicles among the pontine nuclei of the pons proper, and in the pyramid of the medulla. Most of its fibers (85 to 90 percent) cross over in the lower medulla as the decussation of the pyramidal tract (Chap. 5; see Figs. 5-26 and 8-5).

CRANIAL NERVES AND THEIR NUCLEI

Some basic structural and functional aspects of the cranial nerves are outlined in Chap. 7.

The *general somatic efferent cranial nerves* (oculomotor, trochlear, abducent, and hypoglossal nerves) have their nuclei of origin adjacent to the midline, ventral to the cerebral aqueduct and fourth ventricle, and adjacent to the medial longitudinal fasciculus (see Figs. 7-4, 8-7, 8-11, and 10-11). The *oculomotor nuclear complex*, including the parasympathetic accessory oculomotor nucleus of Edinger-Westphal and the several subdivisions of the somatic efferent nuclei, is located in the midbrain (see Figs. 7-4 and 8-12). Each oculomotor nerve consists mainly of uncrossed and a few crossed fibers that pass through the medial tegmentum and leave the brainstem in the interpeduncular fossa. Each *trochlear nucleus*, located in the lower midbrain, gives rise to the trochlear nerve that curves dorsally through the edge of the periaqueductal gray, decussates in the roof, and then emerges from the midbrain tectum (see Figs. 8-11, A-8, and A-20). Each *abducent nucleus*, located in the lower pons, gives rise to the uncrossed abducent nerve, which passes through the medial brainstem and emerges at the pontomedullary junction (see Fig. 8-9). Each elongated *hypoglossal nucleus*, located in the medulla, gives rise to the uncrossed hypoglossal nerve which emerges from the brainstem as a series of rootlets in the anterior lateral sulcus (preolivary) between the pyramid and the olive (see Figs. 8-6 and 8-7).

The *vestibulocochlearis nerve* enters the dorsolateral aspect of the upper medulla. The *four vestibular nuclei* (superior, medial, lateral, and inferior) are located in the dorsolateral tegmentum in the lower pons and the upper medulla (see Figs. 8-8, A-4, A-5, A-15, and A-16). The *dorsal and ventral cochlear nuclei* are located on the external aspect of the inferior cerebellar peduncle in the upper medulla.

The *visceral arch*, or the *branchiomeric cranial* nerves, emerge from the brainstem on its lateral aspect; the trigeminal nerve leaves in the pons; and the facial, glossopharyngeal, vagus, and spinal accessory (cranial portion) nerves leave in a line (posterior lateral) along the entire medulla just dorsal to the olive (see Figs. 1-14 and 7-3). The *nuclei of the trigeminal nerve* form a column extending throughout the entire brainstem and upper two cervical levels of the spinal cord. The *mesencephalic nucleus of the fifth nerve* (see Figs. 8-10, A-7 and A-8), located in the lateral periaqueductal gray of the midbrain, is an elongated nucleus receiving proprioceptive impulses from the head (see Figs. 7-6 and 8-17). The *motor nucleus of the fifth nerve* is located in the lateral tegmentum of the midpons just medial to the principal sensory nucleus of the fifth nerve (see Figs. 8-10, A-7 and A-18). The trigeminal nerve sends descending fibers in the lateral tegmentum as the spinal tract of the fifth nerve as far down as the second cervical spinal cord level. These fibers terminate along its entire course in the adjacent *spinal nucleus of the fifth nerve* (see Figs. 8-4 through 8-9 and A-1 through A-6). The caudal third of the nucleus is concerned with pain, temperature, and light touch. The nuclei oralis and interpolaris of the fifth nerve (see Fig. 7-6)

project to the reticular formation and to the cerebellum.

Three cranial nerve nuclei are associated with the facial nerve. The *motor nucleus of the facial nerve*, located in the midtegmentum in the low pons, projects its fibers dorsomedially to the medial aspect of the nucleus of the abducent nerve, where they hook around the nucleus as the genu of the facial nerve and continue ventrolaterally through the tegmentum to their exit from the brainstem at the lateral pontomedullary junction (see Figs. 7-7, 8-9, A-5, A-6, and A-17). Parasympathetic fibers from the *superior salivatory nucleus* in the lateral tegmentum (parvicellular reticular nucleus; see Figs. 8-8 through 8-10) join the facial nerve. The visceral afferent fibers, including those of taste, enter the fasciculus and *nucleus solitarius* (rostral half of the nucleus in the middorsal tegmentum of the medulla) (see Figs. 7-7 through 7-9 and A-2 and A-3). The fasciculus (tractus) solitarius is a bundle of descending fibers from cranial nerves VII, IX, and X (the cell bodies are in the sensory ganglia of these nerves.)

The cranial nerve nuclei (see Figs. 7-7 through 7-9 and A-2 through A-4) associated with the glossopharyngeal nerve, vagus nerve, and the cranial part of the accessory nerve are the nucleus solitarius, dorsal nucleus of the vagus nerve, and inferior salivatory nucleus (all located in the medullary dorsal tegmentum), the spinal nucleus of the fifth nerve (located in the lateral tegmentum), and the nucleus ambiguus (located in the medullary central tegmentum). The taste and general visceral sensory fibers in these nerves enter and descend in the fasciculus solitarius before terminating in the *nucleus solitarius*. The superior and inferior salivatory nuclei are actually diffuse and confluent groups of cells located within the parvicellular reticular nucleus (Chap. 8; see also Figs. 8-8 and 8-9).

The rostral portion of the nucleus solitarius, with its input of nerves VII, IX, and X, primarily functions as a gustatory center and possibly as a feeding center (see Figs. 7-7 through 7-9). The remainder of the nucleus, with its primary input from nerves IX and X, has a major role in the regulation of cardiovascular, respiratory, and general visceral functions; it receives inputs from the pressoreceptors in the carotid sinus and aortic arch, chemoreceptors in the carotid body, and sensory endings in the lungs, heart, and other viscera.

The *spinal nucleus of the fifth nerve* receives the few general somatic sensory fibers from the facial nerve, glossopharyngeal nerve, and vagus nerve. The *inferior salivatory nucleus* supplies the parasympathetic fibers to the glossopharyngeal nerve, and the dorsal vagal nucleus supplies the parasympathetic fibers to the vagus and spinal accessory nerve. The *nucleus ambiguus* supplies the motor innervation of the glossopharyngeal and vagus nerves to the pharyngeal (swallowing), palatal, and laryngeal muscles (vocal cords).

FUNCTIONAL CONSIDERATIONS AND LESIONS IN THE BRAINSTEM

The human newborn infant is essentially a brainstem–spinal cord organism that may be said to function without a telencephalon. Anencephalics, infants born without a cerebral cortex, have behavioral and physiologic patterns of expression essentially similar to those of normal newborn infants. By 1 month of age the normal infant has its visual pathways sufficiently developed so that a moving object will be followed, if only for short periods of time. Anencephalics at this age do not react at all.

In general, the tracts passing through and within the brainstem are oriented in a longitudinal plane parallel to the long axis of the brainstem (e.g., spinal trigeminal tract, medial lemniscus, and pyramidal tract). The cranial nerves course through a coronal plane perpendicular to the long axis (e.g., facial nerve). These orientations should be kept in mind in the following account.

Lesions of the following pathways within the brainstem result in signs on the opposite side of the body and back of the head because they are crossed tracts: spinothalamic (decussates in the spinal cord), medial lemniscus (decussates in the low medulla), and corticospinal (decussates in the low medulla). In their courses through the brainstem, (1) the spinothalamic tract is located in the lateral tegmentum; (2) the medial lemniscus shifts as it ascends from its location in the

anteromedial tegmentum in the medulla to the posterolateral tegmentum in the midbrain before terminating in the ventral posterior lateral thalamic nucleus; and (3) the corticospinal tract descends through the anterior and anteromedial aspects of the basilar part of the brainstem.

A unilateral lesion of the auditory pathway (lateral lemniscus and brachium of the inferior colliculus) results in the diminution of hearing in both ears that is more marked in the opposite ear (each auditory pathway conveys influences from both ears, but mainly from the contralateral ear). A lesion of the anterior trigeminothalamic tract (i.e., a lesion above the level where the fibers cross in the medulla) is accompanied by loss of pain and temperature sense on the forehead, face, nasal cavity, and oral cavity on the opposite side (see Fig. 8-17).

Because the cranial nerves are oriented at right angles to the long axis of the brainstem, they can be helpful in localizing the level of a lesion. Nerves III (midbrain), VI (pons-medulla junction), and XII (medulla) emerge on the anterior aspect of the brainstem in close proximity to the massive corticospinal tract. Injury to one of these nerves and the corticospinal tract results in an *alternating hemiplegia*. A lesion to the nerve is accompanied by a lower motor neuron paralysis on the same side, and a lesion to the corticospinal tract by an upper motor neuron paralysis on the opposite side of the body (i.e., a lesion of the corticospinal tract rostral to the level of its decussation).

The branchiomeric nerves (cranial nerves V, VII, IX, X, and XI) pass close to the spinothalamic tract before emerging on the lateral side of the brainstem. Injury to one of these nerves and the spinothalamic tract results in (1) sensory loss of the region and a lower motor neuron paralysis of the muscles innervated by that nerve, and (2) loss of pain and temperature sense on the opposite side of the body and back of the head due to the interruption of the decussated fibers of the spinothalamic tract.

Cranial nerves III, IV, and VI are exquisitely integrated to ensure that the eyes move together; these are called conjugate or coordinated movements (see later discussions of the oculomotor system in Chaps. 10 and 12).

Blood supply The sequence of vertebral arteries, basilar artery, and posterior cerebral arteries forms the main trunk system supplying arterial blood to the medulla, pons, midbrain, cerebellum, and posterior medial cerebrum (see Figs. 1-32 and 1-33). The paired vertebral arteries ascend along the anterolateral aspect of the medulla and join at the pons-medulla junction to form the medial basilar artery, which ascends and then divides in the midbrain region into the paired posterior cerebral arteries. Branches of these arteries supply the brainstem in patterns which may be conceptually summarized as follows: in a general way, the paramedian branches are distributed to a medial zone on either side of the midsagittal plane, the short circumferential branches to an antero-lateral zone, and the long circumferential branches to a posterolateral zone and to the cerebellum (Fig. 8-23).

Medial zone of the medulla (Fig. 8-24A) The occlusion of an anterior spinal artery and its paramedian branches to the medial zone of the medulla may be the cause of a lesion which involves the hypoglossal nerve (N. XII), corticospinal tract of the pyramid, and medial lemniscus. This *alternating hemiplegia* combines a lower motor neuron paralysis of the tongue on the ipsilateral side (N. XII) with an upper motor neuron paralysis and a loss of discriminatory general senses (medial lemniscus) on the contralateral side of the body. During the first few weeks after the lesion, the ipsilateral half of the tongue will fibril-

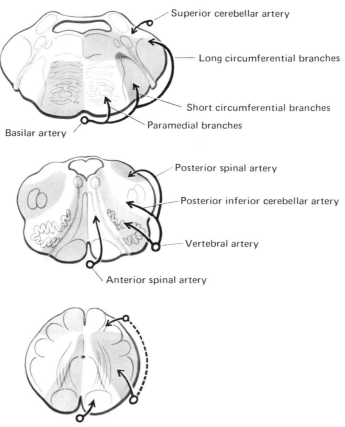

FIGURE 8-23 The patterns of arterial supply of the branches of the basilar artery within the pons (*upper*), mid-medulla (*middle*), and caudal medulla (*lower figure*).

late (denervation sensitivity) and fasciculate; later the muscles atrophy, and that side of the tongue appears wrinkled. When protruded, the tongue deviates to the paralyzed side, primarily because of the unopposed action of the contralateral genioglossus muscle. The contralateral side of the body exhibits the signs of an upper motor neuron paralysis (corticospinal tract) and loss of position, muscle, and joint sense, impaired tactile discrimination, and loss of vibratory sense (medial lemniscus), because the lesion interrupts these tracts above the level of their decussation.

Posterolateral medulla (Fig. 8-24*B*) The occlusion of the posterior inferior cerebellar artery (a long circumferential artery) may be the cause of this lesion, which results in the syndrome of the posterior inferior cerebellar artery (lateral medullary syndrome). Damage to the following structures will produce the symptoms: spinothalamic tract; spinal trigeminal tract and nucleus; fibers and possible nuclei associated with the glossopharyngeal, vagal, and spinal portions of accessory nerves (including the nucleus ambiguus, dorsal vagal nucleus, and fasciculus and nucleus solitarius); part of the reticular formation; portions of the vestibular nuclei; and some fibers of the inferior cerebellar peduncle. The symptoms include:

1 Loss of pain (*analgesia*) and temperature sense (*thermoanesthesia*) on the opposite side of the body including the back of the head (crossed spinothalamic tract).
2. Loss of pain and temperature sense on the same side of the face and nasal and oral cavities in all three trigeminal divisions (uncrossed spinal trigeminal tract and nucleus).
3. Difficulty in swallowing (*dysphagia*) and a voice that is hoarse and weak (damage of nucleus ambiguus produces a lower motor neuron paralysis of the ipsilateral pharyngeal and laryngeal muscles; the normal palatal muscles will deviate the uvula to the normal side).
4. Loss of gag reflex on the ipsilateral side and absence of sensation on the ipsilateral side of the fauces (glossopharyngeal nerve). A transient tachycardia (increase in heartbeat) may result from sudden withdrawal of some para-

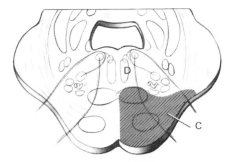

LOWER PONS

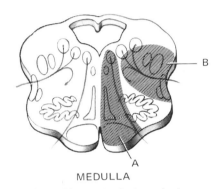

MEDULLA

FIGURE 8-24 Sites of lesions in the lower brainstem, as described in the text. In the medulla, the lesions are located in the medial zone (A) and in the posterolateral zone (B). In the lower pons, the lesions are located in the medial and basal portion (C) and in the medial longitudinal fasciculus (D).

sympathetic innervation; compensatory mechanisms, including influences from the contralateral vagus nerve, will restore the normal heartbeat. The absence of visceral afferent stimulation from some visceral receptors (e.g., carotid body and carotid sinus) to the solitary nucleus is compensated for by the input from similar receptors to the normal contralateral side. The interruption of fibers passing through the inferior cerebellar peduncle results in some signs of cerebellar malfunction on the ipsilateral side of the body— including hypotonia, asynergia, and poorly coordinated voluntary movements (Chap. 9). Irritation of the vestibular nuclei may be expressed by nystagmus or a deviation of the eyes to the ipsilateral side. Horner's syndrome on the same side may occur if many descending fibers of the autonomic nervous system to the thoracic sympathetic outflow are damaged. The tactile and discriminative general senses from the face are normal because the principal sensory nucleus of N. V and its ascending pathways are above the lesion.

Region of the cerebellopontine angle (cerebellopontine angle syndrome) The slowly growing acoustic neuroma, which originates from neurolemmal cells of the vestibular nerve in the vicinity of the internal auditory foramen, may extend into the junctional region of the cerebellum, pons, and medulla near the emergence of cranial nerves VII and VIII, know as the *cerebellopontine angle*. In the early stages, symptoms are refereable to the eighth cranial nerve; they include tinnitus followed by progessive deafness on the lesion side, and abnormal labyrinthine responses such as tilting and rotation of the head with the chin pointing to the lesion side. Later the tumor exerts pressure upon the brainstem and damages the fibers of the inferior and middle cerebellar peduncles, spinothalamic tract, spinal trigeminal tract, and facial nerve.

The cerebellar signs which result from the involvement of the cerebellar peduncles include coarse intention tremor, dysmetria, moderate ataxic gait, adiadochokinesis, and others on the lesion side (Chap. 9). The loss of pain and temperature senses on the ipsilateral side of the face, oral cavity, and nasal cavity and on the contralateral side of the body are a consequence of damage to the spinal trigeminal tract and the spinothalamic tract, respectively. Injury to the facial nerve may result in a lower motor paralysis of the muscles of facial expression (Bell's palsy), hyperacusis, and loss of taste on the anterior two-thirds of the tongue ipsilaterally (Chap. 7).

Medial and basal portion of the caudal pons (Fig. 8-24C) The occlusion of paramedian and short circumferential branches of the basilar artery may result in damage to the following structures within the confines of the lesion: abducent nerve (N. VI), facial nerve (N. VII), pyramidal tract, medial lemniscus, and medial longitudinal fasciculus. The interruption of the fibers of N. VI (lower motor neurons) and the pyramidal tract (upper motor neurons) results in an *alternating abducent hemiplegia*. The transection of N.

VI produces horizontal diplopia (double vision) because of the paralysis of the lateral rectus muscle (an abductor), as a consequence of which the image of an object falls upon noncorresponding portions of the two retinas and is seen as two objects. The diplopia is maximal when the patient attempts to gaze to the lesion side. When the ipsilateral lateral rectus muscle, which is innervated by N. VI, is paralyzed, the subject's ability to abduct the eye (i.e., direct the pupil toward the temple) is impaired. The signs occurring from damage to the corticospinal fibers, seventh nerve, and medial lemniscus are discussed above, and the medial longitudinal fasciculus is discussed below.

Lateral half of the midpons The structures within the region of the lesion (see Fig. 8-25A) include the trigeminal nerve, spinothalamic tract, lateral lemniscus, and middle cerebellar peduncle. Damage to the trigeminal nerve (N. V) results in (1) the loss of all general senses (anesthesia) on the ipsilateral side of the face, forehead, nasal cavity, and oral cavity, including the loss of corneal sensation and corneal reflex; and (2) a lower motor neuron paralysis of the muscles of mastication, with the chin deviating to the lesion side on opening of the mouth. If the lesion is extensive enough to include the corticospinal tract, the combination of the pyramidal tract and N. V produces an *altering trigeminal hemiplegia*. The lesion of the lateral lemniscus may be followed by a diminution of audition, which is more marked on the opposite side (the lateral lemniscus is composed of fibers conveying some auditory influences from the same side but mainly from the opposite side). Interruption of pontocerebellar fibers may be expressed with some cerebellar signs on the same side (Chap. 9) including hypotonia, coarse intention tremor, and tendency to fall to the side of the lesion.

Basal region of the midbrain The occlusion of paramedian branches and short circumferential branches of the basilar and posterior cerebral arteries may produce a *Weber's syndrome* (see Fig. 8-25B) which is a consequence of damage to the oculomotor nerve (N. III), the corticospinal tract, and a variable number of corticobulbar and corticoreticular fibers. The interruption of all the fibers in the oculomotor nerve results in

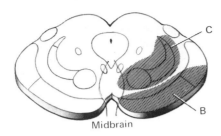

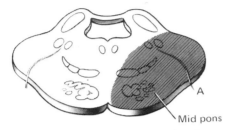

FIGURE 8-25 Sites of lesions in the pons and midbrain, as described in the text. In the midpons, the lesion is located laterally (A). In the superior collicular level of the midbrain, the lesions are located in the basal region (B) and in the midbrain tegmentum (C).

signs restricted to the ipsilateral eye, including drooping of the eyelid (ptosis, or inability to raise the eyelid because of paralysis of the levator palpebral muscle), diplopia, external strabismus (squint) due to unopposed contraction of the lateral rectus muscle; inability to elevate, depress, or adduct the eye; and a fully dilated pupil (the normally acting sympathetic influences are unopposed because of absence of the parasympathetic influences conveyed by the damaged parasympathetic fibers of N. III). The consensual light reflex to the contralateral eye is normal (Chap. 12). An alterating hemiplegia is a consequence of the lower motor neuron paralysis of the oculomotor nerve and the upper motor neuron paralysis of the contralateral side of the body from the damage to the corticospinal tract.

The unilateral interruption of the corticobulbar and corticoreticular (indirect corticobulbar) fibers results in only minimal, if any, effects upon the muscles innervated by the cranial nerves except for the contralateral muscles of facial expression of the lower part of the face. In general, the motor nuclei of the cranial nerves (except for the neurons of the facial nucleus innervating the lower part of the face) receive upper motor neuron influences from both halves of the cerebrum. Hence supranuclear unilateral lesions interrupting the upper motor neurons to these motor nuclei do not produce upper motor neuron paralysis of the muscles innervated by these nerves, except for the weakness of the contralateral muscles of facial expression of the lower part of the face. In some individuals, the interruption of the upper motor neurons results in a tongue and jaw which deviate to the side contralateral to the lesion; the explanation for this observation is that these patients have few, if any, upper motor neurons originating in the ipsilateral cerebral cortex.

The bilateral, diffuse involvement of the corticobulbar and corticoreticular fibers results in a *pseudobulbar palsy*. In this syndrome there is a bilateral paralysis or weakness without atrophy of many muscles innervated by cranial nerves. The muscle groups affected control chewing, swallowing, speaking, and breathing. Unrestrained crying and laughing occur in many subjects with pseudobulbar palsy. These emotional outbursts may be related to release from influences derived from the cerebral cortex and subcortical centers in the telencephalon and diencephalon.

Upper midbrain tegmentum A unilateral lesion in the midbrain tegmentum (see Fig. 8-25C) limited to the region including the fibers of the oculomotor nerve, red nucleus, superior cerebellar peduncle, medial lemniscus, and spinothalamic tract results in *Benedikt syndrome*. The damage to the red nucleus and the fibers of the superior cerebellar peduncle (decussated dentatorubral and dentatothalamic fibers) results in such signs of cerebellar damage as coarse intention tremor, adiadochokinesis, cerebellar ataxia, and hypotonia on the contralateral side of the body (Chap. 9). Experimental evidence indicates that no signs in this syndrome are definitely attributable to a lesion of the red nucleus. The injury to the third cranial nerve results in a lower motor neuron paralysis of the ipsilateral extraocular muscles and in a dilated pupil (mydriasis) from absence of parasympathetic influences (see "Basal Region of the Midbrain," above). The interruption of the crossed spinothalamic tract, anterior trigeminothalamic tract, and medial lemniscus results in the loss of sense of pain, temperature, light-touch, vibratory, pressure-touch, and other discriminatory senses on the opposite side of the body and head. The retention of touch and other discriminatory senses on the contralateral side of the head may occur when the uncrossed posterior trigeminothalamic tract is intact.

Cranial nerves of the brainstem A *lesion of one oculomotor nerve* results in outward deviation of the ipsilateral eye, drooping of the upper eyelid (ptosis), and a dilated pupil of the eye (unopposed action of sympathetic innervation because of lack of parasympathetic innervation). *Lesion of one trochlear nerve* results in impaired ability to turn the eye downward; *lesion of one abducent nerve* results in an inwardly turned eye (internal strabismus), because of pull of the medial rectus muscle unopposed by the paralyzed lateral rectus muscle. Double vision is a consequence of paralyzed eye muscles because the visual images on the two eyes are not properly fused. Patients turn and tilt their heads to one side to minimize and prevent the diplopia (thereby fusing the images by causing the visual axes of the eyes to become parallel to each other). A *lesion of one hypoglossal nerve* results in an ipsilateral paralysis of the tongue muscles; because the tongue is pulled forward when protruded, it will deviate to the paralyzed side when voluntarily protruded (the paralyzed side acts as a pivot).

Lesions of the corticospinal tract at the levels where the oculomotor nerve (midbrain level), the abducent nerve (pontomedullary junction), or the hypoglossal nerve (medulla) emerges on the ventral aspect of the brainstem may be combined with the interruption of one of these cranial nerves. This combination of the interruption of an uncrossed cranial nerve and the corticospinal tract (and a portion of tegmentum to include other motor tracts) may result in an *alternating hemiplegia*—an ipsilateral lower motor paralysis of the muscles innervated by the cranial nerve and the contralateral upper motor neuron paralysis of the muscles on the opposite side of the body.

A *lesion of the trigeminal nerve* results in the complete loss of the general senses of pain, temperature, touch, and proprioception on the ipsilateral side of the head and in the lower motor neuron paralysis of the muscles of mastication (when voluntarily protruded, the jaw deviates to

the paralyzed side). The *functional interruption of the facial nerve* results in the total paralysis of the ipsilateral muscles of facial expression and in the loss of taste on one side of the anterior two-thirds of the tongue. This paralysis (*Bell's palsy*) is expressed as the ipsilateral sagging of the face, inability to close the eyelid (the patient may wear an eyemask to prevent drying out of the cornea), and drooping of the side of the mouth (saliva may drip from the corner of the mouth). Many patients with Bell's palsy recover after several months. The face is actually drawn to the normal side by the contraction or tone of unaffected muscles of facial expression.

Impairment of the nucleus ambiguus and its efferent fibers in the glossopharyngeal and vagus nerves results in difficulty in swallowing (dysphagia) and in forming vocal sounds (dysphonia). A nasal quality of sounds (dysarthria) and hoarseness may follow.

BIBLIOGRAPHY

Andén, N. E., A. Dahlström, K. Fuxe, K. Larsson, L. Olson, and U. Ungerstedt: Ascending monoamine neurons to the telencephalon and diencephalon. Acta Physiol Scand, 67:313–326, 1966.

Azmatia, E. C., and M. Segal: An autoradiographic analysis of the differential ascending projections of the dorsal and medial raphe nuclei in the rat. J Comp Neurol, 179:641–668, 1978.

Beckstead, R. M., and R. Norgren: An autoradiographic examination of the central distribution of the trigeminal, facial, glossopharyngeal and vagal nerves in the monkey. J Comp Neurol, 184:455–472, 1979.

Beckstead, R. M., J. R. Morse, and R. Norgren: The nucleus of the solitary tract in the monkey: Projections to the thalamus and brainstem nuclei. J Comp Neurol, 1980 (in press).

Beidler, L. M. (ed.): "Taste," in *Handbook of Sensory Physiology*, vol. IV, sec. 2, Springer-Verlag, Berlin and New York, 1971, pp. 1–410.

Brodal, A.: *The Reticular Formation of the Brain Stem: Anatomical Aspects and Functional Correlations*, Charles C Thomas, Publisher, Springfield, Ill., 1957.

Brodal, A.: *Neurological Anatomy in Relation to Clinical Medicine*, Oxford University Press, London, 1969.

Burton, H., and A. D. Craig, Jr.: Distribution of trigeminothalamic neurons in cat and monkey. Brain Res, 161:515–521, 1979.

Cedarbaum, J. M., and G. K. Aghajanian: Afferent projections to the rat locus coeruleus as determined by a retrograde tracing technique. J Comp Neurol, 178:1–16, 1978.

Fields, H. L., and A. I. Basbaum: Brainstem control of spinal pain transmission neurons. Ann Rev Physiol, 40:217–248, 1978.

Ganchrow, D.: Intratrigeminal and thalamic projections of nucleus caudalis in the squirrel monkey (*Samiri sciureus*). A degeneration and autoradiographic study. J Comp Neurol, 178:281–312, 1978.

Garver, D. L., and J. R. Sladek, Jr.: Monoamine distribution in primate brain. I. Catecholamine-containing perikarya in the brain stem of *Macaca speciosa*. J Comp Neurol, 159:289–304, 1975.

Gobel, S.: Golgi studies of the neurons in layer II of the dorsal horn of the medulla (trigeminal nucleus caudalis). J Comp Neurol, 180:395–413, 1978.

Graybiel, A. M.: Direct and indirect preoculomotor pathways of the brainstem: an autoradiographic study of the pontine reticular formation in the cat. J Comp Neurol, 175:37–78, 1978.

Jacobowitz, D. M., and P. D. Maclean: A brainstem atlas of catecholaminergic neurons and serotonergic perikarya in pygmy primate (*Cebuella pygmaea*). J Comp Neurol, 177:397–416, 1978.

Jasper, H. H., and L. O. Proctor (eds.): *Reticular Formation of the Brain*, Little, Brown and Company, Boston, 1958.

Loewy, A. D., and C. B. Saper: Edinger-Westphal nucleus: projection to the brain stem and spinal cord in the cat. Brain Res, 150:1–27, 1978.

Moore, R. Y., and F. E. Bloom: Central catecholamine neurons systems: anatomy and physiology of the dopamine systems. Ann Rev Neurosci, 1:129–169, 1978.

Moore, R. Y., and F. E. Bloom: Central catecholamine neuron systems: anatomy and physiology of the norepinephrine and epinephrine systems. Ann Rev Neurosci, 2:113–168, 1979.

Norgren, R.: Taste pathways to hypothalamus and amygdala. J Comp Neurol, 166:17–30, 1976.

Olszewski, J., and D. Baxter: *Cytoarchitecture of the Human Brain Stem*, S. Karger, Basel, 1954.

Pfaffmann, C., M. Frank, and R. Norgren: Neural mechanism and behavioral aspects of taste. Ann Rev Psychol, 30:283–325, 1979.

Pierce, E. T., W. E. Foote, and J. A Hobsen: The efferent connections of the nucleus raphe dorsalis. Brain Res, 107:137–144, 1976.

Ramón-Moliner, E., and W. J. H. Nauta: The isodendritic core of the brainstem. J Comp Neurol, 126:311–336, 1966.

Siggins, G. R., B. J. Hoffer, A. P. Oliver, and F. E. Bloom: Activation of a central noradrenergic projections to cerebellum. Nature, 233:481–483, 1971.

Synder, S.: Opiate receptors and internal opiates. Sci Am, 236:44–56, 1977.

Ungerstedt, U.: Stereotaxic mapping of the monoamine pathways in the rat brain. Acta Physiol Scand Suppl, 367:1–48, 1971.

Weisberg, J. A., and A. Rustioni: Cortical cells projecting to the dorsal column nuclei of rhesus monkeys. Exp Brain Res, 28:521–528. 1977.

CHAPTER NINE

CEREBELLUM

The cerebellum has an essential role in the coordination of group muscle activities. It is not the initiator of motion but acts (1) as a monitor of ongoing dynamics of stretch and tension within the muscular system, (2) as the great modulator and control system of motor activities and (3) as a preprogrammer of a movement (Chap. 14). The cerebellum plays no part in the appreciation of conscious sensations or in intelligence.

The cerebellum is integrated with the vestibular system in the maintenance of muscle tone and equilibrium and with other motor systems in such phasic movements as locomotion. This suprasegmental structure functions primarily in smoothing out and synchronizing the delicate timing between the muscles of a group, and between groups of muscles, whether the activities are at the reflex, automatic, or conscious level. A patient with a cerebellar lesion is capable of carrying out the general outlines of movements, but each movement is usually executed with an inadequacy of the finer muscular coordination.

In common with neural structures that are derived from the embryonic alar plate, the cerebellum is basically a somatic afferent organ, often called the *head ganglion of proprioceptive and exteroceptive systems*. The cerebellum receives and processes unconscious afferent stimuli from general proprioceptive receptors (primarily from receptors in muscles, joints, and tendons) and exteroceptive receptors in the body and from the vestibular, auditory, and visual systems. This information is then utilized by the motor systems.

GROSS DIVISIONS OF THE CEREBELLUM

Several general schemas of dividing the cerebellum are useful (see Figs. 9-1 and 9-2). The classic subdivisions of the cerebellum into numerous lobes and lobules is not described in this account, for they are based on descriptive criteria with limited special functional significance.

The cortex of the cerebellum is the thin layer of gray which covers it. The cortex is unusual because it is one of the few neuronal structures that are continuous across the midline. Deep to the cortex is the medullary core of white matter, which consists of fibers projecting to and from the cerebellar cortex. Deep in the medullary core are four pairs of the deep cerebellar nuclei (see Fig. A-5): fastigii, globosus, emboliformis, and dentatus (from medial to lateral). These nuclei consist of neurons that project the cerebellar output to other portions of the brain.

The cerebellum is connected to the brainstem by the three cerebellar peduncles or pillars: the inferior cerebellar (restiform body), the middle cerebellar (brachium pontis), and the superior cerebellar (brachium conjunctivum). The *inferior cerebellar peduncle* is the bridge between the medulla and the cerebellum, with fibers projecting both to and from the cerebellum. The *middle cerebellar peduncle* is the bridge between the pons and the cerebellum, with fibers projecting to the cerebellum. The *superior cerebellar peduncle* is the bridge between the midbrain and the cerebellum, with fibers largely

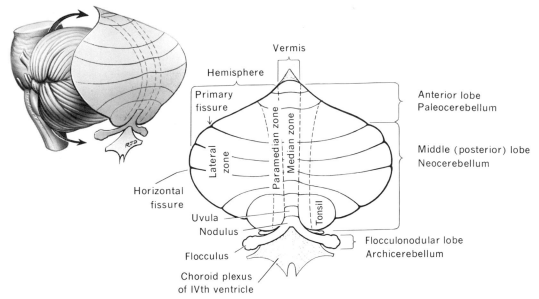

FIGURE 9-1 The surface of the cerebellum after it is unfolded and laid out flat.

projecting from the cerebellum toward the midbrain and the thalamus.

Sagittal subdivisions

Classically, the cerebellum is divided into two large bilateral *cerebellar hemispheres* and the narrow median *vermis*. This standard sagittal organization can be modified into a structural and functional schema based on the relation of the cerebellar cortex, the deep cerebellar nuclei, and their projections into three zones: (1) medial (vermal) zone, (2) paramedian (paravermal) zone, and (3) lateral (hemispheric) zone (see Fig. 9-1). The output from the entire cerebellar cortex is primarily to the deep cerebellar nuclei.

Median zone The median zone comprises the cortex of the vermis, anterior lobe, and flocculonodular lobe and the nucleus to which it projects—the fastigial nuclei (see Fig. 9-4; see also 8-8, A-5, and A-6). Some fibers from this cortex project directly to the vestibular nuclei (see Fig. 9-6). The fastigial nuclei project primarily to all vestibular nuclei and some reticular nuclei in the pons and medulla (see Fig. 9-6; see also Fig. 10-13). Some fibers course rostrally via the superior cerebellar peduncle to the ventral lateral and centromedianum nuclei of the thalamus.

The main output from the median zone is primarily directed to the spinal cord via (1) the lateral vestibulospinal tract (from lateral vestibular nucleus) to all spinal levels, (2) median vestibulospinal tract (from medial vestibular nucleus) to cervical and upper thoracic levels, and (3) reticulospinal tracts to all spinal levels (Chaps. 5 and 10). These pathways exert their influences either directly or indirectly through spinal interneurons on the alpha and gamma motor neurons. These pathways have a crucial role in the automatic motor actions of standing, walking, equilibrium, and gait. This includes balancing of the head (cervical region innervates cervical musculature to the head) and the extensor muscle tone of truncal musculature (entire vertebral column or axial muscles) involved with posture.

Paramedian zone The paramedian zone comprises the paravermal cortex and the nucleus to which it projects—the emboliform and globose nuclei (see Figs. 8-8, A-5, and A-6). The output of these nuclei is directed primarily to the contralateral caudal two-thirds of the nucleus ruber and to a slight degree to the ventral lateral thalamic nucleus and to some brainstem reticular nuclei (Figs. 9-5, 10-13). The major projection from

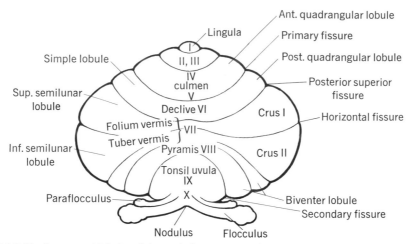

FIGURE 9-2 The fissures and lobules of the cerebellum. Regions of the vermis are designated by Roman numerals. In this figure, the paleocerebellum (anterior lobe) is located rostral to the primary fissure, and the archicerebellum (flocculonodular lobe) lies caudal to the posterolateral fissure. The neocerebellum is located between the primary fissure and the secondary fissure.

the nucleus ruber (magnocellular portion) is via the crossed rubrospinal tract that terminates in all spinal levels (see Fig. 9-5; see also Figs. 5-27 and 8-21 and Chaps. 5 and 8). The paramedian zone exerts its influences at spinal levels with a role in posture and stance.

Lateral zone The lateral zone comprises the bulk of the cerebellar hemispheres and the nucleus to which it projects—the dentate nucleus. This nucleus projects to the ventral lateral nucleus of the thalamus (main target nucleus), intralaminar thalamic nuclei, rostral third of nucleus ruber, and the reticulotegmental (pons) and paramedian (medulla) reticular nuclei. These connections are mainly involved in two pathway systems: (1) one directed to the motor and premotor (areas 4 and 6) cerebral cortex and (2) one in the feedback to the cerebellum (see Figs. 9-4 and 9-5; see also Figs. 5-27 and 8-21), the pathway to areas 4 and 6, areas from which the corticospinal, corticoreticulospinal, and corticorubrospinal tracts originate. Thus, the lateral zone directs its influences to the spinal cord via the cerebral cortex, nucleus ruber, and brainstem reticular nuclei. This zone is involved with the complex fine manipulative skills.

Functionally, the vermis and the flocculonodular lobe are involved with truncal movements and the hemispheres with coordination of movements involving the limbs.

Transverse subdivisions

The cerebellum may be divided into three transverse divisions: archicerebellum, paleocerebellum, and neocerebellum (see Figs. 9-1 and 9-2). These lobes, based partially on phylogenetic criteria, are not defined in precisely the same way by different investigators. The *archicerebellum* (flocculonodular lobe) consists of the paired flocculi of the hemispheres and possibly the unpaired nodulus and uvula of the vermis. This *flocculonodular lobe* is phylogenetically the oldest lobe of the cerebellum. It is actually a specialized portion of the somatic afferent column that is dominated by direct, indirect, and feedback connections with the vestibular system. It receives direct input via fibers from the vestibular nerve and the medial and inferior vestibular nuclei. The archicerebellum subserves a significant role in muscle tone, equilibrium, and posture through its influences of the trunk muscles.

The *paleocerebellum* consists of most of the vermis and the anterior lobe in front of the primary fissure. This phylogenetically old lobe is primarily associated with the proprioceptive (spinocerebellar, cuneocerebellar, and rostral spinocerebellar tracts) and the exteroceptive input from the head and body, including some from the vestibular system. The primary role of the paleocerebellum involves the regulation of muscle tone. This is associated with its input from the muscle spindles and Golgi tendon organs.

The *neocerebellum* (posterior lobe) consists of the main bulk of the cerebellar hemispheres and part of the vermis. This phylogenetically new lobe (essentially a mammalian structure) is functionally associated with the neocortex of the cerebrum, pontine nuclei, and the principal inferior olivary nucleus of the medulla. Input is also derived from visual, auditory, and cutaneous senses. It has an essential role in the muscular coordination of phasic movements.

In a general way, the archicerebellum and paleocerebellum subserve significantly in muscle tone, equilibrium, and posture through the neck and trunk (axial) musculature. The neocerebellum has a role in the coordination of musculature involved with phasic movements related to fine manipulative skills.

DEEP NUCLEI OF CEREBELLUM

The four paired deep cerebellar nuclei are located in the white matter of the cerebellum (see Figs. 8-8, A-5, and A-6). From medial to lateral these are the fastigial, globose, emboliform, and dentate nuclei. The globose and emboliform nuclei are collectively called the interposed nucleus (nuclei interpositus) in mammals other than humans. The globose nucleus is equivalent to the posterior interposed nucleus and the emboliform nucleus to the anterior interposed nucleus.

These nuclei receive projections from the cerebellar cortex (specifically from the Purkinje cells, Fig. 9-3). The vermis (medial zone) projects its fibers to the fastigial nuclei. The paravermis (paramedial or paravermal zone) project primarily to the globose and emboliform nuclei and to a portion of the dentate nucleus. The hemispheres (lateral or hemispheric zone) project to the dentate nucleus and caudal portions of the globose nucleus. The deep nuclei also receive afferent input from extracerebellar sources via collateral branches of the climbing and mossy fibers. These deep nuclei have critical dual roles in the initial selection of the cerebellar input and in the final processing of cerebellar output.

THE CEREBELLAR CORTEX

Folia

The cerebellar surface is corrugated into numerous parallel, long "gyri" called *folia* (see Fig. 9-3). The folia are separated from one another by cerebellar fissures that are equivalent to the sulci of the cerebral cortex. Although the cerebellum is much smaller than the cerebrum, its total cortical surface area, because of the increased surface formed by the folia, is actually three-fourths that of the cerebral cortex. Only 15 percent of the cerebellar cortex is exposed to the outer surface, whereas 85 percent faces the sulcal surfaces between the folia. When flattened, the unfolded cortex of a human has a surface area of about 120 by 17 cm. The branching of the white matter and the treelike appearance of the folia in sections of the cerebellum at right angles to the long axis of the folia suggested the name *arbor vitae*. All folia have the same histologic structure.

Cytoarchitecture and intrinsic cerebellar circuits

The cerebellar cortex is organized in a precise, geometrically ordered pattern. Its neuronal elements are oriented along axes resembling a Cartesian coordinate system; some neurons are arranged in planes perpendicular to the long axis of a folium (stellate cells, basket cells, and dendritic arborization of the Purkinje cells), while the granule cell and its axonal branches are oriented in a plane parallel to the long axis of a folium (see Fig. 9-3). Knowledge of this geometric organization is fundamental to an understanding of the cerebellar circuits.

The cerebellar cortex is divided into three layers: the *inner* or *granular layer* (200 to 300 μm thick) in which are located the cell bodies of granule cells and the glomeruli; the thin *middle layer* composed of the cell bodies of the Purkinje cells; and the *outer* or *molecular layer* (about

400 μm thick) in which are located the stellate and basket cells. Deep in the cerebellum are the cerebellar nuclei: *fastigii, emboliform, globose, and dentate*. The cerebellum is constructed of (1) two types of input axons: climbing fibers and mossy fibers; (2) five types of intrinsic neurons: granule cells, stellate cells, basket cells, Golgi type II cells, and Purkinje cells; and (3) one type of output neuron: cells of the deep cerebellar nuclei. Some Purkinje cells are output neurons projecting to the lateral vestibular nucleus.

The number of neurons of the cerebellar cortex is enormous. In fact more neurons are present in the cerebellar cortex than in the cerebral cortex. In humans, there are said to be from 34 to 45 billion granule cells, 45 million stellate and basket cells, and 15 to 30 million Purkinje cells. The fibers within the cerebellar cortex are unmyelinated (Zagon et al.).

Input fibers The *climbing fibers* originate from cells of the inferior olivary complex (olivocerebellar fibers) and other brainstem nuclei.

Each main myelinated climbing fiber divides into several branches in the white matter that are distributed into several adjacent Purkinje cells in a limited portion of the cortex. Each myelinated branch loses its myelin when it reaches the Purkinje cell layer; the unmyelinated branches "climb" and coil like ivy around the dendrites of the Purkinje cell. They make excitatory monosynaptic axodendritic synapses with the smooth (nonspinous) segments of the dendrites. Bergmann glial cells insulate the smooth portions from the parallel fibers of the granule cells that synapse with the spines. The Purkinje cells express the largest excitatory postsynaptic potentials because such numerous dendritic expanses on each cell are stimulated all at once by the excitatory climbing fiber.

Collateral branches of the climbing fibers synapse with all other neuronal cell types of the cerebellum, including neurons of the deep cerebellar nuclei, granule cells, Golgi cells, stellate cells, and basket cells.

The *mossy fibers* originate from many nuclei of the brainstem and spinal cord; they course to the cerebellum via spinocerebellar, cuneocerebellar, vestibulocerebellar, and pontocerebellar tracts and other small tracts. Each of the mossy fibers branches many times before terminating in hundreds (or even thousands) of mossy-fiber rosettes. Each *rosette* is the central element of a *cerebellar glomerulus* (cerebellar island). Each *glomerulus* is composed of (1) one mossy-fiber rosette, (2) dendritic terminals of many granule cells, and (3) axonic terminals of several Golgi cells. The basic functional units of a glomerulus (see Fig. 9-3) are considered to be (1) two presynaptic elements—the mossy-fiber rosette and several axonic terminals of Golgi cells—and (2) one postsynaptic element—dendrites of many granule cells. Each glomerulus is ensheathed by the lamella of a glial cell. Another type of glomerulus receives its input from a climbing fiber instead of a mossy fiber.

Essentially all climbing and mossy fibers have collateral branches that terminate in excitatory synapses in the deep cerebellar nuclei.

The locus coeruleus, located in the brainstem, has fibers that project to and extend throughout all the layers of the cerebellar cortex (see Fig. 8-19 and Chap. 8). These noradrenergic fibers are presumed to exert modulatory influences and to have a role in cerebellar activities during sleep rhythms and wakefulness.

The *Purkinje cells* are the sole output neurons of the cerebellar cortex. Their espalier-like dendritic trees arborize within the molecular layer *in a plane perpendicular to the long axis of a folium* (see Fig. 9-3; see also Fig. 2-7E). Each Purkinje cell receives input from about 80,000 granule cells and from stellate, basket, and other Purkinje cells. The main axon of each cell makes terminal synaptic connections with the neurons of the deep cerebellar nuclei or of the lateral vestibular nucleus. Each has recurrent axonal collateral branches which synapse with stellate, basket, Golgi, and other Purkinje cells.

The elaborate dendrite tree of the Purkinje cell (see Fig. 9-3; see also Fig. 2-7E) is not simply a morphologic adaptation for the mere summation of excitatory and inhibitory potentials. Rather, it is a complex processing specialized for the generation of (1) dendritic local responses and (2) dendritic or "baby" action potentials. The dendritic action potentials are generated by the summation of local responses at or near a dendritic bifurcation. These branch points act as "hot spots" for the generation of intradendritic "baby" action potentials that spread in a pseudosaltatory fashion from branch point to branch point toward the cell body. At this site they interact to generate an action potential at the initial segment of the Purkinje cell axon (Chap. 3).

Intrinsic neurons (Fig. 9-3)

The cerebellum contains five intrinsic neurons with cell bodies located in the cerebellar cortex. These are granule cells, stellate (outer stellate) cells, basket (inner stellate) cells, Golgi cells, and Purkinje cells. Each *granule cell* has from four to five short dendrites; each dendrite terminates in a different glomerulus. Thus each granule cell receives input from several mossy fibers (an average of four). The unmyelinated axon of each granule cell extends from a cell body, located in the granular layer, into the molecular layer, where it bifurcates as a T into two branches, which extend for about 2 mm in opposite directions *parallel to the long axis of a folium;* these so-called parallel fibers have synaptic connections with the spines of the Purkinje cell dendrites and the dendrites of the stellate, basket, and Golgi cells. The synapses between the parallel fibers and the dendrites of these neurons are called *"crossover" synapses.* As many as 300,000 parallel fibers pass through the dendritic tree of each Purkinje cell, making about 60,000 to 120,000 synapses with each Purkinje cell (each parallel fiber does not synapse with each Purkinje cell it traverses). Each parallel fiber passes through the planes of about 500 Purkinje cells.

The *stellate* (*outer stellate*) *cells* and the *basket* (*inner stellate*) *cells* are interneurons, located within the molecular layer; their dendritic and axonal processes are oriented in a plane perpendicular to the long axis of a folium (see Fig. 9-3). These neurons receive input from the climbing and parallel fibers and collaterals of Purkinje cells; they project their output to the Purkinje cells. The axons of the stellate cells terminate upon the dendrites (axodendritic synapses) of a number of Purkinje cells. The axons of a basket cell terminate in arborizations around the cell bodies (axosomatic synapses) of about 250 Purkinje cells and as terminal collaterals on the dendrites of Purkinje cells (axodendritic synapses). Each Purkinje cell receives input from many stellate and basket cells. The stellate and basket cells exert *feed-forward inhibition* upon the Purkinje cells (Chap. 3).

Each *Golgi cell* has a cell body in the granular layer and a dendritic tree which arborizes in all planes through the granular and molecular layers (see Fig. 9-3). A Golgi cell receives input from the parallel, climbing, and Purkinje cells and conveys output to thousands of glomeruli.

The Golgi cell axons project *feedback type of inhibition* to the granule cells and together with the mossy fiber terminal form the glomerulus, the *basic functional unit* of the granular layer.

In brief, the basket cells and stellate cells receive their input from the granule cells and, in turn, project their feed-forward inhibitory output to the Purkinje cells. These two interneurons together with the third interneuron, the Golgi cells, are now considered to act as modulators of Purkinje cell activity either *directly* through the stellate and basket cells or *indirectly* through the Golgi cells by inhibiting the granule cells in the glomeruli. In other words, these three interneurons serve to set the level of cerebellar cortical activity. This combination of feedback (Golgi cells) and feed-forward (stellate and basket cells) inhibition means that each stream of activity (message) is fast and discrete and is cleared away rapidly. Each message lasts but a brief interval because this inhibitory combination is able to turn neurons off rapidly.

Summary The cerebellar cortex (1) receives input from two main systems, the climbing fiber and mossy fiber systems; (2) is processed, in part, through four sets of interneurons, granule, stellate, basket, and Golgi cells; and (3) projects its output via one neuron, the Purkinje cell.

The neurons within the cerebellum exert excitatory and inhibitory effects.

1. The mossy fibers and climbing fibers convey excitatory influences to the neurons of the deep nuclei and cortex of the cerebellum.
2. The output of the cerebellar cortex is conveyed exclusively by Purkinje cells. This output is inhibitory.
3. The output of the cerebellum to the rest of the brain is conveyed mainly from the deep cerebellar nuclei. This output is excitatory.
4. The granule cells convey their influences, all excitatory, via parallel fibers to the Purkinje,

Golgi, stellate, and basket cells of the cerebellar cortex.

5. The output of the Golgi, stellate, and basket interneurons is inhibitory.
6. The Purkinje cells have recurrent axon collaterals which feed back to cortical cells.

Output neurons

The output cells of the cerebellum are located in the fastigial, emboliform, globose, and dentate nuclei (see Figs. 9-3 through 9-6). They receive excitatory input from climbing and mossy fibers and inhibitory input from Purkinje cells. Their axons course to the brainstem and thalamus via the superior cerebellar peduncle and juxtarestiform body and also have collaterals which project to the neurons of the cerebellar cortex.

NEUROTRANSMITTERS OF NEURONS WITHIN THE CEREBELLUM

The putative neurotransmitters associated with some of the neurons and nerve fibers within the cerebellum have been identified. α-Aminobutyric acid (GABA) is the transmitter of the inhibitory Purkinje, basket, stellate, and Golgi neurons. Glutamate is presumed to be the excitatory transmitter of the granule cells. Norepinephrine is the neurotransmitter of the fibers of the locus coeruleus terminating in the cerebellar cortex. As yet, the identity of the transmitters of the climbing fibers, mossy fibers, and neurons of the deep cerebellar nuclei is unknown.

Intrinsic circuitry (Fig. 9-3)

Although the input fibers (climbing and mossy) convey excitatory influences to the cerebellum, the *entire output of the cerebellar cortex is inhibitory*. Of the five interneurons with cell bodies in the cerebellar cortex, four exert inhibitory influences—they act to reduce the excitability of the neurons on which their axons synapse. These *inhibitory neurons* include the stellate, basket, Golgi, and Purkinje cells. The excitatory cortical neuron is the granule cell. The role of the inhibitory intracortical neurons—Golgi, stellate, and basket cells—is to regulate and focus (a process called *sharpening of the focus* or *focusing effect* or

lateral inhibition) the excitatory influences conveyed by the input fibers upon the Purkinje cells. The entire output of the cerebellar cortex is inhibitory because the inhibitory Purkinje cells are the sole output neurons of the cerebellar cortex. This should not be equated with the final output from the cerebellum, which is conveyed to the rest of the brain by the excitatory neurons of the deep cerebellar nuclei.

The Purkinje cells are (1) stimulated by the excitatory influences of the climbing fibers and of the parallel fibers of the granule cells and (2) modulated by the inhibitory influences of the stellate and basket cells. The activated Purkinje cells convey inhibitory influences to the output neurons of the cerebellum located in the deep cerebellar nuclei (and to some neurons in the vestibular nuclei).

These *output neurons of the deep cerebellar nuclei normally convey excitatory influences* from the cerebellum; the degree of this excitatory activity can be modulated by the inhibitory influences from the Purkinje cells. The output neurons of the deep cerebellar nuclei generate their excitatory activity (1) by excitatory influences received from the collaterals of climbing and mossy fibers and (2) by a pacemaker mechanism which generates action potentials "spontaneously" without extrinsic excitatory sources. In effect, the degree of the frequency of the output of action potentials to the rest of the brain is modulated by the inhibitory activity of the Purkinje cells upon the deep cerebellar nuclei.

The inhibitory activity of the Purkinje cells is regulated and focused by the inhibitory and excitatory inputs received following the activity of the other neuronal circuits within the cerebellum. These will be outlined. The excitatory climbing fibers stimulate the inhibitory stellate and basket cells to exert inhibitory influences upon the Purkinje cells. This inhibition from the stellate and basket cells partially suppresses the excitatory activity resulting from the facilitatory influences exerted by the climbing fibers on the Purkinje cells. The mossy fibers, through their rosettes within the glomeruli, excite the granule cells to exert facilitatory influences via the parallel fibers upon the stellate, basket, Purkinje, and Golgi cells. In effect, granule cells convey (1) excitatory influences directly to the Purkinje cells through the "*crossover*" *synapses* on the spines

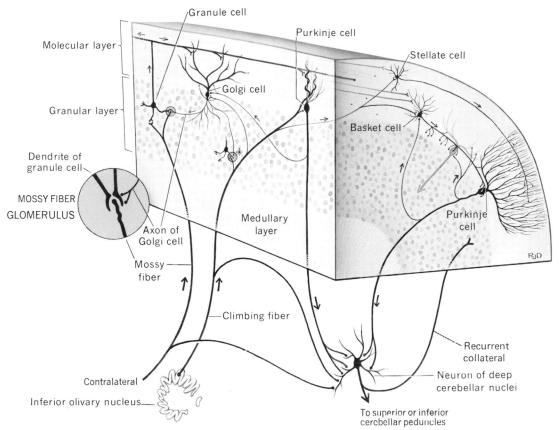

Granule cell
Molecular layer
Purkinje cell
Stellate cell
Golgi cell
Granular layer
Basket cell
Dendrite of
granule cell
MOSSY FIBER
GLOMERULUS
Axon of
Golgi cell
Medullary
layer
Purkinje
cell
Mossy
fiber
RjD
Climbing fiber
Recurrent
collateral
Neuron of deep
cerebellar nuclei
Contralateral
Inferior olivary nucleus
To superior or inferior
cerebellar peduncles

FIGURE 9-3 The neuronal organization within a cerebellar folium. *Right,* transverse section through a folium; *left,* longitudinal section (long axis). The nerve processes of the stellate cells, basket cells, and Purkinje cells are oriented parallel to the transverse plane, the axonal branches of the granule cells are oriented parallel to the longitudinal plane. Note the mossy fiber glomerulus (insert) and climbing-fiber glomerulus (*). The main circuits (thick lines) exerting excitatory influences on the Purkinje cells include (1) mossy fiber→granule cell→ Purkinje cell; (2) climbing fiber→granule cell→Purkinje cell; and (3) climbing fiber→Purkinje cell. The Golgi cells, stellate cells, and basket cells are interneurons integrated into circuits exerting inhibitory influences on the main circuits. Note recurrent collateral fiber supplying feedback from deep cerebellar nuclei to cerebellar cortex.

of dendrites and (2) inhibitory influences indirectly to the Purkinje cells by facilitating the inhibitory stellate and basket cells. This circuit of the mossy fibers to granule cells to stellate and basket cells to Purkinje cells is a *feed-forward* (or *ongoing*) *inhibitory control system.*

The excitatory influences conveyed by the granule cells can be modulated by a *negative feedback control circuit* which helps to sharpen the focus by conveying inhibitory influences upon the granule cell dendrites within the glomeruli. This circuit is composed of granule cell to Golgi cell to granule cell dendrite in a glomerulus; the granule cell facilitates the Golgi

cells to convey inhibitory influences (via an inhibitory presynaptic element of the glomerulus) to the granule cells. The Golgi and granule cells can also be facilitated by collateral branches from the climbing fibers. Additional inhibitory influences can be exerted upon these cortical neurons by collaterals of the Purkinje cell axon, which synapse with the stellate, basket, Golgi, and other Purkinje cells. Some inhibitory influences are conveyed from the locus ceruleus (noradrenergic neurons) to the dendrites of the Purkinje cells (Chap. 8).

The intracerebellar circuits do not act to stop the operation of the system. Rather they act by altering the level of operation of the cerebellum.

The cerebellar cortex has been conceived as an elaborate neuronal complex capable of applying precisely timed inhibitory control upon the processing within the central nervous system through their influences upon the deep cerebellar nuclei. An indication of the precise connectivity within the cerebellum is illustrated by its relations with the inferior olivary nuclei. Olivary fibers terminate on cells of deep cerebellar nuclei that receive input from Purkinje cells which, in turn, receive their climbing fiber input from the same cells of the inferior olivary nuclei.

The basic functional units of the circuitry within the cerebellar cortex are the *sagittal zones* (with each zone oriented at a right angle to the long axis of a felium) of about 1 mm wide and up to more than 100 mm long. In turn, each zone can be subdivided in *sagittal microzones*, each with a width of 200 μm or less. These microzones coupled with their efferent relay neurons located in the deep cerebellar nuclei are considered to be the operational units of the cerebellum (Oscarsson). In a sense, these units correspond with the cell columns of the cerebral cortex (Chap. 16).

PHYSIOLOGIC PROPERTIES OF THE CEREBELLAR CORTEX

The widely accepted concept of the functional property of mossy fiber and climbing fiber systems are that these two systems are elements of an overall interactive system integrated at the Purkinje cell level. Two other hypotheses on the properties of the cerebellar cortical circuitry have been proposed (Llinas).

1. *The two-channel concept.* In this formulation the climbing fiber system and the mossy fiber system represent *two* totally separate channels to the cerebellar cortex, with the two systems "time sharing" a given Purkinje cell. Thus, at any one moment the Purkinje cell may be involved either with a mossy fiber or a climbing fiber generated pattern. Each of these systems conveys both excitatory and inhibitory influences to the Purkinje cells.

2. *The two-dimensional representational state concept.* The mossy fiber afferent system is conceived as utilizing (*a*) the cerebellar cortex as an ongoing, continuous representation of the functional states and positions of the voluntary musculature, joints, limbs, and head and trunk axis at any given instant and (*b*) the general functional state of the cerebellar cortex. In this formulation, the new motor instructions from the body are blended with the "state of readiness" in the cerebellar cortex. In turn, the motor command is modified in the context of the total motor stance of the organism. Therefore, the information conveyed from the periphery via the mossy fiber system, rather than being a true feedback, may serve more to reset the state of readiness of the cerebellar cortex into a "continuously upgraded mirror of the motor functional state."

THE CEREBELLAR PEDUNCLES AND PATHWAYS

Cerebellar afferent connections

There are approximately three times as many cerebellar afferent fibers as cerebellar efferent fibers. Each of the cerebellar peduncles (see Fig. 1-15) contains afferent fibers projecting to the cerebellar cortex (see Figs. 9-4 through 9-6).

The *inferior cerebellar peduncle* (restiform body) conveys "unconscious" exteroceptive and proprioceptive information to the cerebellum from the spinal cord, medulla, and vestibular system. The *posterior spinocerebellar tract* projects ipsilaterally in the paleocerebellum (lobules I to IV) and the caudal vermis. The *cuneocerebellar fibers* from the lateral cuneate nucleus terminate in lobule V of the ipsilateral vermis. The *lateral reticular nucleus* receives input from the spinoreticular, spinothalamic, and rubrobulbar (red nucleus) fibers and projects its output to the neocerebellum. This nucleus is somatotopically organized, with the rostral and caudal parts receiving input from the upper and lower extremities, respectively. The *paramedian reticular nuclei of the medulla* are integrated in a cerebellar-brainstem-reticular-cerebellar feedback circuit.

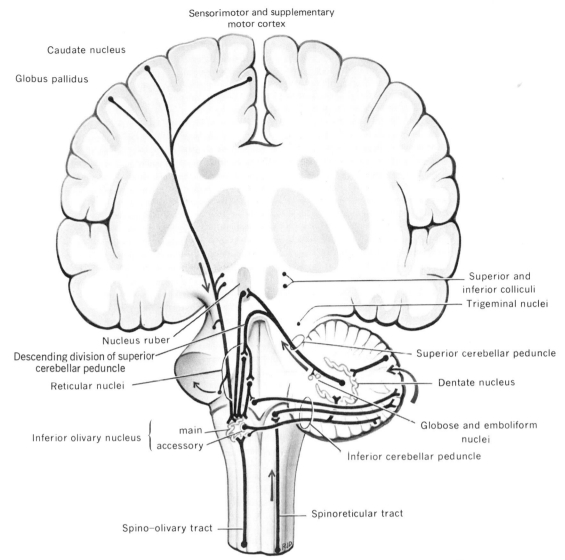

Sensorimotor and supplementary
motor cortex

Caudate nucleus

Globus pallidus

Superior and
inferior colliculi

Trigeminal nuclei

Nucleus ruber

Superior cerebellar peduncle

Descending division of superior
cerebellar peduncle

Reticular nuclei

Dentate nucleus

Inferior olivary nucleus { main
accessory

Globose and emboliform
nuclei

Inferior cerebellar peduncle

Spinoreticular tract

Spino-olivary tract

FIGURE 9-4 Neocerebellar connections with the brainstem. Illustration outlines some cerebellar connections with the brainstem nuclei. Note (1) the circuit from cerebellum to brainstem reticular nuclei (including nucleus ruber and inferior olivary nucleus) back to cerebellum and (2) the input into this circuit from the sensorimotor and supplementary motor cortices, superior and inferior colliculi (visual, auditory, somatosensory systems), and trigeminal nuclei.

The *inferior olivary nuclear complex* projects climbing fibers topographically organized point-to-point to the contralateral deep nuclei and cortex of the cerebellum. The accessory olivary (paleoolivary) nuclei are connected with the vermis and flocculonodular lobe. The principal olivary (neoolivary) nucleus is connected with the cerebellar hemisphere. The inferior olivary nuclei receive afferent input from a variety of sources via crossed and uncrossed projections. Descending topographically organized corticoolivary fibers from the sensorimotor and supplementary motor cortices are derived from the telencephalon (see Fig. 9-4). Mesencephalically derived projections originate in the red nucleus, periaqueductal gray, superior colliculus, and midbrain reticular nuclei. Other fibers originate in the lateral cervical nucleus and the posterior horn and lamina VII of the spinal cord and in the nuclei gracilus and cuneatus and pars caudalis of the spinal trigeminal nucleus.

The input from the vestibular system to the cerebellum is conveyed via the *juxtarestiform body of the inferior cerebellar peduncle* (see Fig. 9-6; see also Fig. A-5). Some direct (first-order) vestibulocerebellar fibers are distributed to the ipsi-

lateral archicerebellum (nodules, uvula, and flocculus). Secondary vestibular fibers from the medial and inferior vestibular nuclei are distributed bilaterally, but mainly ipsilaterally, to the nodulus, uvula, and flocculus and, additionally, to the fastigial nuclei.

The *middle cerebellar peduncle* (brachium pontis) conveys information primarily from the pons (see Fig. 9-5; see also Fig. 1-15). The pontocerebellar tract projects fibers from the pontine nuclei primarily to the contralateral neocerebellum (with some to the contralateral paleocere-

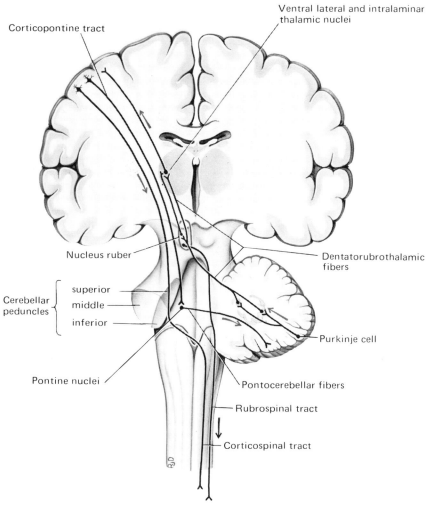

FIGURE 9-5 Neocerebellar connections with the cerebral cortex, thalamus, nucleus ruber, and pontine nuclei. Note (1) the sequence of cerebellum→nucleus ruber→thalamic nuclei→cerebral cortex, and (2) the connections of this sequence with the corticospinal tract, rubrospinal tract, and corticopontine-pontocerebellar pathway.

bellum). A few projections are also conveyed from the pontine nuclei to the ipsilateral neocerebellum. Fibers from the reticulotegmental nucleus pass through the middle cerebellar peduncle on their way to most of the vermis.

The *superior cerebellar peduncle* (brachium conjunctivum) has a few afferent fibers. The anterior spinocerebellar tract projects from the spinal cord to the contralateral paleocerebellum (lobules I to IX).

Visual influences to the cerebellum are derived from retinotectal fibers via the accessory optic pathway to the midbrain (accessory optic nuclei). From midbrain sources descending fibers project to brainstem nuclei and the inferior olivary nucleus (see Fig. 9-4). Mossy fibers and climbing fibers terminate in lobules VI and VII of the vermis. Additional input to these lobules comes from the nuclei of the auditory pathways via reticular nuclei and the inferior olivary nucleus. Trigeminocerebellar fibers to the neocerebellum convey general afferent stimuli from the head. Noradrenergic fibers from the locus ceruleus pass via the superior cerebellar peduncle and white matter before terminating in the cerebellar cortex (see "Locus Ceruleus," Chap. 8).

Cerebellar efferent connections

No direct cerebellospinal pathways exist. The influences from the cerebellum on motor activity are mediated through indirect pathways. The efferent pathways of the inferior cerebellar peduncle are associated primarily with the vestibular system (archicerebellum and the nuclei fastigii); those of the superior cerebellar peduncle, primarily with the neocerebellum and paleocerebellum (dentate, emboliform, and globose nuclei). Efferent fibers are not present in the middle cerebellar peduncle.

The cerebellar cortex projects its influences (all inhibitory) via Purkinje cell axons to the deep cerebellar nuclei and to the lateral vestibular nucleus. The *vermal cortex* projects directly to the fastigial nuclei. Many Purkinje cells of the flocculonodular lobe and anterior portions of the vermis project directly (bypass deep cerebellar nuclei) to the vestibular nuclei. The *paravermal cortex* projects primarily to the interposed nuclei (globose and emboliform nuclei) and slightly to the dentate nucleus. The *cerebellar hemispheric cortex* projects to the dentate nucleus and portions of the interposed nuclei.

Collateral branches of the output fibers of the neurons of the deep cerebellar nuclei project to the cerebellar cortex in a precise and orderly fashion. The corticonuclear axons of the Purkinje cells and the nucleocortical collateral axons of the deep cerebellar nuclei to the cortex are reciprocally organized with groups of neurons of the deep nuclei projecting back to the cerebellar cortical regions from which they receive input (Gould). This output of the deep nuclei is presumably involved in feedback control of the cerebellar cortical neuronal activity.

The *juxtarestiform body* (*medial bundle of the inferior cerebellar peduncle*) consists of fibers associated with the vestibular system, archicerebellum, and nuclei fastigii. The fibers from the fastigal nuclei project via two pathways by way of the juxtarestiform body to all the vestibular nuclei and the brainstem reticular formation: an uncrossed direct fastigiovestibular tract and a crossed and uncrossed uncinate fasciculus (Fig. 9-6; see also 10-13). The *uncinate fasciculus* (*hooked bundle*) is a bundle of fastigiovestibular fibers which arch rostrally around the superior cerebellar peduncle before joining the juxtarestiform body. These fastigiovestibular fibers exert facilitatory influences upon ipsilateral extensor muscle tone. The fastigioreticular projections probably influence the medullary reticulospinal pathways.

The *superior cerebellar peduncle* consists primarily of the efferent fibers from the dentate, emboliform, and globose nuclei (dentate nucleus used to designate efferent tracts) via the dentatorubral, dentatothalamic, and dentatoreticular fibers. The entire outflow completely crosses over in the lower midbrain as the decussation of the superior cerebellar peduncle. Most fibers from the dentate nucleus project rostrally to the ventral lateral thalamic nucleus and the rostral intralaminar (reticular) nuclei of the thalamus with some fibers to the rostral third of the nucleus ruber. The globose and emboliform nuclei project mainly to the caudal two-thirds of the nucleus ruber.

Some efferent fibers from the dentate and interposed nuclei, after crossing in the decussation of the superior cerebellar peduncle, project

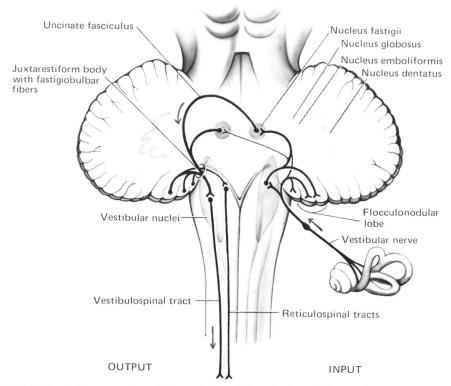

Uncinate fasciculus

Juxtarestiform body
with fastigiobulbar
fibers

Nucleus fastigii
Nucleus globosus
Nucleus emboliformis
Nucleus dentatus

Vestibular nuclei

Flocculonodular
lobe

Vestibular nerve

Vestibulospinal tract

Reticulospinal tracts

OUTPUT

INPUT

FIGURE 9-6 Cerebellar connections of the vestibulocerebellum (archicerebellum and fastigial nucleus) with the vestibular nerve and vestibular nuclei.

caudally as the descending division of the superior cerebellar peduncle. These fibers terminate in the reticulotegmental nucleus, paramedian reticular nuclei of the medulla, and inferior olivary nuclear complex. These fibers and nuclei are integrated into feedback systems projecting back to the cerebellum. The fibers of the reticulotegmental nucleus course through the middle cerebellar peduncle and terminate in the vermis (except for the nodulus). The paramedian reticular nuclei of the medulla also receive a major input from the corticoreticular systems; the fibers from these nuclei pass through the ipsilateral inferior cerebellar peduncle before terminating in the vermis. The fibers of the inferior olivary nuclear complex cross and pass through the inferior cerebellar peduncle and terminate in the contralateral neocerebellum.

General overall circuitry

The neuronal circuits to and from the cerebellum are (1) the source of the polysensory input to

the cerebellum, (2) output from the cerebellum, and (3) links in complex feedback loops.

Polysensory input   The unconscious polysensory input projects to the cerebellar cortex and deep cerebellar nuclei. The impulses derived from these various sources are projected to regions of the cerebellar cortex designated as the somatosensory, visual, auditory (audiovisual), and vestibular areas (archicerebellum). In the rostral neocerebellar cortex is a somatotopic representation of the entire body plan, while in each of the bilateral caudal areas is a somatotopic representation of the ipsilateral half of the body. There is a large overlap of somatic inputs. Each small region receives inputs from many sources. The general proprioceptive endings have an essentially similar representation in these somatosensory areas. Somatotopic projections from the cerebral somesthetic cortex are also represented in these somatosensory areas. Photic and click stimuli send influences, via the optic pathways and auditory pathways, to the midbrain tegmen-

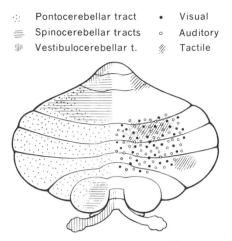

:∴: Pontocerebellar tract   • Visual
≡   Spinocerebellar tracts   ○ Auditory
⫼   Vestibulocerebellar t.   ▨ Tactile

FIGURE 9-7 Projection areas on the cerebellar cortex that receive influences from outside the cerebellum. (*Adapted from Snider.*)

tum and from there to lower brainstem nuclei that, in turn, project to the coextensive audiovisual area of the neocerebellar cortex (see Fig. 9-7). Vestibular influences are conveyed to the archicerebellum in the vestibular pathways (Chap. 10).

The influences from the neuromuscular spindles from the extraocular muscles, a nonvisual source of information about eye position, are relayed to lobules VI and VII of the vermis.

The patterns of distribution of mossy fibers and climbing fibers and of the geometric relations of the granule and basket cells to the Purkinje cells are organized to produce certain functional effects. Each climbing fiber and its branches terminate on several Purkinje cells in a limited region of the cortex. Each Purkinje cell receives input from only one climbing fiber. In contrast, each mossy fiber and its branches project diffusely to granule cells whose parallel fibers are distributed to extensive regions of the cortex. The spread is increased through the connections with the stellate and basket cells whose axons are aligned at right angles to the parallel fibers and plane of arborization of the dendritic tree of Purkinje cells. This orientation of the stellate and basket cells results in inhibitory processing in effecting some macroeffects of contrast inhibition (Chaps. 3 and 12) between rows of Purkinje cells. The effect can be explained in relation to the geometric patterns of

these neurons. Within each folium, the Purkinje cells and their dendritic trees are lined up in adjacent rows parallel to the long axis of each folium. The stellate and basket cells are oriented so that their cell bodies are located within a row of Purkinje cells while their axons extend and cut across the Purkinje cell plane into the territory of an adjacent row of Purkinje cells. Assume the circuitry excites through the parallel and climbing fibers all the Purkinje, stellate, and basket cells in one of these rows. The turned-on stellate and basket cells can through their cutting across axons exert inhibitory effects on Purkinje cells in adjacent rows. This inhibition on adjacent parallel rows on either side of the excited row results in contrast inhibition (Chap. 3 and 12). This is one of the means by which the cerebellar cortex is stimulated differentially.

The noradrenergic fibers from the locus coeruleus (Chap. 8) to the cerebellar cortex are presumed to exert a modulatory effect on the cerebellum.

Output In a general way, the output of the cerebellum, except for the feedback loops, may be conceived as being integrated into three pathway systems involved with somatic motor activity.

1. The *cerebellar vermal zone*, including the flocculonodular lobe through its main connections with the fastigial and vestibular nuclei, exerts its influences via the vestibulospinal tracts upon spinal reflexes (see Fig. 9-6). This system has a role in facilitating extensor muscle tone.

2. The *cerebellar paravermal zone*, through its main connections with the ipsilateral nucleus interpositus and contralateral nucleus ruber, exerts its influences via the crossed rubrospinal tract upon spinal reflexes (see Fig. 9-5). This system has a role in facilitating flexor muscle tone on the side ipsilateral to the paravermal zone.

3. The *cerebellar hemispheric zone* (*neocerebellum*), through its connections with the dentate nucleus and the ventral lateral (VL) nucleus of the thalamus, exerts powerful effects upon the motor cortex (see Figs. 9-4 and 9-5). In turn this input from the cerebellum to the motor cortex influences the activity of the cor-

ticospinal, corticorubrospinal, and corticore-ticulospinal systems. These pathways are essential in the coordination of somatic motor activity.

Feedback loops The cerebellum is integrated into a number of circuits and feedback loops (see Figs. 9-3 through 9-6).

1. The short *intracerebellar loops* include (*a*) the recurrent inhibitory pathway of granule cells to Golgi cells back to the dendrites of the granule cells in the glomeruli (negative feedback loops); (*b*) the inhibitory pathways of granule cells via basket cells and stellate cells to the Purkinje cells (feed-forward or ongoing inhibitory control circuits); and (*c*) pathway of the recurrent collaterals of Purkinje cells back to cerebellar interneurons and either to the same or other Purkinje cells (see Fig. 9-3).
2. *The long intracerebellar loop* includes (*a*) Purkinje cells to deep cerebellar nuclei and (*b*) recurrent collaterals from axons of deep cerebellar nuclei that feed back to the cerebellar cortex. These recurrent collaterals are referred to as *nucleocortical projections*.
3. The *vestibular-archicerebellar loop* (see Fig. 9-6; see also Fig. 10-13) includes the connections from the vestibular nerve and vestibular nuclei to the archicerebellum and fastigial nuclei, and the output from the latter through the juxtarestiform body to the vestibular nuclei and reticular nuclei of the brainstem. This loop is an integral part of the vestibular system (Chap. 10).
4. The *cerebrocerebellar loop* (see Figs. 9-4 and 9-5) interconnects the cerebrum and the cerebellum. It includes, in order, the corticopontine tracts (from wide areas of the cerebral cortex to the ipsilateral pontine nuclei), the mainly crossed pontocerebellar tracts to the contralateral cerebellar cortex, the Purkinje cell axons of the cerebellar cortex to the deep cerebellar nuclei, and the dentatorubrothalamic cortical pathway that projects to the cerebral cortex. The latter pathway has neural processing stations in the nucleus ruber and ventral lateral thalamic nuclei of the opposite side (crossing occurs at the decussation of the superior cerebellar peduncle) before projecting topically to the cerebral motor cor-

tex. This circuit interrelates the cerebral cortex of one side and the cerebellar cortex of the opposite side, and it is a significant system in phasic locomotor acitvities. Volitional movements initiated in the cerebrum utilize this feedback system to modulate coordinated movements. The corticopontine and pontocerebellar tracts are the pathways by which the auditory, visual, general somesthetic, and motor areas of the cerebral cortex transmit their influences to the cerebellum. Much of the cerebral neocortex evolved together with the cortex of the neocerebellum.

5. *Cerebellar-brainstem-reticular-cerebellar loops* (see Fig. 9-4) comprise, in order, (*a*) deep cerebellar nuclei (fastigial, emboliform, and globose nuclei); (*b*) nucleus ruber and lower brainstem nuclei (reticulotegmental, paramedian reticular nuclei of medulla); (*c*) nucleus ruber projections to inferior olivary nucleus and reticular nuclei pedunculopontine, pontis oralis, pontis caudalis, and gigantocellularis; and (*d*) projections via mossy and climbing fibers from these nuclei to the deep cerebellar nuclei and cerebellar cortex.

These "loops" should be thought of not as self-contained circuits but rather as sequences of tracts which are indicative of the complexities of the interconnections of the cerebellum with other centers of the brain. Of significance are the numerous influences upon these loops from other centers and the influences of these loops upon other centers. For example, collaterals from the corticospinal tract have connections with the ventral lateral nucleus of the thalamus, nucleus ruber, pontine nuclei, lateral reticular nucleus, and inferior olivary nuclear complex.

FUNCTIONAL ASPECTS OF THE CEREBELLUM

The cerebellum is the great modulator subserving the coordination of groups of muscles (synergy). Its significant background role is expressed in the simple and complex movements associated with standing, walking, sitting, running, and dextrous finger and hand manipulations. The cerebellum smooths out the actions of muscle groups by delicately regulating and grading muscle tensions. It has been conceived as an organ which is continuously receiving input from the neuromuscular and Golgi tendon sensors in the muscles and tendons regarding the moment-to-moment status of the tension within the muscular system. This information is utilized by the motor pathway systems.

The cerebellum acts as a servomechanism in a negative feedback system, functioning to prevent oscillations (tremor) during motion and thereby maintaining stability in a movement (Chap. 3). Marked injury to the cerebellum releases other regions of the nervous system from cerebellar influences. The resulting *release phenomena* illustrate the loss of the effects of the negative feedback system. In the motion of moving the upper extremity to touch an object with the tip of the finger, an intention tremor results, with the extremity oscillating in a series of rhythmic movements as the object is approached. This resembles the automatic pilot and automatic antiaircraft control systems, in which each correction is followed by an overshoot. In normal cerebellar activity the negative feedback activity reduces the overshoot to insignificance.

The unconscious *polysensory input* from the tactile, proprioceptive, vestibular, auditory, visual, and visceral sources is processed by the cerebellum and utilized in the activities of the cerebellum. The functional expression of the cerebellum is channeled into (1) equilibration and tonus and (2) voluntary movements. Equilibration and tonus are utilized in the static and postural activities of standing, sitting, and balancing. *Muscle tone* (hypotonus and hypertonus) is influenced and modified by the archicerebellum and paleocerebellum. The facilitation of extensor muscle tone is mediated through connections with the lateral vestibular nucleus (vestibulospinal tract) and reticular nuclei of the brainstem (medullary reticulospinal tract); its inhibition is mediated through connections with other reticular nuclei. The phasic or locomotive movements involved in the voluntary movements are mediated largely through the cerebrum-to-neocerebellum-to-cerebrum feedback circuit, with the corticospinal tract as the major pathway for the expression of the neocerebellum. The paravermal cortex is particularly involved with facilitatory influences on extensor

muscle tone, whereas the vermal cortex has a role in flexor muscle tone.

Much of the information fed into the cerebellum relates to activity that precedes the generation of movement, rather than to activity that serves as a feedback corrective signal (Llinás). Thus, the cerebellum is utilized for the generation of new movements inasmuch as the cerebellum automatically takes dynamic as well as static parameters into account when applying corrective measures to a motor command. In this sense, the cerebellum acts to serve as more than a feedback when the afferent information is utilized for motor error correction. In addition, the input fed in from the periphery serves to upgrade the state of readiness of the cerebellar cortex into a continuously modified mirror of the motor functional state.

Posture control

Posture control is coordinated and regulated by processing centers located in all levels of the central nervous system. An understanding of the structural and functional interrelations of several of these centers explains a number of the phenomena associated with the complex control mechanisms of posture. The nodal regions comprise the sensorimotor cortex, pontine reticular nuclei (nuclei reticularis, pontis oralis, and caudalis; reticular extensor facilitatory area), medullary reticular nuclei (nucleus gigantocellularis, bulbar reticular inhibitory area), vestibular nuclei of the anterior lobe of the cerebellum, and neuronal motor parts in the gray matter of the spinal cord (see Fig. 9-6; see also Figs. 5-28 and 5-29). Each of these regions is, in turn, integrated into special subcircuits.

Two of the critical features in this organization are the roles of (1) the spinal neuronal pools and (2) the three brainstem centers projecting influences to these spinal pools. The spinal pools are organized to regulate muscle activity through the alpha and gamma motor neurons. The brainstem centers comprise the pontine reticular, medullary reticular, and vestibular nuclei. The pontine reticular nuclei, acting through the pontine reticulospinal tract (see Fig. 5-29), facilitate extension and inhibit flexion. The medullary reticular nuclei, acting through the medullary reticulospinal tract, inhibit extension and facilitate flexion. These two pathways operate mainly through the gamma motor neurons. The lateral vestibular nucleus, acting through the lateral vestibulospinal tract, facilitates extension; this pathway does have direct connections with the alpha motor neurons.

These brainstem nuclear complexes are, in turn, influenced by inputs from other centers. The pontine reticular nuclei are excited by sensory input from the joints and muscle receptors from ascending pathways in the spinal cord and brainstem. The medullary reticular nuclei are excited by influences from the sensorimotor cortex. The lateral vestibular nucleus is excited by input from the vestibular end organs and is inhibited by influences from the anterior lobe of the cerebellum.

These inputs can explain a number of experimentally observed phenomena. For example, the decerebrate animal (transected at the midbrain level), displays extensor rigidity—an increase in the middle tone of agonist and antagonist musculature. This may be explained by the decrease in inhibitory influences following the removal of the excitatory influences from the sensorimotor cortex to the medullary reticular nuclei. In this condition the excitatory influences from the pontine reticular nuclei and lateral vestibular nuclei are presumed to dominate.

When the dorsal roots to a limb of a decerebrate animal are cut, the rigidity is lost and the denervated limb becomes flaccid. This indicates that the rigidity has a reflex component and is largely mediated through the activity of the gamma motor neurons with the gamma loop activating the alpha motor neurons. Thus, in rigidity the alpha motor neurons are made more active by (1) direct effects from the vestibulospinal tract and (2) indirect effects of medullary reticulospinal tract on the gamma loop. The severance of the dorsal roots reduces the rigidity because the gamma loop is interrupted. Rigidity in the decerebrate animal can also be lost following ablation of the lateral vestibular nuclei. This occurs because the vestibular system furnishes background facilitation directly to the alpha motor neurons. The role of the vestibular system in rigidity is in enhancing muscle tone. The decerebrate animal exhibits even more rigidity following ablation of the anterior lobe of the cerebellum. This results because the inhibitory influences normally projected to the lateral vestibular nuclei are removed. In effect, the vestibular nuclei are released. The concomitant increase in the flow of excitatory influences to the alpha motor neurons further enhances the rigidity—such an animal is called an alpha neuron preparation. The ablation of the lateral vestibular nucleus in alpha neuron preparations produces an animal with "normal" rigidity. In this condition the medullary reticular nuclei are active in driving the gamma motor neurons and the gamma system—such an animal is called a gamma motor preparation.

CEREBELLAR DYSFUNCTION

Lesions of the cerebellum or of its input or its output result in a characteristic constellation of symptoms expressed on the motor side. The disturbances are actually the result of the activity of other units (such as the lateral ventral thalamic nucleus) of the nervous system that are functionally intact. These functional units are released (*release phenomenon*) from cerebellar influences. Following lesions of the cerebellum, volitional motor activity usually results in an excess of motion.

Neocerebellar lesions

Dysfunction of the neocerebellum produces a complex of clinical disorders. These symptoms are primarily the result of the release of cerebellar influences on the thalamic nuclei, for neocerebellar symptoms are abolished or reduced by lesions in the ventral lateral thalamic nucleus and intralaminar nuclei of the thalamus. The tendon reflexes are diminished (*hypotonia*), this effect being expressed at times as a pendular knee jerk that swings freely back and forth. The muscles are weak and flabby and tire easily (*asthenia*). The horizontally extended forelimb will gradually drift downward when the eyes are closed because the proprioceptive sense from the extremity is not being used properly. *Asynergia*, or loss of muscular coordination, is revealed by jerky, puppetlike movements, including *decomposition of movement, dysmetria, past pointing, dysdiadochokinesia*, and the *rebound phenomenon*.

The *decomposition of movement* is the breaking up of the movement into its component parts, as in the finger-to-nose test. Instead of a smooth, coordinated flow of movement in bringing the tip of the finger of the extended upper extremity to the nose, each joint of the shoulder, elbow, wrist, and fingers may flex independently (puppetlike) in an almost mechanical fashion.

Dysmetria, or the inability to gauge or measure distances accurately, results in the overshooting of the intended goal by consistently pointing to the lesion side of the object (past pointing).

Dysdiadochokinesia is impaired ability to execute alternating and repetitive movements, such as supination and pronation of the forearm, in rapid succession with equal excursions. The limb on the lesion side will perform the movements more slowly and clumsily.

The *intention or action tremor* is expressed during the execution of a voluntary movement. It is absent or diminished during rest. These tremors are particularly noted at the end of the movement (terminal tremor).

The *ataxic gait*, or the asynergic activity elicited during walking, is a staggering gait resembling that of drunkenness. (The cerebellum is sensitive to alcohol and to slight circulatory impairment.) The ataxia is due to incoordination of the trunk and proximal shoulder and pelvic girdle muscles. A tendency to veer or to fall to the side of the lesion is apparent. To counteract the unsteadiness, the patient will stand or walk with legs far apart (broad-base stance).

The loss of the normal check of antagonist over an agonist muscle results in the *rebound phenomenon*. When the actively flexed forearm, held within a few inches of the face, is suddenly released, the open hand does not hit the face in the normal individual (normal rebound), because the antagonistic extensor muscles check the flexor muscles immediately. Patients with a cerebellar lesion will hit their faces because the antagonist muscles contract too late.

A *scanning speech*, or *dysarthria*, is a result of the incoordination of the muscles used in speaking. The speech is hesitating, slurred, and explosive in quality, with a telegram-staccato pace (pauses in the wrong places). Nystagmus does not occur following a cerebellar lesion.

Archicerebellar lesions

Lesion of the uvula and flocculonodular lobe may result in ataxia of the trunk muscles without any signs of tremor or hypotonia (archicerebellar syndrome). There are bilateral disturbances of locomotion and equilibrium similar to that accompaning labyrinthectomy. Children with nodular lobe tumors (archicerebellum) have a tendency to fall backward, sway from side to side, and walk with a wide base. They may be unable to maintain equilibrium or an upright balance. This *truncal ataxia* resembles the walk of a drunkard; there is staggering accompanied by a tendency to fall to the side or backward. An experimental animal with ablated nodulus is not subject to motion sickness and can swim upright under water. An animal without semicircular canals of the vestibular system is unable to swim upright under water (Chap. 10).

Paleocerebellar lesions

There is a probable increase in extensor muscle tone and postural reflexes so as to resemble decerebrate rigidity. The experimental ablation of the entire anterior lobe in animals produces a decerebrate rigidity (see "Postural Control").

General comment

Unilateral cerebellar lesions have homolateral effects. The symptoms are expressed on the same side because the pathways from the cerebellum decussate and integrate with systems that in turn cross over to the side of the original cerebellar output, before exerting their effects. For example the crossed dentatorubrothalamocortical ascending pathways have connections with the contralateral nucleus ruber, thalamus, and cerebral cortex. The rubrospinal and corticospinal tracts are crossed descending tracts. In effect the cerebellum exerts its influences primarily through a *double crossing* of (1) the ascending fibers of the superior cerebellar peduncle and (2) the descending fibers of the corticospinal tract.

Lesions of the cerebellum result in inadequacy of certain responses and general symptoms. The disturbance is expressed in the constellation of symptoms and neurologic signs previously noted. Small lesions may produce no symptoms or only transient symptoms, whereas large lesions produce severe symptoms. The cerebellum possesses a good margin of physiologic safety; with time the neurologic symptoms attenuate and the resulting compensation markedly reduces the severity of the deficits. The reasons for this phenomenon are not fully known but are probably related to the polysensory input which is integrated in a cortex that is similar throughout. The reduction of certain input is compensated for by other input sources that become adequate for effective activity. Cerebellar cortical lesions are notable for being associated with attenuating deficits and reduction in severity of the symptoms with time, whereas damage to the deep cerebellar nuclei or superior cerebellar peduncle is accomplished by similar but lasting (nonattenuating) and more enduring deficits.

Of clinical significance is the fact that the cerebellum is bounded on most of its sides by the rigid and taut tentorium and the bony wall of the posterior fossa. As a consequence, the pressure exerted by an enlarging lesion of the cerebellum from a tumor or hemorrhage is directed upon the pons and medulla. The result can be life-threatening because of the effects on the vital cardiovascular and respiratory centers within the lower brainstem.

BIBLIOGRAPHY

Eager, R. P.: "Modes of Termination of Purkinje cell Axons in the Cerebellum of the Cat," in R. Llinás (ed.), *Neurobiology of Cerebellar Evolution and De-velopment,* American Medical Association, Chicago, 1969, pp. 585–601.

Eccles, J. C., M. Ito, and J. Szentágothai: *The Cerebellum as a Neuronal Machine,* Springer-Verlag, New York, 1967.

Fields, W. S., and W. D. Willis: *The Cerebellum in Health and Disease,* Warren H. Green, Inc., St. Louis, 1970.

Fox, C. A., and R. S. Snider (eds.): The cerebellum. Prog Brain Res, 25:1–335, 1967.

Gould, B. B.: The organization of afferents to the cerebellar cortex in the cat: Projections from the deep cerebellar nuclei. J Comp Neur, 184:27–42. 1979.

Larsell, O., and J. Jansen: *Cerebellum: The Human Cerebellum, Cerebellar Connections and Cerebellar Cortex,* The University of Minnesota Press, Minneapolis, 1972.

Llinás, R. (ed.): *Neurobiology of Cerebellar Evolution and Development,* American Medical Association, Chicago, 1969.

Meyer-Lehmann, J., J. Hore, and V. B. Brooks: Cerebellar participation in generation of prompt arm movements. J Neurophysiol, 40:1038–1050, 1977.

Oscarsson, O.: Functional units of the cerebellum-sagittal zones and microzones. Trends Neurosci, 2:143–145, 1979.

Nieuwenhuys, R.: "Comparative Anatomy of the Cerebellum," in C. A. Fox and R. S. Snider (eds.), The cerebellum. Prog Brain Res, 25:1–93, 1967.

Palay, S. L., and V. Chan-Palay: *Cerebellar Cortex: Cytology and Organization,* Springer-Verlag, Berlin, 1974.

Snider, R. S.: Recent contributions to the anatomy and physiology of the cerebellum. Arch Neurol Psychiatry, 64:196–219, 1950.

Zagon, J. S., P. S. McLaughlin, and S. Smith: Neural populations in the human cerebellum: Estimation from isolated cell nuclei. Brain Res, 127:279–282, 1977.

CHAPTER TEN

THE EAR, AUDITORY SYSTEM, AND VESTIBULAR SYSTEM

The ear consists of two functional units: the acoustic apparatus, concerned with the exteroceptive sense called hearing, and the vestibular apparatus, concerned with the special proprioceptive sense involved with posture and equilibrium. The former is innervated by the *cochlear nerve*, the latter by the *vestibular nerve*. These two nerves are collectively known as the *vestibulocochlear, auditory, statoacoustic*, or *eighth cranial nerve*.

THE LABYRINTHS

The sensory receptors of the cochlear system and the vestibular system are located in a complex of canals and vesicles called the *membranous labyrinth* (see Figs. 10-1 and 10-2). The tube of this membranous labyrinth is filled with a fluid called *endolymph*. The membranous labyrinth is in turn surrounded by canals and vesicles filled with a fluid called *perilymph*. The entire complex is encased by a rigid box called the *bony labyrinth*. The endolymph and the perilymph, which have different chemical compositions and electrical potentials, are not continuous with each other.

The endolymph has a high concentration of potassium ions and a low concentration of sodium ions, whereas the perilymph has a high concentration of sodium ions and a low concentration of potassium ions; this is reminiscent of the intra- and extracellular concentrations of these ions.

An analogous structural model would be a closed tube encased by another tube. The inner tube would be the membranous labyrinth containing the endolymph (see Fig. 10-2). The outer tube is within the bony labyrinth. The perilymph fills the cavity of the outer tube and surrounds the inner tube (see Fig. 10-2).

The *membranous labyrinth* consists of the three semicircular ducts, utricle, and saccule, which are associated with the vestibular system, and the cochlear duct (scala media) which is associated with the auditory system (see Fig. 10-3). Each semicircular duct is in open communication at each end of the utricle. By definition, the semicircular ducts are bounded by the membranous labyrinth, and the semicircular canals by the bony labyrinth; the ducts are erroneously called canals. Each semicircular duct has one bulbous portion, the ampulla.

The entire membranous labyrinth (cochlear duct, saccule, utricle, semicircular ducts, and endolymphatic duct and sac) is filled with endolymph. This endolymph is actively formed in both the cochlear and vestibular portions of the labyrinth. The endolymphatic sac is located between layers of a well-vascularized region of the dura mater on the posterior face of the petrous bone (see Fig. 10-2). The perilymphatic space is connected through the narrow cochlear canaliculus to the subarachnoid space near the endolymphatic sac.

There are six specialized sensory epithelial receptor areas in contact with the terminal endings of the eighth cranial nerve. These are the three cristae ampullae (one in the ampulla of each semicircular duct), one macula utriculi, one macula sacculi, and a long ribbonlike spiral organ of Corti in the cochlea.

Within the bony labyrinth of the auditory system are three ducts: the scala vestibuli, scala

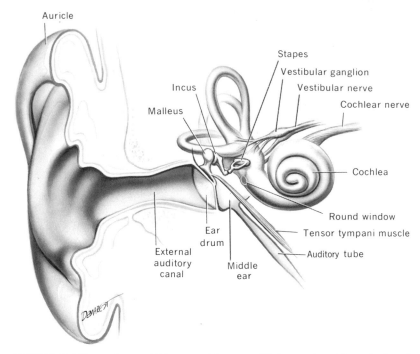

FIGURE 10-1 External ear, middle ear, and inner ear. (Right ear viewed from the front.)

tympani, and cochlear. The ducts, arranged in parallel, ascend in a spiral 2¾ times around the bony core, or modiolus.

The cochlear duct of the membranous labyrinth extends between the two scalae. Its roof is the vestibular (Reissner's) membrane, adjoining the scala vestibuli. Its floor is the basilar membrane, bordering the scala tympani. Resting on the basilar membrane is the spiral organ of Corti, the organ of hearing. The surface of the spiral organ is bounded by the reticular membrane (see Fig. 10-3). The last two membranes together with the spiral organ itself comprise the cochlear partition. The term *cochlea* refers to the cochlear duct, with the spiral organ of Corti and the scalae vestibuli and tympani.

The cochlear duct, like the entire membranous labyrinth, is filled with endolymph. The reticular membrane prevents endolymph from entering the spaces of the spiral organ. The scalae vestibuli and tympani, like the rest of the bony labyrinth, are filled with perilymph.

The vestibular organs lie superiorly in the inner ear; the cochlea lies inferiorly.

THE AUDITORY SYSTEM

The auditory system is organized to detect several aspects of sound: frequency (pitch), intensity (loudness), and spatial location (direction).

Outer ear and middle ear

Airborne vibrations may be perceived as sounds by our auditory system or as vibrations by our sense of 'touch." The vibrations that are heard are conveyed successively through the outer ear, middle ear, and inner ear before reaching the sensory receptors of the spiral organ of Corti (see Figs. 10-1 and 10-2). Sounds can also reach the ears through solids or liquids.

The *outer ear* consists of the auricle and the *external acoustic meatus* (auditory canal); it ends at the oval-shaped tympanic membrane (eardrum). The canal acts as a resonator, especially at the frequencies of greatest acuity (2000 to 5500 Hz), and as a buffer against temperature and humidity changes which can alter the elasticity of the drum. The tympanic membrane is a

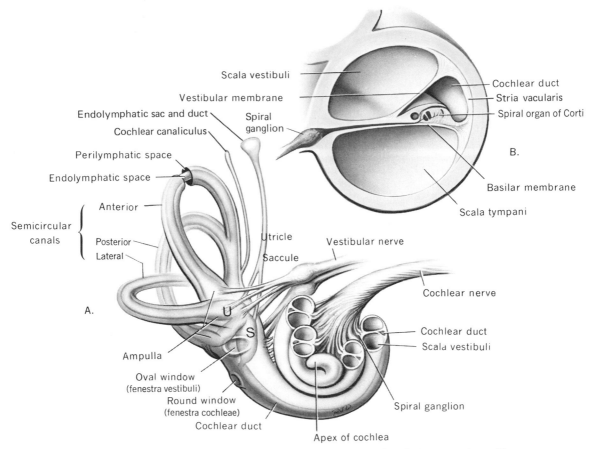

FIGURE 10-2 The labyrinth. *A*. Right labyrinth, from the front. The perilymphatic space is located between the bony labyrinth and the membranous labyrinth; it extends as the cochlear canaliculus. The endolymphatic space is located within the membranous labyrinth, which includes the three semicircular ducts, utricle, saccule, cochlear duct, and endolymphatic duct and sac. *B*. Cross section through the cochlea. The scala vestibuli and scala tympani are connected through a passage called the helicotrema, located at the apex of the cochlea.

thin, slightly stiff cone (like a paper-cone loudspeaker) sensitive to airborne vibrations. The remarkable sensitivity of the tympanic membrane offers an example of extreme biologic miniaturization, for air movements in ordinary conversation produce inward and outward displacements of the membrane of about the diameter of the hydrogen atom. This atomic displacement is almost at thermal Brownian movement level. The most sensitive frequency in the region of 3000 Hz is on the order of one-tenth of one angstrom unit (0.1 Å).

Because the threshold of hearing is low, the transfer of the vibratory energy from the com-

pressible atmospheric air (low impedance) to the incompressible perilymphatic fluid (high impedance) of the inner ear must be accomplished without any appreciable loss of energy. The impedance matching device that effects this efficient energy transfer includes the sequence from the tympanic membrane to the solid levers (ear bones), to the liquid perilymph, to the (solid) sensory hair cell receptors in the spiral organ of Corti. The device works at 99.9 percent transmission efficiency. The ear is considered a more efficient energy converter than the eye.

The *middle ear (tympanic cavity)* is a small chamber located between the tympanic membrane and the inner ear. The three ear ossicles (malleus, incus, and stapes) are located in the middle ear, which is continuous with the throat via the auditory (eustachian, pharyngotympanic) tube (see Fig. 10-1).

The ear bones of the middle ear form the lever chain extending from the tympanic membrane to the inner ear. The bones are the malleus (hammer), incus (anvil), and stapes (stirrup), in that order. The oval foot of the stapes fits into the oval window (fenestra vestibuli in the bony labyrinth) which is the site of the functional contact between the stapes and the perilymph of the inner ear. The efficiency of the energy transfer from the tympanic membrane to the oval window is enhanced (1) by the arrangement of the connective tissue fibers within the tympanic membrane and (2) by the fact that the tympanic membrane has an area which is about 18 times greater than that of the oval window. This real difference accounts for the great hydraulic piston thrusts of the stapes on the perilymph (even though the total force exerted in the tympanic membrane and the oval window is about equal). The lever action of the ear ossicles contributes only slightly to the energy transfer. Therefore the middle ear is an efficient transformer; it converts the large-amplitude, low-force vibrations of the sound in the air at the tympanic membrane to the low-amplitude, large-force vibrations at the oval window with a net increase in force.

These bony levers are important; airborne vibrations are almost impossible to hear when these ear ossicles are fused and become immobilized. This condition, called *otosclerosis,* also occurs following the formation of new bone around the round window. Use of a hearing aid, which utilizes bone conduction, can make hearing essentially normal in persons with fused bony ossicles. In hearing by bone conduction, the vibrations are conducted through the bones of the skull (bypassing ear ossicles) to the cochlea. Bone conduction plays little part in hearing ordinary sounds, except by adding resonance and body to one's voice. This is why our voices sound different to us than to others, and why a tape recording of our voices sounds different from our voices when we are speaking.

Adjustments to sounds are afforded by the two tiny muscles that are inserted into two of the ear ossicles—the tensor tympani muscle into the arm of malleus, and the stapedius muscle into the neck of the stapes. The tensor tympani and the stapedius muscles are innervated, respectively, by branches of the trigeminal and facial nerves. The tensor tympani and the stapedius respond primarily to sound stimuli and are synergistic with actions opposite to each other on the bones of the chain. The *stapedial reflex* involves the sequence of cochlear nerve (spiral ganglion), cochlear nuclei, superior olivary nucleus, to nucleus and fibers of facial nerve to the stapedius muscle. The tensor tympani responds to stimuli produced by vocalization, yawning, and swallowing by the sequence of afferent fibers in the trigeminal nerve and via the efferent fibers from the motor nucleus of the trigeminal nerve to the tensor tympani muscle. The contractions of the stapedius muscle have a dampening effect, especially to loud sounds, by exerting tension on the stapes. Sustained loud sounds can cause damage. In addition, weak sounds may be magnified and amplified as much as 50 times by decreasing the tension on the ear ossicles by the relaxation of these muscles. The tensor tympani regulates the stiffness of the tympanic membrane. In effect, these muscles increase the range of loudness we hear through dampening and magnification. The contraction of these muscles provides a protective mechanism, producing a significant attenuation of cochlear excitation for frequencies less than 1000 Hz. This attenuation can reach 40 dB. This *acoustic reflex* is analogous to the pupilloconstrictor reflex of the eye to bright and dim light. The cochlea is not protected by the stapedial reflex when subjected to a sudden explosion (e.g., a gunshot) or to a sustained loud noise; this occurs because the latent period is relatively long and the muscle adapts.

The middle ear is connected to the pharynx through the normally closed auditory tube. Discomfort from the differential pressure on the tympanic membrane results from changing atmospheric pressures (e.g., during ascent or descent in an elevator). This discomfort can be alleviated by opening the auditory tube by swallowing movements, because this permits the atmospheric pressure in the pharynx to force air to enter (or leave) the middle ear cavity and equalize the atmospheric pressure on the outside of the tympanic membrane. The air pressure within the middle ear would not be maintained without the presence of an auditory tube; the pressure would fall because gases within enclosed body cavities are naturally absorbed by the vascular system.

Inner ear

The vibrations of the stapes are converted at the oval window into pressure waves in the perilymph of the inner ear. These pressure waves travel up through the perilymph of the scala vestibuli to the helicotrema at the apex of the cochlea and, along the way, are transmitted across the vestibular membrane to the endolymph of the cochlear duct. After passing through the helicotrema, the vibrations travel down the perilymph of the scala tympani and are transmitted to the basilar membrane and the spiral organ of

Corti, and finally to the thin resilient membrane of the round window at the base of the cochlea. This membrane at the round window accommodates the vibratory motions of the perilymph originally generated at the oval window. The inward (or outward) thrust of the stapes is accompanied, after a fraction of a second, by the outward (or inward) compensatory movement of the membrane at the round window.

The spiral organ of Corti and the basilar membrane are attached on either side of the bony labyrinth, along the entire 35-mm length of the cochlear coil. The membrane gradually widens as it ascends; it broadens from 0.08 mm wide at the base to 0.52 mm at the apical end (Fig. 10-6). The spiral organ of Corti is an organized complex of supporting cells and hair cells (Fig. 10-3). Hair cells (neuroepithelial sensory end organs) are arranged in rows along the

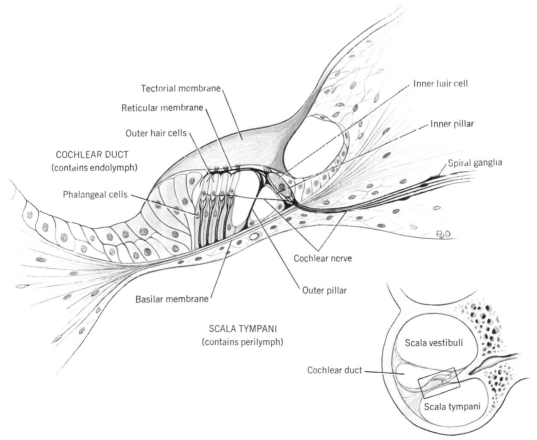

FIGURE 10-3 Cross section through the spinal organ of Corti. Because of angle of section four hair cells may be present.

length of the coil. The outer hair cells are arranged in three rows. The inner hair cells are in a single row. There are about 3500 inner hair cells and roughly 12,000 to 13,000 outer hair cells.

Although differences exist between the inner and outer hair cells, the similarities are important. Both have bristlelike *sensory hairs* (see Fig. 10-4), which are specialized microvilli; these sensory hairs, or stereocilia, are similar to those of the vestibular hair cells described later in the chapter and shown in Fig. 10-9. Each outer hair cell has from 80 to 100 sensory hairs, while each inner hair cell has from 40 to 60 sensory hairs. They are arranged in each hair cell in rows that form the letter W or U, with the base of the letter directed laterally (see Fig. 10-5). The tips of many hairs are embedded within and firmly bound to the tectorial membrane or one of its specialized portions. The tectorial membrane is an acellular protein structure similar to epidermal keratin. One of its specialized portions, on

its undersurface, is *Hardesty's membrane.* The tips of many hairs of the outer hair cells are embedded within it. Another specialized area on the underside of the tectorial membrane is *Hensen's stripe.* The tips of many of the hairs on the inner hair cells may be in contact with it.

Because the basilar membrane and the rigid tectorial membrane are hinged to different sites, a shearing (tangential) motion develops when these structures vibrate, and as a result the sensory hairs of the hair cells are displaced. The hairs are probably stiff levers that do not bend. Rather, the stiff bundle of hairs of a cell may depress or elevate the basal body (see Fig. 10-4). This distortion of the basal body region is presumed to be the event that triggers the generation of the receptor potential. The basal body is a remnant of a kinocilium like that associated with the hair cells of the vestibular receptors (see Fig. 10-9). (A kinocilium is a true cilium, not a microvillus.)

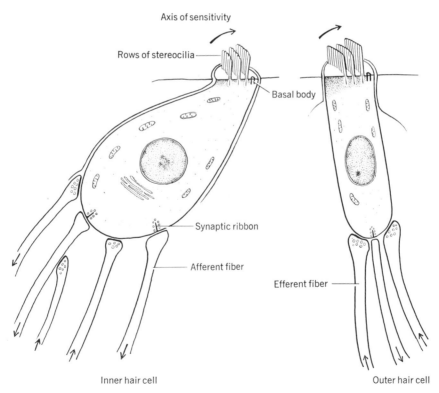

FIGURE 10-4 The hair cells of the spiral organ of Corti. The axis of sensitivity of a cochlear hair cell is in the direction of the basal body. (*After Wersäll and Flock.*)

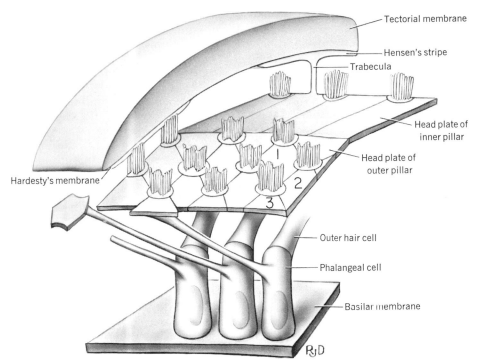

FIGURE 10-5 The spiral organ of Corti viewed from the outer rim of the tectorial membrane. The tips of the long hairs of the outer hair cells are embedded in the tectorial membrane; those of the inner hair cells probably are not. Along with the head plates of the inner and outer pillars, the expanded phalanges (1, 2, 3) of the processes of the phalangeal cells form the bulk of the reticular membrane. (*From Rivera-Dominquez, Agate, and Noback, Brain Research, Elsevier Publishing Company, Amsterdam, The Netherlands, 1974.*)

The hair cells are the mechanoreceptors in which transduction of the mechanical energy of the sound waves into the generator potentials of the cochlear nerve endings occurs. The response in the hair cell and nerve terminals is graded. Each hair cell is innervated by several neurons. The nerve terminals of the myelinated cochlear nerve fibers are naked fibers (unmyelinated and without neurolemma cell sheaths) that conduct with decrement. In total, there are about 15,000 to 16,000 hair cells in the spiral organ of Corti and approximately 30,000 neurons and fibers in the cochlear nerve of humans.

The hairs act both as transducers and as biologic amplifiers (Khanna and Tonndorf). Whereas the displacement amplitude of the tympanic membrane can range to atomic dimensions, the displacement of the basilar membrane is even smaller and, in turn, the deflection of the hairs is still less.

Of the fibers of the cochlear nerve 90 to 95 percent are in synaptic contact with inner hair cells while 5 to 10 percent are in contact with outer hair cells. Each "inner hair cell fiber" extends straight out from modiolus to only one inner hair cell. In turn, each inner hair cell receives up to 20 fibers. Each "outer hair cell fiber" enters the organ of Corti and runs down the cochlear coil about 0.5 cm and supplies about 10 outer hair cells in a "random" fashion. In effect, the outer hair cells are associated with a convergent innervation pattern and the inner hair cells with a divergent innervation pattern.

The nature of the perilymph and endolymph may be significant in the genesis of the receptor and action potentials. The *perilymph* resembles an ultrafiltrate of blood similar in composition to other extracellular fluids, including the cerebrospinal fluid. Perilymph has high Na^+ and low K^+ concentrations. In contrast, endolymph resembles intracellular fluids in having high K^+ and low Na^+ concentrations.

The *endolymph* within the cochlea is located in the cochlear duct, including the space between the tectorial membrane and reticular membrane of the spiral organ of Corti. Note that the sensory hairs of the hair cells are bathed in endolymph. Endolymph is produced, and its ionic composition maintained, by active transport and secretion from blood plasma in the area vascularis (see Fig. 10-2). Excess endolymph is presumed to be lost, in part, by diffusion out of the endolymphatic sac located within the dural layers (see Fig. 10-2).

A fluid called *cortilymph* is in the spaces of the spiral organ of Corti between the reticular membrane and the basilar membrane and surrounding the hair cells and unmyelinated nerve fibers. Cortilymph resembles perilymph, not endolymph; it has high Na^+ and low K^+ concentrations. The ionic composition of cortilymph is maintained by the porous basilar membrane acting as a "sieve" for ions passing from the perilymph of the scala tympani; in contrast, the reticular membrane acts as an ionic barrier preventing exchange between the endolymph and cortilymph. The high Na^+ and low K^+ concentrations of cortilymph form a normal physiologic ionic environment for the excitable cells; the rich K^+ levels of the endolymph would be incompatible with the generation and transmission of excitatory impulses of the unmyelinated portions of the cochlear nerve fibers passing through to the spiral ganglia (see Fig. 10-2).

Because the spiral organ of Corti has no blood vessels of its own, its oxygen supply is presumably precarious. Most of its nourishment apparently comes via the cortilymph from the perilymph. Short periods of diminished oxygen supply are in part compensated for by the high concentration of enzymes in the cortilymph. These enable anaerobic glycolysis to satisfy the organ's energy needs.

A relationship exists between the pitch of a tone (frequency of vibration) and the region of maximal vibratory displacement of the basilar membrane. The highest tones (high pitch, high frequency, and short waves) are "heard" at the base of the cochlea near the stapes, and the lowest tones (low pitch, low frequency, and long waves) are "heard" at the apex. The basilar membrane acts as a low-pass filter (i.e., high fre-

quencies are filtered out), and thus low frequencies progress farther along the membrane than do higher ones.

The *tonotopic localization* described above formed the basis of the *place theory* of Helmholtz, in which the basilar membrane is considered a string resonator like the strings of a harp, with a specific place on the basilar membrane vibrating for each tone. However, it now seems likely that the basilar membrane is not a string resonator; it appears to exert no tension in any direction. Yet it displays a stiffness gradient from the base to the apex, the membrane being 100 times more compliant at the apex than at the base. It vibrates as a unit with the vestibular (Reissner's) membrane.

The *traveling-wave*, or *telephone*, *theory* of Rutherford was based on the thesis that the entire basilar membrane vibrates to a degree for each tone. The displacement of the membrane "travels" continuously up the cochlea from the base to the apex.

The modern *duplex theory* combines elements of the place theory and the traveling-wave theory. The vibrating stapes sets up traveling waves successively in the perilymph and basilar membrane. For each tone, the wave height of the vibrating basilar membrane, as it moves up the cochlea, increases to a maximum and then drops off rapidly. Each site of maximal displacement of the basilar membrane is correlated with a specific frequency of a sound wave. The sites of lesser displacement along the basilar membrane have as yet unknown functional roles that are probably associated with some of the qualities of each tone.

Loudness or intensity discrimination depends on the length of the basilar membrane set into maximal motion (amplitude of vibration); a longer portion activates more receptors and, in turn, more neurons than a short one. Musical sounds, chords, and harmonics are the result of the several frequencies vibrating in simple numeric oscillations. These are rhythms. Noises and background sounds are the result of frequencies not in periodic oscillation. These may be unpleasant discords.

The intensity of sound is expressed as a logarithmic scale called decibels (dB). The threshold of hearing is at 0 dB, a whisper is under 20 dB, average office noise is about 40 dB, boiler shop noise is about 100 dB, and permanent damage to the hearing apparatus can occur at 140 dB.

The human ear is used most often at frequencies ranging from 300 to 3000 Hz, the approximate range of the human voice (middle C is 256 Hz). Humans are most sensitive to vibration of about 2000 Hz, with little useful hearing occurring below 50 or above 16,000 Hz, although some individuals can hear sounds with frequencies of from 16 to 30,000 Hz. High frequencies are best perceived in early childhood, with a gradual decrease after 30 years of age, a loss that may be related to a change in the stiffness of the basilar membrane. Vibrations can be sensed as vibrations of the joints (vibratory sense) when the stem of a vibrating tuning fork is placed in contact with the joint.

The input codes conveyed by the fibers in the cochlear nerve are significant to loudness and to pitch. The loudness code is related to the frequency of nerve impulses (up to a maximum of 1000 Hz) transmitted in each nerve fiber. The arrangement is not that each sound is conveyed by only one specific fiber in the cochlear nerve; neither does each sound stimulate the firing of all the fibers of the nerve. Rather, the code for a sound is transmitted over the cochlear nerve by a compromise between these two extremes. Apparently the pitch code for each of the many thousands of different pitches heard by humans is relayed via the cochlear nerve by different combinations of nerve fibers. The response of the specific nerve fibers of the cochlear nerve to a pure tone is to increase the firing rate over the level of the spontaneous firing rate of these fibers.

One theory suggests that the outer hair cells are involved with the initial processing that results in loudness or volume discrimination, and that the inner hair cells are involved in pitch discrimination. The auditory input is conveyed via the cochlear nerve. It averages about 1 million or so impulses per second.

The detection of the location of low-frequency sounds (less than 2000 Hz) depends primarily on the differences in the time of the arrival of the sound to the two ears (interaural time difference) and the sound pressure differences on the tympanic membranes of the two ears. The localization of high-frequency sounds is based on the differences in the intensities of the sound source striking the two ears (interaural intensity difference). The bitufted dendritic cells of the medial superior olivary nucleus are involved in sound localization in space (see later on in chapter). The source of the sound is directly in front, behind, or above when the sound reaches each ear with the same intensity. Low-frequency sound location is based on the capacity of the subject to detect interval differences as small as 10 ms (0.01 s) in the arrival of a sound at the two ears. It is difficult to localize a sound heard only by one ear.

Auditory pathways

General features The ascending pathway of the auditory system is composed of sequences of neurons which are organized both in series and in parallel. Some neurons extend from one nucleus to the next, the neurons forming "sequences in series," whereas other neurons, arranged in parallel, extend from one nucleus and bypass a nucleus before terminating in another nucleus. This organization does not permit a precise designation of second-order, third-order, and fourth-order neurons. In general, the following sequence may be considered as basic (see Figs. 10-6 and 10-7):

1. *Neurons of the first order*, with cell bodies in the spiral ganglion of the cochlear nerve, extend from the spiral organ of Corti and terminate centrally in the dorsal and ventral cochlear nuclei.

   The cochlear nuclei comprise a dorsal cochlear nucleus (dorsal division) and a ventral cochlear nucleus (ventral division); the ventral nucleus is divided into an anterior ventral nucleus and a posterior ventral nucleus (Fig. 10-6).

   The cochlear nerve enters the cochlear nuclei in its ventral division with all nerve fibers terminating in the cochlear nuclear complex. After entering, each fiber divides into two main branches within the ventral division (ascending and descending branches). The ascending branch innervates the anterior ventral nucleus and the descending branch innervates the posterior ventral nucleus and dorsal nucleus (see Fig. 10-4). The cochlear fibers are arranged tonotopically with the low-frequency fibers from the apex of the cochlear coil located on the superficial aspect of the nuclei and with the high-frequency fibers from the base of the cochlear coil penetrating and locating on the deepest aspect of the nuclei. Thus, each of the fibers of the cochlear nerve innervates in all three cochlear nuclei in a tonotopic organization. The neurotransmitter of the cochlear nerve is probably glutamate.

2. *Neurons of the second order,* with cell bodies in the dorsal and ventral cochlear nuclei, extend from these nuclei and ascend as crossed fibers in the lateral lemnisci to the inferior colliculus.

3. *Neurons of the third order,* with cell bodies in the inferior colliculus, have axons which pass through the brachium of the inferior colliculus to the medial geniculate body (parvocellular or dorsal portion) of the thalamus.

4. *Neurons of the fourth order,* with cell bodies in the medial geniculate body, pass from there via the auditory (geniculocortical) radiations to the primary auditory cortex (transverse temporal gyri of Heschl, areas 41 and 42).

Several nuclei are intercalated in the auditory pathways between the cochlear nuclei and the inferior colliculus. These include the superior olivary nuclei, the nucleus of the trapezoid body, and the nucleus of the lateral lemniscus. These nuclei receive input from the cochlear nuclei, interconnect with one another, and project to the inferior colliculus (see Fig. 10-7).

The cochlea converts the acoustic signals into neural signal codes that are then further processed within the nuclear stations along the auditory pathways. As previously noted, there is a linear spatial distribution from the base to the apex of the cochlear coil in the selective responsiveness of the spiral organ of Corti to different frequencies (tone). In this sense *frequency coding* of auditory input is basically initiated and determined in the spiral organ. This tonotopic organization within the spiral organ is preserved within the cochlear nuclei and inferior colliculi. A neuron within these processing stations has a characteristic frequency response to a tone of a certain frequency over its spontaneous firing rate.

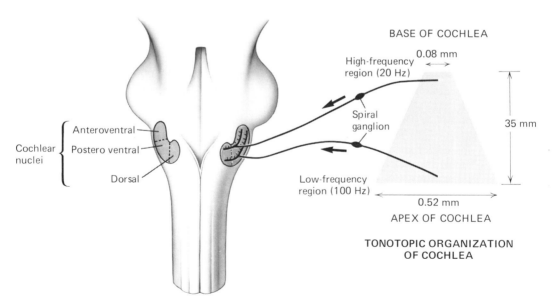

FIGURE 10-6 Diagram illustrating the tonotopic projections of the fibers of the cochlear nerve from the basilar membrane of the cochlea to the cochlear nuclei. These nuclei consist of a dorsal cochlear nucleus and a ventral cochlear nucleus. The latter is subdivided into an anterior ventral nucleus and a posteroventral nucleus. The dimensions of the uncoiled basilar membrane are indicated.

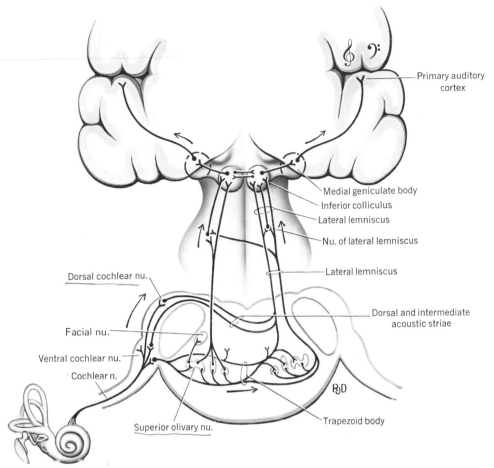

FIGURE 10-7 The ascending auditory pathways. <u>The cross section is through the junctional zone between the pons and medulla</u>. The nuclei comprising the superior olivary nuclear complex include from lateral to medial: lateral superior olivary nucleus (labeled), medial superior olivary nucleus, and nucleus of the trapezoid body. An accessory olivary nucleus is located just dorsal to the superior olivary nuclei (not illustrated). The ventral acoustic stria contributes to the trapezoid body. The connection with the facial motor nucleus involved with the stapedial reflex is not indicated.

The relay nuclei and primary auditory cortex of the central auditory pathways appear to be tonotopically organized. These are (1) each of the cochlear nuclei, (2) both the central nuclei and the dorsally located cortex of the inferior colliculus, (3) parvocellular portion of the medial geniculate body, and (4) primary auditory cortex (area 41). This tonotopic organization is often difficult to discern. However, a laminar pattern of the "best" frequencies forms complex yet orderly configurations within these processing auditory stations. These laminae, identified by their isofrequency bands, are consistent with the laminar patterns that are formed by the neurons as observed in Golgi preparations. Many details of this tonotopic organization remain to be uncovered and understood.

Recent studies suggest that the tectal component (inferior colliculus), thalamic component (medial geniculate body), and cerebral cortical component of the auditory pathway may be composed of two subsystems, the core subsystem and the fringe subsystem, or more. The *core subsystem* consists of the central nucleus of the inferior colliculus, portions of the medial geniculate body, and regions of the auditory cortex.

This subsystem is considered to be the direct auditory pathway, which is tonotopically organized in some degree throughout its course. The *fringe subsystem* consists of the capsule of the inferior colliculus, part of the medial geniculate body, and peripheral regions of the auditory cortex. This polymodal subsystem receives input from nonauditory as well as auditory sources and is less tonotopically organized at successive higher levels. The details of these subsystems in humans and other primates are incompletely understood. The functional relation of these ascending pathways to the descending (reflected) fibers (see later on) further complicate an understanding the precise role of each subsystem.

Specific features The displacement of the sensory hairs of the hair cells produced by the shearing motion generates the receptor potentials (see Fig. 10-4). The neurons of the cochlear nerve have their bipolar cell bodies in the spiral ganglion, which forms a spiral following the inner portion of the cochlear coil.

The nerve fibers of the cochlear nerve comprise a homogeneous nerve population of lightly myelinated axons 4 to 6 μm thick. The unmyelinated dendritic terminal branches of each neuron synapse directly with from several to many hair cells. The central axons of the cochlear nerve terminate in the ventral and dorsal cochlear nuclei, which are located on the lateral surface of the inferior cerebellar peduncle.

Each of the fibers of the cochlear nerve bifurcates into branches which are precisely distributed within each cochlear nucleus in a tonotopic organization.

The neurons of the cochlear nuclei have axons which project to several nuclei of the same and/or the opposite sides, as follows (see Fig. 10-6):

1. The fibers from the dorsal cochlear nucleus decussate through the posterior tegmentum as the *dorsal acoustic stria*, ascend in the contralateral lateral lemniscus, and terminate in the nucleus of the lateral lemniscus and the inferior colliculus.
2. The fibers from the dorsal part of the ventral cochlear nucleus pass dorsal to the inferior cerebellar peduncle, decussate through the in-

termediate tegmentum as the *intermediate acoustic stria*, ascend in the contralateral lateral lemniscus, and terminate in the nucleus of the lateral lemniscus and the inferior colliculus.
3. The fibers from the ventral cochlear nucleus pass through the anterior tegmentum as the large *ventral acoustic stria* (part of the trapezoid body); these fibers (*a*) terminate in the ipsilateral and contralateral reticular formation, superior olivary nuclei, and nuclei of the trapezoid body, and (*b*) ascend in the contralateral lateral lemniscus and terminate in the contralateral nucleus of the lateral lemniscus and the inferior colliculus. The decussating fibers of the ventral acoustic stria and from the superior olivary and trapezoid nuclei are collectively called the trapezoid body.

The *superior olivary* and *trapezoid body nuclei* give rise to third-order fibers, which ascend in both lateral lemnisci to the nucleus of the lateral lemniscus and the inferior colliculus.

The superior olivary complex consists of the S-shaped lateral superior olivary nucleus, medial (accessory) superior olivary nucleus, periolivary nuclei, and nucleus of the trapezoid body (see Fig. 10-7). Functional correlates have not been fully established for all these nuclei. The *medial superior olivary nucleus* probably has a role in localizing sounds in space. It consists of bitufted dendritic spindle-shaped cells, each with a medially directed dendrite and a laterally directed dendrite. The medially directed dendrite receives input from the contralateral cochlear nuclei, while the laterally directed dendrite receives input from the ipsilateral cochlear nuclei. These neurons project their axons rostrally in the ipsilateral lateral lemniscus. These differential sources of input are, in part, the basis for the concept that these neurons are exquisitely sensitive for detecting differences in the time of arrival of auditory stimuli from the two ears and thereby important for localizing sounds in space. The *lateral superior olivary nucleus* receives input only from the ipsilateral cochlear nuclei in tonotopic fashion; it projects some axons to the ipsilateral lateral lemniscus and some to the contralateral lateral lemniscus. This *lateral nucleus* and the *periolivary nuclei* have neurons that give rise to cochlear efferent fibers (see later on). Some cells of the superior olivary complex project to the neurons of the nucleus of the facial nerve innervating the stapedius muscle (stapedial reflex) and are involved with hyperacusis (see Fig. 10-7).

The *inferior colliculus* is composed of a large central nucleus and a thin, laminated, gray mantle of cortex adjacent to the dorsal surface. A pericollicular tegmentum containing fibers passing to and from the nucleus and cortex is located on all except the dorsal sides. Most of the cells in the central nucleus receive a biaural input and exhibit a laminated and orderly tonotopic orientation. The orientation of these isofrequency laminae appears to be consistent with the patterns of the neurons and their dendritic planes (Fitzpatrick).

The inferior colliculus is centrally located within the auditory pathways with ascending and descending direct input from neurons in essentially all nuclei of the auditory pathways including the auditory cortex. The cells of the subcollicular auditory nuclei have axons terminating in both the ipsilateral and contralateral inferior colliculi. Evidence indicates that the cochlear nuclei projections are largely contralateral and that the superior olivary complex and nuclei of the lateral lemniscus projections are largely ipsilateral. Commissural fibers interconnect the inferior colliculi and other neural levels, including the cerebral cortex. The inferior colliculus projects fibers rostrally to the parvocellular portion of the medial geniculate body via the brachium of the inferior colliculus.

The *medial geniculate body* is composed of bipolar and stellate cells. The bipolar cells are organized in sheets. These sheets correspond to the isofrequency bands of tonotopic localization. *Fibers from the medial geniculate body* pass via the sublenticular portion of the posterior limb of the internal capsule to the transverse gyri of Heschl (areas 41 and 42) as the auditory radiations.

The *primary auditory cortex* (area 41) receives from the medial geniculate body the geniculotemporal fibers (auditory radiation). These fibers pass through the sublenticular portion of the internal capsule. Area 42 receives some fiber projections. Some fibers in the auditory radiations project from the area 41 to the medial geniculate body, pulvinar, and inferior colliculus.

The primary auditory cortex is located in the two transverse temporal gyri of Heschl (see Fig. 1-4). The auditory cortex exhibits a relatively precise tonotopic organization. The auditory association cortical areas are located in area 42 and some of area 22 (Chap. 16). The pattern of projections to and from the laminae of the primary auditory cortex is presumed to be similar to that for the primary visual cortex (Chap. 12). Laminae II and III project to the association auditory areas. Lamina IV receives input from the medial geniculate body. Lamina V projects to the inferior colliculus and the pulvinar, and lamina VI feeds back to the medial geniculate body.

Decending (reflected) efferent fibers within the auditory pathways

Parallel to the ascending fibers of the auditory pathways are *centrifugal* (*descending*) *fibers* (see Fig. 10-8). These centrifugal projections comprise (1) *corticogeniculate fibers*, from temporal cortex to medial geniculate body; (2) *corticocollicular fibers*, from temporal cortex to the inferior colliculus; (3) *geniculocollicular fibers*, from the medial geniculate body to the inferior colliculus; (4) *collicular efferents*, from the inferior colliculus to the nuclei of the superior olivary complex and lateral lemniscus and to the dorsal and ventral cochlear nuclei; and (5) the *efferent cochlear bundle* of fibers, from the superior olivary complex to the hair cells of the spiral organ of Corti. These centrifugal fibers are integrated in the feedback control of auditory input. They are involved with processing and sharpening the ascending auditory influences by channeling the essential neural information (*signal*) and inhibiting and suppressing unwanted neural activity (*noise*).

Cochlear efferent fibers Cochlear efferent fibers arise from cells in the superior olivary complex and form the *olivocochlear bundle* (see Fig. 10-8). The bundle consists largely, about 80 percent, of fibers arising from the contralateral periolivary cells and partly, about 20 percent, of fibers from the ipsilateral superior olivary nucleus. It passes near the abducent nucleus before leaving the brainstem within the vestibular nerve. The efferent fibers course through the vestibular nerve to the labyrinth region, where they pass through the vestibulocochlear anastomosis (Oort's bun-

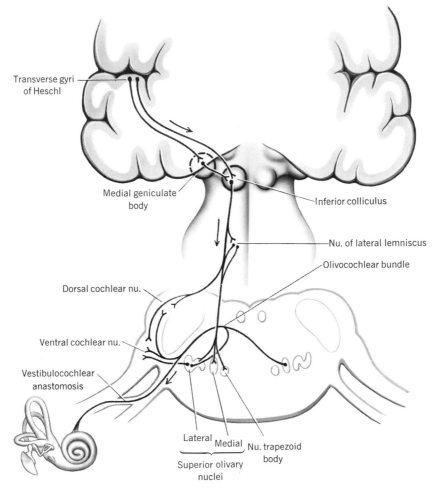

Transverse gyri
of Heschl

Medial geniculate
body

Inferior colliculus

Nu. of lateral lemniscus

Olivocochlear bundle

Dorsal cochlear nu.

Ventral cochlear nu.

Vestibulocochlear
anastomosis

Lateral Medial   Nu. trapezoid
body

Superior olivary
nuclei

FIGURE 10-8 The descending auditory pathways. The fibers of the olivocochlear bundle emerge from the medulla through the vestibular nerve and then pass via the vestibulocochlear anastomosis into the cochlear nerve.

dle) to the cochlear nerve and then to the outer hair cells but not to the inner hair cells (see Fig. 10-8). Although the precise role of these efferent fibers is said to be unresolved, they are presumed to act as a feedback that inhibits the receptivity of the cochlea.

Structural and functional correlations

The fact that the impulses from the ear largely ascend on the opposite side of the brain explains why sounds perceived by the right ear result in neural activity in the auditory cortex of the left cerebral hemisphere. Lesions interrupting the ascending auditory pathways result not in com-

plete deafness in either ear but rather in diminished hearing, especially on the opposite side. The bilateral composition of the auditory projections helps to explain these findings.

Although meaningful conscious hearing requires the neural activity of the cerebral cortex, the cortex is not essential for the auditory reflexes. "Listening" and reacting to cochlear input can take place with only the lower brain stations intact. A decorticate animal (one without a cerebral cortex) or even a decerebrate animal (one without a cerebrum) will respond to sounds; a sound can induce a decerebrate cat to mew and to turn its head toward the sound, which may not be subjectively heard. The nucleus of the inferior colliculus and the brainstem reticular formation may be the integrative center for this reflex.

The ascending and descending fibers and the several nuclei of the auditory pathways are involved with complex integrative mechanisms. The anatomic expressions of (1) one neuron synapsing with many other neurons, (2) many neurons converging on one neuron, (3) descending pathways among the ascending auditory pathways, (4) cross connections, and (5) the increasing number of neurons as the pathway ascends are indicative of the complex neuronal networks forming the substrates for physiologic mechanisms involved in hearing.

Cruder responses to various frequencies are primarily the function of the first station, the spiral organ of Corti. The transmission of stimuli from the spiral organ of Corti to the cerebral cortex is far more than just the relaying of neural impulses to the cortex. Fine discrimination of pitch, timbre, intensity of sound, and volume are the products of complex processing and interactions in and among the various nuclear stations in the auditory pathways. *Pitch coding* is in part a function of the combination of neurons stimulated and conducting and the frequency of neural impulses.

Active processing in the nuclei of the auditory pathways accounts for such contrasting expressions as the dampening and even loss of the conscious perception of extraneous background noises and the heightened awareness of sounds demanding attention. The filtering out of background noises and the enhancement and intensification of attention-directing sounds are expressions of the *focusing effect* (*sharpening effect, lateral inhibition,* or *mutual inhibition*), which is the equivalent of the simultaneous brightness-contrast effect in the visual system (Chap. 12). Theoretically the vibration produced by the flow of blood in the ear should be heard, but it is not. Blood flow can be heard as a hum when we concentrate and tense the jaw muscles or magnify the sounds with the cupped hand (sea shell) over the ear. Actually, blood vessels are absent in the vicinity of the organ of Corti. Usually these "weak, unheard" vibrations are filtered out, in part, by lateral inhibition in the nuclei of the ascending pathways. In theory, a sound may commence to ascend by several subpathways.

The optimal path is sustained and reinforced, and the others are inhibited along the way.

Presbycusis is the gradual impairment of ability to perceive or to discriminate sounds in old age. This increasing difficulty in hearing high-pitched sounds during aging is associated with the degeneration of the hair cells near the base of the cochlear coil.

There are times when the parent of a totally deaf child thinks that the child shows evidence of hearing. In fact, the child is only reacting to vibrations felt. This is related to the overlap between the auditory frequencies heard (from 20 to 20,000 Hz) to frequencies felt through proprioceptive receptors in the joints (fraction of a hertz to several hundred hertz).

Ringing in the ears (tinnitus) does occur in certain individuals who are sensitive to caffeine or aspirin. Hair cells can be destroyed in certain patients treated with such antibiotics as kanamycin or streptomycin.

THE VESTIBULAR SYSTEM

The purpose of the vestibular system is to signal changes in the motion of the head (kinetic) and in the position of the head with respect to gravity (static). The information from the periphery required by the nervous system to perform these roles is obtained from three afferent sources: the eyes, the general proprioceptive receptors throughout the body, and the vestibular membranous labyrinth. These three afferent sources are integrated into three systems—visual, proprioceptive, and vestibular systems—known as the *equilibrial triad*.

The vestibular system is actually the special proprioceptive system that functions to maintain equilibrium, to direct the gaze of the eyes, and to preserve a constant plane of vision (head position), primarily by modifying muscle tone. The specific receptors in the membranous labyrinth that sense the critical stimuli are the *cristae in the ampullae of the semicircular ducts, the macula of the utricle,* and *the macula of the saccule* (see Fig. 10-9). The vestibular system receives its input from environmental frequencies ranging from a fraction of a hertz to several hertz, with an optimum of 0.3 Hz. This range overlaps that sensed by the proprioceptive sys-

CRISTA AMPULLA

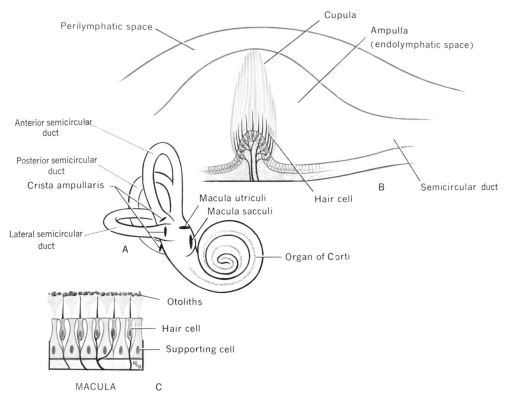

FIGURE 10-9 Vestibular and auditory receptors. *A.* The right membranous labyrinth as viewed from the front. Neuroepithelial areas are in black. These include a crista ampullaris in the ampulla of each semicircular duct, the macula of the utricle, the macula of the saccule, and the spiral organ of Corti of the cochlear duct. *B.* The crista ampullaris of an ampulla. Note that the free border of the crista is in contact with the wall of the ampulla. *C.* The macula. Note that the tips of the hairs of the hair cells are in contact with the otoliths embedded in the gelatinous mass.

tem which can sense frequencies from a fraction of a hertz to several hundred hertz.

Hair cells

The hair cells are specialized receptor cells of the vestibular sense organs; they act as transducers characterized by a high degree of directional sensitivity, wide dynamic range, and slow adaptation and high sensitivity to mechanical stimulation. Two types of sensory hairs are present in the hair cells: *stereocilia*, which are modified microvilli; and *kinocilia*, which are modified cilia. Each hair cell has about 100 stereocilia (called sensory hairs) and 1 kinocilium. The hairs are arranged in parallel rows. At one side of the cell

is the long kinocilium and the row of longest sensory hairs; the length of the hairs in a row decreases successively with increasing distance from the kinocilium. This is known as a morphologic polarization. The bending of the hairs alters the conductance to sodium and potassium ions; in turn, this affects the receptor potentials in the hair cells and in the afferent neurons. The action potentials are triggered at the first node of Ranvier. Normally the vestibular afferent fibers have a spontaneous pulsing rate. When the hairs are deflected kinopetally (toward the kinocilium), the firing rate increases, and when the hairs are bent kinofugally (away from the kinocilium), the firing rate is reduced below the normal rate. Another means by which the firing rate

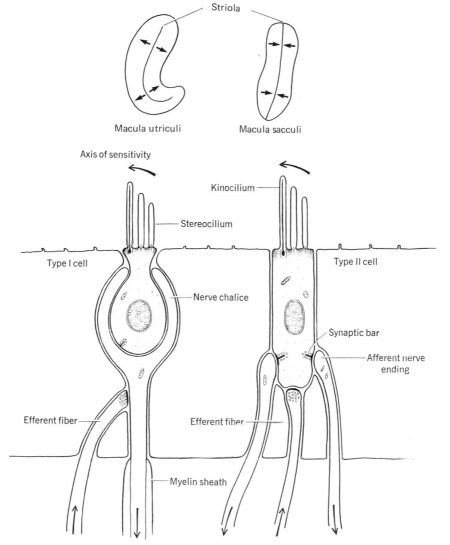

FIGURE 10-10 Schematic drawing of type I and type II vestibular hair cells in the maculae of the saccule and utricle and in the crista ampullaris of each semicircular duct. The afferent nerve envelops the type I hair cell in a cuplike ending. The axis of sensitivity of a vestibular hair cell is in the direction of the kinocilium. The maculae of the saccule and utricle have a central band called a striola (upper figures). In these maculae, the axis of sensitivity of the hair cells is polarized toward the striola in the macula utriculi and away from the striola in the macula sacculi. This is indicated by the arrows. (*Upper part of figure after Wersäll and Flock.*)

of the vestibular afferents can be modulated is via vestibular efferent fibers from the vestibular nucleus to the hair cells (see later on in chapter).

The vestibular sensory receptors consist of two types of sensory cells and some supporting cells (see Fig. 10-10). The *sensory cell type I* is a flask-shaped cell with a round base and constricted neck enclosed by a chalice-shaped affer

ent nerve ending. Vestibular efferent fiber synapses are associated with the afferent nerve ending.

The *sensory cell type II* is a thin, cylindric, columnar cell with a basally located synaptic region. Several afferent and efferent nerve terminals synapse with the hair cell. Within both types of hair cell are synaptic bars, which resemble synaptic ribbons in the retinal neurons. Each vestibular end organ has synaptic connections with both afferent and efferent fibers.

With respect to the location of the stereocilia, the kinocilium of each hair cell of the crista ampullaris of the lateral semicircular duct is oriented on the utricle side, while the kinocilium of each hair cell of the anterior and posterior semicircular ducts is oriented toward the semicircular duct (away from the utricle).

The cristae of the semicircular ducts are organs of *angular acceleration;* they are bidirectional accelerometers monitoring angular acceleration and deceleration, i.e., change in the direction of movements of the head. The cristae of the utricle and possibly of the saccule are organs of gravitation; these position recorders respond to *linear acceleration* (i.e., movement of the head in a straight line—forward, backward, up, or down), gravitational forces, and tilting of the head. The role of crista of the saccule is unknown; destruction of the saccule in animals produces no obvious defects in locomotion or equilibrium. The crista of the saccule may be an organ of vibration monitoring low-frequency vibrations.

Vestibular membranous labyrinth

The *three semicircular ducts* are arranged at right angles to one another in the three orthogonal planes as are the three sides in the corner of a cube (see Figs. 10-1, 10-2, and 10-8). The lateral (horizontal) duct is in the horizontal plane when the head is tilted forward at an angle of 30°. The posterior (verticle) duct forms a 55° angle with the midsagittal plane of the head. The inferior (anterior) duct is at right angles to the posterior duct. The lateral ducts of the two ears are in the same plane. The anterior duct of one side is parallel to the posterior duct of the opposite side. Each duct is but 0.1 mm in diameter and 10 to 15 mm long.

The ampulla (1 mm in diameter) of each duct contains the crista ampullaris, which is the sensory receptor. The crista contains hair cells and supporting cells. The cupula, a gelatinous, soft, and compliant wedge of sulphomucopolysaccharides in which the hairs of the hair cells are embedded, acts like a swinging door. The hinge is the crista, and the free edge of the cu-

pula brushes firmly against the curved wall of the ampulla. Any movement of the endolymph displaces the cupula slightly and consequently bends the hairs, thereby setting up transduction. The ampullae of the semicircular ducts are sensors detecting the movements involved with the change of direction of the head (angular movement or angular rotation) associated with acceleration and deceleration.

The crista of each duct is stimulated by the rotation of the head in its own plane. Although the hair cells can quickly detect the direction of acceleration by the deflection of the sensory hairs, it takes roughly 15 s for the velocity of the endolymph to attain that of the ducts. Once the endolymph is rotating at a speed equal to that in the ducts, the endolymph and ducts rotate at similar speeds. The *cupula-endolymph system* acts like a dampened spring-loaded torsion pendulum. The cupula and the sensory hairs return to their resting positions when the acceleration or deceleration is replaced to a constant velocity rotation. The cristae are especially geared to detect the common *angular movements*—those which are transient and end abruptly. The movement in one directly results in a discharge of a greater number of impulses than in the resting rate, while a movement in the opposite direction results in a discharge of a lesser number of impulses than in the resting rate. Each ampulla is bidirectionally active; this is expressed by an increase or decrease in the ongoing spontaneous activity, which is the resting rate of discharge from the receptor. This tonically active resting rate is roughly between 100 and 300 action potentials per second. Changes from the resting state mean that this end organ can be finely tuned.

Rotation as slow as 2° per second can be recognized and interpreted as direction. The semicircular ducts do not sense movement at slow uniform speeds, because the duct and the endolymph move at the same rate. During an angular (not straight-line) movement the ducts move with the head, but through inertia the endolymph lags and thereby forces the cupula of the ampulla to bend in a direction opposite to that in which the head moves. When the head stops quickly, the momentum of the endolymph forces the cupula to move in the direction of the original head movement (i.e., to reverse the bend of the hairs). In an analogous situation, a car rider (endolymph) is thrown back in the seat as the car accelerates and is thrown forward when the car suddenly stops. In a specific movement the stimulated crista is the one associated with the duct in the plane of the motion. Endolymph can set up currents if it is warmed or cooled by placing a warm or cold tube in the outer ear. Such caloric tests are used diagnostically to test vestibular function.

A ridge or macula composed of hair cells and supporting cells is the receptor in the utricle and in the saccule. The hairs are embedded in the mucopolysaccharide mass containing minute concretions of calcium carbonate and protein (ear dust, otoliths, statoconia, or otoconia) located near the tips of the hairs. The long axis of the macula in the utricle is oriented in the horizontal plane roughly parallel to the base of the skull and that of the macula in the saccule is in a vertical plane roughly parallel to the sagittal plane and facing laterally.

To perform its role in equilibrium, the utricle is specialized to respond to linear acceleration and deceleration in any one of several directions but primarily in the horizontal plane and, in addition, to a variety of tilts of the head (from the vertical plane). The role of the saccule is not clearly understood. It may function as an auditory receptor of low frequencies or may be involved with sensing vibratory stimuli. In these end organs, the hair cells with kinocilia are the transducer elements. In both the utricle and the saccule are some cells that are polarized in one direction and the other cells that are polarized in the opposite direction. All hair cells are polarized in relation to a curved central band passing through the macula utricle and the macula saccule called the *striola* (see Fig. 10-10). In the utricle, the hair cells on either side of the striola are polarized with their axes of sensitivity directed toward the striola. In the saccule, the hair cells on either side of the striola are oriented with their axes of sensitivity directed away from the striola.

The *macula utriculi* is maximally stimulated when the head is bent either forward or backward and is minimally stimulated when the head is erect. The utricle is a slowly adapting position recorder concerned with static equilibrium; it responds to changes in quantal force

and to linear acceleration. The *macula sacculi* is said to be maximally stimulated when the head is bent to the side. The utricle and saccule are not such efficient static sensors in humans as they are in other animals. The failure of these sensors to function reliably explains why an airplane pilot, when flying through clouds in a small plane without instruments, may fly upside down without realizing it. The delayed response of a standee in a bus to a sudden stop by the bus has been attributed to the delay of the utricle in registering the deceleration. The vomiting reflex may be initiated by utricular stimulation.

Vestibular pathways

The vestibular tracts consist of suprasegmental pathways that are distributed to the brainstem, spinal cord, cerebellum, and cerebral cortex (see Fig. 10-13).

The 19,000 nerve fibers of each vestibular nerve have their cell bodies in the vestibular (Scarpa's) ganglion near the membranous labyrinth. The *vestibular ganglion* is divided into the pars superior and pars inferior. The nerves from the receptors of the anterior and lateral semicircular ducts and the utricle have their cell bodies in the pars superior; the nerves from the posterior semicircular duct and the saccule have their cell bodies in the pars inferior.

The primary vestibular fibers from the vestibular nerve pass deep into the upper medulla to the inferior cerebellar peduncle, bifurcate into short ascending and descending branches, and terminate in specific regions (1) in each of the four vestibular nuclei—lateral, medial, superior, and inferior— in the upper lateral medulla and (2) in the uvula, nodule, and flocculonodular lobe (vestibulocerebellum) and fastigial nuclei of the cerebellum.

The primary vestibular fibers from the cristae of the semicircular ducts are distributed mainly to portions of the superior and medial vestibular nuclei, whereas the primary vestibular fibers from the maculae of the utricle and saccule terminate mainly in portions of the medial and inferior vestibular nuclei. They receive input primarily from the labyrinth and the archicerebellum. Influences from the fastigial nuclei to the vestibular nuclei are facilitatory; those from the cerebellar cortex (vermis and flocculonodular lobe) are inhibitory. The vestibular nuclei project *secondary vestibular fibers* to (1) the upper brainstem (pons and midbrain) via the medial longitudinal fasciculus, (2) cervical spinal segments via the medial longitudinal fasciculus (medial vestibulospinal tract), (3) the full length of the spinal cord via the (lateral) vestibulospinal tract, (4) the archicerebellum and fastigial nucleus of the cerebellum via the juxtarestiform body (medial part of inferior cerebellar peduncle), (5) brainstem reticular formation, and (6) hair cells of the maculae and crista of the membranous labyrinth via the vestibular nerve as the vestibular efferent fibers. All contralateral projections from the vestibular nuclei to the medial longitudinal fasciculus decussate at the level of the vestibular nuclei.

The *medial longitudinal fasciculus* is composed of many ascending and descending fibers from the vestibular nuclei; this association bundle is important because it conveys influences which integrate the vestibular system with the movements of the eyes, head, and neck (see Fig. 10-11 and "The Oculomotor System," and "Neural Basis for Nystagmus" later on).

The *lateral vestibular nucleus* is the major source of vestibular projections to the spinal cord. Its influences are conveyed via the uncrossed (lateral) vestibulospinal tract that facilitates extensor muscle tone through both the alpha and gamma motor neurons with some direct connections on alpha motor neurons. These extensor muscles include the antigravity axial and appendicular muscles. The lateral vestibular nucleus receives major and powerful excitatory input from the utricle (receives macular signals) and from both the ipsilateral and contralateral fastigial nuclei. The anterior lobe of the cerebellum exerts (1) indirect influences by inhibiting the fastigial nuclei and (2) direct influences by the monosynaptic Purkinje cell projections to the lateral vestibular nucleus. The

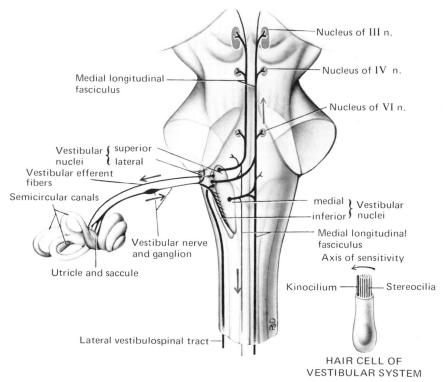

FIGURE 10-11 Vestibular pathways comprising the vestibular nerve, vestibular nuclei, medial longitudinal fasciculus, and lateral vestibulospinal tract. The connections of the vestibular system with the vestibulocerebellum are illustrated in Fig. 9-6.

role of the cerebellum is primarily to dampen the facilitory output of the lateral vestibular nucleus (refer to "Postural Control" in Chap. 9).

The *medial vestibular nuclei* receive powerful input from the semicircular canal receptors (receive canal signals). These nuclei project via the medial vestibulospinal tracts in the MLF bilaterally to the cervical and upper thoracic levels; they convey both excitatory and inhibitory influences to the axial musculature (see Fig. 10-11).

Vestibular system and the cerebral cortex

The vestibular system apparently does have cortical representation in the temporal lobe near the auditory cortex. Vestibular influences are said to be projected contralaterally via (1) a pathway to the medial geniculate body from where fibers ascend to the superior temporal gyrus or (2) a pathway to the ventral posterior inferior (VPI) thalamic nucleus (small subdivision of the ventral posterior nucleus) that projects to the postcentral gyrus near the junction of areas 2 and 5. The latter may be the primary vestibular cortex. Either pathway may account for some objective sensations (dizziness) associated with active vestibular end organs. Other cortical areas with probable vestibular representation include the frontal lobe and the parietal lobe near the head region of the postcentral gyrus. The vestibular nuclei do *not* receive direct projections from higher centers including the cerebral cortex and superior colliculus.

THE OCULOMOTOR SYSTEM
(see Chap. 12)

The oculomotor system comprises the many neuronal substrates associated with the control of coordinated movements of the eyes. Eye movements are essentially responses to a variety of sensory inputs including vestibular, auditory, visual, and proprioceptive stimuli and nonspecific inputs from alerting and orienting reflexes. A critical staging and coordinating region for the oculomotor system is presumed to be the *paramedial pontine reticular formation (PPRF)*. Anatomically it consists of several magnocellular pontine nuclei—nuclei pontis oralis, nucleus

pontis caudalis, and rostral portion of nucleus gigantocellularis (see Figs. 8-7 and 8-8). Adjacent nuclear complexes are often included—such as the perihypoglossal nucleus and periventricular and periaqueductal gray matter.

Input to the PPRF is derived from many regions. In turn, the PPRF integrates input and, after processing, projects influences via two coordinating "linkage pathways" to motor nuclei III, IV, and VI. These two longitudinally oriented pathways are (1) the medial longitudinal fasciculus (MLF) and (2) the more loosely organized neuronal circuitry in the medial tegmental reticular formation adjacent to the periventricular gray matter.

The input to the PPRF is derived from the cerebral cortex, superior colliculus and other tectal nuclei, vestibular and auditory systems, cerebellum, and spinal cord. The cortical sources include the frontal eye (area 8) and occipital eye (area 19) fields (Chap. 16) and others. The projections descend and follow a paramedian course through the ventral thalamus and the median brainstem reticular formation to the PPRF. Many of these descending fibers from widely separated areas of the cerebral cortex decussate before entering the PPRF. This differs from the more lateral course of the direct corticobulbar pathways. Input from visual system is derived from the superior colliculus and other tectal nuclei. Projections from the vestibular nuclei and some nuclei of the auditory pathways are thought to be directed to the caudal PPRF. Cerebellar influences are derived via the brainstem reticular formation from lobules VI and VII of the vermis. These vermal areas receive their input from the auditory, visual, and tactile pathway systems. The visual input to the cerebellum comes from retinotectal system of the so-called accessory optic pathway (to accessory optic nuclei). From midbrain sources (1) one route (possibly direct) via mossy fibers terminates in the cerebellar cortex and (2) another route passes to the inferior olivary nucleus and then via climbing fibers to the cerebellar cortex. Another nonvisual source of influences is derived from the neuromuscular spindles of the extraocular muscles; the fibers innervating these spindles have cell bodies in the mesencephalic nucleus of nerve V that relays information to the PPRF.

The precise organization of the neuronal circuitry of the PPRF and its relation with the medial longitudinal fasciculus (MLF, Chap. 10) and the loosely organized medial tegmental circuits remains to be worked out in sufficient detail to understand the entire repetoire of eye movements. The PPRF is most likely to be composed of several interconnected zones which can be characterized by their inputs and by their output responses.

Vestibular system and eye movements

Nystagmus The phenomenon of nystagmus is related to the imbalance of synchronized impulses from vestibular sources. *Nystagmus* refers to rhythmic to-and-fro movements of the eyes, with a rapid movement in one direction (called a saccade) followed by a slow movement in the opposite direction. This forms the basis for the whirling sensation that follows after rapidly spinning in one direction and suddenly stopping. The impulses from the vestibular source stimulate the eye movements, and the visual impulses from the eyes, in turn, create the conscious spinning sensation (vertigo).

Nystagmus in the normal individual has the following basis. As the head and body pivot and circle, the eyes attempt to fix on an object in space (slow component); as the head and body continue to circle, the eyes snap quickly in the direction in which the head is circling (fast or quick component or compensatory movement). The action is similar to what happens when one is watching telegraph poles from a moving train —the fast component is in the direction in which the train is moving. These eye movements repeat throughout the duration of the circling. By convention, *nystagmus is named by the direction of the fast saccade component.*

Neural basis for nystagmus The slow and fast components of nystagmus are activated from at least two sources: (1) hair cells in the cristae ampullae of the vestibular system and (2) the paramedian pontine reticular formation (PPRF). A portion of the PPRF may be the pontine gaze center and parabducent nucleus of clinical neurology. The influences from the vestibular system are instrumental in driving the *slow component*, while those from the pontine center trigger and maintain the *fast (saccade) component*. The

latter is accomplished by two types of units (neurons) in the PPRF: (1) fast-component burst units that discharge before and throughout the duration of the saccade and (2) pause units that cease firing and remain silent during the saccade.

The following account outlines the neural basis for horizontal nystagmus (see Fig. 10-12). When the head along with the body in a standing individual accelerates (angular movement) in a spin, the endolymph within a semicircular duct lags slightly behind the semicircular duct (owing to inertia of the fluid), or when the head stops moving after rotating the endolymph overshoots slightly (again owing to inertia). As the standing individual turns in a clockwise direction to the right, the endolymph lags behind and exerts pressure on the cupulae of the ampullae of the horizontal semicircular ducts. The cupulae and the hairs on the hair cells are deflected toward the utricle (utriculopetal) in the right ampulla and are deflected away from the utricle in the left ampulla. The result of these deflections is that the eyes move conjugately in a slow, smooth horizontal deflection to the left. At the point of maximal desplacement a quick saccade to the right returns the eyes conjugately to the right. This activity repeats over and over again. The kinopetal deflection of the hairs of the right ampulla evokes excitatory influences that are conveyed via the right vestibular nerve to the right superior and medial vestibular nuclei, and, in turn, influences are then conveyed from the vestibular nuclei via the medial longitudinal fasciculus (MLF) to facilitate the contraction of the ipsilateral medial rectus muscle (nerve III) and the contralateral lateral rectus muscle (nerve VI). Synchronized with these activities are the inhibitory influences from the kinofugal deflection of the hair cells in the left ampulla. These inhibitory influences are relayed via vestibular fibers to the left superior and medial vestibular nuclei and then via the MLF to inhibit the contraction of the ipsilateral (left) lateral rectus muscle and the contralateral (right) medial rectus muscle. The total effect is to direct the slow component to the left (see Fig. 10-12). In essence, the right and left horizontal canals act reciprocally (equal and opposite), with one exerting facilitatory influences on the agonist eye muscles and the other exerting inhibitory influences on the antagonist eye muscles. The subjec-

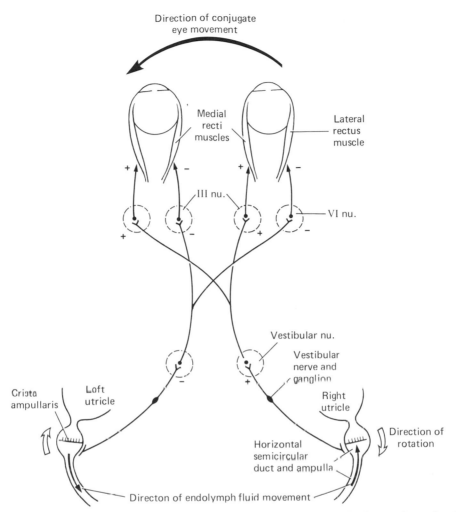

Medial
recti
muscles

Lateral
rectus
muscle

III nu.

VI nu.

Vestibular nu.

Vestibular
nerve and
ganglion

Crista
ampullaris

Left
utricle

Right
utricle

Direction of
rotation

Horizontal
semicircular
duct and ampulla

Direction of endolymph fluid movement

FIGURE 10-12 Conjugate eye movement associated with the horizontal semicircular ducts and ampullae. The short parallel lines directed toward the utricle in the cristae ampullares indicate the axis of sensitivity (direction of polarization) of the hair cells of the cristae ampullares. Rotational acceleration of the head in a clockwise direction (to the right; outlined arrows outside the ampullares) results in the relative movement of endolymph in the paired semicircular ducts to the left (solid arrows in the ducts). Movement of the endolymph toward the utricle results in excitatory activity (+) in the hair cells of the right ampulla and away from the utricle results in inhibitory activity (−) in the hair cells in the left ampulla. These activities result in excitation (+) and inhibition (−) in the medial and superior vestibular nuclei and fibers of the medial longitudinal fasciculi; this produces excitatory and inhibitory influences in appropriate motor neurons in the abducent (lateral rectus muscles) and oculomotor (medial rectus muscles) nuclei to stimulate conjugate eye movement to the left (solid arrow).

tive sense of turning (vertigo) is to the left (direction of the slow component).

In some as yet unknown circuit, influences are fed back to the PPRF, where the fast component burst units fire and the pause units cease firing and thereby activate the saccade component. According to one concept, "a pulse generator" mechanism stimulates burst neuronal circuitry. This mechanism, said to be located in the rostral PPRF, provides the critical signals for saccadic movement that is triggered by the integrator mechanism, said to be located in the caudal PPRF. The latter contains the essential circuitry projecting influences to the nuclei of the extraocular muscles. Some of the control and regulation of the pulse generator is presumably exerted by the pause (omnopause) units. The saccade is immediately followed by the dominance of vestibular activity with the suppression of the burst units and activation of neurons controlling the slow component to the left.

When the spin to the right is suddenly stopped, the nystagmus is reversed because the momentum of the endolymph persists and now deflects the cupulae in the opposite direction—away from the utricle in the right ampulla and toward the utricle in the left ampulla (postrotation nystagmus). This is accompanied by a reversal of the vertigo.

To test for functional activity of the semicircular canals, a caloric test is used in which warm (or cold) water is placed in the external auditory meatus. With the head placed in an appropriate position, the application of warm water in the right ear causes a shift of endolymph to deflect the cupula toward the utricle and produce a nystagmus to the right side (side of fast component). Warm water produces a nystagmus to the same side and cold water to the opposite side. To obtain optimal results warm water at 44°C and cold water at 30°C is used and the ear is irrigated for about 30 s with about 250 mL of water.

Cerebellum and eye movements The cerebellum can, through its projections to the vestibular nuclei, exert powerful inhibitory influences on the vestibulooculomotor reflex activity. In addition it can through projections from the vermal lobules VI and VII facilitate the production of saccadic eye movements. These lobules receive afferent input from visual, auditory, and tactile sources and especially from the neuromuscular spindles in the extraocular muscles. The PPRF is integrated into this reflex (Chap. 9); its purpose is to produce compensating eye movements during head rotation so as to stabilize retinal images of the visual field surround.

The vestibulocerebellum operates as a control system acting through (1) the vestibuloocular reflex and (2) the vestibulospinal reflex. The vestibuloocular reflex is a reflex activating compensating eye movements that are directed to maintaining the constancy of the visual field on the retinas (preventing retenal slip). The vestibulospinal reflex is a reflex directed to the control

of head position through coordinating the activity of the neck musculature so that the vestibuloocular reflex can be effective within its range of movement.

Vestibular connections with the cerebellum and with the reticular formation

Primary fibers of the vestibular nerve and secondary fibers mainly from the inferior and medial vestibular nuclei pass through the juxtarestiform body (medial portion of the inferior cerebellar peduncle) and course as mossy fibers mainly to the ipsilateral flocculonodular lobe and uvula (see Fig. 10-13). The *flocculonodular* lobe and the adjacent cerebellar cortex are often called the *vestibulocerebellum*. In addition, fibers from these vestibular nuclei project to the fastigial nuclei. The maculae of the utricle and saccule are the major source of vestibular input to the cerebellum. Influences from these receptors are conveyed to the inferior and medial vestibular nuclei. The Purkinje cells of the vestibulocerebellum and vermis relay inhibitory influences to the fastigial nuclei and the lateral vestibular nucleus. The fastigial nuclei project fibers conveying excitatory influences to parts of each vestibular nucleus and to the reticular formation (lateral reticular nucleus and nucleus reticularis pontis caudalis). As noted in Chap. 9 the anterior lobe of the cerebellum has a functionally significant connection with the lateral vestibular nucleus. It is through this projection that the cerebellum inhibits and dampens the discharge rate of the neurons of this nucleus. This includes a powerful influence through the PPRF on the vestibuloocular connections. Stimulation of the vermal lobules VI and VII can evoke saccades; these lobules receive inputs from the visual, auditory, and tactile systems and from the neuromuscular spindles of the extraocular muscles.

Vestibular efferent pathway to the membranous labyrinth

Efferent fibers from the brainstem pass through the vestibular nerve and terminate in the vestibular receptors of the membranous labyrinth. The nuclei of origin and the role of these vestibular efferent fibers are controversial. They arise from

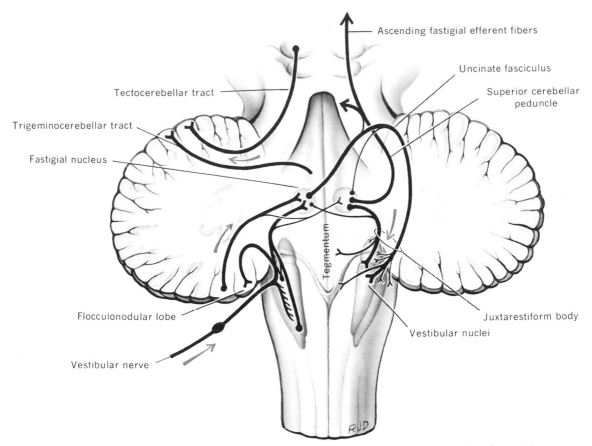

FIGURE 10-13 The vestibulocerebellar pathways. Left, input to the cerebellum; right, output from the cerebellum.

cells in the reticular formation and vestibular nuclei. Some fibers terminate directly on sensory cells type II and on the afferent fibers innervating sensory cells type I (see Fig. 10-10). These fibers are similar to the efferent fibers of other systems, including the cochlear efferent fibers. These vestibular efferent neurons probably modulate the spontaneous firing rate of the vestibular nerve fibers and may ameliorate the effects of motion sickness and its aftersensations and nystagmus.

Functional features of the vestibular system

The role of the vestibular system is to monitor the orientation of the head in space. In response, the eyes and head move in space to compensate and to maintain the visual axis that is stable with respect to the environment. This is analogous to a shipboard radar system with tracking devices (radar or eyes) mounted on a moving platform (ship or head).

The influences from the labyrinth have significant roles in the maintenance of head and neck position and body posture. Tightrope walkers rely on vestibular and other proprioceptive cues to sustain their performance. A cat held up in the air, back down and feet up, turns with incredible speed and lands on its feet when dropped. Labyrinthine activity is critical to this complex maneuver. When the cat is released, its neck musculature reacts to vestibular stimulation by twisting the head to the normal position of eyes parallel to the ground. Differential tension is now exerted on the neck muscles of the two sides. The resulting proprioceptive imbalance of these muscles sends impulses that activate the spinal reflexes that twist the trunk to its normal relation with the neck. The sequence repeats, and finally the hindquarters are properly positioned. The rapid sequence from head to tail is initiated by the vestibular sensors. A falling person does not respond so rapidly nor so deftly. We utilize the less effective cues from the visual and the proprioceptive receptors for our righting reflexes. A cat can right itself by utilizing vestibular cues or visual cues exclusively.

Labyrinth activity is integrated into many natural postures, actions, and positions, as seen in the boxer's pose, with the left arm and forearm partially flexed, the right upper extremity cocked and forearm partially flexed, left thigh and both legs partially flexed, and the right thigh partially extended; the performance of the high diver, who utilizes the position and movements of the head and neck as the key to his or her dive, with the rest of the body following naturally; or the coordination of a runner or marcher, who uses all four extremeties rhythmically.

Vertigo dizziness or the sensation associated with lack of equilibrium involves the subjective sense of rotation, either of the surroundings or of the person. It is a cardinal sign of labyrinthine and vestibular dysfunction. Vertigo may occur in the normal subject; excessive stimulation of the semicircular ducts gives the sensation of vertigo, with objects appearing to move in a circular pattern because of compensatory movements of the eyes (nystagmus). In vestibular disease nystagmus occurs; it is a consequence of influences conveyed from the vestibular system via the medial longitudinal fasciculus to the extraocular muscles.

The vestibular system is geared to signal changes in the motion of the head (acceleration and deceleration) and in the position of the head with respect to gravity. A clinical expression states that the vestibular input from one ear opposes similar activity from the opposite ear. A unilateral lesion results in relative overactivity in the vestibular output from the unaffected ear. Thus when the head is erect and vestibular end organs are activated, the eyes deviate away from the unaffected ear and a sense of rotatory vertigo is toward the side of the unaffected ear.

Pirouetting ballet dancers prevent vertigo by periodically snapping their heads as they break up, as far as the head is concerned, the continuous movement of the spin. This minimizes the flow of the endolymph. In addition they learn to compensate by practice, and complete the pirouette by coming to a broad-based stance.

Dizziness, headache, nausea, and vomiting are symptoms of motion sickness (seasickness, carsickness, and airsickness). *Motion sickness* is primarily due to the excessive stimulation of the utricle and saccule. The vestibulocerebellar projections are involved; following the removal of the flocculonodular lobe, experimental animals do not show evidence of motion sickness. The conflict of sensory cues from the labyrinth, the body, and the eye may contribute. Deafmutes, who lack labyrinthing receptors, do not experience motion sickness. Drugs like Dramamine raise the threshold of vestibular stimulation and thereby help to prevent motion sickness. Because the labyrinth is not functional during the first year of life, infants do not get motion sickness.

Ménière's disease is a disorder probably resulting from an abnormal circulation of the vestibular endolymph or excessive amount of endolymph. *Tinnitus* (ringing in the ear), violent attacks of vertigo, pallor, vomiting, nausea, and increased respiration occur. The cristae ampullaris are entirely normal. Symptoms of Ménière's disease may be partially alleviated by pharmaceutic agents that block motion sickness.

The human being is not so dependent on the vestibular system as on the visual and general proprioceptive systems. Injury to the labyrinths, the vestibular nuclei, or the vestibular pathways may result in nystagmus, tendency to fall to one side, past pointing, and some difficulty in maintaining erect posture. However, these symptoms will attenuate and finally disappear as other proprioceptive cues are more fully utilized. Astronauts experience motion sickness, including nausea, dizziness, and unsteadiness, during the first few days of exposure to the weightlessness of outer space, and again for a few days after returning to earth and its gravitational forces.

Loss of both labyrinths is not followed by vertigo or nystagmus. Normal locomotion and posture will then require the utilization of visual cues. The difficulties of walking and performing postural movements will lessen with time, but walking, for example, will always be accomplished with a broad base. A swimmer who has lost the use of the labyrinths may navigate down instead of up to reach the surface unless adequate visual cues are available.

Syndrome of medial longitudinal fasciculus (MLF) (Fig. 8-24 D)

Horizontal gaze of the eyes to the right or left involves the coordinated contractions of the lateral rectus muscle of one eye (abductor innervated by nerve VI) and of the medial rectus of the other eye (adductor innervated by nerve III). The integration of this action depends upon the functional integrity of the PPRF. Projections from the PPRF along with those from vestibular and cerebellar sources from one side are conveyed to the ipsilateral abducent nucleus and via the contralateral MLF to the opposite oculomotor nucleus. A unilateral lesion of the MLF rostral to the abducent nucleus results in a disturbance of horizontal conjugate gaze movements called *internuclear ophthalmoplegia*. In such a lesion there is impairment or loss of adduction of the ipsilateral eye (paresis of horizontal gaze to the side opposite the lesion) accompanied by nystagmus of the abducting eye (cause uncertain). In contrast, a unilateral lesion of the PPRF may result in a horizontal gaze paresis or paralysis of lateral gaze to the same side because the PPRF projects to the ipsilateral abducent nucleus and the contralateral oculomotor nucleus.

BIBLIOGRAPHY

Adams, J. C.: Ascending projections to the inferior colliculus. J Comp Neurol, 183:519–538, 1979.

Békésy, G. von: *Experiments in Hearing*, McGraw-Hill Book Company, New York, 1960.

Brodal, A., O. Pompeiano, and F. Walberg: *The Vestibular Nuclei and Their Connections, Anatomy and Functional Correlations*, Charles C Thomas, Publisher, Springfield, Ill., 1962.

Celesia, G. G.: Organization of auditory cortical areas in man. Brain, 99:403–414, 1976.

De Reuck, A. V. S., and J. Knight (eds.): *Hearing Mechanisms in Vertebrates*, Ciba Foundation Symposium, Little, Brown and Company, Boston, 1968.

Engström, H., H. Ades, and A. Anderson: *Structural Pattern of the Organ of Corti*, Almqvist and Wiksell, Stockholm, 1966.

Fields, W., and B. Alvord (eds.): *Neurological Aspects of Auditory and Vestibular Disorders*, Charles C Thomas, Publisher, Springfield, Ill., 1964.

Fitzpatrick, K. A.: Cellular architecture and topographic organization of the inferior colliculus of the squirrel monkey. J Comp Neurol, 164:185–207, 1975.

Furato, S. (ed.): *Submicroscopic Structure of the Inner Ear*, Pergamon Press, New York, 1967.

Khanna, S. M., and J. Tonndorf: "Physical and Physiological Principles Controlling Auditory Sensitivity in Primates," in C. R. Noback (ed.), *Sensory Systems of Primates*, Plenum Press, New York, 1978, chap. 2, pp. 23–52.

Lim, D. J.: Fine morphology of the tectorial membrane: Its relationship to the organ of Corti. Arch Otolaryngol, 96:199–215, 1972.

Lindemann, H. H.: Studies on the morphology of the sensory regions of the vestibular apparatus. Adv Anat Embryol Cell Biol, 42:1–113, 1969.

Morest, D. K.: Synaptic relationships of Golgi type II cells of the medial geniculate body of the cat. J Comp Neurol, 162:157–193, 1975.

Moskowitz, N.: Comparative aspects of some features of the central auditory system of primates. Ann NY Acad Sci, 167:357–369, 1969.

Precht, W.: Vestibular mechanisms. Ann Rev Neurosci, 2:265–289, 1979.

Raphan, T., and B. Cohen: Brainstem mechanism for rapid and slow eye-movements. Ann Rev Physiol, 40:527–552, 1978.

Rasmussen, G. L., and W. F. Windle (eds.): *Neural mechanisms of the Auditory and Vestibular Systems*, Charles C Thomas, Publisher, Springfield, Ill., 1961.

Smith, D. E., and N. Moskowitz: Ultrastructure of layer IV of the primary auditory cortex of the squirrel monkey. Neuroscience, 4:349–359, 1979.

Spoendlin, H.: The innervation of the organ of Corti. J Laryngol, 81:717–738, 1967.

Stein, B. M., and M. B. Carpenter: Central projections of portions of the vestibular ganglia innervating specific parts of the labyrinth in the rhesus monkey. Am J Anat, 120:281–318, 1967.

Strominger, N. L.: "The Anatomical Organization of the Primate Auditory Pathways," in C. R. Noback (ed.), *Sensory Systems of Primates*, Plenum Press, New York, 1978, chap. 3, pp. 53–91.

Tonndorf, J.: "Cochlear Mechanics and Hydrodynamics," in J. V. Tobias (ed.), *Foundations of Modern*

Auditory Theory, vol. 1, Academic Press, Inc., New York, 1970, pp. 203–254.

Wersäll, J., and A. Flock: "Functional Anatomy of the Vestibular and Lateral Line Organs," in W. Neff (ed.), *Contributions to Sensory Physiology*, Academic Press, Inc., New York, 1965.

Whitfield, I. C.: *The Auditory Pathway*, The Williams and Wilkins Company, Baltimore, 1967.

Wilson, V. J.: Physiological pathways through the vestibular nuclei. Int Rev Neurobiol, 15:27–82, 1972.

CHAPTER ELEVEN

HYPOTHALAMUS

LOCATION AND GENERAL FUNCTION

The hypothalamus is the phylogenetically ancient region at the base of the diencephalon. It is flanked medially by the third ventricle and laterally by the subthalamus (Fig. 13-2). It is bordered rostrally by the lamina terminalis, dorsally by the anterior commissure and the hypothalamic sulcus [which extends from the interventricular foramen (foramen of Monro) to the cerebral aqueduct of Sylvius], and caudally by the midbrain. Its ventral part consists (from the rostral aspect to the caudal) of the preoptic region, optic chiasma, median eminence, hypophysis, tuber cinereum, and the mamillary bodies (see Fig. 11-1). The median eminence is a subdivision of the tuber cinereum.

The hypothalamus has a vast array of functional correlates in both the visceral and the somatic sphere in its mere 4-g mass. It functions in two broad areas: the maintenance of a relatively constant internal body environment (homeostasis) and behavior patterns. For example, the hypothalamus has (1) a homeostatic role in the regulation of body temperature and (2) a role in behavioral expressions ranging from calm to rage and in such feeling patterns as hunger, thirst, and sexual affect.

NEUROANATOMY OF THE HYPOTHALAMUS

Nuclei of the hypothalamus

The *hypothalamus* may be anatomically divided into four areas, arranged from the lamina terminalis to the midbrain: the *preoptic area* (telencephalic portion), the *supraoptic area* dorsal to the optic chiasma, the *tuberal area* dorsal to the tuber cinereum, and the *mamillary area* dorsal to and including the mamillary bodies (Figs. 11-2, 11-3).

Each of the four principal areas may be schematically subdivided into three zones of nuclei arranged mediolaterally into (1) the *periventricular zone* adjacent to the third ventricle, (2) the *medial zone*, and (3) the *lateral zone*. In the following schema the numbers 1, 2, and 3 correspond to the zones as numbered above; only some of the hypothalamic nuclei in these zones are noted. The *preoptic area* includes (1) the periventricular zone, (2) the medial preoptic zone, and (3) the lateral preoptic zone. The *supraoptic area* includes (1) the periventricular zone, (2) the paraventricular nucleus and other nuclei of the medial hypothalamic zone, and (3) the supraoptic nucleus and other nuclei of the lateral hypothalamic zone. The *tuberal (infundibular) area* includes (1) the periventricular zone, (2) the dorsal medial and the ventral medial nuclei, and (3) the nuclei of the lateral zone. The *mamillary area* includes (1) the periventricular zone, (2) the nuclei of the mamillary body as well as the posterior hypothalamic zone, and (3) the lateral hypothalamic zone.

Basic circuits of the hypothalamus

General The neural circuits associated with the hypothalamus are numerous and complex. The named fiber pathways have reciprocal connections with widespread regions of the cerebrum and the brainstem. These intricate interrela-

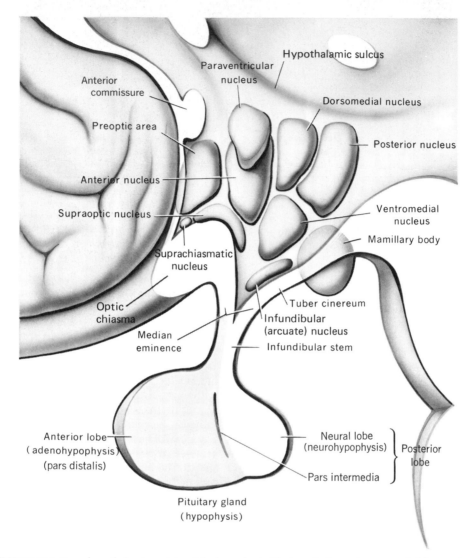

FIGURE 11-1 Some hypothalamic nuclei and the hypophysis. The hypothalamus is composed of four nuclear areas: (1) nuclei of the preoptic area (telencephalic region); (2) nuclei of the supraoptic or anterior area, including the paraventricular nucleus, anterior nucleus, and supraoptic nucleus; (3) nuclei of the tuberal or middle areas: (1) nuclei of the preoptic area (telencephalic region); (2) nuclei of the supraoptic or anterior area, including the posterior nucleus and the mamillary body.

tions, in which are intercalated numerous synaptic stations, are consistent with the multifaceted functions of the hypothalamus. In addition, extensive intrahypothalamic connections exist.

In general, the hypothalamus is thought of as deriving its major input either directly or indirectly from the nonspecific reticular system and little, if any, input from the specific lemnis-

cal system (Chap. 8). The sites of hypothalamic input and output include the brainstem reticular formation, the limbic lobe (including the hippocampal region and the amygdaloid body; see Chap. 15), neocortex, thalamus, and the olfactory system. Significant neural and vascular connections are made with the hypophysis.

Many of the basic anatomic features of the

hypothalamus (e.g., isodendritic neurons) are similar to those of the brainstem reticular formation. Thus the hypothalamus may be considered to be a rostral extension of the reticular formation, especially that of the medial midbrain tegmentum and the periaqueductal gray matter. The preoptic area of the hypothalamus and the septal regions of the telencephalon are the most rostral extensions of the reticular formation. This may be called the septopreopticohypothalamic component of the reticular formation.

Most of the ascending sensory input is derived from the multisynaptic pathways of the mesencephalic reticular formation and from the thalamic reticular nuclei (tegmentohypothalamic pathways, medial forebrain bundle, dorsal longitudinal fasciculus, and thalamohypothalamic pathways). The major fiber connections with the limbic lobe are mediated through the median forebrain bundle, fornix system, and stria terminalis pathway (Chap. 15). The influences from the neocortex are relayed either directly to the hypothalamus or indirectly via the limbic lobe or the thalamus.

The effector role of the hypothalamus is mediated via neural pathways and via endocrine (humoral, hormonal, or neurosecretory) agents. The pathways of the autonomic nervous system (primarily) and the somatic motor system are both instrumental in the expression of hypothalamic activity. Behavioral and psychic manifestations are mediated via the pathways to the limbic lobe and neocortex. The neurosecretions elaborated in the hypothalamus are the humoral agents that influence (1) the anterior lobe of the hypophysis (pituitary gland) via the hypophyseal (hypothalamohypophyseal) portal blood vessels (see Figs. 11-2 and 11-3) and (2) the neurophyphysis via the supraopticohypophyseal pathways (see Figs. 11-2 and 11-3).

In brief, the hypothalamus is strategically located between the cerebrum and the brainstem and spinal cord.

Pathways of the hypothalamus

Input (Fig. 11-4) The *input to the hypothalamus* is conveyed via (1) ascending fibers from the brainstem tegmentum and periaqueductal gray matter, (2) descending fibers from the forebrain, and (3) other sources. Most of these fibers are ac-

companied by fibers projecting influences in the opposite direction. These fiber groups are thus reciprocally directed.

ASCENDING FIBERS FROM THE BRAINSTEM TO THE HYPOTHALAMUS These include the following: (1) fibers originating in the dorsal and ventral tegmental nuclei which pass in the mamillary peduncle to the lateral mamillary nucleus; (2) fibers originating in the periaqueductal gray matter which pass in the dorsal longitudinal fasciculus of Schütz to several hypothalamic nuclei; (3) fibers originating in the midbrain tegmentum which pass in the medial forebrain bundle to the lateral hypothalamus; and (4) the ascending catecholamine pathways (Chap. 8) and fibers from a number of brainstem tegmental and raphe nuclei (see Figs. 1-10, 8-14, 8-19, 8-20, and 15-3).

The input to these brainstem tegmental nuclei and the periaqueductal gray matter is derived from (1) cerebral levels largely through descending fibers accompanying the ascending fibers (reciprocal connections) and (2) ascending fibers from the nuclei of the lower brainstem tegmentum (ascending reticular pathways). In turn, these pontine and medullary reticular nuclei receive their input from (1) spinal levels via spinoreticular fibers and collaterals of the spinothalamic tract and (2) brainstem levels via cranial nerves and their nuclei. Many ascending signals from the nucleus solitarius are relayed to the hypothalamus.

DESCENDING FIBERS FROM THE FOREBRAIN These include: (1) Fibers of the fornix originating in the hippocampus and the septal nuclei of the limbic system which terminate in the medial hypothalamus (preoptic region, anterior hypothalamus, and medial mamillary nucleus). The subiculum of the hippocampus is a significant channel for sensory and neocortical input to the hypothalamus (Chap. 15). (2) Fibers originating in the pyriform cortex, olfactory tubercle, and amygdaloid body project via the stria terminalis and the ventral amygdalofugal pathway to the medial hypothalamus (see Fig. 15-3). These neural pathways provide the route of access of olfactory influences to the hypothalamus. These influences are conveyed from the olfactory nerve to the olfactory bulb to the primary olfactory cortex and to the corticomedial group of the amyg-

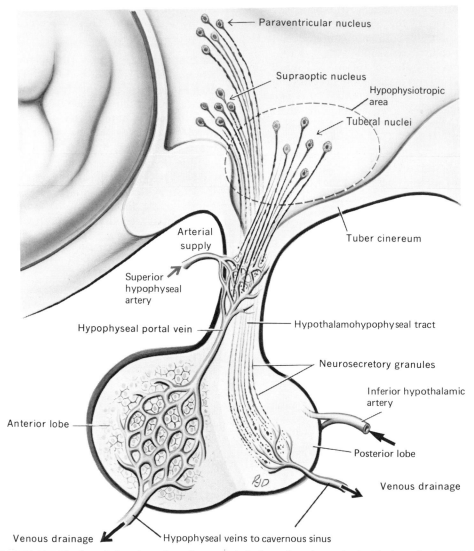

Paraventricular nucleus

Supraoptic nucleus

Hypophysiotropic area

Tuberal nuclei

Tuber cinereum

Arterial supply

Superior hypophyseal artery

Hypophyseal portal vein

Hypothalamohypophyseal tract

Neurosecretory granules

Inferior hypothalamic artery

Anterior lobe

Posterior lobe

Venous drainage

Venous drainage

Hypophyseal veins to cavernous sinus

FIGURE 11-2 The hypothalamohypophyseal tract and the hypophyseal portal vein. The hypophysiotrophic area (shaded area) comprises those hypothalamic cells which project to the median eminence.

daloid body. The primary olfactory cortex projects to the lateral hypothalamus via the medial forebrain bundle. The olfactory system is the only sensory system with a major direct route to the hypothalamus (fibers from the retina project to the suprachiasmatic nucleus of the hypothalamus). The input from the olfactory system to the hypothalamus is not involved with the subjective interpretation of odors but rather with behavior and emotional expression (Chaps. 6 and 15). (3) Fibers from the orbitofrontal neo-

cortex (corticohypothalamic fibers) and septal nuclei may pass along with the medial forebrain bundle to the lateral hypothalamus (see Fig. 11-4). (4) Some thalamohypothalamic fibers from the magnocellular portion of the dorsomedial nucleus and midline thalamic nuclei pass to the lateral hypothalamus and rostral portions of the amygdaloid body. (The dorsomedial nucleus has reciprocal connections with the prefrontal neocortex.) The several possible routes from the neocortex to the hypothalamus are important as the

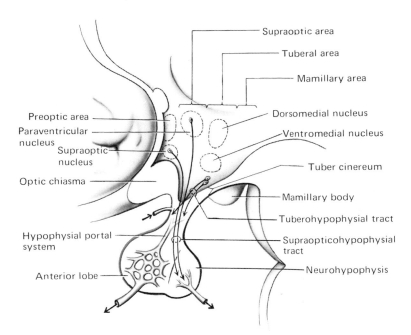

FIGURE 11-3 Some hypothalamic nuclei and the hypophysis (pituitary gland). The supraopticohypophyseal tract extends from the supraoptic and paraventricular nucleus to the capillary bed of the neurohypophysis. The hypophyseal portal system is a vascular network extending from the base of the hypothalamus and upper neurohypophysis to the anterior lobe of the hypophysis.

channels by which the affective states of being can elicit the unconscious autonomic responses and endocrine activities.

THE BLOOD VASCULAR SYSTEM This system conveys influences to which the hypothalamus may respond, including hormones, temperature of the blood, and osmolality of the blood plasma.

Output (Fig. 11-5) The *output from the hypothalamus* is conveyed via (1) ascending fibers to the forebrain, (2) descending fibers to the midbrain, and (3) pathways of fibers and blood vessels to the hypophysis (endocrine effector projections).

ASCENDING FIBERS FROM THE HYPOTHALAMUS TO THE FOREBRAIN These include the following: (1) fibers originating from the lateral hypothalamus, which pass with the medial forebrain bundle to the septal region, septal nuclei, amygdala, bed nucleus of the stria terminalis (see Figs. 1-10 and 15-3), and olfactory tubercle. These fibers are integrated in the limbic pathways (Chap. 15). (2) Fibers originating from the medial mamillary nucleus, which course via the mamillothalamic tract to the anterior thalamic nuclear group.

Reciprocally connecting fibers are included in this tract, which is a link in the so-called Papez circuit of the limbic pathways (see Chap. 15, Fig. 15-4). (3) Several hypothalamic nuclei are reciprocally connected via periventricular fibers with the magnocellular portion of the dorsomedial thalamic nucleus. This suggests a functional relation to the prefrontal cortex (Chap. 16), which has reciprocal connections with the parvocellular portion of the dorsomedial nucleus.

DESCENDING FIBERS FROM THE HYPOTHALAMUS TO THE MIDBRAIN These are paralleled by ascending fibers as reciprocally connecting pathways. Some of these fibers are incorporated in the pathways of the limbic system, discussed in Chap. 15. Many of these descending fibers are the significant links in the activity of the autonomic nervous system. In general, the medial hypothalamic system is involved through the hypophysis with neuroendocrine functions. The lateral hypothalamic system and its major pathway, the medial forebrain bundle, are associated with visceral (autonomic nervous system) and somatic (somatic nervous system) responses. This lateral

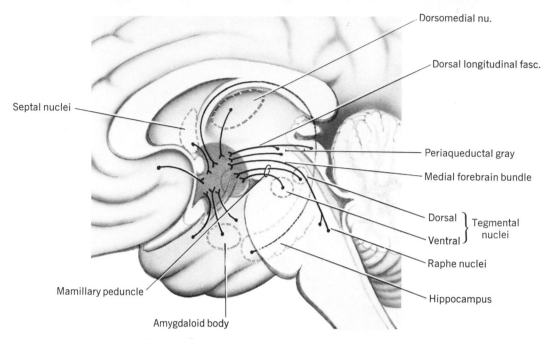

FIGURE 11-4 The major tracts conveying input to the hypothalamus.

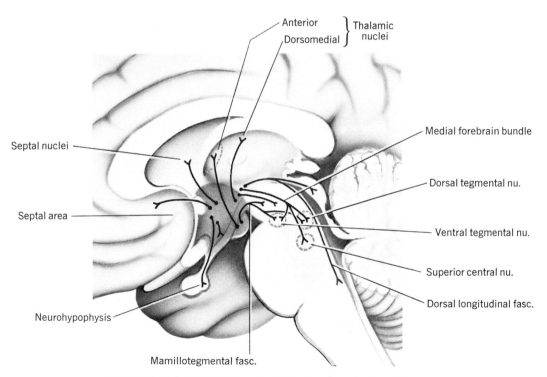

FIGURE 11-5 The major tracts conveying output from the hypothalamus.

system is interconnected with the medial system.

Fibers originating in the lateral hypothalamus form the medial forebrain bundle, which terminates primarily in paramedian cell groups of the midbrain tegmentum (limbic midbrain area) and in several mesencephalic raphe nuclei —superior central nucleus and the dorsal and ventral tegmental nuclei. The fibers of the mamillotegmental fasciculus from the mamillary bodies descend in the midbrain tegmentum and terminate in the dorsal and ventral tegmental nuclei. Some fibers terminate in the lateral midbrain tegmentum. These descending hypothalamic pathways are the most rostral links conveying hypothalamic influences to the peripheral neurons of the autonomic nervous system. Interneurons convey influences to the accessory oculomotor nucleus. A second link in this descending autonomic pathway extends from these mesencephalic nuclei to the rhombencephalic tegmentum, which contains the nuclei of origin of the pontine reticulospinal and medullary reticulospinal tracts. These are the third in the chain of linkages to the interneurons of the spinal gray matter which synapse with the preganglionic autonomic neurons.

The medial hypothalamus is interconnected by reciprocally connected fibers of the dorsal longitudinal fasciculus of Schütz with the ventral half of the periaqueductal gray matter of the midbrain and the dorsal tegmental nucleus. From this mesencephalic source, other fibers convey influences caudally to rhombencephalic reticular nuclei and, probably, to such parasympathetic nuclei as the dorsal vagal nucleus and the superior and inferior salivatory nuclei of the seventh, ninth, and tenth cranial nerves.

NEURONS IN THE MEDIAL BASAL HYPOTHALAMUS, INCLUDING THE MEDIAN EMINENCE   These neurons apparently synthesize neurohormones called *hypothalamic releasing hormones* (RH) or releasing factors (RF). These neurohormones are transported from the cell bodies in the tuber cinereum as neurosecretory substances via axons of the so-called *tuberohypophyseal tract* (*tuberoinfundibutract*), which terminates in pericapillary loops in the median eminence and the infundibular stem. This region is known as the *hypophysiotropic* or *neurohaemal area*, where the neurally derived hypothalamic releasing hormones are released and transferred to the *hypophyseal portal system*.

The hypophysiotropic area and the hypophysis receives its blood supply from several arteries. A pair of *inferior hypophyseal arteries* from the internal carotid arteries furnishes the blood supply to the neurohypophysis (neural lobe, infundibular process) and, to a lesser degree, to the sinusoids of the anterior lobe. Several *superior hypophyseal arteries* from each internal carotid artery form a capillary plexus in the pars tuberalis median eminence, and infundibular stem (see Fig. 11-3). This *capillary plexus* collects into the hypophyseal portal veins, which, in turn, arborize into the sinusoidal capillary plexus of the pars anterior. In essence, these portal veins are intercalated between the capillaries of the former and the sinusoidal capillaries of the latter. Functionally, this *hypophyseal portal system* is the neurovascular bridge or link between the hypothalamus of the brain and the pars anterior of the hypophysis, an endocrine gland. This portal system forms a conduit by which hypothalamic releasing hormones and factors (hypophysiotropins, hypophysiotropic factors) are conveyed from the tuber cinereum and infundibular stem to the anterior lobe of the hypophysis. The *venous drainage* of the pars anterior and pars nervosa is via hypophyseal veins that drain into the cavernous sinus.

The hypophyseal portal system is the vascular pathway through which the neural language from the hypophysiotropic area, in the form of releasing hormones and factors, is transferred and conveyed to the pars anterior to trigger the endocrine language of the pituitary gland. More specifically, the hypothalamic nerve fibers of different types liberate the releasing hormones from these nerve endings into the capillary plexuses of the median eminence and infundibular stem; these hormones are conveyed through the hypophyseal portal vessels to the adenohypophysis, where they stimulate or inhibit the release of a number of the hypophyseal hormones.

Neurosecretory systems

Many functional roles of the hypothalamus are mediated through two neurosecretory efferent systems acting upon the hypophysis. These are the parvicellular and magnocellular neurosecretory systems. The *parvicellular system* consists of small neurons producing neurohormones that regulate the anterior pituitary gland. The *magnocellular system* is composed of large cells in the supraoptic and paraventricular nuclei producing neurohormones that are conveyed by the hypothalamoneurohypophyseal tract to the posterior pituitary gland.

Each system consists of morphologically typical neurons, in that each neuron consists of dendrites, cell body, axon, and axon terminals. Functionally each neuron synthesizes a neurohormone (transmitter substance, neurotransmitter, hypothalamic neurohormone), conducts an action potential, and, after being triggered by calcium ions, releases the neurohormone by exocytosis. Unlike the typical neuronal synapses in which the neurotransmitter is released into a synaptic cleft, the neurohormone is released into a perivascular space and then into the capillaries of the vascular system for distribution to a target organ. The capillaries at this "synaptic site" are highly fenestrated endothelial cells (Fig. 2-18). Presumably, transport across these cells is more effective. Thus, the neurosecretory neurons are neurons that do not synapse with another neuron but instead form close contacts ("synapsis") with capillaries.

Parvicellular neurosecretory system   The neurons of the parvicellular system synthesize polypeptide neurohormones, called *hypophysiotropins*, that regulate the release of the hormones of the anterior lobe of the hypophysis. The cell bodies of these hypothalamic neurons are located in the medial basal hypothalamus and comprise the infundibular nucleus (arcuate nucleus in nonprimates), periventricular zone, and portions of the ventromedial nucleus; the region containing these cells is called the *hypophysiotrophic area* (see Fig. 11-2). The axons of these neurons terminate amid the perivascular spaces and complex network of fenestrated capillaries of the hypophyseal portal plexus located within the median eminence of the tuber cinereum. The region containing this neurovascular link is called a *neurohaemal organ*. The hypothalamic neurons in which these hypophysiotropins are found are the site of synthesis of these substances.

The hypophysiotropins are also known as *hypothalamic releasing hormones* and *hypothalamic releasing factors*. Those hypophysiotropins whose biologic and biochemical identity is firmly established are called releasing hormones, whereas those whose identity has not been fully established are called releasing factors. At present there are *three* known hypothalamic releasing hormones. (1) The decapeptide *luteinizing hormone–releasing hormone* (LHRH) regulates the release of luteinizing hormone and follicula-stimulating hormone from the anterior lobe of the pituitary gland. Most of the neurons containing this hormone are located in the infundibular nucleus and a few are in the medial preoptic–anterior hypothalamic region. LHRH, as well as other peptides, is present in other regions of the brain as structures associated with the limbic system. (2) The tripeptide *thyrotropic hormone–releasing hormone* (TRH) regulates the release of thyrotropin (thyroid-stimulating hormone, TSH). TRF is located in neurons of the periventricular, infundibular, ventromedial, and dorsomedial hypothalamic nuclei. It has been located in the thalamus, brainstem, cerebral cortex and cerebellum, lateral septal nuclei, and some motor cells of the brainstem and spinal cord. (3) The tetradecapeptide *somatostatin* (SS) acts to inhibit the release of growth hormone from the pituitary gland. It is also called *somatotropin release–inhibiting hormone* (SRIH), and it can block the TRH-induced release of TSH. Somatostatin is found in the ventromedial and periventricular hypothalamus and, additionally in the hippocampus, amygdala, and spinal cord. These three peptides are widely distributed throughout the brain; their precise biologic role in the brain has not been resolved.

The following are four recognized hypothalamic releasing factors: The *corticotropin-releasing factor* (CRF) regulates the release of adrenocorticotropin (adrenocorticotropic hormone, ACTH). The precise location in the hypothalamus where this factor is synthesized is not known. The *prolactin-inhibiting factor* (PIF) acts to inhibit the release of prolactin. This factor may be dopamine and may be synthesized in the infundibular nucleus. Two possible releasing factors are *growth hormone–releasing factor* (CRF) and *prolactin-releasing factor* (PRF), which are presumed to stimulate the release of growth hormone and prolactin, respectively. Another is a *melanocyte-stimulating hormone–inhibiting factor* (MIF), which acts to inhibit the release of melanocyte-stimulating hormone (MSH).

In reality, *the hypothalamus is the master gland*, because through the releasing hormones and factors it regulates the activity of the pituitary gland.

Magnocellular neurosecretory system The magnocellular system comprises the supraoptic and paraventricular nuclei of the hypothalamus, the hypothalamoneurohypophysial tract, and the neurohypophysis (posterior lobe of the pituitary gland).

The *hypothalamohypophyseal* (*supraopticohypophyseal*) *tract* is a bundle of about 50,000 to 100,000 unmyelinated fibers originating in the supraoptic and paraventricular nuclei of the hypothalamus. Its fibers pass through the median eminence and infundibular stem and terminate in palisades around the capillaries of the neurohypophysis. The median eminence, infundibular stem, and neurohypophysis are often considered to be a unit (see Fig. 11-1). The cells of these nuclei are neurosecretory cells, which synthesize the neurohypophyseal hormones *oxytocin* and *vasopressin* (*antidiuretic hormone, ADH*). These hormones are incorporated into dense-core vesicles, which are transported down the axonal fibers by *axoplasmatic flow* to the nerve endings. The neurosecretory material accumulates within the axoplasm of these fibers as the so-called Herring bodies. These axon terminals contain granules about 2000 Å in diameter and synapticlike vesicles about 400 Å in diameter. The *vasopressin* and *oxytocin* are probably formed in the supraoptic and paraventricular nuclei. The neurohypophysis serves as both a storage and release center for these hormones. They pass through the neurolemma, perivascular space, and fenestrated endothelium into the capillaries, which drain into the systemic circulation. Evidence indicates that vasopressin is also released into the hypophyseal portal system and conveyed to the pars anterior, where it exerts an influence on the activity of this gland.

Within the cell bodies of these nuclei, each of these neurohormones is combined with a specific "carrier protein" called a *neurophysin*. Each neurohormone and its neurophysin are synthesized in the same neuron in the rough endoplasmic reticulum, packaged in the Golgi complex, and incorporated in large membrane-bound dense-core vesicles (neurosecretory granules). The neurons forming vasopressin and those forming oxytocin are located in both the supraoptic nucleus and the periventricular nucleus. The neurons containing vasopressin are activated by such stimuli as dehydration, salt-loading, hypovolemia (decreased blood volume), and stress. The neurons containing oxytocin are stimulated by estrogen elevation and by suckling on the nipples of mammary glands.

Tanacytes

Specialized cells called *tanacytes* (probably modified astrocytes, Chap. 2) are located in the median eminence. Processes from the "cell body" of these cells extend to the third ventricle (contact cerebrospinal fluid), to the capillary plexuses of the hypophyseal portal plexus, and to some neurosecretory neurons in the median eminence. It has been suggested that tanacytes act as a functional window or interface between the parvicellular neurosecretory system and the ventricular cerebrospinal fluid.

Reflex arcs of the hypothalamus

The hypothalamus is integrated into a number of complex reflex arcs, many of which vary considerably from the classic reflex arcs. Several examples follow.

Neural reflex arc utilizing a peripheral receptor
To perform its role as a modulator of the rate of the heartbeat, the hypothalamus utilizes the classic reflex arc patterns. The peripheral receptors in the carotid sinus and the aorta (Chap. 6) relay stimuli via the glossopharyngeal and vagal nerves and brainstem tegmentum nucleus solitarius to the hypothalamus, which in turn projects efferent impulses to the cardiovascular centers in the medulla and eventually by the vagus nerve (autonomic nervous system) to the heart.

Neural reflex arc utilizing an intrinsic hypothalamic receptor To permit the hypothalamus to perform in its role as the integrator of body temperature, an intrinsic receptor within the hypothalamus monitors the temperature of the blood flowing through the capillaries of the hypothalamus itself. The efferent arms of this arc include (1) descending autonomic pathways to the sweat glands and peripheral blood vessels and (2) descending somatic pathways to the trunk musculature (used in panting).

Neurohumoral reflex This arc utilizes both the *nervous system* (*neuro-*) and the *blood vascular system* (*humoral*). To perform its role in water metabolism, the hypothalamus utilizes an intrinsic hypothalamic receptor to monitor the osmotic pressure of the blood flowing through the brain. This receptor is stimulated to put forth a neurosecretion which is conveyed via the neural pathways to the neurohypophysis, where it is released into the blood system and conveyed to its target structures in the kidney. Further examples of this type of reflex arc are noted further on in this chapter under "Hypothalamus and the Hypophysis."

In the analyses of the functional roles of the hypothalamus below, it should be borne in mind that the reflex arcs are integrated into negative-feedback, closed-loop servomechanisms (Chap. 3). The nervous system and the endocrine system have reciprocal interrelationships. Not only does the nervous system modify the functional activities of the endocrine glands, but the endocrine system, acting through the hormones in the blood circulation, influences the nervous system. This effect of the endocrine system on the nervous system may be expressed through both (1) the secretory activity of the hypophysis and (2) the behavioral patterns of the animal. For example, female sex hormones in the bloodstream may act upon hypothalamic receptors, which, in turn, "secrete" pituitary releasing hormones (factors) into the hypophyseal portal system. These factors influence the secretory activity of the anterior lobe of the hypophysis. When the blood titer of a sex hormone is elevated, the reacting hypothalamus can act to depress the secretion of gonadotropic hormones by the hypophysis; when the titer is low, the hypothalamus can act to elevate the secretion of gonadotropic hormones. The seasonal behavioral activity of mammals "in heat" or "in rut" appears to be determined, at least in part, by the response of the central nervous system to the stimulation of gon-

adal hormones (see "Hormonal Effects on Development of Behavior Patterns," Chap. 4).

FUNCTIONAL ROLE OF THE HYPOTHALAMUS

Hypothalamus and the autonomic nervous system

The hypothalamus has a significant role in the regulation of autonomic activities. Essentially it acts as a modulator (Chap. 3), influencing the autonomic centers in the brainstem and spinal cord. For example, anxiety generates neocortical activity that may be projected to the hypothalamus. In turn, the hypothalamic output to the cardiovascular integrative center in the medulla has a modulatory effect which may increase the rate and force of the heartbeat and raise the blood pressure.

The anterior (anterolateral) hypothalamus has an excitatory parasympathetic (inhibitory to sympathetic activity) role. The stimulation of this region may produce a decrease in the force and rate of the heartbeat, decrease of the blood pressure, dilatation of the visceral blood vessels, increase in peristalsis and digestive juice secretion in the alimentary canal, constriction of the pupils of the eyes, sweating, and increased salivation.

With regard to the modulation of the cardiovascular system, the hypothalamus contains neurons that respond directly to an increase in arterial blood pressure (pressure receptors) and other neurons that respond to influences from the pressoreceptors in the carotid sinus, atrium of the heart, and aortic arch.

Activity in this region produces a *parasympathetic (vagal) tone*. As a consequence, lesions of this region often result in the production of sympathetic effects. Stimulation may also produce somatic responses such as panting (increased activity of the voluntary muscles of the chest).

The posterior (posteromedial) hypothalamus has an excitatory sympathetic role. The stimulation of this region may produce an increase in the force and rate of the heartbeat, increase in blood pressure, decrease in peristalsis and in secretion of digestive juices into the alimentary canal, dilation of the pupils, and erection of hair.

Stimulation of this region often results in the production of a *sympathetic tone*. A lesion in this region may reduce both the sympathetic and parasympathetic effects of the hypothalamus upon other centers, because in addition to destroying the hypothalamic "sympathetic" centers, the lesion interrupts the caudally projecting pathways from the "parasympathetic" centers. In addition, stimulation of the posterior hypothalamus may produce such somatic activities as shivering, running, and struggling.

Vertebrates, including human beings, have a direct pathway of retinohypothalamic fibers which convey information from the retina to the hypothalamus. Through this pathway, influences from light stimulation exert a physiologic role in the activity of the hypothalamus and the hypophysis (*photoneuroendocrine system*), especially in nonmammalian vertebrates (see "Pineal Body" later on). Evidence suggests that this system may have a role in some of the metabolic activities of the organism (e.g., light may influence water balance and carbohydrate balance). The daily cycle of light and dark and the seasonal variations of this daily cycle may exert a role on the reproductive cycle. Drastic experimental modification of the light and dark environment of rats may produce demonstrable changes in their estrous cycles, uteri, ovaries, hormonal levels, sexual drives, and psychic behavioral patterns. The diurnal light-dark rhythm of the environment ("external clock") may thus act through the eye, the hypothalamic-ohypophyseal system, and the hypothalamic-oautonomic system to correlate some internal cycles ("internal clocks," circadian systems). Other aspects of this subject are noted later on in the chapter, under "Pineal Body."

Hypothalamus and temperature regulation

The hypothalamus has an essential role in the maintenance of body temperature within the narrow ranges vital to warm-blooded animals. Impairment of hypothalamic activity may give rise to either hyperthermia (hyperpyrexia) or hypothermia, because the hypothalamus contains the integration center for the homeostatic regulation of temperature. More specifically, the hypothalamus houses thermal detector neurons

(receptors) that monitor the blood temperature and the *thermostat* that regulates the heat-producing and the heat-conserving control systems. The specific function of the hypothalamus is to utilize its monitor for making the continual fine adjustments which maintain a constant body temperature. In addition the cerebral cortex (conscious recognition), after processing the environmental information from peripheral sensors in the skin, for example, operates to effect crude adjustments against environmental heat and cold (use of clothes, furnaces, and air conditioners).

The anterior hypothalamus contains a neuronal organization that acts to prevent a rise in body temperature. Some basic elements in the complex circuitry of the hypothalamic neurons associated with thermoregulation may be schematized in the following way. Warmth detector neurons monitoring an elevated hypothalamic arterial blood temperature excite circuits innervating the so-called heat loss neurons and inhibit circuits with so-called heat production-conservation neurons. These warmth detector neurons can be influenced from input derived from warmth thermoreceptors in the skin and warmth detector neurons in the cervical spinal cord. These hypothalamic circuits activate, through the autonomic nervous system, those processes favoring heat loss. These include sweating (evaporation of water for cooling), vasodilation of cutaneous blood vessels, behavioral heat loss responses, and panting. During periods of heat loss, reciprocal neuronal connections act to inhibit the cold detector and heat production-conservation neurons. Destruction of the "heat-dissipating region" may result in highly elevated body temperature (hyperthermia). Animals with this condition may survive in a cold environment, for they can then dissipate excess heat; however, they are hyperthermic in normal and warm environments. An animal with a lesion in the rostral hypothalamus cannot lose heat efficiently; death may result from hyperthermia even at room temperature.

The posterior hypothalamus contains a neuronal organization that triggers those activities concerned with heat production and heat conservation. Cold detector neurons monitoring a lowered hypothalamic arterial blood temperature excite circuits innervating the so-called heat loss neurons and the heat production-conservation neurons. These cold detector neurons can be influenced by input derived from cold thermoreceptors in the skin. These circuits activate, through the autonomic nervous system primarily, those processes favoring heat production and conservation. These include metabolic heat-producing systems (oxidation of glucose); vasoconstriction, especially of cutaneous blood vessels; erection of hair (goose pimples), and shivering. During periods of heat production, reciprocal neuronal connections act to inhibit the warmth detector and heat loss neurons. Destruction of this region may produce a cold-blooded mammal (poikilothermic) that cannot sustain a uniform body temperature. Such a lesion destroys not only the heat-conservation center but also the caudally projecting pathways from the heat-dissipating center.

Pyrogenic substances produced in some diseases affect the hypothalamus. A fever known as *neurogenic hyperthermia* results.

The precise topography and degree of dichotomy of this dual hypothalamic thermostat concept has still to be resolved. A dual chemical thermostat has been proposed; it is said to be interposed between the two thermal regions of the hypothalamus.

Hypothalamus and feeding responses

The primitive drive to ingest food for the survival of the organism is generally associated with true hunger. A more sophisticated urge to ingest food is called *appetite*, which is a drive regulated largely by the cerebral cortex. Appetite does not necessarily have any relationship to the need for food for survival. The stimulus for appetite comes from such diverse sources as stomach distention, glucose concentration in the blood, and such psychic associations as the smell, sight, and taste of food.

The hypothalamic region involved with feeding responses has been called the *appestat*, with the ventral medial hypothalamic nucleus called the *satiety center* and the lateral hypothalamic nucleus called the *hunger* or *feeding center*. Stimulation of the ventral median nucleus inhibits the animal's urge to eat. Destruction of this nucleus produces an animal exhibiting decreased physical activity and a voracious appetite (not true hunger) with a two- to threefold increase in food intake. The animal becomes excessively obese. Stimulation of the lateral hypothalamic nucleus induces the animal to eat, whereas its destruction produces an animal that refuses to eat until severe emaciation or death from starvation ensues. These hypothalamic nuclei apparently respond to the blood glucose levels.

Other humoral and nonhumoral factors that modify the firing patterns in these nuclei include fatty acids, olfactory and gustatory inputs, and the motivational state of the individual. When the level is low, the hypothalamus discharges impulses to the brainstem. Such responses as salivation, gastric contractions, chewing motion, and swallowing reflexes follow. Stimuli from the cerebrum (orbital cortex, hippocampus, and amygdaloid body) to the hypothalamus influence feeding responses. Animals with lesions in the postorbital cortex have a low food intake; those with frontal lobe lesions may have an increased food intake. Animals with small lesions of the amygdaloid body may experience transient aphagia; those with large lesions may experience hyperphagia.

Hypothalamus and the hypophysis (pituitary gland)

The hypothalamus (see Table 11-1 and Figs. 11-2 and 11-3) exerts its influences on the hypophysis and thus on endocrine activity. These routes from the hypothalamus to the hypophysis comprise (1) the neural pathway from the supraoptic and paraventricular nuclei to the neurohypophysis (hypothalamoneurohypophyseal system) and (2) the combination of a neural pathway from the hypophysiotrophic area to the capillary loops of the hypothalamohypophyseal portal system to the anterior lobe of the hypophysis.

The *hypophysis* is divided into the adenohypophysis, derived embryologically from the oral ectoderm, and the neurohypophysis, derived from neural ectoderm. The *adenohypophysis* consists of the pars tuberalis; the pars anterior, which is the largest subdivision of the hypophysis; and the pars intermedia, which is a lamina located adjacent to the pars nervosa. The *neurohypophysis* comprises three parts: (1) the median eminence, which is a continuation of the

Table 11-1
Divisions of the hypophysis (Fig. 11-1)

Adenohypophysis	Pars tuberalis Pars anterior (pars distalis, anterior lobe) Pars intermedia (intermediate lobe)	Posterior lobe
Neurohypophysis	Pars nervosa (neural lobe) (Processus infundibula)	Posterior lobe
	Infundibulum (neural stalk)	Infundibular stem Median eminence of the tuber cinereum

tuber cinereum of the hypothalamus; (2) the infundibular stem; and (3) the pars nervosa, which is the distal end of the neurohypophysis. The pars intermedia and pars nervosa form the *posterior lobe*. The *infundibulum* of the neurohypophysis consists of the median eminence of the tuber cinereum and the infundibular stem; it is a ventral projection of the hypothalamus.

The *hypothalamoneurohypophyseal system* displays features of an endocrine gland and the nervous system: a locus for the formation of secretory products (nuclei), a route for transporting the products (nerve tract), and an end organ for the storage and release of the hormonal secretions. These hormones are the octapeptides vasopressin (antidiuretic hormone, ADH) and oxytocin. *Vasopressin* has roles in the regulation of water balance through its action in the kidney as the antidiuretic hormone and in the contraction of the smooth muscles in the walls of small blood vessels (it raises blood pressure). *Oxytocin* causes the contraction of uterine smooth muscle during coitus and during parturition, and the contraction of the myoepithelial cells of the mammary gland alveoli; this mediates the milk ejection reflex (response to suckling in lactating mammals). (See "Regulation of Water Balance," below.)

The hypothalamus influences the adenohypophysis through the *hypothalamohypophyseal portal system*. Commencing as a capillary bed in the hypothalamus (median eminence of the tuber cinereum), this portal blood system collects into several main channels before arborizing as a capillary (sinusoidal) bed in the anterior lobe of the hypophysis. This portal system reaches its highest state of development in human beings and the other higher mammals. No neural connections exist between the hypothalamus and the anterior lobe of the hypophysis. In fact the anterior lobe has been de-

scribed as a gland without an innervation, yet under the control of the nervous system (through the hypophyseal portal system).

The hypophyseal portal system may be thought of as the final common and only pathway between the hypothalamus and the anterior lobe. The secretion of the humoral agents into this portal system is stimulated (or inhibited) by neural and humoral input to the hypothalamic neurons, which, in turn, project axons to the capillary bed in the median eminence. The pituitary-releasing hormones (or their precursors) may be liberated from axon terminals at the neurovascular contacts (synapses) in the median eminence; the nerve terminals on these capillaries are filled with presynaptic vesicles. These vesicles contain the neurosecretions that are liberated into the portal system through which they are conveyed to the anterior lobe. In addition, inhibiting hormones are also produced in the hypothalamus and transported via the hypophyseal portal system to the anterior lobe.

The structural and functional (neurohypophyseal hormones) relations of the hypothalamus and the neurohypophysis are discussed above, under "Pathways of the Hypothalamus."

These activities are indicative of the role of the hypothalamus in the integration of the nervous system and the endocrine system. Although seemingly different, these two systems show many basic similarities in their role in the regulatory processes of the organism. The nervous system is the rapidly reacting coordinator; the endocrine system is the slower, more general integrator. The distance between the site of origin of the chemical transmitter (neurosecretions and hormones) and its site of action (synapse) are only several hundred angstrom units in the nervous system; the distances are much longer in the endocrine system (the bloodstream is interposed between the endocrine organ and the target organ). Temporally, the nervous system acts in the time scale of milliseconds, and the endocrine system in hours and days. The nervous system and the endocrine system are functionally linked both in the suprarenal medulla (Chap. 6) and in the hypothalamohypophyseal complexes.

The synthesis and release of many hypothalamic releasing hormones may be regulated and influenced through several feedback mechanisms to the neurons in the basal hypothalamus. Both negative (inhibitory) and positive (stimulatory) feedback mechanisms have been demonstrated. These include (1) the *long feedback loop* in which the hormones are synthesized and released in the peripheral target glands (e.g., estrogens, testosterone, corticoids) and fed back to the basal hypothalamus and (2) the *short feedback loop* in which the tropic hormones synthesized and released by the adenohypophysis (e.g., follicle- and thyrotropin-stimulating hormones) are also fed back to the basal hypothalamus, and (3) the *short short feedback loop* in which the releasing hormones released in the tuber cinereum may feed back to the neural receptors of the hypothalamus involved with regulating the synthesis of releasing hormones and factors.

Regulation of water balance

The hypothalamus contains the integration center concerned with the regulation of water balance. In fact, this most highly vascularized region in the brain is essentially an osmoreceptor sensitive to the osmotic pressure (concentration of sodium chloride level, osmolarity) of the blood in the capillaries that bathe these nuclei. As a consequence, this general region has been called the "drinking center." An animal with a lesion in the region of the ventral median nucleus and the lateral hypothalamic area may consume little water even when dehydrated, while an animal in which this region is stimulated will consume prodigious amounts of water even when already "saturated" with it.

Other stimuli such as mechanical stretch of the left atrium of the heart may influence water intake. The stimulation of peripheral receptors in the mouth resulting from dryness of the mucous membranes creates the sensation of thirst. The sight of beverages and the smell of aromatic coffee can produce psychic responses (limbic system) that affect fluid consumption.

The role of the hypothalamus in water metabolism is focused on the magnocellular neurosecretory system, namely the supraoptic nucleus and paraventricular nucleus, the hypothalamohypophyseal pathways, and the posterior lobe. The supraoptic and paraventricular nuclei respond to the fluctuations in the osmotic pressure of the blood.

Hyperosmotic blood, present during dehydration of the water stores of the body, stimulates *osmoreceptor* cells of the hypothalamus to initiate the sequence that releases the *antidiuretic hormone* (*ADH*, vasopressin) into the bloodstream in the neurohypophysis. In turn, the ADH acts upon the kidney (distal convoluted and collecting tubules) to increase the reabsorption of water back into the bloodstream. Water is thereby conserved, not excreted in the urine. Thirst also follows, with water intake increased by drinking. Whether the neurons elaborating ADH are also the osmoreceptors or whether the osmoreceptors are specialized cells has not been resolved.

If the blood is hypotonic, as in a hydrated animal, ADH is not released. Water is not conserved, because it is reabsorbed in lesser quantities by the kidney tubules. Normally only 1 to 2 L of urine is excreted each day because 14 to 18 L is reabsorbed into the bloodstream each day, largely by the distal convoluted tubules. The more ADH released, the more water is conserved; the less ADH released, the more water is excreted. Individuals with a lesion of the supraoptic nuclei drink excessive amounts of water to quench their thirst, because the lack of ADH may result in the excretion of equal amounts of urine per day (diabetes insipidus). This condition may be transitory because the hypothalamohypophyseal tract is capable of regeneration. Cholinergic fibers terminating in the supraoptic and paraventricular nuclei stimulate the release of vasopressin, whereas the noradrenergic terminals can inhibit vasopressin release. Water balance is also influenced by the renin-angiotensin system in the kidney. Angiotensin is a polypeptide with a direct effect on the hypothalamic neuronal organization subserving thirst and drinking behavior. A circumventricular organ, the subfornical organ (see later on in chapter), has a role in mediating the effects of angiotensin on drinking activities.

Hypothalamus and the anterior lobe of the hypophysis

The hypothalamus acts as a regulatory center capable of modifying the secretory activity of the anterior lobe through hypothalamic neurosecretions (pituitary hormone-releasing hormones) which are transported via the blood vessels of the hypophyseal portal system to the anterior lobe. These humoral (blood-conveyed) substances activate the secretion of such anterior lobe hormones as growth hormones, gonadotropins (ovary and testis), corticotropin (suprarenal cortex), and thyrotropin (thyroid gland); these pituitary hormones are then conveyed through the bloodstream to their target organs.

Ovulation (extrusion of the ovum from the ovary) in the cat offers an example of an physiologic process which is influenced by the nervous system acting through the hypothalamus and the hypophysis. The activity generated in the limbic lobe cortex following sexual excitement stimulates the hypothalamus to secrete luteinizing hormone-releasing hormone (factor) into the hypophyseal portal circulation. The resulting release of luteinizing hormone by the anterior lobe into the systemic bloodstream induces ovulation in the ovary.

The interplay and interdependence between the nervous system and the endocrine system are illustrated in the maintenance of lactation. The sucking of the mother's nipple by the infant results in the generation of neural impulses from tactile receptors which are conveyed by peripheral nerves to the spinal cord and ultimately to the mother's hypothalamus (tuberal region), where neurosecretions are released into the hypophyseal portal system. This neurosecretion stimulates the anterior lobe to release the hormone lactogen into the bloodstream. In turn, the lactogen activates the cells of the mammary gland to secrete milk. The distended mammary gland apparently feeds back information to the paraventricular nucleus of the hypothalamus, which acts, via the hypothalamohypophyseal tract, upon the neurohypophysis. The resulting

release of oxytocin by the posterior lobe into the circulation stimulates the myoepithelial cells of the mammary glands, resulting in their contraction and the ejection of milk from the glandular cells into the ducts of the mammary gland, so that the infant may successfully suckle its mother's milk. The cycle is thereby completed and sustained.

Hypothalamus in emotion and behavior

The behavioral patterns associated with our emotional experience are of two general types: subjective "feelings," or inward expression, and objective physical expressions, or consummatory behavior. The subjective aspects of emotion, from depression to euphoria, are more intimately bound up with the cerebral cortex. Many of the physical expressions are largely mediated through the hypothalamus and the autonomic nervous system under the influences of the cerebral cortex, limbic system (Chap. 15), thalamus, and brainstem. Many of these objectives expressions are recognizable as the enhanced activity of the autonomic nervous system. They include alterations in the heartbeat (palpitations) and the blood pressure, blushing and pallor of the face, dryness of the mouth, clammy hands, dilatation of the pupils (glassy eye), disturbances of secretory activity and motility of the digestive system, cold sweat, tears of happiness or sadness, and changes in the concentration of the blood sugar. Some of the expressions of emotional stress that utilize the somatic nervous system include such voluntary muscle activities as facial grimaces, shrugging of the shoulders, and the movements accompanying nervousness, crying, escaping, and fighting.

The primitive expressions of emotional behavior may be evoked by ablating or stimulating portions of the hypothalamus. Bilateral destruction of the ventromedial nuclei (or stimulation of the dorsomedial nuclei) can transform a gentle animal into one exhibiting varying degrees of wildness. If mildly provoked, an animal whose hypothalamus has been injured may attack savagely and hiss, or may attempt to escape. Such an animal exhibits a sham (simulated) rage, for when the provoking stimulus is removed, the animal immediately becomes seemingly placid. In a sham rage, an animal immediately becomes seemingly placid. In a sham rage, an animal demonstrates objective signs of rage but does not have the corresponding subjective feelings. Some investigators claim that the provoked rage is not a true sham rage, for these outbursts are often directed at a specific object or goal and are not actually aimless. Stimulation of the hypothalamus in human beings is said to evoke changes in the blood pressure and rate of heartbeat without any psychic manifestations.

An animal with portions of its new and old cerebral cortices removed exhibits the explosive behavior patterns of sham rage. Under these conditions, the sham rage is a form of *release phenomenon* as the hypothalamus, autonomic nervous system, and other regions are released from the regulatory influences of the cortex. In a decorticate cat, for example, a mildly noxious stimulus, such as pinching the tail, may evoke such sympathetic effects as pupillary dilatation, elevated blood pressure and faster heartbeat, piloerection, and such somatic effects as arching of the back, snarling, and striking with protracted claws. The entire reaction ceases immediately when the tail pinching is stopped.

The hypothalamus has a central role in many expressions associated with sexual behavior. The sources of powerful influences upon the hypothalamus are the olfactory system, neocortex, limbic system, and hormones. Many of the functional aspects of these influences are obvious. The output from the hypothalamus for these expressions utilizes primarily (1) the descending autonomic pathways and (2) the hypophyseal portal system to the hypophysis in order to mobilize the autonomic nervous and endocrine systems.

Hypothalamus and the sleep-wake cycle

The hypothalamus is associated with the state of awakeness, but precisely how this structure is integrated into the sleep-wake cycle is not known. In contrast to the agitated reactions of the "sham rage" evoked in an animal with a tuberal lesion, the bilateral ablation of the regions dorsolateral and caudal to the mamillary bodies produces a tame, apathetic, and often somnolent monkey or cat. Stimulation of the hypothalamus of the cat may induce drowsiness and sleep. The ascending reticular activating system which projects to the hypothalamus and the diffuse projections from the hypothalamus to the cerebral cortex are among the neural substrates for the sleep-wake cycle.

Hypothalamus and the "pleasure" and "punishing" centers

The region of the lateral hypothalamus in the median forebrain bundle near the feeding center is incorporated into the "pleasure-center" complex discussed in Chap. 15. Electric stimulation of this area drives the animal to seek more of such stimulation. The medial hypothalamus is integrated into the "punishing-center" complex (Chap. 15). Electrical stimulation of this area is apparently unpleasant, because the animal attempts to avoid further stimulation.

SOME CLINICAL CONSIDERATIONS

Degenerative changes of the hypothalamohypophyseal tract result in a deficiency of the antidiuretic hormone (vasopressin, ADH); this condition may be accompanied by *diabetes insipidus, polydipsia* (compulsive water drinking), and *polyuria* (excessive excretion of urine). Some lesions of the hypothalamus, often in the region of the tuber cinereum, give rise to severe gastric disturbances associated with erosion, ulceration, and hemorrhaging in the mucosa of the stomach; this condition may involve areas involved with the secretion of hydrochloric acid in the stomach preparatory to the ingestion of food.

Lesions in the tuberal region, including the adjacent ventral medial nuclei, result in *adiposogenital dystrophy*—characterized by obesity and gonadal atrophy. The obesity is a consequence of the damage to the ventral medial nuclei; the gonadal atrophy is probably due to the malfunctioning of the tuberoinfundibular tract, which is involved with the hypophysiotropic region. Tuberal lesions may give rise to hyperglycemia and distrubances in heat regulation.

THE CIRCUMVENTRICULAR ORGANS OF THE CENTRAL NERVOUS SYSTEM (Fig. 11-6)

Adjacent to the median ventricular cavities (third ventricle, cerebral aqueduct, and fourth ventricle) are several specialized regions called *circumventricular organs*. The common vascular, ependymal, and neural organization of these structures differs from that found in typical brain tissue. They are referred to as "being in the brain but not of it," in part because they lack a blood-brain barrier. In humans, the circumventricular organs include (1) the median eminence of the tuber cinereum, the neurohypophysis, and the pineal body, which are considered to be sites of neuroendocrine activity, and (2) the organum vasculosum of the lamina terminalis, subfornical organ, subcommissural organ, and the area postrema (see Fig. 11-6), the functional roles of which have not, as yet, been clearly defined. The ependymal cells of the circumventricular organs and choroid plexus are nonciliated.

Median eminence of the tuber cinereum

The *median eminence of the tuber cinereum* is that portion of the floor of the third ventricle where the releasing and inhibiting hormones are released from the axon terminals into the capillary loops of the hypophyseal portal system. In essence, it is site of a neurovascular link between the nervous system and the adenohypophysis. The secretion of the releasing hormones from the axon terminals may be influenced by a system of dopaminergic and noradrenergic neurons.

Neurohypophysis

As previously noted, the *neurohypophysis* is the site for the storage and release of vasopressin and oxytocin, which are synthesized in the supraoptic and paraventricular nuclei. The nerve terminals of the supraopticohypophyseal tract containing these neurohormones are intermingled among cells called pituicytes, which are modified glial cells.

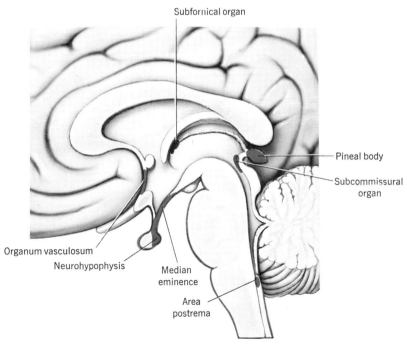

FIGURE 11-6 Midsagittal view of the brain illustrating the location of the circumventricular organs. (*After Weindl.*)

Pineal body (Figs. 11-5 and A-37)

The *pineal body*, or *epiphysis cerebri*, in mammals is a midline cone-shaped structure located in the caudal epithalamus just above the midbrain tegmentum. Descartes called the pineal body, "the seat of the soul." It is a highly vascular organ consisting of parenchymal cells (*pineocytes*), astrocyte-like glial cells, and calcareous granules (corpora arenacea). The parenchymal cells have processes which terminate on the basal lamina of the perivascular space surrounding the fenestrated capillaries. It is probable that the only innervation to the pineal body is by postganglionic sympathetic fibers from the superior cervical ganglion. Vesicles are present in the nerve endings and the parenchymal cells. These vesicles contain melatonin, serotonin, and other "pineal hormones," and norepinephrine.

Theories regarding the functional significance of the pineal body vary from its being a functionless vestigial organ to its being a significant endocrine organ. Much evidence suggests that the pineal body has a neuroendocrine role in the modulation or regulation of rhythmic activities of the endocrine system as expressed, for example, in seasonal reproductive cycles. In turn, these rhythms are in a large measure influenced by the environmental light diurnal cycles of night and day (circadian cycles) and their graded differences during the seasons.

Environmental light exerts its influences upon the pineal body through the following presumed circuitry. Photostimulation of the retina is projected directly from the eye to the suprachiasmatic nucleus of the hypothalamus (see Fig. 11-1). From this nucleus a multineuronal pathway descends and terminates in the upper thoracic intermediolateral cell column—the site of the preganglionic sympathetic neurons. The axons of these neurons course through the white rami in the sympathetic chain to terminate and synapse in the superior cervical ganglion with postganglionic neurons whose axons terminate in the pineal body. It is likely that the pineal body is innervated exclusively by the sympathetic system. In some way these postganglionic sympathetic influences modulate the release of melanotonin from the pineal body into the vascular system. One of the targets for melatonin is the serotoninergic raphe nuclei of the brain, which through their rostral projections may feed back to the suprachiasmatic nucleus and may influence limbic structures including the hypothalamus. Melatonin seems to have an active role in light-influenced reproductive cycles in many mammals and birds. In addition, the pineal body and the suprachiasmatic nucleus are said to exhibit cyclic activity in their sensitivity and reactivity to stimulation.

Organum vasculosum of the lamina terminalis (Fig. 11-5)

The *organum vasculosum* (*supraoptic crest*, "*prechiasmatic gland*") is a highly vascular region of the lamina terminalis. Structurally it is similar to the median eminence. Its loops of fenestrated capillaries are surrounded by wide, fluid-filled perivascular spaces. This structure contains neurons whose axons project to the supraoptic nuclei. Its probable role is in drinking behavior (osmoregulation), secretion of antidiuretic hormone, and physiological control of body fluid balance.

Subfornical organ (Fig. 11-5)

The *subfornical organ* (*intercolumnar tubercle*) is an elevation located between the diverging columns of the fornix at the level of the interventricular foramina (of Monro). It is partially covered by choroid plexus. This organ may be a neuroendocrine structure. Its sinusoid and glomerular loops are supplied by adjacent blood vessels. The nerve endings synapsing with the parenchymal cells of the organ have synaptic vesicles which may contain acetylcholine. Neurons of the subfornical organ project to the supraoptic nuclei and the organum vasculosum. This structure is thought to have a similar role as the organum vasculosum.

Subcommissural organ (Fig. 11-5)

The *subcommissural organ* is located in the roof of the cerebral aqueduct just rostral and ventral to the posterior commissure and fairly close to the pineal body. It is composed of specialized ependymal cells and some associated glial cells in a capillary bed of nonfenestrated endothelium. The ependymal cells are secretory. They release a product directly into the ventricular fluid, which condenses to form Reissner's fiber—a neutral mucopolysaccharid protein complex. Reissner's fiber can be traced through the cerebral aqueduct, fourth ventricle, and central canal of the spinal cord to the coccygeal levels. Although the functional role the subcommissural organ is unknown, several proposals include thermoregulation, regulation of water and electrolyte balance, and responses to change in illumination.

Area postrema (Fig. 11-5)

The *area postrema* is one of a pair of small rounded eminences on either side of the fourth ventricle just rostral to the obex at the junction of the ventricle and the central canal (see Fig. 11-6; see also Fig. A-15). The area is deep to the nonciliated ependymal cell lining the ventricle. It is composed of modified neurons (its parenchymal cells), astrocyte-like cells, and rich overlapping arterial and sinusoidal network. The synaptic terminals within the area postrema are derived from the nucleus solitarius and from ascending spinal fibers. It is possible that the area postrema monitors certain changes in the composition of the blood and, in addition, releases neurosecretory substances into the systemic circulation. This would be in line with some of the suggested functional roles ascribed to other circumventricular organs. These include regulating blood pressure and functioning as a chemoreceptor for CO_2 in the regulation of respiration; these roles may be expressed through nearby medullary areas involved with blood circulation and respiration. The area postrema or an adjacent region of the medulla may act as an osmosensitive zone or a chemoreceptor emetic trigger zone involved with the vomiting reflex.

BIBLIOGRAPHY

Ganong, W. F., and L. Martini (eds.): *Frontiers in Neuroendocrinology*, Raven Press, New York, 1980.

Harris, G. W., and B. T. Donovan (eds.): *The Pituitary Gland*, University of California Press, Berkeley, 1966.

Haymaker, W., E. Anderson, and W. J. H. Nauta: *The Hypothalamus*, Charles C Thomas, Publisher, Springfield, Ill., 1969.

Hess, W. R.: *The Functional Organization of the Diencephalon*, Grune & Stratton, Inc., New York, 1958.

Knigge, K. M., D. E. Scott, and A. Weindl (eds.): *Brain-Endocrine Interaction. Median Eminence: Structure and Function*, Karger, Basel, 1972.

Knigge, K. M., and A. J. Silverman: "Anatomy of the Endocrine Hypothalamus," in R. O. Greep and E. B. Astwood (eds.), *Handbook of Physiology: Endocrinology*, American Physiological Society, Washington, D.C., 1974, chap. 1, pp. 1–32.

Martini, L., M. Motta, and F. Fraschini: *The Hypothalamus*, Academic Press Inc., New York, 1971.

McEwen, B. S.: Interactions between hormones and nerve tissue. Sci Am, 235:49–58. 1976.

Moore, R. Y.: Retinohypothalamic projection in mammals: a comparative study. Brain Res, 49:403–409, 1973.

Olds, J.: Hypothalamic substrates of reward. Physiol Rev, 42:554–604, 1962.

Page, R. B., and R. M. Bergland: The neurohypophyseal capillary bed. I. Anatomy and arterial supply. Amer J Anat, 148:345–357, 1977.

Pfaff, D. (ed.): *Hormonal Factors in Brain Function*, M.I.T Press, Cambridge, Mass., 1975.

Weindl, A.: "Neuroendocrine Aspects of Circumventricular Organs," in W. F. Ganong and L. Martini (eds.), *Frontiers in Neuroendocrinology*, Oxford University Press, New York and London, 1973.

CHAPTER TWELVE

THE OPTIC SYSTEM

Sight is our most dominant sense; we live primarily in a visual world. The rods and cones in the retinas of the eyes comprise about 70 percent of the receptors of the entire body. About one-third of all the afferent nerve fibers projecting information to our central nervous system are the approximately 2 million nerve fibers in both optic nerves.

Out of the engulfing sea of radiation in the electromagnetic spectrum, from the minute gamma rays one million-millionth nanometer in length to radio waves several miles in length, *our eyes are sensitive only to that narrow band of radiation known as the visual spectrum of from 400 nm (millionth part of a millimeter) to 700 nm (from blue to red).* We do not see in or beyond the infrared band, because our visual receptors cannot be stimulated by these wavelengths. The *ultraviolet radiations from 365 to 400 nm are capable of being "seen" but are normally absorbed by the lens.* An individual without a lens (*aphakic*) can literally see in ultraviolet light. In one respect we are fortunate that the entire electromagnetic spectrum does not supply the stimulus energy to produce a visual image. Otherwise we would literally see everything. Because our sense of sight is restricted to but one-seventieth of the spectrum, we are selective. If we perceived all radiation we should be in a perpetual daylight; even at night we would not see the stars for the glare. Human beings have devised instruments (radios and oscilloscopes) that are capable of bringing invisible forms of radiation (e.g., radio waves) to our selective receptors (e.g., radio to our auditory sense, oscilloscope to our visual sense).

Some of the waves outside the visual spectrum may affect an organism. The invisible short-wave radiation can induce a chemical reaction in living tissues—ultraviolet light can produce a sunburn, and the ionizing radiation of x-rays and cosmic rays can damage tissues. Infrared rays, at the other end of the spectrum, can be felt as heat. Ultraviolet rays and infrared rays can be seen if presented to the eye in very high intensities.

It is essential to understand that the optic system performs in several areas: (1) light and dark, (2) color, (3) image reproduction or form vision, (4) visual acuity, (5) spatial or depth sense, (6) motion perception or resolution of images in time, (7) appreciation of brightness or intensities of light, and (8) recognition and comparison of images with previous experience.

The visual process may be subdivided into five phases: (1) the refraction of light rays and focusing of images on the retina, (2) the transduction of light quanta by photochemical activity, (3) the processing of neural activity in the retina and transmission of coded impulses through the optic nerve, (4) the processing in the brain culminating in perception, and (5) the reflexes associated with the visual system (e.g., accommodation).

ANATOMY OF THE EYE
(Figs. 12-1 through 12-3)

The eye is a sphere that is analogous to the common camera obscura (see Fig. 12-1). It is constructed to perform both optical and sensory

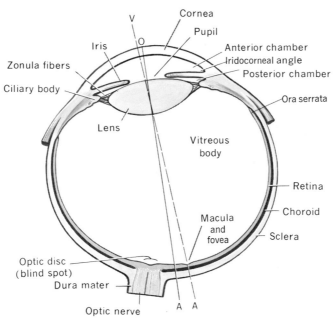

FIGURE 12-1 Diagram of a horizontal meridional section through the human right eye. VA, visual axis; OA, optical axis.

functions. Its optical role is to gather light rays and to focus them onto the retina. To do this, the eye has (1) a variable aperture system—the iris and its opening, the pupil—which regulates the amount of light passing to the retina, and (2) a lens system—cornea and lens—which produces a two-dimensional image of the object on the retina. Its sensory roles are to respond to and to process environmental influences and to transmit coded messages to the brain. These roles are performed by the retina. The fibers of the optic nerve, which originate in the retina, convey the output of the retina to the brain. The sclera corresponds to the frame of the camera; the pigment epithelium of the retina and the choroid layer correspond to the black interior lining of the camera; the cornea and lens to the camera lenses; the aqueous humor of the anterior and posterior chambers and the vitreous humor of the vitreous body to the air spaces within the camera; the iris corresponds to the diaphragm; the pupil to the opening in the diaphragm; the eyelid to the lens cap; and the retina to the film. The television camera is an even better analogue; it not only focuses light and forms coded messages of images but also relays these messages to "transmitters."

The eye is composed of three coats: the *outer* or *fibrous tunic* comprises the *sclera* and *cornea*; the *vascular tunic*, or *uveal tract* (*uvea*), consists of the *choroid, ciliary body*, and *iris*; and the *inner tunic*, or *retina*, includes the photosensitive portion in the back of the eye, the unpigmented epithelium of the ciliary body, and the pigmented epithelium of the posterior iris (see Figs. 12-1 and 12-2). In describing the anatomic locations within the eye, the terms *outer* and *inner* are used with reference to the center of the eye. Thus the fibrous tunic is an outer layer and the retina is an inner layer. The same terms apply to the retina structures (e.g., the rods and cones are "outer" to the bipolar cells). The transparent biconvex *lens* is located behind the iris and the pupil. It is suspended by fine "guy ropes" called the *zonular fibers*, which are anchored in the 70 or more ciliary processes of the ciliary body located in the vicinity of the corneoscleral junction. The ocular chamber is the fluid-filled space between the cornea and vitreous body, which is partially divided by the iris into an anterior chamber and a posterior chamber. Both chambers are filled with clear, watery fluid called the *aqueous humor*. The *anterior chamber* is located between the cornea, iris, and front of the lens;

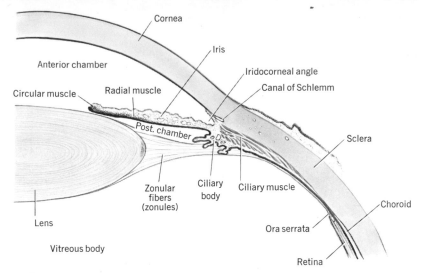

FIGURE 12-2 Horizontal meridional section through a portion of the human eye.

the *posterior chamber* is bounded by the iris, ciliary body, lens, and vitreous body. The large *vitreous chamber* is located between the posterior surface of the lens and ciliary body and the posterior wall of the eyeball. This chamber, comprising about five-sixths of the eye, is filled with a transparent gelatinous material.

The adult human eyeball is roughly a globe approximately 24 mm in diameter and 6.5 mL in volume; it consists of the segments of two spheres which are unequal in size. The smaller sphere comprises the anterior one-sixth of the eyeball; this forms the *corneal curve*. The larger sphere comprises the posterior five-sixths; its outer coat forms the *scleral curve*. The anterior segment has a greater curvature than the posterior segment. The anterior pole is located in the center of the corneal curve, and the posterior pole in the center of the scleral curve. The *geometric (anatomic) axis* is a line from the anterior pole through the posterior pole. The *optical axis* is a theoretical line passing through the center of the optical centers of the principal refracting surfaces of the cornea and lens (see Fig. 12-1). The *visual axis* forms a line passing from the fixation point (center of the object in focus) through the nodal point near the posterior surface of the lens and the fovea centralis (spot of most acute vision). The optical axis differs from the visual axis because the lens is decentered slightly

downward and nasally with respect to the optic axis. This decentration does not alter the visual role of the eye.

Two planes—the vertical and horizontal meridians—are important. The plane of the *vertical meridian* passes through the fovea and divides the eye into a *nasal (medial)* and a *temporal (lateral) half*. The plane of the *horizontal meridian* passes through the fovea centralis and divides the eye into upper and lower halves. The planes divide the eye into four quadrants—*upper nasal, upper temporal, lower nasal,* and *lower temporal.* The associated divided retinal segments are respectively called the *nasal hemiretina, temporal hemiretina, upper nasal retinal quadrant,* etc.

The retina near the posterior pole of the eye is modified into three concentric regions (see Fig. 12-1), namely, the *central part of the retina* (5 to 6 mm in diameter), the *macula or macula lutea* (3 mm in diameter), and the *fovea centralis (central fovea,* 0.4 mm wide). The *macula,* or *yellow spot,* is yellowish because of the carotinoid and xanthophyll pigments in the neurons of the region. The *fovea centralis* is a small, funnel-shaped pit in the macula formed by the spreading and deviation of the inner layers of the retina from the center of the region. Cones are the only photoreceptors found in this region of most acute vision. Medial to the macula is the *blind spot,* where no image is registered. The blind spot is the site of the nerve head at the emergence of the optic nerve; it is called the *optic disk*. This bulging disk has a central depression or excavation. A precise positional relationship exists among the posterior pole, fovea centralis, and optic disk. The fovea centralis is about 1 mm temporal and 1.8 mm inferior to the posterior pole (see Fig. 12-3). The center of the optic disk is located 3 mm nasal and 1 mm inferior to the posterior pole. The blind spot can be located in the following way: place two large dots a few inches apart on a piece of paper, close the left eye, and continually focus on the left dot with the right eye. Move the head toward (or away from) the paper. Note that while you are looking at the left dot, the right dot is not seen at a certain distance from the paper. At this distance the right dot is focused on the blind spot. The blind spot is located in the lower nasal retinal quadrant, which means that it appears in the upper temporal quadrant of the visual fields (see "Fields of Vision and the Retina," later on in this chapter).

The optic nerve is surrounded by the meninges and their spaces up to the junction of the nerve with the eye (see Figs. 12-1 and 12-3). The dura matter is continuous with the sclera. Because the subarachnoid space surrounds the optic nerve, changes in the cerebrospinal fluid pressure can be registered in the optic disk. A high cerebrospinal fluid pressure, such as one caused by a space-occupying lesion, exerts a force which is transmitted to the optic nerve and exerts the central depression of the optic disk to produce a *swollen optic disk* or *choked disk*. The retina and optic disk can be observed with an ophthalmoscope, an instrument which enables a doctor to look into the eye. In such an examination of a patient with a choked disk, the living retina appears red (because of vessels in the choroid layer) except for the pale, circular swollen optic disk. This result of an increased intracranial pressure is also called *papilledema*.

The collagenous *corneoscleral tunic* is a slightly elastic skeleton of the eye, which, with the help of the intraocular pressure, maintains the shape of the eye. It is comparable to a balloon filled with a fluid. This tough coat is composed of 94 percent sclera and 6 percent cornea. The sclera, or white of the eye, is relatively avascular. It is structurally continuous with the cornea. The extraocular muscles are inserted into

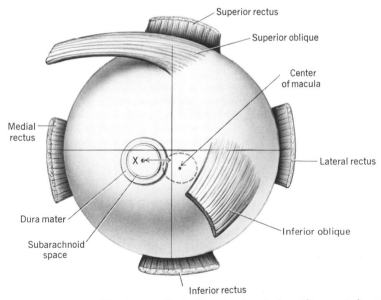

FIGURE 12-3 A posterior view of the right eye. The horizontal and vertical meridians are indicated by the two lines which intersect at the posterior pole of the eye. The center of the optic nerve is 3 mm nasal to the posterior pole of the eye and 1 mm below it. The center of the macula is located 1 mm temporal to the posterior pole and 1.8 mm below it. The circular outline of the 3-mm-diameter macula lutea is indicated by the broken-line circle. (*Adapted from Hogan, Alvarado, and Weddell.*)

the sclera. The boundary between the opaque sclera and the transparent cornea is called the limbus. Of the lenses of the eye, the cornea is nonadjustable, whereas the lens is adjustable. Both are, of necessity, avascular because blood vessels, if present, would scatter light. The first refractile surface is actually the tear film on the cornea.

The *transparency of the cornea* results from (1) the regularity of its epithelial surface, (2) its avascularity, (3) the regular pattern of its collagen fibers and ground substance, and (4) the chemical composition and the state of hydration of its stroma. The basis for this transparency is considered to be physiologic and not anatomic. Its optical homogeneity is primarily maintained by the metabolic activity of its cells, which are continually pumping out interstitial fluid against the normal tendency of the cornea to become hydrated. In this way the cornea is kept in a deturgescent state. The ionic pump is located in the endothelial cell layer adjacent to the aqueous humor.

In contrast, the sclera possesses a higher water content. The sclera can become transparent if it is partially dehydrated locally. Following the cessation of metabolic pumping, after death, the cornea becomes opaque. The sensitivity of the cornea is due to rich and extensive innervation by sensory fibers of the ophthalmic division of the trigeminal nerve.

The cornea is most resistant to infection. Because of the mitotic potential of its surface epithelium, it can effectively heal penetrating wounds. The cornea is one of those few structures that can be readily transplanted (*corneal transplants*) from the eye of a donor to the eye of a host. This resistance of the cornea to rejection when in the host is related to several factors, chiefly its avascularity, but including the absence of lymphatics and the barrier effect of the aqueous humor supplying its metabolic needs. In the transplants that "take," the epithelial surface cells are quickly lost; within days the layers are replaced by the migration and mitotic activity of cells from the host. Apparently the intrinsic cells of the bulk of the cornea (substantia propria) may survive for years; ultimately they are replaced by the host tissue.

The *choroid layer* is the highly vascularized, richly black-pigmented layer of the uveal tract, extending forward about two-thirds of the distance toward the pupil. It is coextensive with the photoreceptive retina, which it supplies with nutriment and oxygen. The pigment absorbs light.

The *ciliary body* is located between the *ora serrata* (anterior edge of the photoreceptive retina) and the corneoscleral junction (see Fig. 12-3). It subserves three roles: accommodation, production of the aqueous humor of the anterior and posterior chambers, and restoration of the mucopolysaccharides of the vitreous body.

The delicate adjustment altering the shape and thereby the refractive power of the lens is called *accommodation*. This adjustment results from the state of contraction of the ciliary muscles—the circular muscle, radial muscle, and meridional muscle—which have a role in adjusting the tension exerted on the lens through the zonular fibers comprising the suspensory ligaments of the lens. The precise manner in which the ciliary body regulates the curvature of the lens is often misunderstood. When the eye is relaxed, as in viewing distant objects, the ciliary muscles are relaxed; in this state the tension exerted by the ring of the ciliary body through the ciliary processes on the zonular fibers is maximal and, as a result, the lens is flattened. To view objects close to the eye (near vision) a rounder lens is necessary, so that the light rays will be refracted more. To accomplish this, the ciliary muscles (longitudinal, circular, and tangential muscle groups) contract and pull the ciliary body slightly forward and inward, narrowing the ring of the ciliary body and thereby reducing the tension on the zonular fibers; these protein zonular fibers are inserted into the lens capsule, a modified basement membrane on the outer surface of the lens. Because the lens has an inherent resiliency, it rounds up on its own when the tension is reduced. The refraction of light is greater with a rounder lens; this occurs with the shift of one's gaze from a distant to a close object.

The *lens* is a transparent biconvex disk with an elliptical shape. It is surrounded by a thin *lens capsule*. The lens is held in position and suspended by hairlike zonular fibers which extend in a radial pattern from the lens capsule to the ciliary body. Nourishment and oxygen for the lens are derived from the aqueous and vitreous humors. The cells constituting the lens have a metabolic role in forming lens crystalline protein and maintaining its optical transparency. Reduction in the nutritional status and metabolic efficiency of the lens cells is an expression of normal aging. One consequence is a decrease in the accommodation power of the lens in middle age. The molecular weight of the lens protein increases with age—and, the protein may become opaque (cataracts). Poor nourishment of the lens during various metabolic and aging diseases can lead to cataracts. For example, abnormal sugar metabolism, as in diabetes, may have an effect on the vitality of the lens. *Cataracts* are the presumed consequence for all who reach extreme old age.

The ability to accommodate gradually decreases with age; it is lost sometime between the early fifties and the early sixties. The normally pale yellow lens becomes more intensified in the sixth decade. This explains why older people often see as green what may be actually blue because some blue and violet light is filtered out.

The lens continues to grow throughout life, with the addition of new cells at the lens equator. The lens has no nerve supply.

The *muscular iris* surrounds the pupil, resulting in an adjustable optic diaphragm which is a variable aperture. Dilating or constricting the iris causes the pupil to be enlarged or reduced, thereby regulating the amount of light passing into the depths of the eyeball (see "The Visual Reflexes," further on). As compared to the f-stop in a camera, the eye operates in the range of f2 to f22. The pupillary size is increased by the radial muscle cells of the iris (contraction of these muscles results in a pupillary dilation) and is decreased by the circular muscle cells of the iris (contraction results in pupillary constriction). The posterior epithelial layer of the iris (iridial portion of the retina) is pigmented. The bulk of the iris is composed of loose, pigmented, highly vascular connective tissue. The color of the eye is related to the amount of pigment in the melanocytes of the iris. Blue eyes have a slight amount of pigment; brown eyes have a moderate amount; and black eyes a great amount. The blue color results from stromal absorption of long wavelengths, with the blue waves returning to the observer's eyes. The red appearance of the eyes of an albino is produced by the blood in a pigmentless iris.

The anterior and posterior chambers are filled with *aqueous humor*—a thin, watery fluid which is essentially an ultrafiltrate of blood resembling cerebrospinal fluid. It is largely responsible for the intraocular pressure and provides such essential nourishment as oxygen, glucose, and amino acids for the avascular lens and cornea. The aqueous humor is formed primarily by the ciliary body, passes into the posterior chamber, and slowly circulates through the pupil to the anterior chamber. At the *iridocorneal (filtration) angle* at the lateral circular border of the anterior chamber, the aqueous humor leaves through the spaces of a trabecular meshwork before diffusing through a thin, nonperforated wall of tissue into the *canal of Schlemm* (an aqueous vein) which drains into the veins of the blood system (see Fig. 12-2). The aqueous humor flows from the posterior chamber to the anterior chamber, not in the reverse direction, because of the ball-valve effect produced by the contact of the pupillary margin with the lens.

Glaucoma results when there is too much aqueous humor, usually because of defective drainage by the outflow channels at the iridocorneal angle. Under such conditions, the intraocular pressure increases above its normal 15 to 20 mm Hg above atmospheric pressure. If untreated, increased intraocular pressure can result in destructive effects on the retina.

The maintenance of the eye as an optical instrument is due in part to the pressures exerted by the blood and aqueous humor; when these pressures drop at death, a partial collapse of the eye occurs. The cornea receives its main, but insufficient, supply of oxygen for its metabolic requirements from the aqueous humor. Additional oxygen is obtained by diffusion from the air in contact with the cornea. The metabolic activity of the cornea is impaired if the cornea is unable to maintain some intermittent contact with the air.

The large *vitreous chamber*, occupying about five-sixths of the eye, is filled with a transparent gelatinous material which is a hydrated mucoprotein enmeshed in some collagenous fibrils. Except for the addition of collagen and hyaluronic acid, the chemical composition is similar to that of the aqueous humor. It contains no blood vessels, and its few cells may be microglia from the retina. The vitreous humor is formed by the ciliary body; it provides a passageway for the nourishment of the lens and possibly of the retina. The turnover of the vitreous water is rather rapid; approximately half the vitreous water is replaced every 10 to 15 min. The slow movement of "fibrous" materials in the vitreous body is supposed to be the source of stimulus for the common experience of threads and spots floating before the eyes.

RETINA

General organization of the retina

The retina is a mobile portion of the brain, because the retina is a central nervous system structure which moves as the eye moves. In fact, the retina is an extension of the forebrain, which reaches forward from the optic nerve into the eye (1) as the photoreceptive layer (neuroretina) and the pigment epithelium to the ora serrata, (2) as the unpigmented epithelium (ciliary retina) over the ciliary body, and (3) as a pigmented epithelium (iridic retina) over the posterior iris. The *neuroretina* is about the size of a square postage stamp and only slightly thicker. The entire retina is embryologically derived from the two-layered outgrowth of the neural tube, called the optic cup (see Fig. 12-4). The outer layer of the cup gives rise to the pigment epithelium of the retina, and the inner layer to the remainder of the retina. The embryonic cavity between the layers—called the optic ventricle—is obliterated during development by the interdigitation of extensions of the pigment epithelium with those of the rods and cones.

A cleavage of the retina (*detached retina*) may occur at the interface between the pigment epithelium and neuroretina. It is a common cause of partial blindness. This retinal detachment, which "recreates" the cavity of the optic vesicle, results, in part, because no tight morphologic connection ever develops between the neuroretina and the pigment epithelium except at the ora serrata and the optic disk, where the retina is firmly attached to the choroid layer.

In common with all other vertebrates, humans have an inverted retina. In this type of retina, the photoreceptive rods and cones lie in

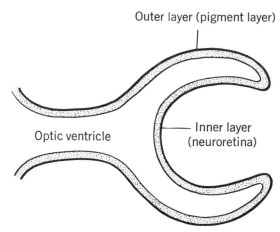

FIGURE 12-4 The optic cup, an outgrowth of the forebrain, comprises an outer layer and an inner layer. The outer layer differentiates into the pigment epithelium of the retina. The inner layer differentiates into the neuroretina. Note the optic ventricle, which, in the embryo, is continuous with the ventricular system.

an outer layer and the neuronal cells involved with processing and transmitting neural information to the brain are in the inner layers. In effect, light must pass through all retinal layers (except at the fovea) before reaching the rods and cones (see Figs. 12-5 through 12-8). In the fovea the inner layers are spread to the sides, so that light has only to pass through the outer nuclear layer before reaching the photoreceptive

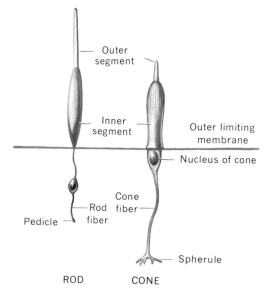

FIGURE 12-5 A rod and a cone of the human eye.

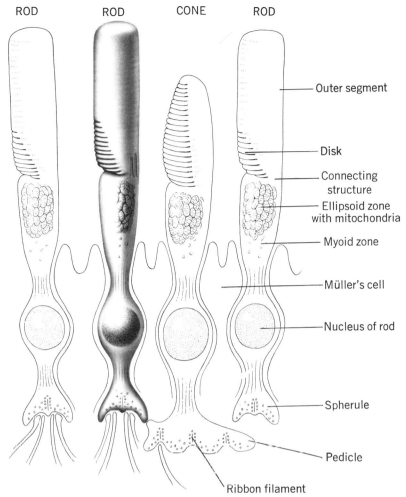

ROD   ROD   CONE   ROD

Outer segment

Disk

Connecting structure

Ellipsoid zone with mitochondria

Myoid zone

Müller's cell

Nucleus of rod

Spherule

Pedicle

Ribbon filament

FIGURE 12-6 Ultrastructure of a cone and three rods. The new disks of the rods are continually formed by the repeated infolding of the cell membrane at the base of the outer segments. The disks of the cones are not continually replaced. (*Adapted from Young, courtesy of Reader's Digest Association.*)

elements (see Fig. 12-8). The output of the retina is projected via ganglion cells and their axons located in the nerve fiber layer. These fibers converge toward the optic disk to form the optic nerve, which terminates in several processing nuclei of the brain.

Cells (neurons) of the retina

Layers of the retina Except at the fovea centralis and the optic disk and its peripheral margins near the ora serrata, the neuroretina is conventionally divided into the following layers, from "outer" to "inner" (see Figs. 12-7 and 12-8).

1. Pigment epithelium.
2. Layer of the outer and inner segments of the rods and cones.
3. External limiting membrane: junctional complexes (tight junctions) between Müller's cells with rods or cones.
4. Outer nuclear layer: cell bodies and fibers of rods and cones.
5. Outer plexiform layer: synapses among rods, cones, bipolar cells, and horizontal cells.
6. Inner nuclear layer: cell bodies of bipolar cells, horizontal cells, amacrine cells, and Müller's cells.

7. Inner plexiform layer: synapses among bipolar cells, amacrine cells, and ganglion cells.
8. Ganglion cell layer: cell bodies of ganglion cells and synapses as in the inner plexiform layer.
9. Nerve fiber layer: axons of ganglion cells.
10. Inner limiting membrane: junctional complexes of expanded ends of Müller's cells at vitreal surface.

The *fovea centralis* is a zone of high density of photoreceptors, in which numerous slender cones and no rods are present. A few cell bodies of the outer nuclear layer are located within the fovea. The other retinal layers and blood vessels are displaced away from the fovea. As a result light rays pass almost directly from the vitreous body without interference to the foveal cones, which are involved with fine visual acuity. The

optic disk contains only the axons of the ganglion cells.

Pigment epithelium (Fig. 12-7)   The cells of the pigment epithelium contain a black melanin pigment which is known as fuscin and is concentrated in granules. These pigment granules are located mainly in the inner portions of the cells and in their cytoplasmic processes. These processes interdigitate between the outer segments of the rods and cones. The pigment epithelium absorbs the light rays ("mops up light") which were not successful in activating the photopigments in the rods and cones. If excess light were not absorbed, it would backscatter, activate photopigments in other rods and cones, and thus blur sharp resolution. In addition, these cells provide metabolic (e.g., active transport of ions) and functional support for the rods and cones.

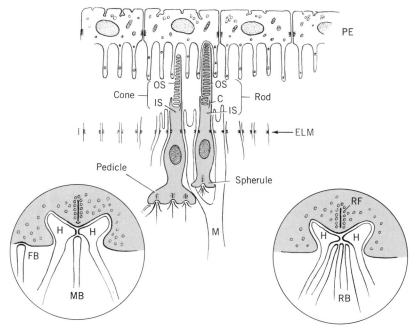

FIGURE 12-7 The ultrastructural organization of a part of the retina, illustrating the relationship of the rods and cones to the pigment epithelial cells (PE) and the processes of Müller's cells (M). A cone terminates in a "synaptic" expansion called a pedicle, whereas a rod terminates as a knoblike "synaptic" ending called a spherule. *Lower left:* the synaptic contacts of a pedicle with processes of midget bipolar cells (MB), flat bipolar cells (FB), and horizontal cells (H). *Lower right:* the synaptic contacts of a spherule with the processes of rod bipolar cells (RB) and horizontal cells (H). The electron-dense line in the presynaptic terminal is called a ribbon filament (RF). The processes of Müller's cells extend outward almost to the level of the connecting stalks (C) located between the outer segments (OS) and inner segments (IS) of the rods and cones. The external limiting membrane (ELM) of light microscopy is actually formed by tight junctions (desmosomes) at the borders of the apposing cell membranes of Müller's cells with those of the rods and cones (ILM). (*Adapted from Dowling and Boycott, 1966, by Noback and Laemle, in The Primate Brain, Appleton-Century-Crofts, Inc., New York, 1970.*)

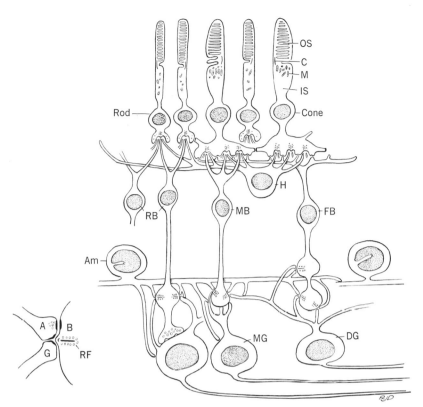

FIGURE 12-8 The ultrastructural organization of the retina, illustrating the relationship of the rods, cones, and intraretinal neurons. The rod spherules have synaptic contacts with rod bipolar cells (RB) and horizontal cells (H). The cone pedicles have synaptic contacts with midget bipolar cells (MB), flat bipolar cells (FB), and horizontal cells (H). The processes of the amacrine cells (Am) have synaptic contacts with the three types of bipolar cells, midget ganglion cells (MG), and diffuse ganglion cells (DG). *Insert at lower left:* synaptic contacts between an amacrine cell terminal (A), ganglion cell process (G), and a bipolar cell process (B); this is called a dyad synaptic complex. The ganglion cells give rise to axons of the optic nerve, chiasm, and tract. Note mitochondria (M) within the inner segments (IS), cilia within connecting stalks (C), and the disks of the outer segments (OS) of the photoreceptors. RF, ribbon filament. (*Adapted from Dowling and Boycott, 1966, by Noback and Laemle, in The Primate Brain, Appleton-Century-Crofts, Inc., New York, 1970.*)

For example, the pigment epithelium may be essential to the survival of the photoreceptors, because when it is severely damaged, the adjacent rods and cones degenerate. This nonrenewable layer (does not exhibit mitosis) acts as a phagocyte in that its cells remove debris from the rods and cones.

Rods and cones: The photoreceptors (Figs 12-5 through 12-9) The rods (rod cells) and cones (cone cells) are elongated photoreceptors which are polarized and segmented into subregions with different functional roles. The *rods* are slender; in the central part of the retina the rods are about 2 μm in diameter, whereas in the more peripheral regions they are about 4 to 5 μm in diameter. The *cones* vary from those in the fovea centralis, with a diameter of 1.5 μm, to those in regions peripheral to the central part, with diameters of about 5 to 8 μm. Each photoreceptor consists of an outer segment, a connecting structure (connecting stalk), an inner segment, a fiber with a cell body, and a synaptic base (see Figs. 12-5 and 12-6).

The *outer segment* of a rod is a slender cylindric structure, and that of a cone has a relatively short conical or tapered shape (see Fig. 12-6). Each outer segment is a stack of hundreds of flattened membranous disks (sacs), which are oriented at right angles to the long axis of the cell. All the disks of a cone retain their continuity with the cell membrane. Although some portions of the disks of a rod retain a similar continuity, most of the rod disks have no attachment to the cell membrane. The lamellar membranes of the rod and cone disks are about 50 Å thick, which is roughly the diameter of a rhodopsin molecule (a visual pigment).

The narrow connecting stalk between the outer and inner segments is a cytoplasmic bridge enclosing a *cilium* (see Fig. 12-6). The latter extends from a complex basal body in the apex of the inner segment into the outer segment. In fact, each outer segment is considered to be a modified shaft of specialized cilium.

The *inner segment* is divided into an outer portion, called the *ellipsoid zone*, and an inner portion, called the *myoid zone*. The outer portion is filled with mitochondria, and the inner portion contains the Golgi complex and an extensive endoplasmic reticulum. The cytoplasmic organelles of this latter myoid segment—the metabolic center of the cell—are the *synthesizers of new proteins, including photoreceptor proteins.* After being synthesized, they are conveyed through the connecting structure to the base of the outer segment, where the double-membrane disks of the outer segments are formed (Fig. 12-7). The lamellae of the new disks of the rods are continually being formed at the level of the connecting structure by the successive infoldings of the cell membrane. The visual pigment molecules are incorporated and precisely aligned as integral structures of the membrane lamella. The disks are displaced in a choroid direction as newly formed disks are added. The disks lose their attachment to the cell membrane and become closed membrane sacks. Eventually, about 3 weeks after being formed, the disks reach the tip of the outer segment where they are shed and incorporated within the pigment cells for disposal (digested by phagosome). In the case of the cones, the newly synthesized proteins from the inner segment diffuse throughout the outer segment and become incorporated in all disks of the cone.

The *visual pigments* of the rods and cones are constructed on a similar pattern. They are composed of a specific type of protein—called an *opsin*—which is bound to a chromophore with a special configuration—called *retinal* (vitamin A

aldehyde, retinaldehyde, retinene). Rhodopsin is the photopigment of the rods in humans; it has a maximum scotopic sensitivity of about 500 nm. Rhodopsin comprises a protein called opsin and a light-absorbing chromophore called retinal. Retinal, the light sensitive moiety, is closely related chemically to vitamin A (retinol).

The cones of humans contain three photopigments, each cone containing one pigment, with peak maximum *electrical responses* at approximately 440 nm (blue), 535 nm (green), and 580 nm (red). The cones are called *blue cones*, *green cones*, and *red cones*. The cone pigments include *cyanolabe* (blue-sensitive pigment), *chlorolabe* (green-sensitive pigment), and *erythrolabe* (red-sensitive pigment). These three cone pigments act as the basis for color discrimination. All four photopigments possess the 11-*cis*-retinal as the chromophore and are united to four different opsins. The light-trapping efficiency of the outer segment is made optimal by the orientation of the chromophores of the photopigment molecule in the plane of the disk. The rods and cones are oriented axially to the incident illumination. It is within this segment that the transduction and genesis of the generator (receptor) potential takes place. In snow blindness, the rhodopsin is being split at a faster rate than it can be regenerated.

The axonlike fiber is a cytoplasmic extension which includes a cell body with the nucleus of the cell. Each fiber terminates in a specialized synaptic body, which is in complex synaptic contact with the nerve fibers of bipolar and horizontal cells. The body of a cone is called a *pedicle*, or *end foot*, because its synaptic surface has a flat base; that of a rod is called a *spherule*, or *end bulb*, because it is small and rounded (see Figs. 12-5 and 12-7).

Neurons and their synaptic connections The human retina contains several types of cells: photoreceptive cells, bipolar cells or neurons, interneurons, and ganglion cells or neurons (see Figs. 12-7 and 12-8). It contains one type of glial cell, called Müller's cell. The photoreceptive cells are the rods and cones. The bipolar cells may be classified into three types: rod (mop) bipolar cells, with moplike tuft endings observed in the light microscope; midget bipolar cells; and flat bipolar cells. The interneurons include the horizontal cell and the amacrine cell (anaxonic neuron, cell without an axon). The two types of ganglion cells are the midget ganglion cell and the diffuse ganglion cell.

The cell bodies of the retinal cells are found in the three nuclear layers. Those of the rods and cones are in the outer nuclear layer; those of the horizontal, bipolar, and amacrine cells are in the inner nuclear layer; and those of the ganglion cells are in the ganglion cell layer (see Fig. 12-8). The main bulk of the synapses are located in two synaptic regions called the plexiform layer and the ganglion cell layer. Synaptic interactions occur among the photoreceptors, horizontal cells, and bipolar cells in the outer plexiform layer. Similar activities take place among the bipolar cells, amacrine cells, and ganglion cells in the inner plexiform layer and ganglion cell layer.

In a general way, the sequence of receptor cells to bipolar cells to ganglion cells conveys neural influences in an axial (vertical) direction within the retina and then to the brain via the axons of the ganglion cells. The horizontal cells and the amacrine cells, with their wide horizontal spread within the plexiform layers, may act to mediate lateral interactions within the retina. The nerve fibers of these cells may be capable of both receiving and transmitting stimuli; it is not possible, as yet, to determine whether each process is a dendrite or an axon.

Müller's cells (Fig. 12-7) These specialized astroglial cells of the retina have radially oriented processes which fill the interstices among the neurons of the retina, including portions of the rods and cones. In a sense these cells envelop these retinal neurons. In addition to their supportive and insulator rods, Müller's cells are a reservoir for glycogen—a source of energy.

Synaptic organization of the cone pedicles and rod spherules (Figs. 12-7 and 12-8) The flat base of each pedicle has from several to as many as 25 invaginations. The region of each invagination represents a synaptic complex composed of a precise arrangement of processes (see Fig. 12-8). The lateral elements are the processes of horizontal cells; the central elements are the processes of one or more bipolar cells. These synaptic complexes are called *ribbon synapses*, because, in addition to presynaptic vesicles, a dense ribbon or bar is located in the presynaptic pedicle of a cone. Ribbon synapses are organized to function as feedback loops. The base of each pedicle has individual superficial synaptic contacts with the dendrites of several bipolar cells.

Each spherule has from one to several ribbon synapses. Within each invagination are the central processes of one or more bipolar cells and the lateral processes of several horizontal cells. In addition, contacts between pedicles, between spherules, and between spherules and pedicles are present.

Bipolar cells (Fig. 12-8) The three types of bipolar cell make the following synaptic connections. Each *rod bipolar cell* is involved with (1) ribbon synapses with from several to many rods and horizontal cells within the outer plexiform layer and (2) axosomatic, axodendritic, and ribbon synapses with diffuse ganglion cells and amacrine cells within the inner plexiform layer and ganglion cell layer. In general, each *midget bipolar cell* (located in the fovea centralis) has several ribbon synapses in the pedicle of but one cone. In turn, each midget cell makes numerous axodendritic and ribbon synapses with amacrine cells and one midget ganglion cell, and, possibly, with some diffuse ganglion cells. Each *flat bipolar cell* makes synaptic contacts with the bases of many cones within the outer plexiform layer, and axodendritic and ribbon synapses with diffuse ganglion and amacrine cells within the inner plexiform layer.

Ganglion cells, horizontal cells, and amacrine cells (Fig. 12-8) Ganglion cells receive their input from bipolar cells and amacrine cells and project their output to the midbrain and lateral geniculate body. Some of the synaptic contacts include regular synapses with presynaptic vesicles and ribbon synapses with the ribbon filament located in the terminals of bipolar cells.

Each *midget ganglion cell* makes several synaptic contacts with but one midget bipolar cell and several amacrine cells. Each *diffuse ganglion cell* makes synaptic contact with many of the three types of bipolar cells and amacrine cells.

The processes of the *horizontal cells of the outer plexiform layer* and those of the *amacrine cells of the inner plexiform layer* are oriented paralled to the retinal surface and at right angles to the axis of receptor cells to bipolar cells to ganglion cells.

The plexiform layers are the synaptic zones of the retina. The *outer plexiform layer* is the lamina where the interactions among the processes of the receptor, bipolar, and horizontal cells occur. In the antagonistic center-surround response, the center seems to be mediated by direct receptor cell–bipolar synaptic activity, while the surround seems to be due to the antagonistic horizontal cell input. This is discussed later on with respect to center-surround. The *inner plexiform layer* is completly organized. The precise functional significance of the synaptic arrangements of the bipolar, amacrine, and ganglion cells is not understood at present. Evidence indicates that the amacrine cells are a critical element through their serial and reciprocal connections with each other and bipolar cell terminals. Two types of amacrine cells and an interplexiform cell have been described (Dowling). The *transient amacrine cell* responds actively when light is turned either on or off, whereas the sustained amacrine cell responds actively while light remains on. The interplexiform cell with cell body in the inner plexiform layer extends to the outer plexiform layer and has a wide spread within it. This cell may exert inhibitory effects on the horizontal cells (an expression of disinhibition).

Functional aspects of the retina

Rods and cones The spatial relations and synaptic connectivity of the neurons of the retina are such that many functionally organized patterns of neurons are possible. In a general way, these cells are geometrically oriented in two planes: one perpendicular to the curve of the retina and the other parallel to the curve of the retina. The sequence of rods and cones to bipolar cells to ganglion cells forms *columns* of cells or *signal pathways* oriented in an axial direction to the retinal curve. The horizontal cells of the outer plexiform layer and the amacrine cells of the inner plexiform layer are oriented parallel to the retinal curve; these cells permit interactions among the cells of the "columns." In addition, the "signal pathways" of the retina are organized for convergence; the approximately 120 million rods and 7 million cones process their influences within these "columns" and then project their output to the brain via only 1 million ganglion cells. Thus there are but 1 million channels of output from the retina. Each ganglion cell is the funnel through which certain rods, cones, and bipolar cells may exert their influences following stimuli from a circumscribed region in the field of vision.

The cones and rods of the retina are the photoreceptor cells which are responsive to the amount of radiant energy and to the wavelengths. Those light rays which do not react with the photopigments are absorbed by the pigment in the pigment epithelium of the retina and in the choroid layer.

The functional activities of the photoreceptive rods and cones are divided into (1) transduction and (2) generator potential. *Transduction* consists of the photochemical reactions which take place in the membranous disks in the outer segments of the rods and cones. In vision, the only action of light is to isomerize the chromophore retinal from the 11-*cis* to the all *trans* configuration.

One quantum of light supplies the stimulus energy which initiates the reaction in one molecule of visual pigment. The extraordinary sensitivity of the dark-adapted visual system of human beings is demonstrated by the perception of visual sensation from but 5 to 10 quanta of light (5 to 10 rods picking up 1 photon per cell). After being bleached by the light, the molecules of the visual photopigments are regenerated quickly, at the rate of thousands of molecules per second. This reconstitution involves the reisomerization of the retinaldehyde to the 11-*cis* form, which is immediately reattached to opsin.

Rods are the sensors for the subjective perception of black, grays, and white. They respond to all radiations in the visual spectrum and even to radiation in the ultraviolet band. Unlike cones, rods do not react selectively to different wavelengths. Human beings are not normally aware of the visual experience of ultraviolet rays, because these wavelengths are absorbed by the lens. Ultraviolet light can activate the photopigments of the rods in a patient whose lens has been removed in treatment of cataracts. Such a person, called an aphakic, can see in an environment "illuminated" exclusively by ultraviolet light. Rhodopsin (visual purple) is the photopigment initiating the train of events leading to black and white vision.

Color vision depends upon (1) the receptor activity of three types of cones and (2) the processing within the central nervous system. Cones are involved in color vision and brightness discrimination. Much is known about the first process and relatively little about the second. In some way, the chemical steps triggered by the light waves in the photopigments are involved in *influencing the receptor (generator) potential in the rods and cones.* The resulting potentials influence changes in the plasma membranes of the synaptic bodies of rods and cones. Presumably, the presynaptic membranes of the ribbon synapses and other synapses associated with the synaptic bodies are depolarized. In turn, neurotransmitters are released from the photoreceptors to stimulate the postsynaptic membranes of the bipolar cells and the horizontal cells. The *ribbon synapse* is considered to be a feedback circuit. The rods, cones, horizontal cells, bipolar cells, and amacrine cells respond to stimulation with slow, graded potentials. These cells exhibit varying degrees of depolarization and hyperpolarization. They do not have all-or-none action potentials.

Response of rods and cones to stimulation by light   Paradoxically, the effect of the conformational changes of the opsins associated with stimulation by light is to produce a slow *hyperpolarizing (inhibitory) potential* in the plasma membrane of the receptor cells (rods and cones). The specific response of rods and cones is to decrease the Na^+ conductance. The paradox is that light does *not* produce excitatory activity in the receptor cells. Some of the effects of this activity may be summarized in the following way. The receptor, horizontal, bipolar, and amacrine cells of the retina convey information by graded (not action) potentials. When stimulated, these cells exhibit hyperpolarizing graded potentials. In the dark or resting state the receptor cells leak ions (primarily Na^+); this leakage keeps the membrane potential low. In this "dark" state the receptor cells are continuously releasing an excitatory neurotransmitter that depolarizes bipolar cells. When the bipolar cells are maintained in a depolarized state (in the dark), they release continuously inhibitory neurotransmitter at the bipolar cell–ganglion cell syanpse and, thereby, *"prevent" the ganglion cells from firing.* On the other hand, light produces other effects. Photostimulation of the rods and cones results in the decrease of release of excitatory transmitter at the receptor cell–bipolar cell synapses (light turns on hyperpolarization and "stimulates" the nonrelease of transmitter). Hyperpolarization of bipolar cells follows. In turn, these hyperpolarized bipolar cells decrease the amount of inhibitory transmitter released at the bipolar cell–ganglion cell synapses. It is thus that the disinhibited ganglion cells increase their rate of action potential discharge. In a sense, the goal of these retinal interactions is to modulate the inhibition on the ganglion cells and the rate of their spontaneous discharge of action potentials from the retina to the brain.

Duplicity theory of vision   The duplicity theory of vision assumes that the retina is a mosaic composed of two fine-grain emulsions: the rods comprise the black and white emulsions, sensitive to low light intensities, and the cones comprise the color emulsion, sensitive to high light intensities. The rods are specialized for dim-light (twilight or night) vision in which low-threshold sensitivity is at a premium. The cones are specialized for color vision and the registering of fine detail. Because cones have a high threshold, they require bright illumination (daylight vision) to be effective receptors. In a way, the retina is a remarkable photographic plate. It is analogous to composite black-and-white and color film. The black-and-white film has the fast emulsion effective in twilight, and the color film has the slow emulsion effective only in broad daylight.

The modern variation of the duplicity theory does not place so much emphasis on the dichotomy of function between rods and cones; it stresses rather the interplay among the rods, cones, and other neurons of the retina.

Receptor fields of the retina   There are roughly 120 million rods and 7 million cones in the retina of each eye, and upward of 1 million ganglion cell nerve fibers to form each optic nerve. The difference between the number of receptors (rods and cones) and the number of ganglion cells is indicative of the convergence operating in the retina.

The rod-free *fovea* contains about 4000 cones and an equal number of bipolar cells and ganglion cells. In essence the functional unit of one cone, one bipolar neuron, and one ganglion neuron forms a "private-line system" that projects through the optic nerve to the brain. Some interaction occurs among these units. Each receptor field in the fovea is narrow. The *receptor field of a bipolar cell* (or of a ganglion cell) is the retinal area from which it is possible to evoke an impulse from stimulation by light. The *receptor field of a foveal ganglion cell* is that of one private-line cone unit (2 μm wide, subtending an angle of only a few minutes of an arc at the cornea). As a result, the fovea is the region of maximal discriminative capacity. In fact, the part of an object seen most sharply is that portion which falls on the fovea.

Proceeding from the fovea toward the rest of the retina, the relative number of rods increases until only rods are present in the periphery of the retina. The nonfoveal retina is composed of receptor fields consisting of many rods converging on one bipolar cell with, in turn, many bipolar cells converging on one ganglion cell; and of receptor fields consisting of many rods and cones converging on one bipolar cell and, in turn, many bipolar cells converging on one ganglion cell. As many as 200 rods converge on one bipolar cell and as many as 600 rods converge to influence (through interneurons) one ganglion cell in the peripheral retina. A receptor field in the peripheral retina may be as large as 1 mm in diameter; this corresponds to an arc of 3° in the 160° visual field.

These nonfoveal receptor fields with multiple receptors (rods and cones) are designed to integrate and pool the stimuli from a "relatively" wide area. Hence this portion of the retina has lower discriminatory power but operates at low thresholds. It is specialized to operate in very dim light. In fact, at night one can identify an object with more certainty by not looking directly at it. In this way the object is focused on the nonfoveal retina, instead of on the fovea. When the object is focused on the nonfoveal retina at night, the rods are permitted to function maximally with their party-line systems.

Receptor field and response field Each bipolar cell and ganglion cell of the retina, neuron of the lateral geniculate body, and pyramidal cell of the visual cortex is wired into a pathway through which it may be influenced by a certain group of photoreceptors. In turn, each photoreceptor or group of photoreceptors is stimulated by light coming from some definable site in the field of vision, i.e., each of these cells has its own "eye view" of the environment. This eye view of a cell is a site in the field of vision which will stimulate the cell either with excitatory or inhibitory stimuli. This site is called the *receptor field* or *response field* of that cell (see Fig. 12-9).

Center-surround The *receptor field* of each ganglion cell is organized into two zones (see Fig. 12-9): a *small circular zone, called the center, surrounded by a concentric zone, called the annular surround (or periphery)*. The center may be likened to the hole in a doughnut, and the surround to the doughnut. On the basis of functional responses to light in the environment, each response field (receptor field) of a ganglion cell is organized into a *center-surround (circular-concentric) configuration*. The term *antagonistic center-surround receptive field* is derived from the contrast in responses between the center and the surround.

Two general types of receptor fields are found in the light-adapted eye: receptor fields with an on-center and an off-surround (excitatory-center, inhibitory-surround), and receptor fields with an off-center and an on-surround (inhibitory-center, excitatory-surround). The on-center, off-surround receptor field of a ganglion cell consists of the center, which fires vigorously when the illumination comes on (or "signs off"), and of a surround which gives a reverse response to a similar stimulus. The off-center, on-surround zones of the receptor field respond in opposite ways. In both types, the two zones are functionally antagonistic, with the surround antagonistic to the center and the center antagonistic to the surround. As a result of the interactions between center and surround, each retinal ganglion cell relays signals concerning the contrast between the intensity of the illumination in the center as compared with that in the surround. In a sense, each neuroretina is a mosaic of about 1 million ganglion cells which relay about 1 million center-surround receptor field transformations via their axons to the lateral geniculate body of the thalamus.

The anatomic basis for the center-surround

receptive field has been proposed. The direct sequence of photoreceptive cells to bipolar cells to one ganglion cell is the basic linkage resulting in an anatomic substrate of the center of a receptive field (see Fig. 12-8).

The sequence is known as the *retinal on-line pathway*. The indirect sequence of photoreceptive cells to horizontal cells to bipolar cells to ganglion cells is the basic linkage of the surround of that receptive field (see Fig. 12-8). This sequence is known as the *retinal off-line pathway*. The summation of the on-center activity with the off-surround activity is resolved by the ganglion cell. The spread of the dendritic tree of each ganglion cell within the inner plexiform layer corresponds with the area of the centers of a receptive field. In summary, the effect of an antagonistic center-surround receptive field is to excite (or to inhibit) a ganglion cell in the center of the field of illumination by the on-line pathway and to inhibit (or to excite) the surround ganglion cells by the off-line pathway.

The center of an antagonistic center-surround receptive field is produced by an on-line sequence of receptor cell(s) to bipolar cell(s) to ganglion cell (see Figs. 12-8 and 12-9). The effect of light is to hyperpolarize receptor cell(s), to decrease the amount of excitatory transmitter released by the receptor cells, and to hyperpolarize the bipolar cell(s). In turn, the bipolar cell(s) reduce the amount of transmitter released at the ganglion cell synapse. This removal of inhibition (disinhibition) results in the increase in the firing rate of the ganglion cell (on-center).

The antagonistic surround is produced by an off-line sequence of receptor cell(s) to horizontal cell(s) to bipolar cell(s) to a ganglion cell. The decrease in the amount of excitatory transmitter released by the receptor cells at the synapse with the inhibitory horizontal cells results in the reduction of the release of inhibitory transmitter at the horizontal cell–bipolar cell synapses. In turn, the bipolar cells increase the amount of inhibitory transmitter released at the bipolar cell–ganglion cell synapses. The result is a decrease in the firing rate of the ganglion cells in the surround (off-surround).

The concept of the receptor field of a ganglion cell applies to color vision responses in the retina. The center of the receptor field would respond maximally to a narrow portion of the

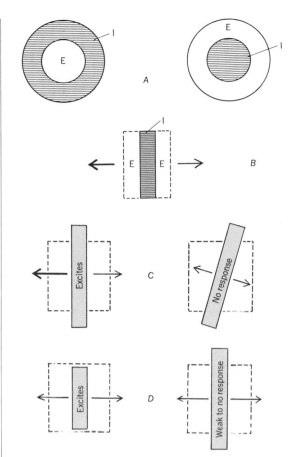

FIGURE 12-9 Receptive fields of neurons of the visual pathway. *A*. The center-surround receptive fields may have an excitatory center (E) with an inhibitory surround (I) or an inhibitory center (I) with an excitatory surround (E). These annular fields are featured by the retinal ganglion cells, neurons of the lateral geniculate body, and some cells of area 17. *B*. The simple receptive field of a neuron of area 17 has linearly oriented excitatory areas parallel to an inhibitory area. *C*. The complex receptive field of neurons of areas 17, 18, and 19 is featured by a moving excitatory slit of light; precise orientation of the slit is critical, but length of slit is not. *D*. The hypercomplex receptive field of neurons of areas 17, 18, and 19 is featured by a moving excitatory slit of light; precise orientation and length of the slit are critical. Arrows indicate direction in which the slit of light moves to obtain response.

visual spectrum (e.g., it may be spectrally sensitive to red wavelengths), whereas the antagonistic surround would respond maximally to another narrow portion of the spectrum (e.g., it may be spectrally sensitive to green wavelengths). The linkage of red cones to bipolar cells to a ganglion cell comprises the red center, while the linkage of green cones to bipolar cells to amacrine cells to a ganglion cell comprises the green surround to the red center. In theory, the receptive fields include fields with (1) a red center with either a green or blue surround, (2) a green center with either a red or blue surround, and (3) a blue center with either a red or green surround. Because these cells and their linkages are color-coded and exhibit a differential sensitivity to different wavelengths of light, they are called *spectrally opponent cells*, and the theory is called the *spectrally opponent concept*.

Ganglion cell systems *Four types of ganglion cell systems* (*sets* or *fibers*) have been described according to the manner in which their discharge is initiated. Some ganglion cells commence to discharge impulses when the light stimulus is *on* and continue to discharge a series of impulses throughout the duration of the photoimpingement on the retina. The firing rate of these units increases under light stimulation. These ganglion cells belong to the *on* system. Other ganglion cells discharge impulses only at the termination of photoimpingement; they belong to the *off* system. Other ganglion cells discharge impulses at the beginning and again at the termination of photoimpingement; they belong to the *on-off* system. Other ganglion cells exhibit a spontaneous steady discharge with no light stimulus acting. The discharge in this *steady-background* system occurs even after the eye has been dark-adapted (kept in the dark) for several hours. Normally the retina is, in fact, discharging at all times, whether it is being photopically stimulated or not. Shadows as well as light can increase retinal activity. In a sense the discharges via the optic nerve are expressed in a frequency modulation (FM) code, with an increase and decrease in the rate of discharge.

FUNCTIONAL ASPECTS OF VISION

Searching movements

The eyes are never still. *Searching movements* are continuously taking place in the pursuit of moving objects. When the object moves, the eye moves. The basic activity is actually a survival legacy from our animal forebears who searched the environment for enemies, food, and shelter. Perpetual, quick, small oscillations are indica-

tive of the high-frequency scanning essential to maintaining a visual image. Actually it is impossible to hold the eyes absolutely still. When an image projected on the retina is held absolutely stationary (which can only be done experimentally), the image fades, its coloration diminishes, and its contours dissolve away.

Contour sharpening and brightness contrast (lateral inhibition)

In the phenomena of perception called contour sharpening and brightness contrast, our subjective sensations are the result of altered comparisons and contrast. For example, a bulb of a certain brightness will appear brighter subjectively in a poorly lighted room than in a well-lighted room. The interactions among neurons are significant in distorting and exaggerating our image of the environment to maintain and to enhance boundaries. The retina utilizes such interactions to sacrifice less significant detail, to emphasize more significant detail, and to bias the representation of the patterns of the objects seen. More specifically, the *eye enhances information about the borders and contours, and this information is transmitted to the brain at the expense of other details*. An artist conveys effects by exaggerating the depth of black at the edge of a shadow and lightening the whiter edge at the border between dark and light. This phenomenon is normally performed by our visual system. For example, place a white sheet of paper on a blackboard; at the junctional edge of the paper and the board, the paper appears whiter and the blackboard blacker. This effect is perceived but does not really exist. The phenomenon is referred to as "contour sharpening" or "simultaneous brightness contrast." It is utilized effectively by the cartoonist.

Contour sharpening is an expression of lateral (*mutual*) *inhibition*. Lateral or cross connections that are inhibitory in their action exist among the neurons of the retina (see Figs. 3-14 and 3-15). The horizontal neurons and amacrine cells (cells oriented parallel to the retinal curve) are important structural substrates for these actions; these cells may inhibit nearby neurons associated with different channels and signal pathways. The lateral inhibition is greater on nearby receptor units than on distant units. Widely separated units have minimal reciprocal inhibitory effects on each other. In effect the efficacy of any receptor unit is modified by the inhibitory influences of neighboring receptor units or by their lack.

The contrast effect in shadows occurs commonly in everyday experience. A careful visual examination of the shadow cast on a white paper on the shaded side of a box (see Fig. 12-10) demonstrates the consequences of lateral inhibition. Recordings by a photometer indicate that each portion of the shadow in the figure reflects essentially the same intensity of light. Thus, if the visual system "sees" the shadow as it really is, then the subjective sensation should be of a relatively uniform dark shadow. However, this is not what is observed. Viewed from the proper perspective, the area of the shadow near the box is actually seen to be relatively lighter than the darker band along the edge of the shadow adjacent to the unshaded white paper. The differences perceived in the shadow are explained as follows:

1. The lighter area of the shadow appears lighter because the neurons stimulated by the shadow area near the box are minimally inhibited (*mutual inhibition*) by influences from the neurons stimulated by the dark side of the box. The result is that the excitatory influences from these neurons are capable of exerting optimal effects in the cerebral cortex.

2. The darker band along the edge of the shadow appears darker because the neurons stimulated by the shadow are maximally inhibited by influences from the neurons stimulated by the unshaded bright white paper. Hence the excitatory influences obtained from the light within the relatively dark band are inhibited sufficiently to yield the subjective experience of appearing darker.

It is obvious that the retina is not like a simple camera film merely registering an image and relaying it to the brain. The retina is actually a movable (since the eyes move) "little" brain that processes stimuli and selects detail, distorts it, and transmits coded information via the optic nerve to the brain. The retina produces neither a photocopy of nature nor a replica. Mutual inhibition contributes to this end by heightening

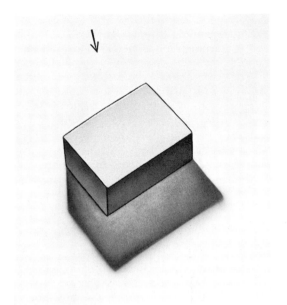

FIGURE 12-10 The phenomenon of *contrast inhibition* explains why certain areas appear lighter or darker than they really are. The shadow adjacent to the box appears lighter than it really is because inhibition from the dark side of the box upon the shadow is minimal. The area of the shadow adjacent to the white unshaded area appears darker than it really is because inhibition from the light area is maximal. Arrow indicates direction from which light is coming.

contrast and discriminating against diffuse light. Information about borders and contours is transmitted at the sacrifice of other details. In a way we create our own personal image of our environment.

Adaptation

The human eye can adapt over a tremendous span of light intensities; it can visually discriminate over a luminance range of about 10 billion to 1. In essence, *adaptation* is an expression of the visual system's attempt to achieve equilibrium with the intensity of environmental light. For example, the completely dark-adapted eye can be stimulated by as much as 1/10,000 less light energy than the light-adapted eye (i.e., the dark-adapted eye is 10,000 times more sensitive to light). Examples of this sensitivity are the change in ability to see during the first half-hour in a darkened motion picture theater and the intense subjective brightness of light upon opening one's eyes after sleeping. The eye which is exposed to good illumination for a time is said to be light-adapted, whereas the eye which has been in darkness for a spell is said to be dark-adapted.

The dark-adapted eye utilizes the pathways involving rods primarily. These sensitive photoreceptors are not sensitive to the longer wavelengths at the red end of the spectrum, because rhodopsin does not absorb red light. If one wears red goggles when in daylight, the eyes can become dark-adapted. Hence a night fighter pilot or a radiologist can attain and retain dark-adapted vision by wearing red goggles in the daylight. One can see because the red light stimulates the red cones. When entering the dark environment, dark adaptation is quickly attained by removing the red goggles.

The ability to become dark-adapted is reduced by anoxia. Reduced oxygen levels in the blood constitute one reason why dark adaptation takes longer to achieve at high altitudes.

Visual acuity

The visual acuity of the eye is a measure of the sharpness with which detail can be distinguished or resolved. In effect, the maximal acuity is the shortest distance by which two lines or two dots can be appreciated without appearing as one line or one dot. When visual acuity is low, fine details are blurred, and outlines and contours become indistinct. Visual acuity can be influenced by such environmental factors as illumination and degree of contrast in detail. In practice, acuity can be measured by the angle of resolution—the angle formed at the retina by the light from any two points in space. The minimal visual angle is slightly less than 1 min.

The "signal pathways" convey information initiated by the rods and cones. They are organized to transmit influences which result in varying degrees of visual acuity. The fovea centralis of the macula is the region of the retina associated with the greatest degree of visual acuity. The cells associated with this zone and its neuronal connections are arranged to ensure this acuity. The fovea centralis consists of a large number of slender cones (no rods) and an outer plexiform layer. The other retinal layers influenced by the foveal cones are displaced ra-

dially away from the fovea. Hence light passes almost directly from the vitreous body to these photoreceptors. The cones are linked by a *"private-line" system* of a cone to a midget bipolar cell to a midget ganglion cell to lateral geniculate body to visual cortex. The communication among these separate channels is minimal and is functionally organized to maintain the identity of each channel. Thus the anatomic basis for visual acuity comprises many separate channels, each conveying its distinct bit of fine-grain datum from a receptive field monitored by one cone and relayed centrally by one ganglion cell.

The degree of visual acuity diminishes the farther away the receptive field of a ganglion cell is from the fovea. In these regions, the receptive field is composed of many photoreceptors to a lesser number of rods and flat bipolar cells to one diffuse ganglion cell. Regions associated with lesser visual acuity are regions in which a greater number of photoreceptors is associated with the receptor field of one ganglion cell. In these regions the grain is coarser. Another factor contributing to lesser acuity in these regions is the fact that each photoreceptor cell (rod in areas of least acuity) is associated with fields of many ganglion cells.

Color vision

The visual system reacts to specific wavelengths of light, and, in turn, this information is processed into the subjective experience of color. The entire visual pathway system is involved. The perception of yellow light from the simultaneous flashing of red light into one eye and of green light into the other is explained as a consequence of cortical processing.

Colors are characterized by hue or tone, brightness, and saturation or purity. The *hue* or *tone* of a color is a measure of the wavelength perceived. Red, yellow, blue, and green are different hues. *Brightness* is the subjective sensation that is determined by the amount of black in the color—the more black, the less brightness. In effect, the more black in the color, the more light is absorbed and the less light is reflected. The *saturation* or *purity* of a color is the subjective sensation that is determined by the amount of white in the color. White alters the hue because it is composed of colors. Thus, the less white in the color, the more saturated or pure is the given hue. Pure colors are pastel colors.

Purkinje effect

The *Purkinje effect* was named after the investigator who noted that light blue flowers are bluer at dawn or twilight than at midday. At dusk, red flowers appear black. An artist realizes that color values vary depending on the quantity and quality of light. Our eyes are more sensitive to reds and blues in dim light than in brighter light. The dark-adapted eye is most sensitive to green; the light-adapted eye is most sensitive to yellow. This Purkinje shift in the sensitivity of our eyes to color at different light intensities is probably related to the shift in the sensitivity of the different light intensities. The Purkinje effect is analogous to the variations of color values that are obtained when color films are overexposed, underexposed, or "correctly" exposed.

THE VISUAL PATHWAYS

The pathways from the eye are involved in two important functional roles: (1) the act of seeing and (2) the numerous reflex activities which either are important to the visual process (such as accommodation) or are a consequence of the visual process (such as ducking on seeing a blow coming).

Fields of vision and the retina

The bounded space of the environment seen by one eye (*monocular vision*) while that eye is fixed upon a stationary or fixation point is known as the field of vision of that eye. The *visual field* of a normal eye outlines an irregular oval; from the fixation point the perimeter of the oval extends roughly 60° nasally (medially), 60° upward, 70° downward, and 90° temporally (laterally).

Normally we see with both eyes, i.e., we have a binocular field of vision formed by the almost complete overlapping monocular fields of both eyes. Without changing the fixation of the eyes, the most lateral peripheral areas of the visual fields are seen by one eye only—this is the *monocular* field or crescent (see Fig. 12-12). The

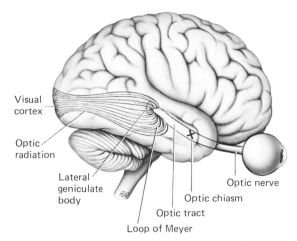

FIGURE 12-11 The visual (retinogeniculocalcarine) pathway as viewed from the right side. Note the loop of Meyer.

accurate mapping of the visual fields of each eye can be determined with a perimeter or mapping screen by a process known as *perimetry*. By this method, the patient's fields can be charted, and sites of functional field defects outlined. With the subject gazing with one eye at a central spot directly in front of the eye (with the other eye covered), a small spot of light is moved back and forth across the field of vision. Subjects indicate when they can or cannot see the spot of light. These indications are recorded on a chart. In such an examination the blind spot of the retina is located approximately 15° lateral to the central point of vision.

The projection of the field of vision upon the retina is inverted and reversed with respect to the object because of the lens (see Fig. 12-12). We do not perceive objects upside down or reversed (right-left reversal), because the mind makes the essential adjustments in some unknown way. The right half of the field of vision of an eye is projected to the left half of the retina (left hemiretina) and the left visual field to the right hemiretina, while the upper half of the field of vision is projected to the lower half of the retina (lower hemiretina) and the lower visual field to the upper hemiretina. The field of vision of an eye or the retina may be divided into quadrants by two lines; a line in the horizontal meridian and a line in the vertical meridian intersecting in the middle of the macula (the fixation point).

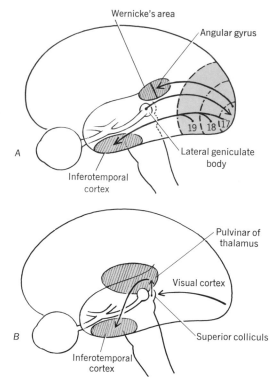

FIGURE 12-12 The two visual pathways. *A.* The geniculo-striate system. *B.* The tectal system. The functional significance of Wernicke's area and the angular gyrus is discussed in Chap. 16.

Thus the upper temporal quadrant of the field of vision is projected to the lower nasal quadrant of the retina, while the lower nasal quadrant of the field of vision is projected to the upper temporal quadrant of the retina. The nasal half of the field of vision of each eye is smaller than the temporal half, because of the shadow of the nose.

The retina may be divided another way. The region of the *macula* is the *macular retina;* this region of most acute sight is called the *central area* of vision. Surrounding the macula is the *paracentral* (*paramacular* or *pericentral*) *retina* or area of vision. This is, in turn, surrounded by the *peripheral retinal area of vision,* the region of least acute vision (see Figs. 12-12 and 12-13).

Relation of visual fields to the organization of the visual pathways Normal vision is mainly *binocular,* with the temporal hemiretina of one eye "seeing" the same half of the field of vision as the nasal hemiretina of the other eye. When the

two hemiretinas do not view precisely the same portions of the visual fields, *double vision (diplopia)* occurs. The visual pathways are organized so that corresponding sites of the images of objects in the real world, which are mapped upon the retina, are matched and fused in the visual cortex in order to obtain binocular vision. To accomplish this, the retinofugal fibers from the nasal hemiretina decussate and terminate in the contralateral lateral geniculate body, while those from the temporal hemiretina do not decussate and terminate in the ipsilateral lateral geniculate body. Thus at the geniculate level the corresponding areas of the two hemiretinas have been projected to the same geniculate body but to different laminae. The fusion of the images from the two hemiretinas into one image occurs at the next level—the visual cortex. To accomplish this transformation the geniculostriate projections to the striate cortex are organized so that corresponding foci terminate with small groups of neurons organized into functional columns. The precision of this connectivity is the means by which the pathways from the two hemiretinas can reinforce one another.

Pathways from the eye

It is through the axons of the ganglion neurons of the retina that the output of the eyes is conveyed centrally. These axons pass through the optic nerves, optic chiasm, and optic tracts in a retinotopic (visuotopic) organization to either the lateral geniculate body of the thalamus or to the tectum of the midbrain. At the present time at least two visual pathways are thought to be involved with visual perception. These are the geniculostriate system and the tectal system (see Figs. 12-11 through 12-13).

The *geniculostriate system,* or *first visual system,* comprises the sequence of retina, to lateral geniculate body, to striate cortex (area 17). In this system the highest processing levels include the primary visual cortex (area 17), association visual cortex (areas 18 and 19), and the inferotemporal cortex (portions of the middle and inferior temporal gyri).

The *tectal system,* or *second visual system,* is difficult to define precisely at the present time. It may comprise the sequence of retina to superior colliculus, to the pulvinar of the thalamus, to the

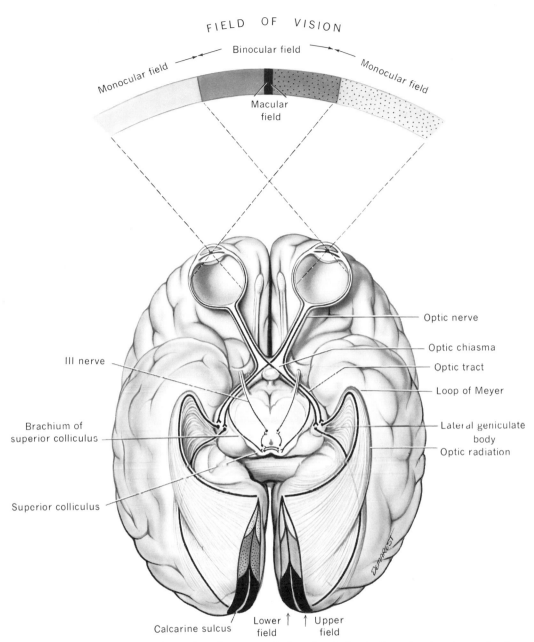

FIGURE 12-13 The visual pathways from the retina to the lateral geniculate bodies and to the primary visual cortex on either side of the calcarine sulcus. The right visual field is projected to the left primary visual cortex (left visual field to right primary visual cortex). The macular field projects to the posterior aspect of the primary visual cortex (solid black). The rest of the binocular field projects to the visual cortex just rostral to the "macular visual cortex." The monocular field projects to the most rostral portion of the primary visual cortex. The upper half of the visual field projects to the primary visual cortex below the calcarine sulcus. The lower half of the visual field projects to the primary visual cortex above the calcarine sulcus.

inferotemporal cortex. The inferotemporal cortex also receives input from the occipital visual areas 18 and 19. This second visual system is said to (1) assist in detecting the position and possibly the contours of objects and (2) be involved with higher levels of visual processing.

Other pathways from the retina include those involved with various reflexes and the pineal gland. The superior colliculus and the pretectum are important nuclear structures intercalated in the pupillary reflex, accommodation, and conjugate movements of the eye.

Retinogeniculostriate pathway (retina to primary visual cortex)

The axons of the ganglion cells of the retina converge to the head of the optic nerve (blind spot, optic disk). After passing through the lamina cribrosa of the sclera at the head, the axons emerge, become myelinated, and form the optic nerve. *The fibers from the temporal hemiretina course via the optic nerve, optic chiasm, and ipsilateral optic tract before terminating in the ipsilateral lateral geniculate body* (see Fig. 12-14). *The fibers from the nasal hemiretina course in the optic nerve, decussate in the optic chiasm, and pass via the contralateral optic tract before terminating in the lateral geniculate body.* Most of the fibers (about 70 to 80 percent) in the optic tracts terminate in the lateral geniculate bodies; the remainder terminate in the midbrain, mainly in the superior colliculi.

The ganglion cells in the retina and their axonal fibers comprise three classes of neurons.

1. *Medium-sized cells with intermediate diameter axons.* Each of these fibers projects exclusively to precisely localized narrow-terminal fields in one of the four parvicellular layers of the lateral geniculate body. Each terminal field forms a glomerulus encased by glial cells. Roughly half of the cells may be of this type.
2. *Small cells with small-diameter, slow-conducting axons.* Each of these axons terminates exclusively as a broad field in the superior colliculus. Slightly less than half of the cells may be of this type.
3. *Large cells with large-diameter fast-conducting axons.* Each of the relatively few cells in this

category has a stem axon that divides into two major branches. One branch projects to the magnocellular layers of the lateral geniculate body and the other to the superior colliculus. These fibers terminate in broad fields.

Although there is some intermingling of the fibers, they are retinotopically localized in their course from the retina to their termination within six laminae of the lateral geniculate body (see Fig. 12-14). The fibers from each temporal hemiretina synapse with neurons in laminae II, III, and V, and those from each nasal hemiretina synapse with neurons in laminae II, IV, and VI of the lateral geniculate body.

Each *optic nerve* is composed of about 1 million axons with the fibers organized into about 800 to 1200 fascicles, each invested by a pial sheath. Actually the optic nerve is not a cranial nerve, but rather it is a tract because its myelin is formed by oligodendroglia (not Schwann cells), and its axons are those of second-order neurons. The bipolar cells of the retina are the first-order neurons. In general, most macular fibers pass through the central region of each optic nerve until they reach the chiasm, where the decussating fibers and the nondecussating fibers ascend and gradually pass into the superior aspect of the optic tracts (see Fig. 12-14). These fibers from the macula project to a wedge-shaped sector in the upper posterior two-thirds of the lateral geniculate body, mainly in the small-celled laminae II, III, IV, V, and VI and only slightly in the large-celled laminae I and II.

The nonmacular fibers from the upper and lower temporal quadrants (those with uncrossed central projections) maintain their superior-inferior temporal positions within the nerve and chiasm; in the chiasm these fibers undergo an inward 90° rotation until (1) the fibers of the upper quadrant shift from their dorsolateral location in the optic nerve to a medial and inferior location in the optic tract, and (2) the fibers of the lower quadrant shift from their ventrolateral location in the optic nerve to their lateral and inferior location in the optic tract.

The nonmacular fibers from the upper and lower nasal quadrants (with crossed central projections) maintain the nerve and chiasm, until they decussate through the chiasm. The fibers of the lower nasal quadrant shift from

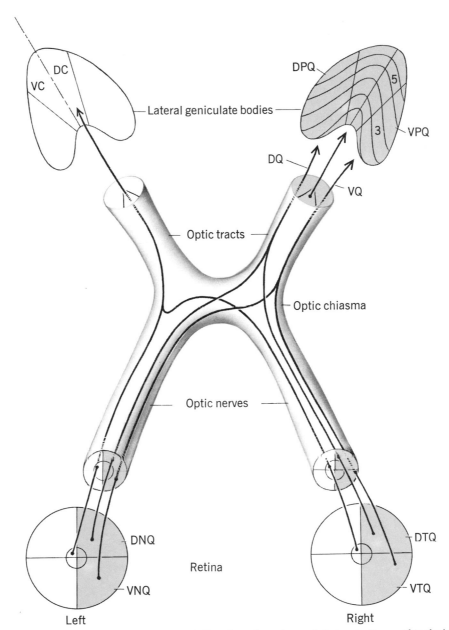

FIGURE 12-14 The course of the ganglion cell fibers from the retina to their terminations within the lateral geniculate bodies. The crossed fibers from the nasal hemiretina (dorsal nasal quadrant, DNQ, and ventral nasal quadrant, VNQ) terminate in laminae I, IV, and VI of the lateral geniculate body (LGB). The uncrossed fibers from the temporal hemiretina (dorsal temporal quadrant, DTQ, and ventral temporal quadrant, VTQ) terminate in laminae II, III, and V of the LGB. The fibers of the dorsal nonmacular quadrants of the retina pass through the medial parts of the optic tracts (DQ) to the medial aspect of the LGB (DPQ). The fibers of the ventral nonmacular quadrants of the retina pass through the lateral part of the optic tracts (VQ) to the lateral aspect of the LGB (VPQ). The fibers from the macular region project to the wedge-shaped *sector* of the LGB; those fibers from the dorsal macula terminate in the medial part of the *sector* (DC); and those fibers from the ventral macula terminate in the lateral part of the *sector* (VC). The retinotopic organization within the optic nerve, chiasma, and tract has been questioned recently. (*Adapted from Hoyt and Luis, 1962, by Noback and Laemle, in* The Primate Brain, *Appleton-Century-Crofts, Inc., New York, 1970.*)

their inferior medial location in the optic nerve to the ventrolateral aspect of the contralateral optic tract, while those of the upper nasal quadrant shift from their superior medial location in the optic nerve to the medial aspect of the optic tract.

In general, fibers from corresponding points in the two retinas course together in the optic tract. The fibers from the upper nonmacular quadrants of the retina project to the medial aspect of the lateral geniculate body, and those from the lower nonmacular quadrants project to the lateral aspect of the lateral geniculate body (Fig. 12-14). Some of the fibers from the inferior nasal retinal quadrant loop slightly (Wilbrand's loop) into the contralateral optic nerve before reentering the chiasm.

The retina has precise point-to-point connections with the lateral geniculate body, which is also called the dorsal lateral geniculate body. In human beings, a small ventral lateral geniculate body, also called the pregeniculate body, is present. The lateral geniculate body consists of six laminae, numbered from I to VI. The two ventral laminae (or magnocellular layers), numbers I and II, contain large cell bodies; the four dorsal laminae (or parvocellular layers), numbers III to VI, contain small cell bodies. The contralateral projection from the optic tract terminates in layers I, IV, and VI, and the ipsilateral projection in layers II, III, and V. More precisely, each fiber in the optic tract projecting to the lateral geniculate body synapses with five to six adjacent neurons within a lamina. Each geniculate cell is monocular, in that it receives input from only one eye. All in all, the number of fibers in the optic tract terminating in the lateral geniculate body is about the same as the number of fibers projecting from the lateral geniculate body to the primary visual cortex.

LATERAL GENICULATE BODY

The lateral geniculate body consists of two types of neurons: (1) principal cells with long axons projecting to the visual cortex and (2) a few local interneurons with short axons terminating within the lamina. The receptive field of each neuron of the lateral geniculate body is similar to that of a retinal ganglion cell (see Fig. 12-9).

The cell's eye view of the visual field is that of an antagonistic center-surround. On the basis of responses evoked following the stimulation of the retina with monochromatic light, two basic types of neurons are indicated: broad-band cells (spectrally nonopponent cells) and spectrally opponent cells. The *broad-band cells* of the lateral geniculate body respond to all wavelengths and white light. The *spectrally opponent cells* are differentially sensitive to light of different wavelengths. These latter cells are associated with black and white vision or with color vision.

Complex interactions and processing probably occur within the lateral geniculate body among the retinogeniculate endings, corticogeniculate endings, and intrageniculate neurons. However, the precise functional role of the lateral geniculate body in the visual system is not known. One certainty is that each neuron of the lateral geniculate body receives direct input from the retina and, in turn, projects directly to the striate cortex (area 17). The body may act (1) to discard certain influences, (2) to modify the input by compressing it into fewer channels, and (3) to modify the code by recoding.

The only output from the lateral geniculate body to the cerebral cortex is via the geniculocalcarine tract to the striate cortex.

GENICULOCALCARINE TRACT (Fig. 12-11)

The *geniculocalcarine tract* (*optic radiation geniculostriate*) is the retinotopically organized pathway from the lateral geniculate body to the primary visual cortex (striate cortex). After it leaves the geniculate body, this tract passes through the caudal aspect of the internal capsule (retrolenticular portion mainly), swings laterally and occipitally as the optic radiation lateral to the atrium and posterior horn of the lateral ventricle, and finally swings medially to terminate in the stellate cell in lamina IV (Fig. 16-9A) of the primary visual cortex (area 17). The fibers carrying information from the macula are located in the center of the optic radiation and terminate in the most occipital part of the visual cortex (see Fig. 12-13). The fibers carrying information from the upper hemiretinas are located in the upper half of the optic radiation and terminate in the visual cortex above the calcarine sulcus. The fibers carrying information from the lower hemi-retinas are located in the lower half of the optic radiation and terminate in the visual cortex below the calcarine sulcus. The fibers that loop into the temporal lobe before heading occipitally with the rest of the optic radiation is known as the *loop of Meyer* (see Figs. 12-11 and 12-13). It conveys impulses originating from the lower peripheral retina (nasal side of the opposite eye, temporal side of the eye on the same side). As a result, interruption of this loop in the right temporal lobe impairs peripheral vision in the upper quadrant of the left field of vision of both eyes.

Some of the fibers in the optic radiations project from lamina VI of area 17 to all layers of the lateral geniculate body and to the inferior pulvinar and adjacent lateral pulvinar. The relation of this geniculate body to visual areas 18 and 19, the so-called circumstriate striate belt, is different. The geniculate body does not project to or receive projections from areas 18 and 19.

Visual cortex

The visual cortex is conventionally divided into the *primary visual cortex* (*visual area I, striate cortex, area 17*), the *secondary visual area* (*visual area II, area 18, parastriate cortex*), and *visual area III* (*area 19, peristriate cortex*). Areas 18 and 19 are often called the visual association cortex or pre-striate cortex.

The primary visual cortex is subdivided into three regions according to the original source of its input from the retina. The *macular (central) fibers* pass from the geniculate body directly through the intermediated part of the optic radiation to the most occipital third of the striate cortex on both sides of the calcarine sulcus. The *paracentral (paramacular) fibers* pass from the geniculate body through the optic radiation just above and below the macular fibers to terminate in the middle third of the striate cortex on both sides of the calcarine sulcus. The *fibers from the peripheral (pericentral) retinal areas* pass to the rostral third of the striate cortex. This most rostral area of the striate cortex is associated with monocular vision; its input is derived from the area of the field of vision which is directed to only one eye. The rest of the primary visual cortex is involved with binocular vision. Note that the small macular area of the retina has a large cortical representation; this is associated with the sharp visual acuity monitored by the macula. The peripheral retinal area, a region registering minimal visual acuity, is represented by a small cortical area.

Each point in the fields of vision is represented only once in the striate cortex, with the neighboring points of the visual field located in neighboring points in the striate cortex. In brief, the points in the visual fields are retinotopically mapped onto the primary visual cortex in a precise and orderly manner.

Of significance is the precise point-to-point retinotopic representation in which the impulses generated by the activity in a small receptor field of the retina are projected to a small discrete group of cells of the lateral geniculate body and in turn to a discrete cortical column. These pathways from the eye to the striate cortex preserve the separate identity of small functional units (center-surround units) of each retina and of one retina from the other. The fibers of the optic radiation terminate and synapse with spiny stellate neurons in lamina IV of the primary visual cortex (see Fig. 16-10). The act of fusion of the visual fields from both eyes commences in the laminae other than lamina IV in the striate cortex. These other five laminae are the site of the initial integration of the information from corresponding points in both eyes. This localized precision and specificity of the optic pathways is neurophysiologically expressed as follows: One specific neuron in the striate cortex can be driven by the activity generated by a small spot of light focused on, and only on, the equivalent site in the other eye. Apparently neurons in laminae II, III, V, and VI of the striate cortex are stimulated by both eyes, suggesting that this is an expression of the *act of binocular fusion*.

The neurons of the primary visual cortex are grouped into thousands of columns, which extend from the pial surface through the entire thickness of the cerebral cortex to the white matter perpendicular to the surface. These columns are physiologically defined; they need not have a regular columnar shape. Each column receives fibers from a small group of lateral geniculate neurons via the optic radiation. Within each column some neurons (approximately 15 percent of them) are stimulated from influences from one eye, either the ipsilateral or the contralateral eye. The other neurons of the column are driven by both eyes, with some neurons being driven equally from both eyes and other neurons being driven more from one eye than from the other. *Most of the cells in lamina IV are driven by one eye only*, with some responding to stimuli from the ipsilateral eye and others to the contralateral eye. *The cells in laminae II, III, V, and VI are driven binocularly*. In general, the contralateral eye is the most effective in firing the striate neurons—this is the phylogenetically older input (see "Ocular Dominance Columns" later on).

The primary visual cortex has connections with other regions of the cortex, mainly with areas 18 and 19 (see Fig. 12-12; see also Figs. 16-1 and 16-2) of the ipsilateral hemisphere. Areas 18 and 19 have direct corticocortical connections through the corpus callosum with areas 18 and 19 of the contralateral hemisphere. Area 17 has no direct connections through the corpus callosum with area 17 of the contralateral hemisphere. In human beings, the inferotemporal area probably receives its main visual input from the geniculostriate pathway through connections with areas 18 and 19. The inferotemporal area may receive significant input from the superior colliculus via a relay in the pulvinar (see Fig. 12-12).

The 2-mm-thick striate cortex (area 17) consists of the six laminae characteristic of the neocortex (Chap. 16). The projections to and from this cortex area are organized with respect to these laminae. Lamina IV is the input terminus receiving projections from the lateral geniculate body. Intracortical processing and connections through stellate cells communicate with the other laminae in area 17. Projections from the other laminae are conveyed via the axons of pyramidal cells. Laminae II and III project to visual association areas 18 and 19 (Chap. 16). Lamina V projects to the superior colliculus and the pulvinar. Lamina VI projects and feeds back to all layers of the lateral geniculate body. This pattern of projections does indicate that the horizontal organization into laminae has functional significance with relation to the flow of information through it.

The various cortical areas involved with the visual system have important connections with subcortical centers. Corticofugal fibers to the midbrain comprise the corticotectal fibers to the superior colliculus and the corticoreticular fibers to the midbrain tegmentum. The corticotectal fibers course in the internal sagittal stratum. This stratum is a sheet of fibers located medial to the geniculocalcarine fibers, which comprise the external sagittal stratum. The influences conveyed by these fibers are integrated (1) in such reflexes as accommodation and extraocular movements and (2) in the tectal system. The corticoreticular fibers are integrated into activities of the midbrain reticular formation. Corticofugal fibers from the visual cortex terminate in such thalamic nuclei as the pulvinar, lateral geniculate body, and lateral dorsal nucleus of the thalamus.

Neurons of the visual cortex The neurons in the binocular regions of the striate cortex (area 17) are responsive to one of four types of receptive field. On the basis of their responses these cells are called *center-surround cells, simple cells, complex cells*, and *hypercomplex cells*. The *center-surround cells* have response features which are basically similar to those found in the ganglion cells of the retina and lateral geniculate neurons. The orientation of an edge or a line is critical to triggering a cell to fire.

Simple cells respond optimally to stimulation obtained from straight lines, bars, or edges having a precise orientation and position in space (see Fig. 12-9). This critically positioned bar is composed of two bands located side by side; one band, an excitatory one, is separated by a straight edge from the other, an inhibitory one. Strong and brisk activity in simple cortical cells is evoked by moving stimuli passing through the excitatory receptive region. In general, each simple cell will respond to stimuli from either eye, but these cells have a preference for influences from one eye over the other.

Complex cells respond optimally to stimulation obtained from moving straight lines, bars, or edges, each having a precise orientation but a variable position in space (see Fig. 12-9). These cells have a definite orientational preference associated with a larger receptive field than a simple cell. The antagonism between the excitatory band and the inhibitory band of the field is not as prominent and the specificity of the position of the stimulus in space is not as critical as for the simple cells.

Hypercomplex cells are detectors of straight lines, bars, or edges that stop to form an angle or corner and that move through the field of vision (see Fig. 12-9). Again the orientation and length are critical. The position of these line segments or corners can vary over a wide range.

In summary, center-surround neurons and simple cells are located in area 17, while complex and hypercomplex cells are found in areas 17, 18, and 19.

These cells are presumed to be organized hierarchically. In the sequence from retina to visual cortex, differences are observed in the sensitivity of the neurons to various stimuli; most of the neurons in the central area of the retina and the lateral geniculate body respond to both form and color stimuli, while many neurons in the striate cortex are sensitive either to form or to color, with only a few responding to both form and color.

The center-surround cortical cells are located only in lamina IV of area 17 (Chap. 16). Each of these neurons is responsive to stimulation from one eye only—either from the contralateral or the ipsilateral eye. Each of these cortical cells has direct connections via the optic radiation from the lateral geniculate body. Some center-surround cells receive their input from the geniculate laminae that have connections with the ipsilateral eye, and the other center-surround cells receive their input from the geniculate laminae that have connections with the contralateral eye; i.e., *these center-surround cortical cells are monocularly driven. The neurons in the other laminae of area 17 are binocularly driven*, in that they are, in varying degrees, responsive to the stimulation from both eyes. This activity is a corollary of the concept that *the act of fusion of the input from corresponding sites of both retinas first occurs in the simple cells of area 17.*

COLUMNAR ORGANIZATION OF THE PRIMARY VISUAL CORTEX (AREA 17)

The functional architecture of the primary visual cortex is the pattern of discrete cortical columns that are oriented perpendicular to the cortical surface extending through all six cortical laminae from pia to white matter. There columns are not cylindrical; rather, they are continuous slabs with thickness and boundaries that extend horizontally for distances through the area 17. The columns receive their input from overlapping receptive fields in the retina. Each column consists of simple, complex, and hypercomplex cells, each with similar receptive fields (see Fig. 16-5). Each column is composed of thousands of neurons, which are characterized by physiologic criteria. The columns in the striate cortex are composed of simple cells, complex cells, and hypercomplex cells, while those in areas 18 and 19 contain only complex and hypercomplex cells. Many neurons in the association visual cortex are not classified as complex or as hypercomplex cells. All neurons in a column, whether simple, complex, or hypercomplex, have similar receptive field orientation (see Fig. 12-9). According to one theory, several cortical neurons with center-surround receptive fields interact with simple neurons. In turn a complex of simple cells interact and supply input to a complex cell, while the activity of a complex of complex cells results in supplying the basic input for the response patterns of hypercomplex cells. Thus many simple cells with similar patterns of orientation are said to synapse with a single complex cell; the latter generalizes a particular contour orientation. Some complex cells are conceived to exert excitatory and others inhibitory influences upon hypercomplex cells. In this way the hypercomplex cells are rendered responsive only to oriented contours of a defined length. Through sequences of serial processing, many orders of hypercomplex cells respond to stimuli from corners, angles, and more complex geometric patterns (Hubel and Wiesel).

Two independent functionally defined columnar units are recognized: (1) *ocular dominance columns* or *columns of eye preference* and (2) *orientation columns*. The slabs of the ocular dominance columns are wider (400 μm) than the orientation columns (25 to 50 μm). These columns have been demonstrated by physiologic and morphologic evidence. The slabs of these two columnar types give the appearance of an irregular honeycomb-like spacing and arrangement. Other columns are indicated, such as color-sensitive columns and direction of movement of the visual stimulus columns. All columns can be conceived as morphologic entities in which neurons are able to interconnect, to interact, and to generate a higher level of abstraction of visual information. Each cortical neuron in area 17 contributes to both columns.

Each ocular dominance column is organized in accordance with the input from each of the eyes. Each primary receptive cell (stellate cell, simple cell) of lamina IV is driven exclusively by one eye with the ipsilateral and contralateral laminae of the lateral geniculate body projecting to separate alternate columns in lamina IV. Most cortical cells (complex and hypercomplex) other than the primary receptive cells in each column respond primarily to the dominant eye and to a lesser degree to the nondominant eye. The preferred eye determines the ocular dominance for each column. To state the matter otherwise, the simple cells in lamina IV are monocularly driven, whereas the cells in the other laminae in the column are binocularly driven—but more by one eye than the other. Each ocular dominance column is about 400 μm wide with each right eye (or left eye) ocular dominance column located between two left eye (or right eye) dominance columns. The result is that one set of adjacent right eye–left eye dominance columns constitutes a hypercolumn of about 800 μm in width.

Each orientation column is organized in relation to its response to specifically oriented lines (linear stimuli) in the visual field. Thus, the neurons in the retina and lateral geniculate body with no orientation preference (actually center-surround response) are connected through the geniculocalcarine fibers to stellate cells in lamina IV; these cortical cells also give a center-surround response and no orientation-preference response; in addition, these cells are virtually all monocular. After the initial stage of visual processing in lamina IV the other cells in the orientation column give optimal responses to similar specifically oriented lines. Thus, each line in the visual field viewed by both eyes is received and processed in an orientation column, where it is registered as a line in a column of from 25 to 50 μm wide. Adjacent to each column are columns with an orientation that differs slightly. In each adjacent column the oriented line changes systematically in small steps clockwise or counterclockwise to the oriented line in the first column at rates such that 180° shift in orientation is covered in about 600 μm or more. The term *hypercolumn* refers to a series of adjacent columns in which the orientation lines have rotated the full 180°.

Areas 18 and 19 have projections to other subcortical structures including the dorsolateral and reticular thalamic nuclei and the superior colliculus, but not to the lateral geniculate body.

Areas 18 and 19 are interconnected with that part of the pulvinar which is connected with the inferotemporal cortex (areas 20 and 21), the cortex associated with the second visual system.

SUPERIOR COLLICULUS

The superior colliculus is a complex laminated cortex consisting of seven alternating white and gray layers. It receives input from diverse, multiple sources and projects output to many neural structures. The superficial laminae contain the axon terminals from visual centers including the retina, lamina V of the primary visual cortex, the pretectum, and the parabigeminal nucleus. The latter is a nucleus located lateral to the lateral lemniscus in the lower midbrain; it receives input from the visual association cortex. These laminae project to the pulvinar, pretectum, and lateral geniculate body. The retinocollicular projections terminate in broad fields exhibiting center-surround organization. The tectogeniculate fibers terminate in the magnocellular layers of the lateral geniculate body.

The deep layers receive multimodal input from a variety of sources including the nonstriate neocortex and numerous subcortical centers. These comprise (1) auditory input from the inferior colliculus, nuclei of the trapezoid body, superior olivary complex, and lateral lemniscus; (2) somatosensory (nonnociceptive) input from all divisions of the trigeminal complex (mainly nucleus oralis), both dorsal column nuclei, and the lateral cervical nucleus; (3) such brainstem catecholamine nuclei as the locus coeruleus and the dorsal tegmental nucleus; (4) deep cerebellar nuclei, (5) such reticular formation structures as the zona incerta, pars reticularis of substantia nigra, midbrain tegmentum, and hypothalamus; and (6) the posterior horn of spinal cord (Edwards et al.). The neurons of the deep layers have axons terminating in the intralaminar nuclei of the thalamus, subthalamus, zona incerta inferior colliculus, brainstem reticular nuclei, inferior olivary nucleus, and the anterior horn of the spinal cord.

Role of superior colliculus

The *superior colliculus* has several roles in (1) the reflex control and regulation of many movements of the eyes and head (noted below) and (2) certain aspects of vision. This subcortical tectal center has a significant function in attention and pattern perception associated with vision. A lesion limited to the superior colliculus modifies visual activity. A monkey (or cat or dog) with one superior colliculus removed does not pay attention to stimuli from the contralateral visual field. Actually the animal is not blind to contralateral stimuli. It is overresponsive to the visual stimuli from the ipsilateral visual fields; in addition, it continually turns its head to the ipsilateral side. In summary, the *superior colliculus is more than a reflex center; it is an integrative center subserving visual perception*. The major role of the superior colliculus is to coordinate responses evoked by a variety of sensory stimuli with behavioral movements that direct the head, eyes, and ears toward the environmental stimulus. Thus the superior colliculus is said to have a critical role in visual localization, orientation, and tracking movements.

The concentration of such diverse and multiple afferents in these deep layers of the colliculus is also a characteristic feature of definition for the brainstem reticular core. This suggests that these deep layers are actually an integral part of the brainstem reticular formation (Edwards et al.).

Higher functional expressions of the visual system The visual system has roles in both the unconscious and conscious spheres. According to some recent findings, the *concept of "two visual systems"*—i.e., *the retinogeniculostriate system* and the *tectal system*—has been utilized to account for many of the physiologic expressions of the entire visual system (see Fig. 12-12). The relative functional contributions of the two systems are incompletely understood. An essential primary difference between the two systems may be that the tectal system answers the question "Where is it?" in terms of visuomotor responses, and the geniculostriate system answers the question "What is it?" in the form of learned and conscious responses (Schneider). The activities of the two systems are integrated through interconnections; they are not independent. Visual information is conveyed via the separate channels of these systems to the visual areas of the cerebral cortex where the perception at the conscious level is completed and unified.

THE VISUAL REFLEXES

Stimulation of the visual system evokes a number of reflex actions of critical significance to vision. Several of these reflexes will be outlined.

Pupillary constriction: the light reflex and the consensual light reflex

When the eyes are exposed to bright light, the pupils contract, thereby reducing the intensity of the light reaching the retina. This *involuntary light reflex* (see Fig. 12-15) is a reflex response to the direct stimulation by light. The involved pathways are as follows: the retinal ganglion cell axons course via the optic nerve, optic chiasma (some fibers decussate), optic tract, and brachium of the superior colliculus (bypassing the lateral geniculate body) to terminate in the pretectum. Interneurons project to the contralateral pretectum through the posterior commissure. Interneurons interact with other interneurons (some probably in the interstitial nucleus), which, in turn, synapse with preganglionic neurons of the oculomotor nucleus. These preganglionic neurons project via the third cranial nerve and synapse in the ciliary ganglion (just behind the eye) with postganglionic neurons which innervate the constrictor muscle of the iris in the eye.

When only one eye is exposed to bright light, the pupils of both eyes will constrict. The crossing of some fibers in the optic chiasma and the interconnections across the midline by inter-

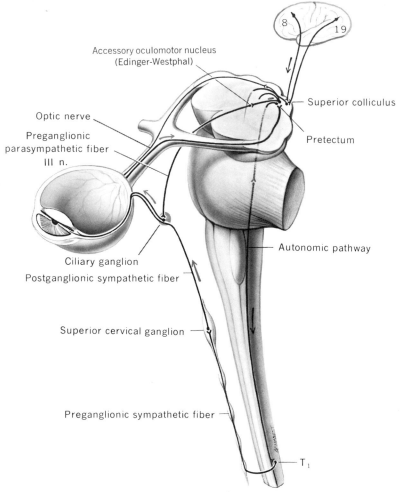

Accessory oculomotor nucleus
(Edinger-Westphal)

Optic nerve

Preganglionic
parasympathetic fiber
III n.

Superior colliculus

Pretectum

Ciliary ganglion

Postganglionic sympathetic fiber

Autonomic pathway

Superior cervical ganglion

Preganglionic sympathetic fiber

T_1

FIGURE 12-15 The light reflex pathways (pupillary reflex) and the accommodation pathway. The light reflex pathways relay (1) through the midbrain pretectum and the parasympathetic outflow of the oculomotor nerve (pupillary constriction), and (2) through the sympathetic pathways of the brainstem, upper thoracic level, and ascending cervical paravertebral sympathetic trunk (pupillary dilation). Accommodation is mediated via a pathway which includes corticocollicular fibers from the cerebral cortex (occipital lobe, area 19, and frontal eye fields, area 8), superior colliculus, and parasympathetic outflow through the oculomotor nerve. (*After Krieg.*)

neurons of the bilateral pretectum account for this consensual reflex. The reflex resulting in the constriction of the stimulated eye is known as the *direct light reflex,* while the reflex resulting in the constriction of the nonstimulated eye is known as the *consensual light reflex.* Constriction of the pupil is more vigorous in the stimulated eye than in the nonstimulated eye.

Pupillary dilatation

When the eye is exposed to dim light, the pupil dilates (see Fig. 12-15). Optic pathways act through the reticular formation and descending sympathetic pathways (in the dorsolateral tegmentum of the brainstem and in the white matter in the anterior half of the cervical spinal cord) to stimulate the preganglionic neurons of the sympathetic intermediolateral cell column of the C8 and T1 spinal levels. The preganglionic fibers ascend in the sympathetic chain and synapse in the superior cervical ganglion (upper part of the neck) with postganglionic neurons, which, in turn, travel adjacent to blood vessels to innervate the dilator muscle of the iris (Chap. 6). Interruption of these fibers may result in Horner's syndrome (Chap. 5).

Accommodation

The process by which the refractory power of the lens is changed is known as *accommodation*. *This reflex action is mediated via the cerebral cortex* (see Fig. 12-15). One can voluntarily focus on a nearby object or a faraway object. The pathways include the optic pathways from the eye to the cerebral cortex; in turn, a projection back from cortical area 19 (and from frontal eye field area 8) via the optic radiation through the brachium of the superior colliculus terminates in the nucleus of the superior colliculus (interneurons interconnect these bilateral nuclei). Through a chain of several interneurons these collicular nuclei are connected to the preganglionic neurons in the accessory motor nucleus of cranial nerve III. These parasympathetic preganglionic neurons project via the third cranial nerve and synapse in the ciliary ganglion with preganglionic neurons, which, in turn, innervate the ciliary muscles in the ciliary body. Pupillary constriction and convergence of the eye accompany accommodation to near vision. In viewing an object close up (near-sight vision) a triad of responses occur: convergence of the eyes, accommodation, and pupillary constriction.

THE OCULOMOTOR SYSTEM AND EYE MOVEMENTS

Eye movements

To obtain true binocular vision the same points in the field of vision common to the two eyes must be focused upon corresponding loci in the two retinas. Optimal visual acuity is attained when the fixation point (center of the visual target) in the field of vision is focused as two images, one on the macula of each retina. The movements of the eyes are exquisitely coordinated to match these corresponding loci. The simultaneous movement of both eyes in the same direction is called a *conjugate movement*. With one exception (convergence), normal eye movements are conjugate. Convergence of the eyes, such as that which occurs during close-up vision (when the maculae are directed to one fixation point), is a *disconjugate movement*.

The system regulating these movements, known as the *oculomotor system*, comprises several central pathways and the lower motor neurons (final common pathway) of cranial nerves III, IV, and VI innervating the extraocular muscles. Each of the three sets of extraocular muscles—medial and lateral recti, superior and inferior recti, and superior and inferior oblique muscles—is reciprocally innervated so that the contraction of one muscle of each pair is synergistically synchronized with the relaxation of the other muscle, in order to direct the gaze to any position (see Fig. 7-5 and 10-12). This delicately balanced muscle system is under continuous tension.

The oculomotor system (see Chap. 10)

The oculomotor system comprises five subsystems directed to place the visual image of regard upon the foveas of both eyes simultaneously and to maintain their position.

1. *The saccadic system.* This system regulates saccadic movements, which the eyes use to acquire new visual targets in the environment. The eyes drift slowly in one direction (called *pursuit* or *searching movements*) and return rapidly to another position in the opposite direction (called *saccadic* or *rapid movements*). Saccadic movements are the flicks of the eyes as they shift from one stationary point to another when reading or viewing a picture. These flicks are so fast that vision is momentarily impaired—a 10° human saccade lasts 45 ms. Saccades may be initiated spontaneously or in response to a visual stimulus. They usually occur when the observer and the object are stationary.

2. *The smooth pursuit system.* This system controls the automatic eye movements which pursue a moving object. In contrast to the saccades during searching, the movements of the eyes when following are smooth. The smooth pursuit system attempts to match eye velocity to target velocity as the eye tracks the moving target in its course through the environment. The saccadic system operates with this pursuit system to correct an error between the target and the macula. Apparently the purpose of pursuit is to allow the visual system to hold the moving object in a stationary position on the retina in order to gain time to perceive the object. The cerebral cortex (areas 17, 18, and 19) and the superior colliculi are integrated into the central pathway involved with the pursuit system—a system which requires visual stimulation for its essentially automatic response. Electrical stimulation of areas 18 and 19—called the occipital eye fields—produces conjugate eye movements to the opposite side. The neurons in the visual cortex and superior colliculus, which are known to respond to direction and velocity of image movements, are probably integrated in the smooth pursuit movements.

3. *The vestibular system.* This system monitors the orientation of the head in space from the information obtained from the receptors in the vestibular sense organs of the inner ear. In response the head and the eyes move in space to compensate and maintain the visual axis stable in the environment. This is analogous to a shipboard-mounted radar system in which the tracking device (radar system or eye) is mounted on a moving platform (ship or head); the tracking device operates efficiently when it is automatically stabilized relative to the movement of the platform. In this activity, the vestibular system monitors and evaluates the motion of the head and then, via influences relayed in the medial longitudinal fasciculus, stimulates the extraocular muscles to move the eyes to compensate for the head movements.

4. *The vergence system.* This system is involved with the control of the degree of convergence and divergence of the visual axes in its role of maintaining the target image on each macula when the target moves in depth through the field of vision. This is the only system that moves the eyes in opposite directions at one time. The vergence system operates during the shift from one fixation point (*X*) at one depth to another fixation point (*Y*) at a different depth. In this shift the eyes follow the sequence of (*a*) a saccade from point *X* to a site in which the two visual axes straddle point *Y* and (*b*) a small vergence movement until the visual axes of both eyes are directed to *Y*. This system is probably influenced via cortical areas 19 and 22, where the information of the slight difference viewed by the corresponding retinal foci is relayed. This activity is directed so that the image of the object viewed can be fused into one—to correct the disparity is to achieve fusion either by convergence or divergence. Otherwise, double vision would occur.

5. *The position maintenance system.* This system acts to maintain eye position vis-à-vis the target. It is driven by visual interest, be it conscious or unconscious. Conscious visual interest is apparently directed from influences projected from the association cortex in the junctional area of the occipital, temporal, and parietal cortices. Unconscious interest is directed from the superior colliculus.

Volitional movements of the eye The voluntary fixation mechanism is the means by which we move our eyes voluntarily to locate an object upon which we wish to focus our attention. The *frontal eye field in area 8* (posterior portion of the middle frontal gyrus) is the cortical center that influences voluntary eye movements mediated through cranial nerves III, IV, and VI (see Fig. 12-15). If this area, called the *voluntary eye field*, is bilaterally damaged, patients either will be unable volitionally to move their eyes or will have extreme difficulty in doing so; they are still able to scan a line on the printed page and to fix on and follow a moving object, probably because area 19 is intact. Patients are unable to "unlock" their eyes from one fixation point and shift them to a second point. The movement to the the second point may occur if the subject blinks the eyes or covers the eyes for a short period.

Automatic eye movements and fixation of the eye Our eyes can, without any volitional effort, scan a line on the printed page or follow a moving object. The neuronal center and pathways involved with locking the eyes upon an object once it has been located are known as the *involuntary fixation mechanism*. These automatic movements include reflex pathways from retina to primary visual cortex to association visual cortex and then via corticotectal fibers to the superior colliculus, from which connections are made with the nuclei of cranial nerves III, IV, and VI. The occipital eye fields in area 19 have a role in controlling the mechanism which may result in the eyes becoming "locked" upon an object. When areas 19 are damaged bilaterally, the patient is unable automatically to follow objects steadily across the visual field or to scan the line on a printed page (see Fig. 12-15).

Accommodation-convergence reaction Immediately after shifting one's attention from a distant gaze to a nearby object (near-point), three ocular adjustments occur. The eyes converge with the contraction of both medial rectus muscles so that the maculae of both eyes are directed to the object to be observed. *Accommodation* for near-sight vision follows, with the rounding up of the lens. Some further sharpening of the image occurs with constriction of the pupils. The convergence may be, in part, the consequence of influences from the frontal eye fields in area 8 which are conveyed via corticobulbar fibers to the superior colliculus and from there, via interneurons, to the nucleus of the oculomotor nerve. The pupillary constriction may result from influences conveyed from the occipital visual association cortex via corticotectal fibers to the superior colliculus, which in turn stimulates, through interneurons, the neurons of the accessory oculomotor nucleus (called the nucleus of Edinger-Westphal).

The so-called *Argyll-Robertson pupil* may occur in syphilis of the central nervous system. In this syndrome, the pupil is small in dim light and does not constrict further when the eye is exposed to bright light. The same pupil will respond by constricting further during the accommodation-convergence reaction. The precise explanation for this differential effect of pupillary constriction is unresolved. The usual stated cause for this dissociation of the pupillary reflex is a lesion in the pretectum.

LESIONS OF THE OPTIC PATHWAYS AND RELATED PHENOMENA

The impairment of a small area of the retina results in a *scotoma* (*blind spot*) in the field viewed by that eye. The optic disk is a natural blind spot, for it contains no rods and cones. A partial defect at a site anywhere along the visual pathway may result in a scotoma.

The complete interruption of the optic nerve results in permanent blindness in one eye-called *monocular blindness* (see Fig. 12-16*A*). However, the blind eye can still accommodate and show the consensual light reflex because the normal eye activates the intact reflex arcs through the pretectum and superior colliculus and oculomotor nerve to the blind eye. A fixed, dilated pupil may be a sign of pressure on the oculomotor nerve.

A midline lesion of the optic chiasm (as from pressure from a tumor of the hypophysis) may interrupt the decussating retinofugal fibers (see Fig. 12-16*B*). The result is loss of reception from the nasal hemiretina of each eye, accompanied by loss of vision in the temporal half of the visual field of each eye, called *bitemporal hemianopia* (*hemianopsia*). Such a defect is *heteronymous*; this means that portions of both retinas which view different areas of the fields of vision are involved. Interruption of the nondecussating fibers on both sides of the optic chiasm produces a *binasal hemianopia*, (loss of reception in the temporal hemiretina of each eye); this is accompanied by loss of vision in the nasal half of the visual field of each eye (Fig. 12-16*C*). In the early stages of its growth, a hypophyseal tumor expands upward to interrupt the lowermost decussating fibers of the optic chiasm first; in this situation impairment of vision occurs in both upper temporal quadrants (fields) initially, because of impairment of fibers from the lower nasal retinal quadrant of each eye. If the disorder is diagnosed correctly at this stage, the chances are favorable that surgical removal of the tumor can save the vision of the patient. A hypophyseal tumor, in addition to interrupting the decussating fibers in the optic chiasm, may damage the anterior hypothalamus. This may result in a persistent *hyperpyrexia* (hyperthermia, elevated body temperature) and diabetes insipidus.

The complete interruption of the optic tract

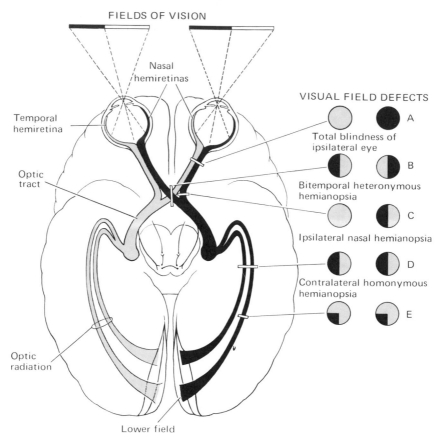

FIELDS OF VISION

Nasal hemiretinas

Temporal hemiretina

Optic tract

Optic radiation

Lower field

VISUAL FIELD DEFECTS

A
Total blindness of ipsilateral eye

B
Bitemporal heteronymous hemianopsia

C
Ipsilateral nasal hemianopsia

D
Contralateral homonymous hemianopsia

E

FIGURE 12-16 Some common lesions at various levels within the visual pathways. The corresponding *visual field defects* are represented on the right side.

or the lateral geniculate body or the optic radiation or the entire primary visual cortex on one (right) side results in a *left contralateral homonymous hemianopia*, or blindness in the field of vision on the side opposite the lesion. *Homonymous* refers to corresponding regions of both retinas, hence to a single visual field. A thrombus of the posterior cerebral artery may result in destruction of the visual cortex, except possibly for that for the macular area; in this condition, central (macular) vision is spared (preserved bilaterally). In some cases of homonymous hemianopia, macular sparing is said to occur after lesions of the optic radiation near or within the visual cortex. This form of macular sparing may be more apparent than actual. This is because the subject with a hemianopia sees with the normal half of the macula and then automatically

shifts the eye with a saccade to view the field previously in the blind area. It is possible to differentiate whether the homonymous hemianopia is caused by a lesion in the optic tract or by a lesion in the optic radiation or visual cortex by testing whether the stimulation of the blinded half of one retina can elicit the pupillary light reflex. This reflex should be evoked if its arc through the optic tract to the pretectum is intact. Light is directed into the blinded half of one retina; if the pupillary reflex can be elicited, the lesion is located beyond the lateral geniculate body, but if the pupillary reflex is absent, the lesion is probably located in the optic tract.

Partial lesions of the visual pathways produce partial defects in the fields of vision. A *lower quadrantic homonymous anopsia* results from a contralateral lesion in the upper (superior) half of the optic radiation or the entire primary visual cortex (area 17) above the calcarine sulcus. This field defect occurs because the pathways from the upper temporal quadrant of the ipsilateral retina and the upper nasal quadrant of the contralateral retina are interrupted. A lesion of the loop of Meyer will produce a *contralateral upper quadrantic anopsia* because pathways from the lower temporal quadrant of the ipsilateral retina and the lower nasal quadrant of the contralateral retina are interrupted.

A blow or an injury that damages the choroid layer of the eye may result in *sympathetic ophthalmia*. In this condition not only may sight be impaired in the affected eye, but the other eye may gradually lose its sight. In some patients the injured eye must be removed to preserve the sight in the normal eye. Apparently, the cause is that the body responds to certain substances released from the injured choroid layer by regarding them as foreign materials. The consequence is an immunologic activity which results in the destruction of both eyes.

True albinos shun light and have difficulty seeing because melanin pigment is absent in the iris, choroid, and retinal pigment layer of their eyes. In these individuals the light passes through the retina, and light which is normally absorbed by the melanin pigment is reflected as scattered light. Hence a discrete spot of light excites more receptors over a wider area than it usually does. In addition, the unpigmented iris permits diffuse light to enter the vitreous body and stimulate many photoreceptors. As a consequence, the visual acuity of albinos is rarely better than 20/100 to 20/200.

BIBLIOGRAPHY

Benevento, L. A., and B. Davis: Topographical projections of the prestriate cortex to the pulvinar nuclei in the macaque monkey: An autoradiographic study. Exper Brain Rs, 30:405–424, 1977.

Brindley, G. S.: *Physiology of the Retina and Visual Pathway*, Edward Arnold (Publishers), Ltd., London, 1970.

Davson, H.: *Physiology of the Eye*. Academic Press, Inc., New York, 1972.

——— (ed.): *The Eye*, Academic Press, Inc., New York, 1969, 1970.

Doty, R. W., and N. Negrâo: "Forebrain Commissures and Vision. Ablation of Visual Areas in the Central Nervous System," in R. Jung (ed.), *Handbook of Sensory Physiology*, vol. VII, part 3, Springer-Verlag, Heidelberg, 1973.

Dowling J. E., and B. B. Boycott: Organization of the primate retina: electron microscopy. Proc Roy Soc Lond (Biol), 166:80–111, 1966.

Dowling, J. E.: "The Vertebrate Retina," in D. B. Tower (ed.), *The Nervous System*, vol. 1, *The Basic Neurosciences*, Raven Press, New York, 1975, pp. 91–100.

Duke-Elder, S., and K. C. Wybar: In S. Duke-Elder (ed.), *The Anatomy of the Visual System; System of Ophthalmolgy*, The C. V. Mosby Company, St. Louis, 1961.

Edwards, S. B., C. L. Ginsburgh, C. K. Henkel, and B. E. Stein: Sources of subcortical projections to the superior colliculus in the cat. J Comp Neurol, 184:309–330, 1979.

Fine, B. S., and M. Yanoff, *Ocular Histology: A Text and Atlas*, Harper & Row, New York, 1972.

Fuortes, M. G. F. (ed.): "Physiology of Photoreceptor Organs," in *Handbook of Sensory Physiology*, vol. VII, part 2, Springer-Verlag, Heidelberg, 1972.

Hogan, M. J., J. A. Alvarado, and J. E. Weddell: *Histology of the Human Eye*, W. B. Saunders Company, Philadelphia, 1971.

Hoyt, W., and O. Luis: Visual fiber anatomy in the infrageniculate pathway of the primate. Arch Ophthalmol, 68:94–106, 1962.

Hubel, D. H., and T. N. Wiesel: Functional architecture of a macaque monkey visual cortex. Proc Royal Soc Lond B 198:1–59, 1977.

———, ———, and M. P. Stryker: Anatomical demonstration of orientation columns in macaque monkey. J Comp Neurol, 177:361–379, 1078.

Kaas, J. H.: "The Organization of Visual Cortex in Primates," in C. R. Noback (ed.), *Sensory Systems of Primates*, Plenum Press, New York, 1978, Chap. 7, pp. 151–179.

Kelly, J. P., and D. C. van Essen: Cell structure and function in the visual cortex of the cat. J Physiol, 238:515–547.

Krieg, W: *Functional Anatomy*, Blakiston Company, Philadelphia, 1942.

Mishkin, M.: "Cortical Visual Areas and Their Interactions," in A. G. Karczmar and J. C. Eccles (eds.), *Brain and Human Behavior*, Springer-Verlag, Berlin and New York, 1972, pp. 187–208.

Noback, C. R., and L. K. Laemle: "Structural and Functional Aspects of the Visual Pathways of Primates," in C. Noback and W. Montagna (eds.), *The Primate Brain*, Appleton-Century-Crofts, Inc., New York, 1970, pp. 55–82.

Palmer, L. A., A. C. Rosenquist, and J. M. Sprague: "Corticotectal Systems in the Cat: Their Structure and Function," in T. L. Frigyesi, E. Rinvik, and M. D.

Yahr (eds.), *Corticothalamic Projections and Sensorimotor Activities*, Raven Press, New York, 1972.

Pettigrew, J. D.: The neurophysiology of binocular vision, Sci Am, 227:84–96, 1972.

Rattliff, F.: *Mach Bands: Quantitative Studies on Neural Networks in the Retina*, Holden-Day, Inc., Publisher, San Francisco, 1965.

Robinson, D. A.: Eye movement control in primates. Science, 161:1219–1224, 1968.

Rughton, W. A. H.: Visual pigments and color blindness. Sci Am, 232:64–74, 1975.

Schneider, G. E.: Two visual systems. Science, 163:895–902, 1969.

Straatsma, B. R., M. O. Hall, R. A. Allen, and F. Crescitelli: *The Retina: Morphology, Function and Clinical Characteristics*, University of California Press, Berkeley and Los Angeles, 1969.

Wald, G.: The receptors of human color vision. Science, 145:1007–1016, 1964.

Young, R. W.: Visual cells. Sci Am, 223:80–91, 1970.

CHAPTER THIRTEEN

THE THALAMUS

THE THALAMUS

General roles of the thalamus

The (dorsal) thalamus is the complex of nuclear processing stations that are coordinators and regulators of the functional activity of the cerebral cortex. Most of the direct input to the cerebral cortex is derived from the thalamus. In turn, the thalamus receives much of its input via direct and indirect connections from the cerebral cortex. Many thalamic nuclei have reciprocal connections with the cerebral cortex.

The thalamus serves four basic roles.

1. *Role in the sensory systems.* All sensory pathways except those of the olfactory system have direct projections to certain thalamic nuclei, which, in turn, convey through their axons influences to restricted sectors of the sensory cerebral cortex. In addition, large sectors of the sensory cerebral cortex have connections with many thalamic nuclei. The conscious awareness of the crude aspects of the sensations pain, touch, pressure, and temperature are probably realized in the thalamus.

2. *Role in motor systems.* The thalamus has a crucial role in projecting critical influences to the cortex involved with somatic motor activities (motor and premotor cortices). Actually, it is intercalated between a number of subcortical structures and the cerebral cortex. The two neuronal circuits which are significant in this regard are the pathway of the cerebellum to the thalamus to the cortex (Chap. 9), and the "feedback" circuit of cortex to corpus striatum to thalamus to cortex (Chap. 14).

3. *Role in general background neural activity.* The thalamus has an essential role in processing through its connections those neural influences which are basic, for example, to the rhythms of the cerebral cortex (as expressed in the electroencephalogram, EEG) and in the phases of the sleep-wake cycle. These activities are fundamental physiologic and behavioral expressions of the activities of the nonspecific thalamic nuclei and the ascending reticular system.

4. *Role in affect and the highest expressions of the cerebral cortex.* The thalamus is involved in some subtle way with affect and many of the expressive aspects of emotion and behavior through its connections with the limbic lobe (Chap. 15) and the prefrontal cortex (Chap. 16). Reciprocal and related circuits act to integrate the thalamus and the association areas of the cerebral cortex, which contain the structural substrates critical to the "highest-ordered" cortical activities, including thought, symbolisms of communication, and creativity.

The general anatomic relations of the thalamus to other cerebral structures are described and illustrated in Chap. 1 and Figs. 13-1, 13-2, 13-4, and 13-8.

Nuclear groups of the thalamus

The thalamus is roughly divided into the *anterior nuclear group*, *lateral nuclear group*, and *medial nuclear group* by a plate of neural tissue called the internal medullary lamina (see Table 13-1 and Figs. 13-2 through 13-5). The anterior nuclear group is flanked between the two arms of

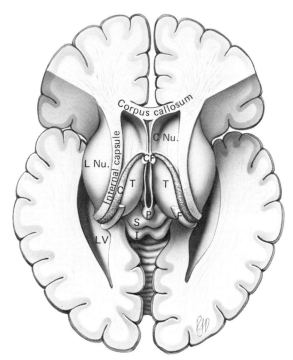

FIGURE 13-1 Dorsal view of a dissection of the cerebrum illustrating the anatomical relations of the thalamus, internal capsule, caudate nucleus, lenticular nucleus, and choroid plexus of the lateral ventricle. C, choroid plexus; CF, column of fornix; C Nu., caudate nucleus; F, fimbira of fornix; I, inferior colliculus; L Nu., lenticular nucleus: LV, lateral ventricle; P, pineal body; S, superior colliculus; T, thalamus. The median region between the corpus callosum and the columns of the fornix contains the two laminae of the septum pellucidum and that between the columns and the pineal body contains the third ventricle. (*Adapted from Netter and Carpenter, chap. 1.*)

* *The ventral posterior nucleus is often called the ventro-basal complex.*

the rostral bifurcation of this lamina. Within the internal medullary lamina is the *intralaminar nuclear group.* On the rostral and lateral surface of the thalamus adjacent to the internal capsule is the external medullary lamina, within which is the *thalamic reticular nucleus.* A narrow lamina on the medial surface of the thalamus, lining the third ventricle, contains several small nuclei called the *midline nuclear group.* The lateral nuclear group is divided into a *ventral tier* and a *dorsal tier.* The *metathalamic group* is the caudal extension of the ventral tier of the lateral nuclear group.

The intralaminar nuclear group has the following anatomic relations. The large centromedian nucleus (CM) is located in the middle third of the thalamus between the medial nuclear

group and the ventral posterior nucleus of the lateral nuclear group. The smaller parafascicular nucleus (PF) is found medial to the CM and adjacent to the fasciculus retroflexus (habenulo-

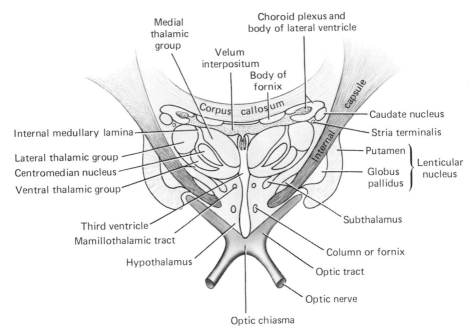

FIGURE 13-2 Schema of a coronal section through the diencephalon and some adjacent structures. The major groups of thalamic nuclei are indicated. (*Adapted from Carpenter.*)

peduncular tract). Rostral to these nuclei are the other intralaminar nuclei; the central lateral and central median nuclei are located caudal to the paracentral nucleus. The former group is referred to as the centromedian-parafascicular nuclear complex (large in humans) and the latter as the rostral intralaminar group (small in human beings).

The *anterior nuclear group* is divided into the anterolateral, anteromedial, and anterodorsal nuclei. The anteroventral nucleus is large.

The *nuclei of the ventral tier* of the lateral nuclear group are arranged roughly in a rostrocaudal order as the ventral anterior nucleus, ventral lateral nucleus, and ventral posterior nucleus. The ventral posterior nucleus is subdivided into the medially located *ventral posteromedial (arcuate, semilunar) nucleus*, the laterally located *ventral posterolateral nucleus*, and the small, ventrally located ventral posterior inferior nucleus. The metathalamic group (metathalamus) comprises the nuclei of the medial and lateral geniculate bodies.

The *nuclei of the dorsal tier* are arranged in a rostrocaudal order as the lateral dorsal nucleus, lateral posterior nucleus, and pulvinar. The

large pulvinar has been subdivided into the medial, inferior, and lateral nuclei.

The medial nuclear group (called *median* or *dorsomedian nucleus*) is divided into a medially located magnocellular part and a laterally located parvocellular part.

Because the dendrites and axons of many neurons of adjacent thalamic nuclei overlap and interdigitate, the precise delineation of each thalamic nucleus may not be critical, considering our present-day knowledge of the precise function of each nucleus.

Some thalamic nuclei according to other terminologies

The description and anatomic delineation of the thalamic nuclei are imprecise because of the indistinct cytoarchitectural boundaries between the "named nuclei." Accordingly, other nuclear groupings have been proposed, especially with regard to the ventral tier of the lateral nuclear group.

The term *ventrobasal complex* is defined on the basis of physiologic criteria. It is the nuclear complex whose cells respond to the stimulation of somatic sensory receptors, particularly those modalities conveyed by the medial lemniscus, spinothalamic tract, and trigeminothalamic tracts. In general the ventrobasal complex corresponds to the ventral posterolateral and ventral posteromedial nuclei. The cells of the ventrobasal complex are excited predominantly by mechanical stimulation, including pressure, touch, vibration, and joint movement. Stimuli associated with thermal sense and possibly pain (nociceptive modality) may activate cells of the ventrobasal complex.

The ventral tier of the lateral nuclear group, exclusive of the metathalamus, has been subdivided into six nuclei by Hassler. In the following list, these six nuclei are noted, along with the probable equivalent portion of the ventral tier:

1. Lateropolaris (LPO) is equivalent to the VA.
2. Ventralis oralis anterior (VOA) is equivalent to the anterior basal region of the VL.
3. Ventralis oralis posterior (VOP) is equivalent to the posterior basal region of the VL.
4. Dorsalis oralis (DO) is equivalent to the dorsal region of VL
5. Ventralis intermedius (VIM) is equivalent to the rostral region of VP.
6. Ventralis caudalis (VC) is equivalent to the remainder of VP.

Specific nuclei and nonspecific nuclei

In the most widely used classification, the thalamic nuclei are grouped as (1) *specific cortical relay nuclei* (specific thalamic nuclei), (2) *specific association nuclei* (association thalamic nuclei), and (3) *nonspecific nuclei* (see Table 13-1).

Specific nuclei   A specific nucleus is one which projects to localized regions of the cerebral cortex. These nuclei can be demonstrated (1) anatomically by the retrograde degeneration of the cell bodies of the thalamocortical fibers following the removal (ablation) of the cerebral cortex and (2) physiologically by stimulating the cells within the nuclei and recording the discharge of the thalamocortical projections within the cerebral cortex. The specific nuclei are often called *"cortically dependent"* nuclei, because their cell bodies exhibit the retrograde degeneration re-

sponse after the destruction of their axon terminals by the cortical ablation. Some cell bodies with axons terminating in the cortex do not exhibit the retrograde degeneration response; they remain normal because their axons have *sustaining axon collateral branches;* these branches project either to several widely dispersed cortical regions or to other thalamic nuclei.

The *specific cortical relay nuclei* are arranged into three groups on the basis of the major sources of their inputs and the objects of their outputs (see Fig. 13-6):

1. The *sensory relay nuclei* include the ventral posteromedial (VPM) nucleus, ventral posterolateral (VPL) nucleus, and the medial and lateral geniculate bodies (nuclei). These nuclei receive their major inputs from the ascending sensory pathways and project their output to the primary and secondary somesthetic, primary visual, and primary auditory cortices.
2. The *"motor" relay nuclei* include the ventral anterior (VA) and ventral lateral (VL) nuclei. They receive their major inputs from the cerebellum, basal ganglia, and substantia nigra and project their outputs to the motor and premotor cortex (Chap. 14).
3. The "limbic" relay nuclei include the nuclei of the anterior nuclear group and the lateral dorsal nucleus. They receive input from the basal diencephalic regions and project to sectors of the limbic cortex (Chap. 15).

The *specific association nuclei* have profuse connections with other diencephalic nuclei with the association areas of the cortex. They receive no direct input or possibly a slight input from the ascending pathways. The lateral nuclear group has connections with the association cortical areas of the temporal, parietal, and occipital lobes, while the medial nuclear group has connections with the prefrontal cortex (Fig. 13-6).

The *nonspecific thalamic nuclei* include the intralaminar nuclear group, midline (periventricular) nuclear group, thalamic reticular nucleus, and the magnocellular part of the ventral anterior (VAmc) nucleus (see Figs. 13-3 and 13-5). The *midline nuclear group* is a rostral extension of the brainstem periventricular gray matter, while the *intralaminar group* and possibly the *thalamic reticular nucleus* are rostral continuations of the brainstem reticular formation. In general, the major connections of these nuclei are apparently (1) reciprocal projections with specific thalamic nuclei and other, nonspecific, thalamic nuclei and (2) afferent projections from the brainstem reticular formation and cerebral cortex. In addition, there are connections with the striatum and globus pallidus (Chap. 14) and from the cerebellum (Chap. 9). The input to the intralaminar nuclei from the brainstem reticular formation is via the fibers of the central tegmental tract. The nonspecific thalamic projection to the entire neocortex is known as the *generalized thalamocortical projection system.* This system has a critical role in the *recruiting response* and other cortical activity associated with the encephalogram, noted later on in this chapter. These responses over the entire neocortex following stimulation of the intralaminar nuclei are the result of influences conveyed (1) by fine collateral axons of intralaminar neurons whose other branches (called sustaining collaterals, Chap. 2) are distributed to other diencephalic nuclei and basal ganglia (especially thalamostriate fibers to the striatum, Chap. 14) and (2) by projections from VAmc to the orbital cortex.

The complexities of the neuronal connections and circuitry of these nonspecific nuclei are such that many essential features are as yet unresolved, and their functional implications incompletely understood.

Duality A duality exists within the thalamocortical systems. The *specific thalamic nuclei* and their projections are primarily organized as precise conveyors and processors of information utilized in the sensory sphere (e.g., touch, sight) and in the motor sphere (e.g., a movement). The *nonspecific thalamic nuclei* and their projections are organized primarily as signal systems subserving an energizing function over wide sectors of the thalamus and cerebral cortex. The powerful internuclear activity within the thalamus modulates, regulates, and modifies thalamocortical activity. The interactions between the thalamic specific nuclei and thalamic nonspecific nuclei are extensive. Much of the internuclear processing is exerted through intense excitatory and inhibitory synaptic activity between the interneurons and neurons of the specific and nonspecific nuclei.

NONSPECIFIC THALAMIC NUCLEI

Intralaminar nuclear group

The intralaminar nuclei are located in the lamina between the medial and lateral thalamic nuclear groups (see Figs. 13-3 to 13-5). The centromedian and parafascicular nuclei are located caudally at the level of the ventral posterior nucleus, with the centromedian nucleus being just lateral to the parafascicular. The habenulointerpeduncular tract (Chap. 15) passes through the parafascicular nucleus. The centromedian-parafascicular nuclear complex is often regarded as a unit; in fact, the centromedian nucleus is a phylogenetically recent specialization of a portion of the parafascicular nucleus. Of the three rostral intralaminar nuclei the paracentral is the most rostral and the central lateral and central medial nuclei are located just in front of the centromedian nucleus. These intralaminar nuclei receive ascending input from the brainstem reticular formation via the central tegmental tract from the spinal cord via fibers associated with the spinothalamic tract from the dentate and fastigial nuclei of the cerebellum and from the tectum of the midbrain. The centromedian-parafascicular complex receives input from the cerebral cortex, with motor area 4 projecting to the centromedian nucleus and premotor area 6 to the parafascicular nucleus. The centromedian receives additional input from the globus pallidus (Chap. 14). The two caudal intralaminar nuclei project to the putamen, while the three rostral nuclei project to the caudate nucleus (Chap. 14).

These projections to the striatum (caudate nucleus and putamen) are called the thalamostriate fibers (Chap. 14). Thin collateral branches from these thalamostriate fibers radiate rostrally and terminate in laminae V and VI primarily, but not exclusively of the entire neocortex. These are most important in relation to the ascending reticular system, recruiting response, sleep phenomena, and the electroencephalogram (Chaps. 8, 15, and 16).

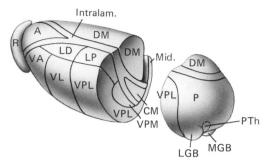

FIGURE 13-3 Schematic representation of the left thalamus illustrating the topographic relations of the major thalamic nuclei. The orientation of the thalamus is similar to that in Fig. 13-4. The reticular nucleus (R) extends along the lateral aspect of the thalamus; only its rostral portion is illustrated. A, anterior nuclear group; CM, centromedianum; DM, dorsomedial nucleus; Intralam., Intralaminar nuclei; LD, lateral dorsal nucleus; LGB, lateral geniculate body; LP, lateral posterior nucleus; MGB, medial geniculate body; Mid., midline nuclei; P, pulvinar; PTh, posterior thalamic zone; R, reticular nucleus; VA, ventral anterior nucleus; VL, ventral anterior nucleus; VPL, ventral posterior lateral nucleus; and VPM, ventral posterior medial nucleus.

The magnocellular portion of the ventral anterior nucleus (VA) exhibits some physiologic characteristics of the intralaminar nuclei. It has widespread projections, apparently via axon collaterals to the frontal cortex, especially to the orbitofrontal cortex. The suggestion has been made that this cortical region may act as a trigger zone involved with the recruiting response.

Thalamic reticular nucleus (Fig. 13-5)

The thalamic reticular nucleus is a thin lamina flanking the rostral and lateral aspect of the thalamus (see Figs. 13-3 and 13-5). It is located adjacent to the posterior limb of the internal capsule. The input to this nucleus is presumed to be derived from (1) the brainstem reticular formation and (2) collateral branches of fibers passing through nucleus into the internal capsule from the intralaminar and specific thalamic nuclei and from descending axons from the neocortex. The thalamic reticular nucleus is presumed to have a critical role in the integration of intrathalamic activities. It is suggested that this nucleus may be related to the synchronized low-frequency, high-amplitude rhythms associated with light sleep and with drowsiness (Chap. 16).

The ventral portion of the thalamic reticular nucleus is continuous with the zona incerta of the ventral thalamus. Both these structures have a common origin from the subthalamus. Because the zona incerta is a rostral extension of the brainstem reticular formation, there is justification for classifying the thalamic reticular nucleus as a part of reticular formation.

Midline nuclear group (Figs. 13-3 and 13-5)

This midline group consists of small nuclei of ancient phylogenetic history located in the periventricular gray matter of the diencephalon. Three of these nuclei—reuniens, rhomboidal, and median central—are in the vicinity of the interthalamic adhesion (massa intermedia) that is present in about 70 percent of human brains (Chap. 1). The cells in these neurons have connections with the periaqueductal gray of the midbrain, the intralaminar nuclei, the magnocellular part of the dorsomedian nucleus, and the hypothalamus. Their functional role is speculative but, because of the connections, involvement in visceral activities is likely.

SPECIFIC THALAMIC (CORTICAL RELAY) NUCLEI (Figs. 13-3 through 13-6)

Anterior nuclear group

The *anterior nuclear group* is intercalated between the mamillary body of the hypothalamus and the cortical areas 23, 24, and 32 of the cingulate gyrus (see Figs. 13-3 to 13-5). The input to this group is conveyed from the mamillary body via fibers of the mamillothalamic tract and from the hippocampus via fibers of the postcommissural fornix (see Fig. 15-4). The medial mamillary nucleus projects to the large anteroventral (AV) and the small anteromedial (AM) nuclei, and the lateral mamillary nucleus projects to the small anterodorsal nucleus (AD) of the group. Some fibers from the anterior nuclear group project back to the mamillary body via the mamillothalamic tract. Reciprocal influences are conveyed between this nuclear group and the cingulate gyrus via thalamocortical and corticothalamic fibers which pass through the anterior limb of the internal capsule. The anterior nuclear group is a processing and relay station in the "Papez circuit" of the limbic system (Chap. 15). Stimulation or ablation of this nucleus results in changes in blood pressure and

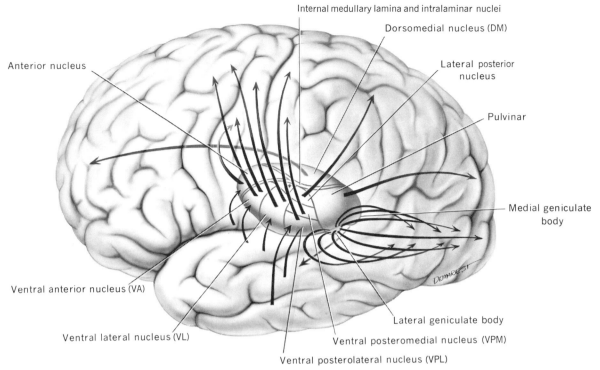

Anterior nucleus

Internal medullary lamina and intralaminar nuclei

Dorsomedial nucleus (DM)

Lateral posterior nucleus

Pulvinar

Medial geniculate body

Ventral anterior nucleus (VA)

Ventral lateral nucleus (VL)

Lateral geniculate body

Ventral posteromedial nucleus (VPM)

Ventral posterolateral nucleus (VPL)

FIGURE 13-4 The thalamus and its major nuclei and cortical projections. [A] Lateral dorsal nucleus.

other expressions of the autonomic nervous system. A cat with a lesion in this nuclear complex is more difficult to excite to anger; it has an elevated threshold for rage. The lateral dorsal nucleus (LD) of the lateral nuclear group may be a posterior extension of the anterior nuclear group.

Lateral nuclear group (ventral tier)

Ventral anterior nucleus (VA) The *ventral anterior nucleus* has a dual role as a specific thalamic nucleus and as a nonspecific thalamic nucleus of the reticular system (Figs. 13-3 to 13-6). Input is derived from the globus pallidus (fibers pass via the ansa lenticularis and lenticular fasciculus to the principal part of VA, VApc), from the pars reticularis of the substantia nigra (fibers terminate in the magnocellular part of the VA nucleus, VAmc), and from the brainstem, intralaminar nuclei of the midline, and collateral branches of descending fibers from the premotor area of the cerebral cortex. VA may receive some input from the cerebellum. The major role of the

VApc in the regulation of somatic motor activity is effected, at least in part, by complex circuits involving the intralaminar nuclei midline nuclear group, dorsomedial nucleus, and basal ganglia, which feed back influences to the VA, VL, and CM (Chap. 14). In turn, this processed information is projected to the cerebral cortex, (Chap. 16). The VAmc is a significant link in the reticular system; its effect upon the elicitation of the recruiting response (noted above under "Nonspecific Nuclei") is thought to be exerted by (1) the projection from magnocellular parts of the VAmc to the orbitofrontal cortex and (2) activation of the nonspecific thalamic nuclei. The VAmc and its projection to the orbitofrontal cortex may act as the trigger zone for the recruiting response and the synchronous electrocortical activity over wide areas of the neocortex (Chap. 16). The mamillothalamic tract passes through the VA nucleus.

Ventral lateral nucleus (VL) The *ventral lateral nucleus* (see Figs. 13-3 through 13-6) is an integral nucleus in the feedback circuits from the

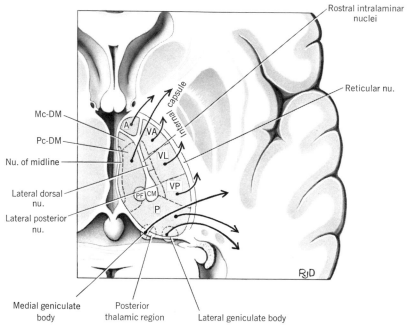

Labels on figure:
- Rostral intralaminar nuclei
- Reticular nu.
- Mc-DM
- Pc-DM
- Nu. of midline
- Lateral dorsal nu.
- Lateral posterior nu.
- Internal capsule
- A
- VA
- VL
- VP
- PF
- CM
- P
- RjD
- Medial geniculate body
- Posterior thalamic region
- Lateral geniculate body

FIGURE 13-5 The major thalamic nuclei in a composite of several horizontal sections through the thalamus. The arrows indicate the general location of the cortical projections within the internal capsule. A, anterior nuclear group; CM, centromedian nu.; P, pulvinar; PF, parafascicular nu.; VA, ventral anterior nu.; VL, ventral lateral nu.; VP, ventral posterior nu.

cerebellum and basal ganglia to the motor cortex (precentral gyrus, area 4). The feedback circuits include (1) cerebral cortex to cerebellum to VL to motor cortex (Chap. 9) and (2) cerebral cortex to basal ganglia to VL to motor cortex (Chap. 14). Through the projection to the motor cortex, *the VL exerts its role as the main gateway to and prime mover of the pathways* (Chap. 14). It receives its main input from the contralateral cerebellar hemisphere (primarily via the dentatothalamic tract and partly from the nucleus interpositus) and the ipsilateral red nucleus via the dentatorubrothalamic tract. Other input comes from the ipsilateral medial segment of the globus pallidus via the thalamic fasciculus and from the substantia nigra. The VL has topographic and reciprocal connections with the precentral and supplementary motor cortex: the medial region of the VL with the face area, the intermediate region with the upper extremity and body area, and the lateral region with lower extremity area of area 4. VL receives some input from some midline nuclei, intralaminar nuclei, and dorsomedial nucleus.

In general, VLo (oral part) receives input from the cerebellum and some from the globus pallidus, and VLm (medial part) receives input from the globus pallidus and substantia nigra. VLo and VLc (caudal part) have reciprocal topographic connections with the motor cortex. The neural processing within the VL of the various inputs, including that from the reticular nuclei, results in the production of the powerful influences exerted by the VL upon motor activity. Thus there appears to be a blending of the afferent input from the basal ganglia and the cerebellum by the overlap of their fiber terminals in VLo. The motor cortex is the source of the fibers of the corticobulbar, corticospinal, corticoreticulospinal and corticorubrospinal tracts. Surgical lesions in the VL may ameliorate the tremors and rigidity on the contralateral side of patients with Parkinson's disease.

The ventral anterior and ventral lateral nuclei

and their projections to the premotor and motor cortices (areas 4 and 6) have been called the *afferent nuclei of the motor cortex, motor thalamus,* prepyramidal *afferents to the motor cortex,* and the *reentry* pathway to the cortex. With respect to a motor act, activity in these nuclei occurs prior to that in the motor cortex. The names relate to their connections and functional relations with the cerebellum and basal ganglia (Chaps. 9 and 14).

Ventral posterior nucleus (VP)   The *ventral posterior nucleus is the primary somatic processing relay nucleus for the general sensory and gustatory pathways* (see Figs. 13-3 through 13-5). The VP nucleus comprises three nuclei: the ventral posterolateral (VPL), ventral posteromedial (VPM), and ventral posterior inferior (VPI). Most of the neurons of the VP respond to one of the following stimulus modalities: tactile sense (e.g., light pressure or bending of hair), mechanical distortion of deep structures (position sense or joint movements), or intense mechanical distortion often associated with pain.

Each neuron is (1) place-specific in that it is excited from a small and precise locus on the body and (2) modality-specific in that it is excited by a single stimulus modality (e.g., bending of a hair). These neurons are arranged somatotopically. Neurons responding to thermal stimulation are few. Some neurons respond to noxious stimuli, but the question as to where specific "pain" cells or even "thermal" cells are located in this nucleus has not been resolved. Cortical projections from lamina VI (corticothalamic fibers) of the primary somatosensory cortex (SSI, areas 1 to 3) terminate in the ventral posterior nucleus (Chap. 16). The relay neurons projecting to the primary somatosensory cortex are subject to recurrent inhibition through feedback via Golgi type II interneurons. The ventral posterior nucleus is often referred to as the ventrobasal complex (VB).

The axons of the ventral posterior nucleus terminate in a dense plexus in lamina IV of the primary somatosensory cortex. They have excitatory synaptic connections with the dendritic spines of the spiny stellate cells and the basilar dendrites of pyramidal cells. Each neuronal terminal contributes to a functionally defined column in the cortex, similar to those in the primary visual cortex (Chaps. 12 and 16). The thalamocortical projections are parcellated so that functionally equivalent neuronal populations in the VP nucleus are connected with neuronal populations (columnar organization) in the primary somatosensory cortex. The same parcellation and equivalence of connectivity apply to body representation, submodality, distribution, and functional properties. In effect, a three-dimensional group of neurons in VP project to a structurally and functionally definable columnar zone in the cortex (see Fig. 16-9).

Ventral posterior lateral nucleus (VPL)   The *VPL nucleus* (see Figs. 13-3 and 13-4) is the nucleus of termination of the lateral spinothalamic tract (pain and thermal sense from the body), medial lemniscus (touch, deep sensibility, and vibratory sense from the body), anterior spinothalamic tract (light touch from the body), and spinocervicothalamic tract (tactile and kinesthetic sense). These ascending pathways terminate somatotopically within the VPL. One schema indicates that the thoracic and lumbar regions are represented dorsally and the distal parts of the limbs ventrally in the VPL; in addition, sacral segments are represented laterally and cervical segments medially in it. Another schema indicates that the pathways from the lower extremity terminate in the posterolateral part, those from the body segments in the intermediate location, and those from the upper extremity in the anteromedial part of the VPL. The sensory homunculus is a distorted image of the body proportional to the innervation density; those parts of the body (e.g., the hand) with great tactile sensitivity occupy a greater volume of the nucleus than those with relatively minimal sensitivity (e.g., the back).

Ventral posterior medial nucleus (VPM)   The *VPM nucleus* is the nucleus of termination of the fibers of the crossed anterior trigeminal tract from the principal and spinal trigeminal nuclei and the uncrossed posterior trigeminal tract from the principal trigeminal nucleus (see Figs. 8-17, 13-3, 13-4). The modalities are topographically localized within the VPM; taste is projected to the medial portion of the nucleus (referred to as the parvocellular part, VPMpc), tactile sense

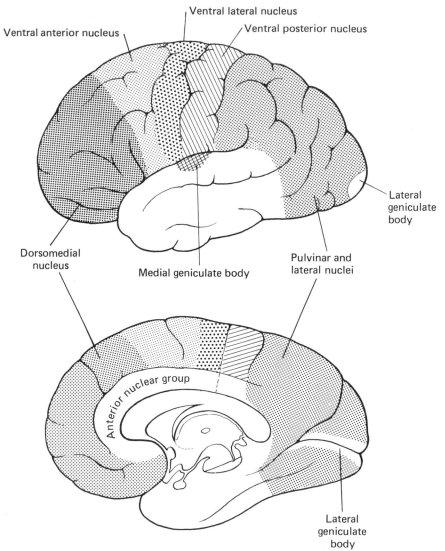

FIGURE 13-6 Lateral and medial views of the left cerebral hemisphere illustrating cortical projection areas of some thalamic nuclei. Much of the temporal lobe does not receive projections from the specific thalamic nuclei. Such an area is known as an athalamic cortex.

to the lateral portion, and temperature to the intermediate portion. The tactile sense from the face and oral cavity is conveyed via crossed and uncrossed fibers to the VPM.

Ventral posterior inferior nucleus (VPI) The *ventral posterior inferior nucleus* is a small nucleus located in ventral VP near the junction of VPL and VPM. This nucleus projects fibers to the postcentral gyrus in the boundary zone between

areas 2 and 5. This region of the parietal lobe is considered to be the primary vestibular area and may be associated with the conscious perception of vestibular sense.

The VP nucleus has precise point-to-point projections to the primary somesthetic cortex (postcentral gyrus, areas 3, 1, and 2). This is consistent with the somatotopic organization of this cortical area and with the modality-specific cortical neurons. Lateral VPL projects to the dorsal sectors of the gyrus, intermediate portions of the VP to the midsector of the gyrus, and the VPM to the lower sector of the gyrus. Although cortical areas 3, 1, and 2 receive projections from the VP, most of the fibers terminate in area 3. In addition, the VP probably has some connections with somatic sensory area II. As in the other ascending systems, descending influences from the postcentral gyrus are projected to the VP.

Posterior thalamic nucleus (zone, region) The posterior thalamic nucleus is located caudal to the VPM and VPL nuclei (see Fig. 13-3). The nucleus includes the magnocellular portion of the medial geniculate body and adjacent midbrain tegmentum.

The general sensory sources are from the cutaneous and deep receptors with the exception of the joint sensors. The posterior thalamic nucleus has direct connections with the secondary somatosensory area (somatosensory area II, SS II) located within the lateral sulcus on the most lateral aspect of the postcentral gyrus. In addition to the bilateral input this SS II area receives from the posterior thalamic nucleus, it receives a strong projection via the corpus callosum from SS II of the contralateral hemisphere.

The *posterior thalamic nucleus* is a significant processing and relay nucleus in the general sensory pathways with a critical role in the perception of painful and noxious stimuli. Bilaterally derived influences from the ipsilateral and mainly from the contralateral sides of the body are conveyed to the posterior thalamic region via the spinothalamic tract, spinocervicothalamic pathway, ascending reticular pathway, and some fibers from the other ascending pathways. In effect, *this complex receives polysensory input* from the auditory, vestibular, and somatosensory systems. Its cells are not modality-specific. Rather they respond to a variety of inputs from tactile, vibratory, and auditory sources.

Metathalamus (metathalamic group)

Lateral geniculate body (nucleus) The nucleus of the lateral geniculate body (LGB) is the thalamic relay nucleus of the visual pathway (see Figs. 13-3 through 13-5). Each LGB (1) receives input from both eyes via the retinofugal fibers of the optic tract and from lamina VI of the primary visual cortex (area 17) via corticogenicu-

late fibers of the optic radiation and (2) projects output to the visual cortex via the geniculocalcarine tract (optic radiation; Chap. 12). Intrathalamic connections are made with pulvinar and other nuclei of the lateral thalamic groups.

Medial geniculate body (nucleus) The nucleus of the *medial geniculate body* (see Figs. 13-3 through 13-5) is divided into the dorsally located parvocellular part (MGpc) and the ventrally located magnocellular part (MGmc, posterior thalamic nucleus). The MGpc is the thalamic relay nucleus of the auditory pathway and of the vestibular system. A vestibular pathway from the vestibular receptors in the membranous labyrinth to the MGpc or to the ventral posterior inferior nucleus (VPI) has been proposed. Vestibular influences are thought to be projected to the face region of the primary somatic sensory cortex. In the sector between areas 2 and 5 of the cortex there are cells which respond to vestibular influences. This system may have a role in our sense of orientation of the head in space. These cells also respond to kinesthetic stimuli in joints.

Each MGpc (1) receives input from the spiral organs of Corti of both ears via the ascending fibers of the brachium of the inferior colliculus and from lamina VI of the primary auditory cortex (area 41) via descending fibers of the auditory radiation, and (2) projects output to the primary auditory cortex (superior temporal gyrus, transverse gyri of Heschl, area 41) via the auditory radiation (geniculotemporal fibers). Intrathalamic connections are made with the pulvinar and other nuclei of the lateral thalamic groups.

Lateral nuclear group (dorsal tier)

The *dorsal tier of the lateral nuclear group* consists, in a rostrocaudal direction, of the lateral dorsal nucleus (LD), the lateral posterior nucleus (LP), and the massive pulvinar.

Lateral dorsal and lateral posterior nuclei (Fig. 13-3) The *lateral dorsal nucleus* is now considered to be a caudal extension of the anterior nuclear group. In common with the latter, the LD has its primary connections with the cingulate gyrus. Reciprocal connections with the cortex of the precuneus have been reported. Information concerning input to LD is wanting. The *lateral posterior nucleus*, located dorsal to the VP, blends into the pulvinar. The input to the LP is apparently derived primarily from the VP and adjacent thalamic nuclei. Its reciprocal connections with the superior parietal lobule (areas 5 and 7) suggest that the LP has a role in processing information of the general somatic sensory system.

Pulvinar (Figs. 13-3 through 13-6) The *pulvinar*, the largest of all the thalamic nuclei, is divided into three subunits—inferior (nucleus), lateral (nucleus), and large medial (nucleus) pulvinar. Although the pulvinar is regarded as a polysensory nucleus, it receives no direct sensory input. Rather, it receives its input from the cerebral cortex and the superior colliculus. The pulvinar has reciprocal interconnections with the cortex of the occipital lobe (areas 17 to 19), superior parietal lobule, posterior temporal lobe, supramarginal gyrus, and angular gyrus. It is integrated in the second visual system (Chap. 12) through its input from the superior colliculus and its projection to the inferotemporal cortex. (It is presumed to have connections with the intralaminar nuclei and the dorsolateral and lateral posterior thalamic nuclei. Interconnections with the specific thalamic nuclei have not been demonstrated.)

The pulvinar is a complex processing nuclear station involved with the normal functioning of the association cortex. It subserves the highest levels of auditory and visual integration (Chap. 16). No functional or behavioral changes in the sensory sphere have been observed in animals or human beings with lesions in the pulvinar. Reduction in the degree of spasticity as indicated by decrease in hypertonus and clonus in certain spastic patients has been reported.

Medial nuclear group

Dorsomedial (medial) nucleus (DM) The massive *dorsomedial nucleus*, located between the internal medullary lamina and the third ventricle, is divided into a *magnocellular* (*large-cell*) part and a larger, *parvocellular* (*small-cell*) part (see Figs. 13-3 through 13-6). This nucleus has extensive intrathalamic connections with the intralaminar nuclei, nuclei of the midline, and the nuclei of the lateral thalamic group. The

dorsomedially and rostrally located magnocellular part of the DM has connections primarily with subcortical structures, while the laterally located parvocellular portion is linked with the prefrontal cortex (areas 9, 10, 11, and 12—all rostral to areas 6 and 32). Via fibers in the inferior thalamic peduncle, the magnocellular part has connections (some of which are reciprocal) with the amygdaloid body, lateral hypothalamus, basal olfactory centers, and temporal and caudal orbitofrontal neocortex. The parvocellular part has massive topically organized reciprocal connections with the prefrontal cortex. A bundle of fibers from the orbitofrontal cortex to the medial dorsomedial nucleus passes through the inferior thalamic peduncle. These fibers and those interconnecting the amygdaloid body and the hypothalamus form the so-called ansa peduncularis (Chap. 15).

The integration and elaboration of this input and its relation with the hypothalamus (Chap. 11) and the prefrontal cortex (Chap. 16) may help to explain why this elaborate nucleus is involved with the affect of an individual rather than with specific sensory activities. The affective tone is expressed as euphoria or as mild depression, as a feeling of well-being or ill-being, or as a pleasant response or an unpleasant response to environmental stimuli. The hypothalamus, as the highest center of the autonomic nervous system, has the expressive role, whereas the prefrontal cortex is a higher elaborator of affect. The ablation of the DM has been used therapeutically, as has prefrontal lobotomy, in certain psychosurgical procedures (Chap. 16). Destruction of the DM in cats produces an animal that has a lower threshold for rage, is easily irritated, and is less adept at solving problems. Ablation of DM in humans can alter the patient's reaction to chronic pain without eliminating the pain. Through its interconnections with the prefrontal cortex and hypothalamus and, in turn, with the amygdaloid nuclear complex and other limbic structures, the dorsomedial nucleus appears to be involved with the neural mechanisms underlying emotional expression (Chap. 15).

Internal capsule

The internal capsule has the shape of an open oriental fan (see Fig. 1-14). The ribs of the fan parallel the course of the fiber bundles (see Figs. 13-7 and 13-8; see also Fig. 16-13). The handle of the fan is analogous to the crus cerebri of the midbrain; the lower half of the fan, to the internal capsule; the upper half of the fan, to the corona radiata (radiating crown) of the cerebral white matter; and the distal margin of the fan, to the gray matter. The pathways of the internal capsule, their sites of origin, and their sites of termination are outlined below. Many fibers do not extend through all portions of the "fan" (e.g., striate fibers and thalamocortical fibers are not found in the "handle").

The *anterior limb of the internal capsule* contains fibers projecting either to or from the frontal lobe (see Figs. 13-7 and 13-8). The reciprocal connections include (1) fibers from the prefrontal cortex to the dorsomedial thalamic nucleus, and from the dorsomedial thalamic nucleus to the prefrontal cortex; and (2) fibers from the cingulate gyrus to the anterior thalamic nuclei, and from the anterior thalamic nuclei to the cingulate gyrus (Chap. 15). The frontopontine fibers to the nuclei located in the pons are integrated into the cerebellar systems (Chap. 9). The orbitohypothalamic fibers of the median forebrain bundle (Chap. 15) and some corticostriate fibers (Chap. 14) to the caudate nucleus (subcallosal fasciculus) pass through this limb.

The *genu of the internal capsule* contains the corticobulbar and corticoreticular fibers (see Figs. 13-7 and 13-8; see also Fig. 16-13). The fibers from the frontal eye fields (Chap. 12) synapse in the brainstem tegmentum with interneurons that innervate the motor nuclei of the eye muscles (oculomotor, trochlear, and abducent motor nuclei) in complex patterns so as to influence the conjugate movements of the eyes. Other corticobulbar fibers terminate in the tegmentum on interneurons that innervate the motor nuclei of the trigeminal nerve, facial nerve, and hypoglossal nerve, nucleus ambiguus, and nucleus of the spinal accessory nerve (Chaps. 7 and 8). Some ascending (sensory) thalamic fibers project to the "motor cortex" of the frontal lobe.

The *posterior limb proper (thalamolenticular portion)* is composed of both motor pathways and sensory pathways (see Figs. 13-7 and 13-8; see also Fig. 16-13) associated with the auditory and visual cortical areas of the temporal and occipital lobes (see Figs. 1-4, 13-7, 13-8, and 16-13). The auditory radiation originates in the medial geniculate nucleus and terminates in the transverse temporal gyri of Heschl. Some descending cortical fibers terminate in the medial geniculate body and in the inferior colliculus. The optic radiation originates in the lateral ge-

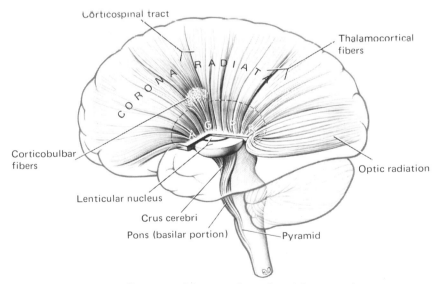

FIGURE 13-7 Some component fiber tracts of the internal capsule and their cortical projections. A, anterior limb; G, genu; P, posterior limb; R, retrolenticular portion of the posterior limb.

niculate body and terminates in the primary visual cortex (area 17). Descending fibers from visual association areas 18 to 20 terminate in the pulvinar of the thalamus, pretectal region, and superior colliculus (Chap. 12), and in the brainstem reticular formation. Ablation of area 20 has been implicated in visual agnosias (Chap. 16). The major corticopontine pathways project from extensive cortical areas to the pontine nuclei (Chap. 9); this includes the frontopontine, parietopontine, temporopontine, and occipitopontine tracts.

The widespread projections from the intralaminar nuclei to the cerebral cortex pass through all the limbs of the internal capsule. Many of the fibers are collateral branches of the thalamostriate fibers (Chap. 14).

Thalamic peduncles

The thalamocortical and corticothalamic fibers between the thalamus and cerebral cortex course through the limbs of the internal capsule (see Fig. 16-13 and Chap. 16) as the *thalamic peduncles* or *thalamic radiation*. Many of these fibers reciprocally interconnect the thalamus and cortex. The *anterior (frontal) peduncle* comprises the fibers in the anterior limb of the internal capsule which connect the DM with the prefrontal cortex and the anterior thalamic nuclear group with the cingulate cortex. The *middle (superior* or *centroparietal) peduncle* comprises fibers in the genu and posterior limb of the internal capsule which connect the VP with the postcentral gyrus, the VL with the precentral gyrus

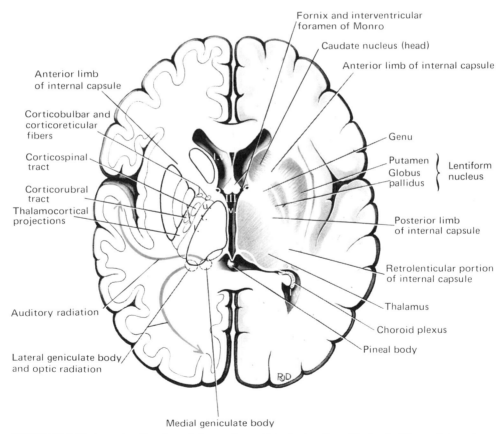

FIGURE 13-8 Horizontal section through the cerebrum. Note the location of the head of the caudate nucleus, lentiform nucleus, and thalamus relative to the ventricles and the internal capsule. The components of the internal capsule are indicated on the left side. The somatotopic organization of the corticospinal tracts is indicated by: U, upper extremity; T, trunk; L, lower extremity.

(area 4), the VA with the premotor cortex (area 6), and the dorsal tier thalamic nuclei with the association cortex of the parietal lobe. The *posterior (occipital) peduncle* comprises fibers in the posterior limb proper and the retrolenticular portion which connect the lateral geniculate body with the visual cortex (area 17) and the dorsal tier thalamic nuclei with the association cortex of the occipital lobe. The *inferior (temporal) peduncle* comprises fibers in the sublenticular portion of the internal capsule which connect the medial geniculate body with the auditory cortex (a few fibers may connect the pulvinar and the association cortex of the temporal lobe).

Some functional aspects of the thalamus

The thalamus is interconnected with the ipsilateral cerebral cortex and with subcortical nuclear complexes, e.g., the hypothalamus and basal ganglia. The ipsilateral thalamus does not have direct connections with any structures on the contralateral side of the brain. Any functional projection of thalamic activity to the opposite half of the brain must take place at other levels through the indirect connections of commissures and decussating pathways.

The thalamus has a significant role in two other types of sensation, viz., affective and discriminative. The "affective" domain of sensory appreciation is apparently mediated through the thalamic reticular system, dorsomedial nucleus, and anterior thalamic nucleus. The affect of an individual relates to emotional tone and somewhat to the phase of the sleep-wake cycle. Well-being, malaise, and a state of contentment are expressions of affect. The degree of agreeableness or disagreeableness of any stimulus depends on the state of an individual. The same objective degree of pain, temperature, or touch can evoke a remarkable variety of subjective degrees of reactivities. This variety is an expression of affective sensory mechanisms. Discriminative sensation is an aspect of sensation mediated through the thalamic specific nuclei. Such sensations include the "objective" appreciation of sensory stimuli from the general somatic and visceral sensors and the special sensors of vision, audition, and taste. The thalamus

has a significant role in the generation of many rhythms, including brain waves (see further on in this chapter, "Rhythms in the Nervous System").

The thalamus has a significant role in the conscious appreciation of sensation. The more general aspects of many sensations (pain, crude touch, vibratory sense, crude temperature discrimination, and possibly general sound detection) are brought to the conscious level in the thalamus. The finer sensory discriminations (those of the somesthetic, visual, auditory, and gustatory senses), which are elevated to the conscious sphere in the cerebral cortex, require the input of the information processed in thalamic nuclei for their final resolution. In brief, the conscious appreciation of sensory input takes place at both thalamic and cortical levels.

RHYTHMS IN THE NERVOUS SYSTEM

Oscillatory activities as expressed in the rhythms of the electroencephalogram (Chap. 16), in the jerky movements of the eye (Chap. 12), in the tremors of cerebellar dysfunction (Chap. 9), and in the respiratory cycles are the products of the functional organization of the neurons resulting from the gaited discharge of nerve cells. The spatial distribution and the timing of the activity at the excitatory and inhibitory synapses of a group of neurons are essential to the phasic discharge of this group of neurons. Some of the neurophysiologic activities suggested as being contributory to these rhythms include an "autorhythmicity" of pacemaker neurons, hyperpolarization of the receptive membranes of neurons, presynaptic inhibition, postsynaptic inhibition, disinhibition, facilitation, and closed self-reexciting neuronal circuits.

Pacemaker neurons exhibiting an "autorhythmicity" may contribute to the genesis of such gaiting; however, experimental documentation for this concept in mammals is inadequate at present. Some neurons are known to become hyperpolarized by a retrograde spread from the initial segment (trigger point) which has just generated an axon potential in the conductile segment. The simultaneous hyperpolarization of the receptive segment of each neuron (dendrites and cell body) of a group places all neurons in the same state of activity. In this hyperpolarized state, each neuron is in the same phase, a probable prerequisite for a rhythm.

Closed self-reexciting chains of neurons have a significant role in generating rhythmic waves. These circuits are feedback loops in which are linked interneurons exerting presynaptic and postsynaptic inhibitory influences. The cortically projecting thalamic neurons, which are associated with brain wave activity, are integrated into these feedback circuits. An axon collateral branch of the cortically projecting thalamic fiber synapses with one or more interneurons, which, in turn, may have axosomatic and axodendritic synaptic connections with several cortically projecting thalamic neurons, or may have axoaxonic synapses with axons terminating on these thalamic neurons. Functionally this is a negative feedback circuit, with the axon collateral branches exciting the interneurons, which, in turn, inhibit the thalamocortical neurons through postsynaptic inhibition (axosomatic and axodendritic synapses) and presynaptic inhibition (axoaxonic synapse). This recurrent inhibitory circuit (functioning mainly through postsynaptic inhibition in the thalamus) tends to suppress the thalamocortical projecting neurons; these neurons are now in phase; all are dampened. These momentarily inactive (for 100 ms or so), cortically projecting neurons now do not feed back information via the feedback circuit to generate new IPSPs on the thalamocortical neurons; hence these previously inhibited cells are now released from inhibitory influences and are phased to receive facilitatory influences to resume the next cycle of the rhythm. The 10-per-second alpha rhythm (Chap. 16) of the electroencephalogram may be generated by such a system. In brief, inhibition has a crucial role in gaiting the rhythms of the nervous system.

Integrative and synchronizing roles of the thalamus

Many of the major pathways interact with one another at many levels of the nervous system, including the cerebral cortex, basal ganglia, diencephalon, and brainstem. This integrative activity is essential to the concept that the pathway systems are interdependent. According to this concept, the thalamus is crucial because (1) many of its nuclei are the final processing stations of systems which project to the cerebral cortex, and (2) the thalamic reticular system apparently acts as a monitor, a modulator, and a modifier of the activity of the thalamic nuclei of the specific system. Through these connections, the thalamus exerts the essential regulatory drive upon the cerebral cortex. This thalamic drive is projected to pools of cortical neurons; these influences are directed through the stellate neurons of the cortex either to subpools of dendrites (axodendritic synapsis) or to subpools of somas (axosomatic synapses). Numerous pieces of neurophysiologic evidence support the concept that the thalamus is the key generator of much of the synchronized activity and rhythms of the nervous system.

The genesis of this recruitment activity is thought to take place in pacemaker cells in the intralaminar nuclei with natural rhythms of between 6 to 12 per second. The stimulation of 8 to 10 per second brings these neurons in synchrony with their pacemaker frequency. This synchrony of the neurons within the thalamic nuclei is brought about by inhibitory circuits. The stimulated cells discharge through axon collaterals to inhibitory interneurons (see Figs. 13-14 and 13-15), which, through their connections, hyperpolarize many other cells within the thalamus for about a 100-ms interval. Then these cells are stimulated, while in the same phase, to fire in synchrony. In turn, these synchronized cells, through their axon collaterals and inhibitory interneurons, hyperpolarize many more cells. This recruitment of more cells continues until the rhythm is established.

The thalamus is essential to such expressions of synchrony as (1) the rhythmic brain wave activity evidenced in the electroencephalogram (Chap. 16) and (2) the phasic and tonic movements mediated by the motor pathways. *The thalamus, through the VA and VL, is considered a "prime mover" of the motor pathways* (Chap. 14). *The nonspecific thalamic reticular system has a major role in the synchronizing effects of the thalamus;* it exerts this role through precise neuroanatomic connections and neurophysiologic inhibitory and excitatory influences on the specific thalamic nuclei. The various brain wave rhythms are apparently set by the thalamic reticular system (see "Rhythms in the Nervous System"). The phasic and tonic movements are largely products of the influences of the thalamic reticular system upon specific thalamic nuclei and thus upon specific systems. These modulatory effects are exerted through (1) the cerebellothalamo- (ventral lateral nucleus) cortical pathway and (2) the basal gangliathalamo (VA and VL nuclei) cortical pathway. Through these integrative and synchronizing activities, the thalamus exerts a major effect upon the motor expressions through the cerebral cortex and its projection pathways, including the corticospinal, corticostriate, and corticoreticular tracts, among others (Chaps. 14 and 16).

Repetitive electrical stimulations (6 to 12 per second) of the nonspecific thalamic nuclei evoke responses with long latency in the cerebral cortex by recruitment through multineuronal chains from these nuclei to the cortex. Neural influences from these nuclei are presumably relayed to (1) the VA thalamic nucleus and then from the VA to the orbitofrontal cortex (presumably serves as a trigger zone for activating the entire cortex) and (2) collateral branches of the thalamostriate fibers (Chap. 14) that radiate to laminae V and VI of all regions of the neocortex. This cortical recruitment response is a type of electroencephalogram (EEG) which is in some way analogous to the normal arousal EEG response (Chap. 16). It is called a *recruitment response because the activity increases in a step-by-step manner as more and more neurons are recruited in the course of this cortical response initiated by the repetitive thalamic stimulation.* No cortical response is obtained from a single stimulus. With a continuous repetitive stimulation the cortical responses increase to a maximum, then decrease, then increase (wax and wane). The phenomena of recruitment, waxing and waning, long latency, and diffuse cortical activity to repetitive stimulation at this frequency are attributable to the multineuronal chain (which favors neuronal interaction) through other thalamic nuclei terminating in numerous axodendritic synapses of the pyramidal cortical neurons. The many inhibitory postsynaptic potentials and excitatory postsynaptic potentials on the cortical cells are the bioelectric responses responsible for much cortical activity recorded by neurophysiologists and electroence-

phalographers (Chap. 16). Destruction of intralaminar nuclei is said to result in temporary somnolence, lethargy, and minimal reactivity to noxious stimuli. Many of the nuclei of the midline have strong connections with the hypothalamus; these nuclei apparently do not influence the cortex. The nucleus centrum medianum has a direct connection with the caudate nucleus and putamen which is integrated into the activity of the somatic motor system (Chap. 14).

Clinical aspects

A change in an individual's reaction to pain can occur following a prefrontal lobotomy or thalamotomy (lesion of the dorsomedial and intralaminar nuclei, or possibly of the pulvinar). Following such surgery, subjects perceive pain but are not unduly disturbed once the fear and dread of the pain and the anxiety about it are gone. This operation is often helpful in alleviating the intractable pain associated with metastatic cancer.

A thrombosis of a branch of the posterior choroidal or posterior cerebral arteries in human beings may produce the *thalamic syndrome.* A transitory contralateral hemianalgesia may be an immediate consequence. Soon painful sensations appear upon the application of noxious stimulation. Later pain is provoked by pressure, touch, and vibration. In time a state of spontaneous constant or paroxysmal pain on the affected (opposite) side is evoked without the application of any external stimulus. In this syndrome, the threshold for pain, temperature, and tactile sensations is usually raised on the opposite side of the body from the lesion. In addition mild stimuli may evoke disagreeable sensations. Stimuli may produce exaggerated and perverted sensations on the affected side of the body. The feelings elicited from a pinprick may be an intolerable, burning, agonizing pain. Heat, ice, cold, and pressure of one's clothes can be exceedingly uncomfortable. Even the sound of melodious music may produce unpleasant sensations on the affected side. Intractable pain which does not respond to analgesics may be a consequence. Affect qualities such as swelling, pulling, compression, and numbness are exaggerated during emotional stress.

In the thalamic syndrome, the symptoms result from a lesion that partially destroys the radiation fibers in the internal capsule and/or substantial portions of the ventral posterior and surrounding nuclei. None of the explanations for this pain has been proved. Collateral sprouting of fibers, denervation sensitivity, an expression of a release phenomenon, or loss of feedback have been suggested as causes of a circuitry with garbled signaling features. Relief from thalamic syndrome pain has been reported following stereotactic placement of electrocoagulation lesions in the dorsomedial nucleus, pulvinar, or intralaminar nuclei.

These highly overactive sensory responses are probably the result of alterations in frequencies and patterns of input to the thalamus, irritation of injured neurons, and changes in the quality of the output to the cerebral cortex. In addition the release (phenomenon) from some cortical influences upon the thalamus may be contributory. Emotional control is modified, as exhibited by forced laughter and sobbing. Mild stimuli may provoke an overresponse with agreeable and pleasant feeling tones. The application of a warm object to the hand may be pleasurable.

Lesions of the ventral posterior nucleus and nuclei of the medial and lateral geniculate bodies produce deficits in the modalities subserved by the pathways associated with these specific nuclei.

The conscious appreciation of crude general sensations occurs in the thalamus. One clinical indication of this phenomenon is that, following lesions of the thalamocortical projections, the sensations of pain and crude touch and some thermal sense are retained.

Lesions in the VLo result in the reduction of muscle tone and rigidity in Parkinson's disease. The probable explanation for the reduced rigidity is that the lesion isolates the processed input of the muscle stretch receptor within the cerebellum, preventing it from being projected to the motor cortex (area 4).

BIBLIOGRAPHY

Carmel, P. W.: Efferent projections of the ventral anterior nucleus of the thalamus in the monkey. Am J Anat, 128:159–184, 1970.

Carpenter, M. B.: "Ventral Tier Thalamic Nuclei," in D. Williams (ed.), *Modern Trends in Neurology*, vol. 4, Butterworth & Co. (Publishers), Ltd., London, 1967, pp. 1–20.

Deeke, L., D. W. F. Schwarz, and J. M. Fredrickson: Nucleus ventroposterior inferior (VPI) as the vestibular thalamic relay in the rhesus monkey. I. Field potential investigation. Exp Brain Res, 200:80–100, 1974.

Ebbesson, S. O. E., J. A. Jane, and D. M. Schroeder: A general overview of major interspecific variations in thalamic organization. Brain Behav Evol, 6:92–131, 1972.

Geldard, F. A.: *The Human Senses*, 2d ed, John Wiley & Sons, Inc., New York, 1972.

Gerard, P. W., and J. W. Duyff (eds.): *Information Processing in the Nervous System*, Proceedings of the International Union of Physiological Sciences. Excerpta Medica Foundation, Amsterdam, 1964.

Graybiel, A. M.: Some fiber pathways related to the posterior thalamic region in the cat. Brain Behav Evol, 6:424–452, 1972.

Hess, W. R.: *Diencephalon: Autonomic and Extrapyramidal Functions*, William Heinemann, Ltd., London, 1954.

Jones, E. G., and R. Y. Leavitt: Retrograde axonal transport and the demonstration of nonspecific projections to the cerebral cortex and striatum from thalamic intralaminar nuclei in the cat, rat and monkey. J Comp Neurol, 154:349–378, 1974.

Mehler, W. R.: The posterior thalamic region in man. Confin Neurol, 27:18–29, 1966.

Partlow, G. D., M. Colonnier, and J. Szabo: Thalamic projections of the superior colliculus in the rhesus monkey. J Comp Neurol, 171:285–318, 1977.

Purpura, D. P., and M. D. Yahr (eds.): *The Thalamus*, Columbia University Press, New York, 1966.

Riss, W., K. Koizumi, and C. M. Brooks (eds.): Basic thalamic structure and function. Brain Behav Evol, 6:1–560, 1972.

CHAPTER FOURTEEN

THE SOMATIC MOTOR SYSTEMS AND THE BASAL GANGLIA

NERVOUS SYSTEM AS AN EFFECTOR

The nervous system may be thought of as a complex assemblage of neural circuits functioning primarily to regulate the activity of the effectors of the body—its muscles and glands. It is only by stimulating muscles to contract (or to relax) and glands to secrete that the nervous system can overtly express itself. The somatic nervous system has the specific role of regulating the activity of striated (voluntary) muscles, while the autonomic (visceral) nervous system (Chap. 6) has the role of influencing the heart, nonstriated (involuntary) muscles, and glandular cells.

Postures are the body poses that are basic to the complex somatic motor activities. Each of the postures is maintained through an elaborate series of reflexes and reactions which utilize continuously acting feedback circuits operating through several segmental levels of control. The smooth flow of striated muscle activities from one posture to another posture is a movement. In this context, postures are the framework for all movements, whether crude, stereotyped, skilled, or volitional.

SEGMENTAL LEVELS FOR THE REGULATION AND CONTROL OF SOMATIC MOTOR ACTIVITY

Input from the peripheral sensors is essential for the nervous system to function as an efficient effector. Most of the vast amount of incoming sensory data is integrated and processed in many neuronal pools of the central nervous system before the resulting influences are transmitted via the somatic motor pathways. These influences from the various levels of the brain and spinal cord are funneled to the pools of motor neurons directly innervating the striated muscles. In addition, the motor pools receive a continuous flow of input directly from peripheral sensors (especially neuromuscular spindles).

The control of muscular activities may be thought of as being regulated from successive segmental levels of the spinal cord and brain. The intrinsic neural patterns in the spinal cord levels are the circuits which are basic for coordinated motor activity (Chap. 5). In the lower brainstem is located the vestibular level, which has a significant role in static reactions, labyrinthine accelerating reactions, and tonic head, neck, and eye movements (Chap. 10). At the pontocerebellar level is located the integrative complex crucial to the synergistic regulation of muscular coordination (Chap. 9). From the processing centers in the midbrain tectum are projected influences from the auditory and optic systems to the other levels. The basal ganglia located at the cerebral level are integrated in the control of automatic movements, while the cerebral cortex is the location of centers involved with volitional movements.

The motor pathways from the brain actually make relatively few direct synaptic connections with alpha and gamma motor neurons of the spinal cord. In fact, descending influences are directed primarily to the spinal interneurons, which, in turn, synapse with the alpha and gamma motor neurons. Stated otherwise, these spinal interneurons are intercalated between the descending pathways from the brain and the lower motor neurons.

FACILITATORY AND INHIBITORY CENTERS

The motor pathways contain many neuronal centers (pools) which are called facilitatory and inhibitory centers. Each of these pools can simultaneously facilitate and inhibit the motor pools essential to an action. For example, the center which evokes the extension of a limb facilitates the motor neurons innervating the extensor muscles and inhibits the motor neurons innervating the flexor muscles. By convention, a *facilitatory center (nucleus or pathway) is one that facilitates extensor reflexes and inhibits flexor reflexes, while an inhibitory center (nucleus, pool, or pathway) is one that inhibits extensor reflexes and facilitates flexor reflexes.* This reciprocal activity on antagonistic muscle groups is essential to integrated action.

It is important to note that the center is defined by the evoked response following its stimulation. This has several implications, because of the interaction among the various centers. For example, *a facilitatory center may, in fact, be the source of inhibitory influences, because it may actually inhibit an inhibitory center (disinhibition) and thereby evoke (facilitate) a response.* In the same way an inhibitory center may also facilitate when it stimulates by inhibiting an inhibitory center.

The interactions of the stimuli from the descending motor pathways with those from the peripheral sensors are crucial to normal muscle activity. The significance can be gauged in the case where all the sensory spinal roots from the upper extremity are transected—in effect, preventing the motor neurons to the limb from receiving sensory data from the limb. The limb after deafferentation, with its motor neurons intact, exhibits a flaccid paralysis; however, the stimulation of the motor cortex can induce movements in it.

In vertebrates, all peripheral somatic efferent (lower motor) neurons are excitatory nerves; when these peripheral nerves are stimulated, the voluntary muscles they innervate contract. There are no peripheral inhibitory somatic efferent nerves. However, in the autonomic nervous system there are inhibitory visceral peripheral nerves that innervate involuntary muscles. These nerves inhibit the activity of the cardiac muscles and the smooth muscles of the many visceral organs, including those of the vascular system and digestive system. Inhibition of the activity of the voluntary muscles is exerted exclusively through the inhibitory activity of the central nervous system (central inhibition). In brief, inhibition is a property of certain neurons of the central nervous system and peripheral autonomic nervous system but not of the neurons of the peripheral somatic efferent system.

THE REGULATION OF POSTURE

Posture, or the attitude of the body, is the product of automatic muscle activity which counters the action of gravity. The various attitudes are not under volitional regulation because they are assumed without conscious effort. Posture is fundamental, for every movement begins from and ends in a posture. A movement may be considered as a change in posture; and a posture, as the point of change in a movement. In addition, all movements are actually reflexes modified by influences from the brain.

Gravity and the proprioceptive receptors are basic to the maintenance of posture. The erect posture is an antigravity response dependent on muscle activity stimulated by the proprioceptors. These antigravity responses are countered by antagonistic muscle groups, so that a balance of tone is maintained between the agonist and the antagonist muscle groups. All muscles are under some continuous tension which is maintained by streams of asynchronous volleys; these volleys are continually being fed to the muscle groups to maintain muscle tonus.

In human beings, the antigravity muscles include the back muscles, posterior neck muscles (which hold the head up), jaw muscles, extensors of the lower extremity (for erect stance), and flexors of the upper extremity (which hold the arms up). The asynchronous discharge from the peripheral sensors is the source of stimulation for the smooth contractions which sustain a static antigravity posture.

The regulation of posture is dependent primarily on the stimuli from muscle and vestibular proprioceptors, their integration in the central nervous system, and their influence on the lower motor neurons. The visual system has a lesser role. The information from muscle receptors is utilized at the spinal level in the spinal reflexes. Much information is transmitted to supraspinal levels, even to the cerebral cortex. The descending pathways from the brain transmit facilitatory and inhibitory influences which have their effects on the spinal reflexes (Chap. 8). A reflex act may be operationally defined as an activity which originates in the peripheral nervous system and is relayed through the central nervous system before stimulating (or inhibiting) lower motor neurons.

The sequence of events in the regulation of posture may be summarized as follows: the upper motor neurons can influence the state of excitability of the neuronal pools in the spinal cord (the control box); this acts to determine the degree (intensity) of muscle tonus. A comparison is made in the neuronal pool between the feedback from the muscle receptors and the state of excitability. After this action, an error-correcting signal is generated in the form of postsynaptic potentials which lead to an increase (or decrease) in the firing rate of the alpha motor neurons. The change in the contractions of the muscle and the subsequent changes in the sensitivity of the muscle receptors are fed back to the neuronal pool for another comparison. This negative feedback loop is important to the maintenance of posture (see Chap. 9).

Regulation of postural tonus as an automatic control system

The interactions leading to the stabilization of the tonic muscular contractions in the postural reflexes utilize the principle of a closed-loop control system with negative feedback (Chap. 3). In this servomechanism, the negative feedback (a fraction of muscle tension acts as a stimulus for feeding back impulses generated by the neuromuscular spindles and Golgi tendon organs; the impulses are transmitted via the sensory nerves to the neuronal pools in the spinal cord) serves to maintain the predetermined goal (tonic muscular contractions) of the control system. This performance (goal) is accomplished through a sequence of self-correcting adjustments which are a consequence of the feedback of the prior performance (tonic muscle contractions) of the system to a control box (neuronal pool in the spinal cord). The feedback is negative because the corrections are in the opposite direction (reduced muscle tonus) to the positive divergence (increased muscle tonus) from the predetermined goal (tonus necessary to maintain posture). Constant surveying, utilizing feedback, is evidenced by the continuous sequences of tiny adjustment movements of muscle groups. The control box in the spinal cord directs the maintenance of the muscle tonus through the alpha motor neurons. The tonus fluctuates about the predetermined tonus set by the activity of the neuronal pools in the spinal cord. The entire system is goal seeking in the attempt to match the predetermined tonus. The intensity of the tonic contractions can be altered (this is comparable to changing the preset temperature in the thermostat) by the descending influences transmitted via the motor pathways from the brain. These descending influences account for the difference in the intensities of the tonic contractions in the upper extremity between holding a 1-lb weight and holding a 10-lb weight. The increase (or decrease) in the excitatory state of the neuronal pool stimulates the gamma motor neurons to increase (or decrease) the firing rate of the neuromuscular spindle; in turn, this increases (or decreases) the degree of muscle tone.

CONCEPT OF PYRAMIDAL AND EXTRAPYRAMIDAL SYSTEMS

By convention, each somatic motor "tract" is classified as belonging to one of two motor systems, pyramidal or extrapyramidal. The pyramidal system includes the corticospinal and the corticobulbar tracts. All other motor systems and the basal ganglia (see Fig. 14-1) influencing the lower motor neurons are collectively grouped into the extrapyramidal system; thus the name *extrapyramidal system* is a term of exclusion.

The concept of a dichotomy between the so-called pyramidal and extrapyramidal systems should be discarded because modern experimental studies demonstrate that the idea of independently functioning pyramidal and extrapyramidal systems is invalid.

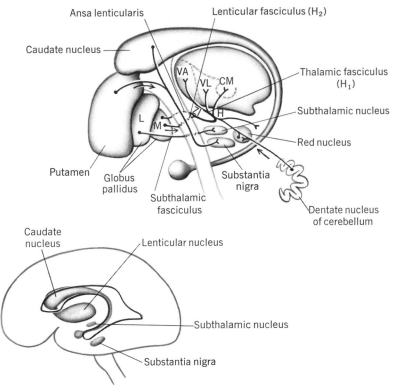

FIGURE 14-1 *Lower:* The location of the basal ganglia with reference to the lateral ventricle. *Upper:* The fields of Forel and some efferent projections of basal ganglia and cerebellum. The pallidofugal fibers pass through three bundles: ansa lenticularis, lenticular fasciculus (H_2), and subthalamic fasciculus. The former two bundles and the cerebellar projections join in the H field of Forel (prerubral field) and continue as the thalamic fasciculus (H_1) to various thalamic nuclei. CM, centromedian nucleus; H, the H field of Forel; L and M, lateral and medial segments of the globus pallidus; VA, ventral anterior thalamic nucleus; VL, ventral lateral thalamic nucleus; ZI, zona incerta.

Pyramidal system

The so-called pyramidal system consists of pathways originating in the cerebral cortex and terminating in the brainstem (corticobulbar fibers) and the spinal cord (corticospinal or pyramidal tract). The corticobulbar tract is a direct tract extending from the cerbral cortex to the brainstem tegmentum, where it innervates, through interneurons and the motor nuclei of the cranial nerves. Those descending fibers from the cerebral cortex with terminals in the brainstem reticular formation are the corticorubral and corticoreticular tracts (see Figs. 5-27 and 5-29). These tracts convey cortical influences to the spinal cord via the rubrospinal and reticulospinal tracts (see Figs. 5-27, 5-29 and 8-21). These corticorubrospinal and corticoreticulospinal pathways may be considered to be an indirect corticospinal system. The only direct tract from the cerebral cortex to the spinal cord is the corticospinal tract (see Fig. 5-26). Within the brainstem, collaterals from the corticospinal fibers branch and terminate in the brainstem reticular nuclei; this is another route by which cortical influences are directed to the reticulospinal tracts. The pyramidal tracts are necessary for skilled voluntary movements. They act as the major pathway through which the individual selects the prime mover of an activity; and they have a role in coordinating the resulting action. The contraction of individual muscles is largely a function of the pyramidal system.

Sectioning the pyramids of the medulla interrupts the corticospinal tracts. A monkey with such a lesion has a paresis, with some hypotonus and no clonus. Gross voluntary movements of the limbs are coordinated, well controlled, and apparently normal. Voluntary finer movements, especially those of the hands and feet, are impaired. The voluntary motor activity exhibited by the animal is presumably conveyed via corticorubospinal and corticoreticulospinal pathways to the motor pools of the spinal cord.

Extrapyramidal system

In general, the circuits of the so-called extrapyramidal system differ significantly from what is depicted in the older literature, where the organization of the system was described as neuronal centers interconnected in linked chainlike sequences extending from the cerebral cortex through subcortical and brainstem nuclei to the spinal cord. Actually, the system consists of complex circuits, some of which feed back to the cerebral cortex; it is from the cortex that the major output fiber pathways arise, namely the corticospinal, corticobulbar, corticoreticular, corticoreticulospinal, and corticorubrospinal pathways (see Figs. 5-26, 5-27, 5-29, and 8-21).

This phylogenetically old system, which has its ancient roots in the nonmammalian vertebrates, is involved in stereotyped motor activity of a postural and reflex nature. These well-coordinated basic motor expressions are regarded as primitive motor reaction.

BASAL GANGLIA IN THE SCHEMA OF MOTOR PROGRAMS

The basal ganglia are integrated with other neural structures in the formulation of motor programs. This account is a brief overview of the relation of the motor control system with the three major interrelated morphological divisions of the brain—namely the cerebral cortex, basal ganglia and cerebellum. The modern conceptualization of the functional role of these structures differs from the older classic view. Formerly the cerebral cortex, especially motor cortex, was hierarchically placed at the highest level for orchestrating motor integration, and the subcortical structures were placed at another level where they functioned in a feedback capacity. The modern view states that both the basal ganglia and the cerebellum are crucial in the initial and early stages of motor programming. Neurons in both the basal ganglia and cerebellum are involved in generating the activity in the motor cortex: They fire well in advance of each volitional movement (DeLong; Thach). The overall circuitry basic to these divisions and the motor program may be epitomized as follows: The entire cerebral cortex has massive projections to the basal ganglia and the cerebellum, and these structures, in turn, have major projections to the ventral lateral and ventral anterior thalamic nuclei; these nuclei act as nodal linkage stations relaying motor programs to the motor cortex. This circuitry has a most significant implication. It is a neural mechanism by which the somatosensory, visual, auditory, and association cortices of the cerebrum exert their influences on the basal ganglia and cerebellum, where transformations of this "sensory" information derived from the cortex are made and then conveyed to the thalamic nuclei, from which a pattern of signals is sent to the motor cortex. The neuronal activity expressed by the ventral lateral thalamic nucleus is intimately related to volitional movements in the human subject. This is in line with the concept that the functional roles of the ventral lateral and ventral anterior thalamic nuclei are essential in processing and relaying motor programs in a topographic manner to the motor and premotor cortex (areas 4 and 6). In fact, the basal ganglia and cerebellum may perform more complex and abstract functions than the motor cortex. In turn, the main role of the motor cortex might be to allow for the refined control of motor activity. This concept does not imply that the function of these subcortical structures is expressed solely through this circuitry. Other roles are expressed through other connections.

Basal ganglia and related centers (Table 14-1)

The nuclear complexes traditionally classified as basal ganglia include the corpus striatum, amygdaloid body, and claustrum. In modern usage the basal ganglia now comprise the corpus striatum, subthalamic nucleus, and substantia nigra. The claustrum is probably a thin sheet of cortex separate from the insula and is not a basal

Table 14-1
Basal ganglia and related centers

Amygdaloid body (archistriatum amygdala, amygdaloid nucleus, amygdaloid complex)†

Corpus striatum
{ Paleostriatum (globus pallidus, pallidum) } Lenticular (lentiform) nucleus
{ Medial segment }
{ Lateral segment }

Neostriatum (striatum) { Putamen
{ Caudate nucleus

Claustrum
Subthalamic nucleus
Substanta nigra
Red nucleus*
Brainstem reticular formation*

Sometimes included.
†*Probably not a basal ganglion (see text).*

ganglion. The amygdaloid body should be grouped with the limbic structures (Chap. 15) because functionally it is associated with the limbic system. Some authors include the red nucleus and the brainstem reticular formation with the basal ganglia. The current classification of basal ganglia is based upon the relation of these structures with somatic motor function.

The corpus striatum is subdivided into the paleostriatum and the striatum (neostriatum). The paleostriatum is also called the globus pallidus or pallidum; the striatum is divided into the putamen (60 percent of the striatum by volume) and the caudate nucleus. The amygdaloid body (archistriatum), striatum, and claustrum are telencephalic structures, while the globus pallidus and subthalamic nucleus are diencephalic derivatives. During development the fibers of the internal capsule insinuate themselves so as to divide some regions of the diencephalon and telencephalon; the result is that the internal capsule separates the subthalamus from the globus pallidus and divides the neostriatum into the caudate nucleus and putamen. The globus pallidus and putamen, both located lateral to the internal capsule, are together called the lenticular (lentiform) nucleus. The globus pallidus is subdivided into a medial (inner or internal) segment and a lateral (outer or external) segment (see Fig. 14-1). The subthalamus is considered to be the rostral continuation of the midbrain tegmentum into the diencephalon. The red nucleus (nucleus ruber) is a major midbrain tegmental nucleus (Chap. 8). The substantia nigra is a large pigmented nucleus located in the midbrain and also separated from the globus pallidus by the internal capsule.

Striatum (neostriatum)

The striatum is a large complex receiving its input from such diverse structures as the cerbral cortex, intralaminar nuclei of the thalamus and the substantia nigra, and some raphe nuclei of the midbrain. As a consequence of its diverse and massive inputs, the striatum is called the receptive segment of the basal ganglia.

In their micromorphology and functional correlates, the caudate nucleus and putamen are similar. They are composed of three types of neurons (Fox).

1. *Spiny striatal neurons* with small cell bodies, spiny dendrites (numerous spines), and short axons. These Golgi type II interneurons terminate within the striatum.
2. *Large aspiny striatal neurons* with large multipolar cell bodies, aspiny dendrites (smooth dendrites), and long, myelinated axons. These neurons are output cells projecting to the globus pallidus and substantia nigra.
3. *Spidery striatal neurons* with small cell bodies, aspiny dendrites, and axons (the axons are not demonstrable with Golgi techniques). These neurons with their smooth, curved dendrites have a *"spidery"* appearance in Golgi preparations.

Estimates indicate that about half or more of the striatal neurons project out of the striatum to

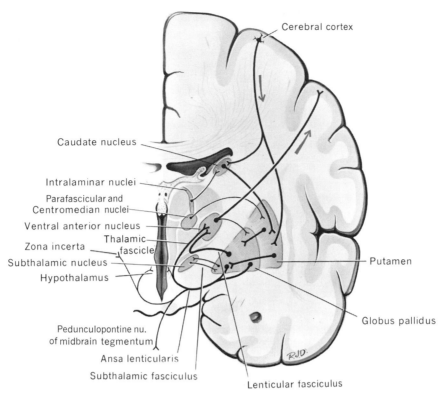

Cerebral cortex

Caudate nucleus

Intralaminar nuclei

Parafascicular and
Centromedian nuclei

Ventral anterior nucleus

Thalamic
fascicle

Zona incerta

Subthalamic nucleus

Hypothalamus

Putamen

Globus pallidus

Pedunculopontine nu.
of midbrain tegmentum

Ansa lenticularis

Subthalamic fasciculus

Lenticular fasciculus

FIGURE 14-2 Some major interconnections of the basal ganglia, thalamus, and cerebral cortex.

both segments of the globus pallidus and to the substantia nigra; it is thus assumed that these spidery neurons are output neurons. These large cells constitute less than 10 percent of the striated neurons. Some striatonigral fibers are presumed to have collaterals terminating in the globus pallidus.

Input to the striatum is derived from pyramidal neurons in lamina V of the cerebral cortex (corticostriate fibers), from the substantia nigra (nigrostriatal fibers), and from intralaminar thalamic nuclei (thalamostriate fibers). The corticostriate fibers terminate on the spines and the small-cell spiny interneurons. The nigrostriatal fibers from the pars compacta of the substantia nigra terminate on cell bodies of spiny striatal cells and dendrites of "spidery" striated cells. The thalamostriate fibers terminate upon the spines of the spiny striatal cells. Of the thalamic nuclei only the intralaminar nuclei project to the striatum.

Globus pallidus

The globus pallidus is partitioned by a medullary lamina into a medial (internal) pallidal segment and a lateral (external) pallidal segment. The pallidal cells are all similar, each with a large cell body, long, smooth dendrites, and a long axon. The input to the globus pallidus is derived from the striatum and the subthalamic nucleus. The striatopallidal fibers from the caudate nucleus and putamen are topographically organized. The subthalamopallidal fibers project primarily to both pallidal segments. The output fibers of the globus pallidus constitute the main projection pathway from the corpus striatum. These pallidofugal fibers form three bundles: (1) ansa lenticularis, (2) lenticular fascicle, and (3) subthalamic fasciculus. The lateral segment of the globus pallidus gives rise to the pallidosubthalamic fibers (within the subthalamic fascicle). Other pallidofugal fibers include

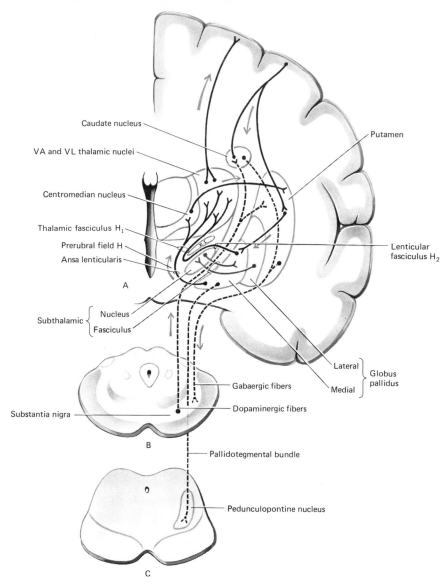

Caudate nucleus

VA and VL thalamic nuclei

Centromedian nucleus

Thalamic fasciculus H₁

Prerubral field H

Ansa lenticularis

A

Subthalamic { Nucleus / Fasciculus

Substantia nigra

Putamen

Lenticular fasciculus H₂

Gabaergic fibers

Dopaminergic fibers

Lateral } Globus
Medial } pallidus

B

Pallidotegmental bundle

Pedunculopontine nucleus

C

FIGURE 14-3 Diagram of the major circuits of the "extrapyramidal system" illustrated (*A*) in a coronal section through the cerebrum and (*B* and *C*) transverse sections through the upper and lower midbrain. Of the pallidofugal projections, the ansa lenticularis is most rostral, the lenticular fasciculus is intermediate, and the subthalamic fasciculus is most caudal in location. Note the pallidofugal fibers (pallidotegmental bundle) to the pedunculopontine nucleus. The nigrostriatal fibers are dopaminergic while the striatonigral fibers are gabanergic (GABA). The corticosubthalamic projection from the motor cortex and the subthalamonigral projection are not illustrated. ZI, zona incerta.

those that terminate in the ventral lateral nucleus (pars oralis and pars medialis), in the ventral anterior nucleus (pars principalis), in the habenular nucleus (pallidohabenular fibers), and in the pedunculopontine nucleus (pallidoteg-mental fibers) in the midbrain (see Fig. 14-3). Some of these projections are topographically organized, especially those to the ventral lateral, ventral anterior, and subthalamic nuclei. Both segments of the globus pallidus are somatotopically organized with regard to active movements in the head, upper extremity, and lower extremity. The pallidofugal fibers are further discussed later on.

Subthalamic nucleus

The subthalamic nucleus is a lens-shaped structure located in the ventral thalamus just medial to the internal capsule (see Fig. 14-5). This nucleus and the globus pallidus are interconnected by reciprocal topographically organized projections. The major sources of input to the subthalamic nucleus are the lateral segment of the globus pallidus and the motor cortex.

The major projections from the subthalamic nucleus are to both segments of the globus pallidus and to the pars reticulata of the substantia nigra (Hartman-vonMonakow et al.) In addition, the subthalamic nucleus may have neurons whose axons terminate in the ventral lateral and ventral anterior thalamic nuclei and in the pedunculopontine nucleus of the midbrain. The subthalamic nucleus is somatotopically organized with respect to active movements of the extremities and topographically organized in its projections to the globus pallidus and substantia nigra. The subthalamic nucleus is thought to act as a modulator of activity in the globus pallidus and substantia nigra pars reticulata (see later on). This activity is possibly exerted through the putative neurotransmitter glycine (an inhibiting agent).

Substantia nigra

The substantia nigra is located throughout the length of the midbrain just posterior to the crus cerebri. It is usually divided into (1) the anteriorly located low-density cell region adjacent to the crus cerebri called the *pars reticulata (reticularis)* and (2) the posteriorly located high-density cell region called the *pars compacta*. Many of the large cells in the latter contain the black pigment melanin, which gives this structure a black appearance in the freshly cut brain. Compacta cells, whether pigmented or not, contain high concentrations of dopamine.

The afferent input to the substantia nigra is derived primarily from the striatum and the subthalamic nucleus. These topographically organized projections terminate in the pars reticu-lata. Some pallidonigral fibers may exist. Corticonigral fibers have not been demonstrated with certainty. The striationigral fibers contain high concentrations of γ-aminobutyric acid (GABA); hence these are gabanergic neurons and fibers (see Fig. 14-3).

The efferent projections from the neurons of the pars compacta terminate topographically in all parts of the striatum, upon cell bodies of spiny interneurons and dendrites of spidery cells. These nigrostriatal cells and their axons contain high concentrations of dopamine and, hence, dopaminergic fibers. The other efferent projections from the nondopaminergic neurons of the pars reticulata terminate in (1) several thalamic nuclei, including the medial part of the ventral lateral (VLm), the magnocellular part of the ventral anterior (VLmc), and the paramedian subnucleus of the dorsomedian thalamic nuclei; (2) superior colliculus (nigrotectal) fibers; and (3) the pedunculopontine nucleus of the midbrain.

Globus pallidus and substantia nigra

The globus pallidus and the pars reticulata of the substantia nigra exhibit many similarities. On gross inspection it can be seen that the medial segment of the globus pallidus is separated from the pars reticulata (rostral portion) only by the fibers of the internal capsule. The few cells within the internal capsule may represent the bridge between them. Among the common features between these two structures are:

1. Both are composed of neurons with essential similar micro- and ultramicroscopic features.
2. Both receive major projections from the striatum.
3. Both receive major projections from the subthalamic nucleus.
4. Both project to the motor thalamus (VA and VL).
5. Both have a somatotopic organization expressed in active movements of the face and the upper and lower extremities (DeLong).
6. Of all the major nuclei of the basal ganglia the medial pallidal segment and the pars reticulata are the only parts to discharge "major" projections to other structures of the central

nervous system—namely VA and VL of the thalamus. These nuclei comprise the so-called motor thalamus projecting prepyramidal afferents to the premotor and motor cortices.

Basic principles

Functional The general role of the basal ganglia is to serve as processing stations linking the cerebral cortex to certain thalamic nuclei; in turn, the latter project to the cerebral cortex. This is indicated by circuitry which conveys influences from widespread areas of the cortex to the striatum to globus pallidus to thalamus. The specific functional roles of the basal ganglia are not, as yet, resolved. According to one concept, the basal ganglia are nuclei where many influences, including those from visual, labyrinthine, and proprioceptive sources, are integrated in activities which involve the initiation and direction of voluntary movements and motor responses. This is based upon some of the symptoms observed in patients with damage to the basal ganglia. Such patients have difficulty in initiating willed movements and have defects in some of the attributes that contribute to normal motor activities.

A most important suggested role for the corpus striatum is that it acts as a nuclear processing linkage between the association cortex (involved in some way with the mnemonic system) and that system of the brain involved with handling this sensory experience properly for meaningful responses. The following statement by Mettler expresses this role: "Without the striatum the animal is quite unable to relate itself to its environment at a satisfactory level of self-maintenance. Without its cortex it is unable to relate itself accurately to its environment but it can still do it. The cat . . . is able to get along reasonably well without much cortex, but if you add a sizable striatal deficit to this, the animal looks at you with vacuous eyes and . . . will walk out of a third story window with complete unconcern."

Circuitry Two subcortical structures are central to the circuits influencing the motor and premotor cortex. They are the corpus striatum and the cerebellum. Two key loops involved with the corpus striatum are (1) wide areas of cerebral cortex to corpus striatum to VA and VL of the thalamus to motor and premotor areas of the cerebral cortex (see Fig. 14-4) and (2) corpus striatum to intralaminar nuclei of the thalamus to corpus striatum (see Fig. 14-4). Two key circuits involved with the cerebellum include (1) wide areas of cerebral cortex to pontine nuclei to cerebellum to the VA and VL of the thalamus to motor and premotor cortex (see Fig. 14-6) and (2) cerebellum to intralaminar nuclei of thalamus (see Fig. 14-6 and Chap. 9).

These circuits and loops apparently have a significant role, supplying input to the motor and premotor areas of the cerebral cortex which give rise to such important motor pathways as the corticospinal, corticorubrospinal, and corticoreticulospinal tracts. Note that there are structures which are common to both the cerebellar and striatal systems. These are (1) wide areas of the cerebral cortex (source of input), (2) VA and VL of the thalamus, (3) intralaminar nuclei, and (4) motor and premotor areas of the cerebral cortex (site of output). This does not imply that the neurons in these structures are all common to both systems. However, many of the neurons are probably functionally integrated into both systems.

CONNECTIONS AND CIRCUITS

The cerebral cortex, basal ganglia, and related nuclei are organized into complex linkages of interconnections, feedback circuits, and descending pathways. The following schemata outline some of the major proposed circuits of the extrapyramidal motor system (Figs. 14-1 to 14-6).

Circuit 1

A major loop is the following: Cerebral cortex →striatum→globus pallidus→thalamus→cerebral cortex (see Fig. 14-4).

Nearly all regions of lamina V of the cerebral cortex project corticostriate fibers in a topographically organized arrangement to the ipsilateral striatum (both caudate nucleus and putamen). The frontal cortex projects to the head of the caudate nucleus while the more posterior parietal, occipital, and temporal areas project to progressively more caudal portions of the body and tail. A variant of this is expressed by area 9 of the prefrontal cortex, which projects

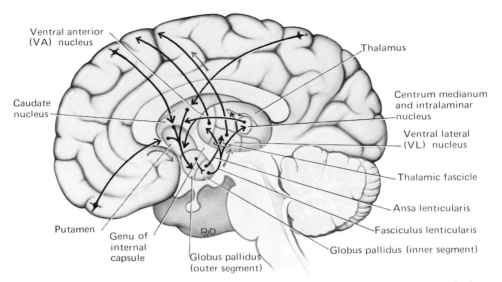

Figure labels:
- Ventral anterior (VA) nucleus
- Caudate nucleus
- Putamen
- Genu of internal capsule
- Globus pallidus (outer segment)
- Thalamus
- Centrum medianum and intralaminar nucleus
- Ventral lateral (VL) nucleus
- Thalamic fascicle
- Ansa lenticularis
- Fasciculus lenticularis
- Globus pallidus (inner segment)

R/D

FIGURE 14-4 Some of the major interconnections of the "extrapyramidal system" involving the cerebral cortex, basal ganglia, thalamus, and brainstem. (Arrows indicate major direction of projections.)

to columnlike clusters arranged throughout the entire length of the nucleus (Goldman and Nauta). The sensorimotor cortex (areas 1 to 4, 6, and 8) projects sparsely to the ipsilateral striatum but does project a significant number of fibers via the corpus callosum to the contralateral striatum.

There are no fibers which interconnect the caudate nucleus with the putamen. In turn, fibers from the striatum terminate topographically in both segments of the globus pallidus. Fibers from the lateral segment of the globus pallidus terminate in both the medial segment of the globus pallidus and the subthalamic nucleus. From the medial pallidal segment fibers course via the *ansa lenticularis* (loops under the internal capsule) and *fasciculus lenticularis* (penetrates through internal capsule); these fascicles join to form the *thalamic fasciculus* before terminating in the VA, VL, and centrum medianum (CM) nuclei of the thalamus. The VA and VL nuclei project somatotopically to the premotor cortex (areas 6 and 8) and to the motor cortex (area 4), respectively.

Other connections of the nuclear centers of this circuit add to the complexity. The CM nucleus (which receives input from the globus pallidus) and other intralaminar thalamic nuclei project to the striatum: the CM projects to the putamen, and other intralaminar nuclei project to the caudate nucleus. The axons of these intralaminar neurons terminate on the spines of the striatal spiny neurons. In a sense the CM is incorporated in a closed circuit relaying back to the striatum. In addition, the globus pallidus projects pallidotegmental fibers to the pedunculopontine tegmental nucleus (see Figs. 8-11 and 14-4) and other brainstem reticular nuclei.

Input to this circuit is also derived from the brainstem via (1) the ascending brainstem reticular projections to the intralaminar thalamic nuclei, (2) projections from some serotonergic cells of the mesencephalic raphe nuclei to the striatum, and (3) projections from the cerebellum.

Circuit 2 (Fig. 14-5)

This circuit involves the substantia nigra. It comprises the following sequences: (1) cerebral cortex to the striatum to the substantia nigra. Some collaterals from the striatonigral fibers terminate the globus pallidus. The striatonigral fibers project to the pars reticularis of the substantia nigra. (2) The projections from the substantia nigra are directed rostrally via (a) nigrostriatal fibers to the striatum or (b) nigrothalamic fibers to the VA and VL thalamic

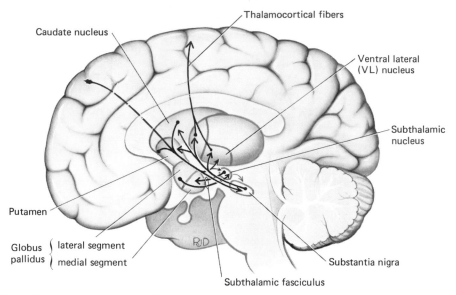

Caudate nucleus

Thalamocortical fibers

Ventral lateral
(VL) nucleus

Subthalamic
nucleus

Putamen

Globus { lateral segment
pallidus { medial segment

Substantia nigra

Subthalamic fasciculus

FIGURE 14-5 Some major circuits of the "extrapyramidal system." The corticosubthalamic projection from the motor cortex and the subthalamonigral projection are illustrated.

nuclei, which project to the motor and premotor cortical areas. Direct corticonigral fibers probably do not exist.

The substantia nigra is divided into the anteriorly located pars reticularis (adjacent to the crus cerebri) and the posteriorly located pars compacta. The *pars reticularis* is rich in iron and lacking in melanin pigment. The *pars compacta* contains neurons rich in dopamine (a catecholamine) and melanin. Topographic projections are the main connections (1) between the pars reticularis and the VA and VL thalamic nuclei and (2) between the pars compacta and the striatum. The striatonigral connections are primarily between the caudate nucleus and the rostral portion of the substantia nigra and between the putamen and the caudal two-thirds of the substantia nigra.

Output projections from the substantia nigra also include (1) the nigrotectal fibers to the deeper layers of the superior colliculus from which arise tectoreticular and tectospinal fibers and (2) nigroreticular fibers to the brainstem reticular formation. The nigral efferent projections to the VA and VL thalamic nuclei terminate in different regions of these thalamic nuclei than those projections from the globus pallidus (slight if any overlap). The nigrostriatal fibers

compose the *dopamine neuronal system;* the substantia nigra, nigrostrital fibers, and striatum are rich in dopamine, which is an active neurotransmitter substance (see discussion of paralysis agitans, below).

Circuit 3

The *subthalamic nucleus* is integrated in the above circuitry (see Figs. 14-1 and 14-5). Fibers from the lateral segment of the globus pallidus terminate in the subthalamus, which, in turn, projects back to the medial segment of the globus pallidus. In addition, the subthalamic nucleus receives somatotopically organized direct input from the motor cortex and projects output fibers to the pars reticularis of the substantia nigra. The putative transmitter of the output neurons is possibly glycine. The subthalamic nucleus is presumed to exert its role by its inhibitory influences upon the globus pallidus and substantia nigra.

Circuit 4

Another circuit includes the following: cerebral cortex→ipsilateral pontine nuclei (corticopontine fibers)→contralateral cerebellar cortex (pontocerebellar fibers)→dentate nucleus of the

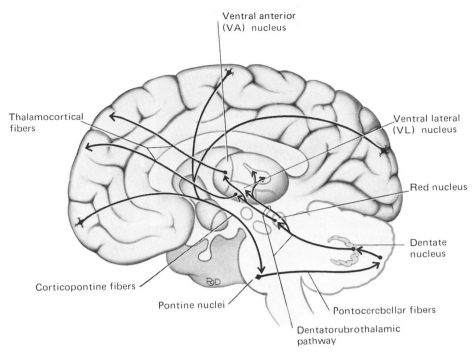

Ventral anterior
(VA) nucleus

Thalamocortical
fibers

Ventral lateral
(VL) nucleus

Red nucleus

Dentate
nucleus

Corticopontine fibers

Pontine nuclei

Pontocerebellar fibers

Dentatorubrothalamic
pathway

RjD

FIGURE 14-6 Some major circuits of the "extrapyramidal system." (Arrows indicate major direction of projections.)

cerebellum→contralateral VL, VA, and intra-laminar thalamic nuclei (dentatothalamic fibers)→cerebral cortex (areas 4, 6, and 8) (see Fig. 14-6; see also Fig. 9-4).

There is an overlapping of the dentatothalamic fibers from the cerebellum and pallidothalamic fibers from the globus pallidus in the VL thalamic nucleus. Some influences from the cerebellum to the thalamus are also conveyed via the dentatorubrothalamic pathway (see Chap. 9).

Circuit 5

The subcortical influences upon the cerebral cortex are, in turn, projected from the cerebral cortex to the brainstem and spinal cord motor nuclei via several descending pathways (see Figs. 8-21 and 8-22). These include the pyramidal pathways (corticospinal and corticobulbar tracts), corticorubrospinal pathway, corticoreticular pathway, and corticoreticulospinal pathway (medial and lateral reticulospinal tracts). The basal ganglia have access to the limbic system via the pallidohabenular fibers from the

globus pallidus to the lateral habenular nucleus (Chap. 15).

NEUROTRANSMITTERS ASSOCIATED WITH THE BASAL GANGLIA

Several putative neurotransmitters have been identified in some of the neurons associated with the basal ganglia. The corticostriate neurons are said to be glutamatergic neurons utilizing glutamate as an excitatory transmitter acting upon the spiny interneurons of the striatum. Nigro-striatal neurons are dopaminergic neurons utilizing dopamine as an inhibitory transmitter acting upon the spiny interneurons of the striatum. The spiny interneurons are cholinergic neurons utilizing acetycholine as an excitatory transmitter acting on the striatonigral and striatopallidal neurons. The striatonigral neurons are gabanergic neurons utilizing GABA as an inhibitory transmitter acting upon neurons in the pars reticulata and possibly on the dendrites of the dopaminergic neurons. The subthalamopallidal and subthalamonigral neurons of the subthalamic nucleus release the inhibitory transmitter glycine, which acts upon the neurons of the globus pallidus and substantia nigra.

Pallidofugal fibers and the H fields of Forel (Fig. 14-1)

The output from the globus pallidus is conveyed via pallidofugal fibers which are organized in three bundles of fibers. These bundles, arranged in a rostrocaudal sequence, are the ansa lenticularis, the lenticular fasciculus (H$_2$ of Forel), and the subthalamic fasciculus.

The *ansa lenticularis* arises from the ventral portion of the medial segment of the globus pallidus, loops ventromedially around the internal capsule near the crus cerebri, curves to pass upward and caudally, and then joins the fibers of the lenticular fasciculus at the H field of Forel (prerubral field) of the subthalamus.

The *lenticular fasciculus* arises from the dorsal portion of the medial segment of the globus pallidus, penetrates as the comb bundle (because it resembles the teeth of a comb) through the posterior limb of the internal capsule (rostral to the subthalamic nucleus), and then courses medially and caudally between the subthalamic nucleus (located ventrally) and the gray matter called the zona incerta (located dorsally). The lenticular fasciculus then joins the ansa lenticularis in the H field of Forel; the fibers of the fasciculus and ansa recurve and project rostrally just dorsal to the zona incerta as the thalamic fasciculus (H$_1$ field of Forel).

The *zona incerta* is the rostral extension of the midbrain reticular formation into the ventral thalamus. It is located within the subthalamus between the subthalamic nucleus and the thalamic fasciculus. The *thalamic fasciculus* is a key bundle. Its fibers convey influences from the cerebellum and globus pallidus to the thalamic nuclei (VA and VL); these nuclei project their output to the motor and premotor cortex.

The *subthalamic fasciculus* consists of fibers passing through the internal capsule as a comb bundle. It consists of pallidosubthalamic fibers passing from the lateral segment of the globus pallidus to the subthalamic nucleus and of subthalamopallidal fibers passing from the subthalamic nucleus to the medial segment of the globus pallidus. Another pallidal projection, consisting of the pallidotegmental fibers, leaves the H field and descends to the pedunculopontine reticular nucleus of the midbrain (see Fig. 14-3).

Physiology

The basal ganglia motor "system" has a significant role in the regulation of sterotype movements. In human beings and primates, this system is capable of stimulating the preformance of complex volitional motor acts, for, as previously noted, such activities are exhibited even when the corticospinal tracts are interrupted in the pyramids of the medulla.

The precise role of each nucleus is not known. The complex connectivity implies that each nucleus expresses its role through facilitatory or inhibitory influences (or both) on several other nuclei and systems. Release phenomena may be expressed when some inhibitory influences are suppressed. Such emotionally triggered gestures as yawning, stretching, and tics may be related to the connections of the basal ganglia with the hypothalamus and the descending reticular system.

SKILLED AND VOLUNTARY MOVEMENTS

All normal movements are to a greater or lesser degree skilled. Even "crude" reflexes are the product of exquisite neural integration. The most skilled acts may range from the contraction (and relaxation) or a few muscles for the execution of each brush stroke by a van Gogh to the continuous muscle flow of an Olympic gymnast. These highest skills may include (1) the unilateral control of finger movements, as in writing and playing a piano, and (2) the bilateral control of word formation by the vocal cords, throat. mouth, tongue, and lips. Inhibition is as significant to skilled movements as is excitation. The inhibition of nonessential movements and of antagonist muscles is essential to each skilled act.

A *voluntary movement is a focal act of which the executor is consciously aware.* The acquisition of the ability to perform these actions takes time. Learning to walk, to write, or to play a musical instrument occurs only after a number of complex motor patterns have been mastered. Persistent efforts and repeated trials are required before such movements are gradually integrated into automatic patterns and into voluntarily controlled actions. The automatic aspect of each movement is subcortically regulated, while the volitional aspect is largely controlled by the cerebral cortex. A voluntary act may be operationally defined as an activity produced by a stimulation originating within the central nervous system. The term "voluntarily controlled act" is not wholly accurate; although the doer is consciously controlling the act, there is no awareness of the means to attain the end. *The focus of a voluntary movement is called the focal act: this expresses the fact that one concentrates on performing one movement at a time.* Trying to perform many acts simultaneously is difficult if not impossible. In executing a voluntary act many movements accompany the focal act. For example typists are conscious of the control of their fingers, but unaware of the whole complex of supporting movements. The latter include the slight adjustment movements of the hand, forearm, and arm; the stabilizing muscle contractions of the shoulder; the maintence of the posture of the body; and the head and eye patterns as the lines on a page are followed.

The corticospinal tracts are essential substrates to volitional actions. These tracts, which are largest in human beings, have a crucial role in the manipulative skills and the independent movement of extremities, particularly of the fingers.

Effects of stimulation and ablation of basal ganglia

In general, stimulation of the neostriatum evokes different effects than does stimulation of the paleostriatum. Apparently the neostriatum exerts inhibitory influences on somatic motor activity (specifically, the inhibition of spontaneous activity, of a motion in progress, or of deep tendon reflexes). Stimulation of the globus pallidus produces a minimum of effects, such as increased muscle tonus. This hypertonus occurs after a long latency, and it outlasts the stimulus. A prolonged stimulus can produce a tremor. Effects evoked by stimulation of the pallidum occur on the contralateral side.

The unilateral ablation of the globus pallidus or of the putamen produces slight, if any, objective signs of malfunction. The bilateral ablation of either structure gives evidence of the release phenomenon. The bilateral ablation of the putamen produces a hyperactive animal that wanders about continuously, with a disregard of its environment. For example, the animal will walk into a wall and continue to push against the obstruction (forced progression), or it will walk across a table and continue until it falls off the edge (labyrinth disregard). In addition, behavioral changes in affect are exhibited. A cat shows no fear and may even purr when confronted by a hostile dog. In contrast, the bilateral ablation of the globus pallidus produces a hypoactive animal, exhibiting hypotonus and somnolence. Such an animal seldom moves about. If placed in a bizarre enforced posture, it can retain the posture for an extended period. For example, a monkey with bilateral ablation of the globus pallidus makes little or no effort to assume a natural posture if the upper extremity is placed behind the neck with the hand touching the opposite shoulder and if a lower extremity is lifted until the foot rests against the back of the neck. The hypoactivity has a resemblance to that in Parkinson's disease. However, these animals do not exhibit any tremor or rigidity.

Violent flinging ballistic movements, especially in the contralateral upper extremity, are exhibited in humans and monkeys with discrete lesions in portions of the subthalamic nucleus (the syndrome is called *ballism* in humans). This hyperactivity is another manifestation of a release phenomenon producing an abnormal movement.

SPASTICITY AND RIGIDITY

Spasticity is the state in which muscles exhibit hypertonus, hyperreflexia, and clonus. These are phasic hyperactive expressions in which the muscle tension increases when the muscle is stretched. This hyperactivity is presumed to be associated with phasic (ballistic) reflex activity. Spasticity is associated with the activity of the spinal reflex loop consisting of the gamma I motor neurons (gamma I fusimotor and dynamic gamma neurons), the nuclear bag intrafusual muscle fibers of the neuromuscular spindles, and the group Ia afferent fibers (see Chap. 5 and Figs. 2-20 and 5-22 to 5-24).

Rigidity is a form of hypertonus in which the muscles are continuously or intermittently firm and tense. This is associated with an increase in muscle tone that has an even or uniform quality throughout the range of the passive movement. The increased tone is present in all muscle groups—flexors, extensors, agonists, and antagonists. This hyperactivity is linked with the tonic reflexes. Rigidity is associated with the activity of the reflex loop consisting of the gamma II motor neurons (gamma II fusimotor and static gamma neurons), the nuclear chain infrafusal muscle fibers of the neuromuscular spindles, and the group II afferent fibers (see Chap. 5 and Figs. 2-20 and 5-22 to 5-24).

FUNCTIONAL AND CLINICAL CONSIDERATIONS

The basal ganglia are functionally organized into an exquisitely "tuned" complex of interconnected nuclei. The role of the basal ganglia and associated nuclei is to modulate motor activities through circuits which directly and indirectly feed back to the motor cortex. In turn, the cortex projects its influences to the brainstem and spinal levels through the descending pathways upon the alpha and gamma motor neurons. The malfunction of various nuclear complexes results in an imbalance in the interactions within the complex circuitry of the extrapyramidal system. This is a plausible explanation for the variety and assortment of symptoms and signs noted in the clinically observed disorders in the control of posture and movements when the harmonious interactions are altered within this system. Posture is modified by an increase in muscle tone to a similar degree in the agonists and antagonists of a muscle group without an accompanying increase in reflex activity; this is *rigidity*. Abnormal involuntary movements, called *dyskinesias*, may be rhythmic or arrhythmic, generally without paralysis of the muscles. The motor disorders resulting from the improper functioning of the extrapyramidal system, the basal ganglia, and associated nuclei include paralysis agitans (Parkinson's disease), athetosis, choreas, and ballism.

Paralysis agitans (*Parkinson's disease*) is characterized by rigidity, tremor, and bradykinesia (difficulty in initiating movements). The rigidity is essentially the same in all muscles; it is accompanied by poverty of movements but with normal deep tendon reflex activity. As a limb is passively forced through flexor or extensor movements, the muscular resistance alternately increases and decreases to give a cogwheel effect. The patient exhibits resistance to passive movements in all directions. From a standing position, patients have difficulty in starting to take their initial steps. Subjects also have the same problem in arresting the movement. During forward locomotion, short, shuffling steps are taken. The masked face has a fixed expression accompanied by no overt spontaneous emotional response. The tremor with its regular frequency and amplitude occurs while the subject is at rest; it is lost or reduced during a movement and is aggravated by emotional tension.

The rigidity is the disabling symptom although the tremor bothers and the bradykinesia restricts the patient. Degenerative changes in the globus pallidus and substantia nigra are present in parkinsonian patients; in addition, dopamine in the striatum and substantia nigra and melanin pigment in the substantia nigra are markedly reduced to absent. Stereotactic lesions in the globus pallidus and ventral lateral thalamic nucleus may reduce the tremor and rigidity but not the bradykinesis. A lesion in the substantia nigra may relieve the bradykinesis. L-Dihydroxyphenylalanine (L-dopa), a precursor of melanine and dopamine, crosses the blood-brain barrier. In low doses it may ameliorate the rigidity and the bradykinesis. Use of L-dopa does not provide much improvement in tone and tremor, although high doses may decrease the tremor. The symptoms of parkinsonism are probably due to the removal of the inhibitory influences which are normally exerted upon the globus pallidus.

Several antipsychotic drugs are utilized in psychiatric medicine which are known to produce parkinsonian-like side effects such as rigidity and poverty of movement. Such drugs as reserpine, chlorpromazine, and haloperidol presumably help alter psychotic states by acting on the dopaminergic neurons of the limbic system. The parkinsonian effects from these drugs are thought to be caused by their action on certain neurons. Reserpine activity results in a depletion of the dopamine in the nigrostriatal neurons. Chlorpromazine is said to block the dopamine receptor sites on the spiny interneurons of the striatum. Haloperidol is presumed to act as a dopamine antagonist.

The movements of *athetosis* are slow and are exaggerated by voluntary movement. Spasticity is characteristic. The slow, writhing character of the involuntary movement of the extremities appears wormlike. The alternating adduction and abduction of the shoulder joint are accompanied by flexion and extension of the wrist and fingers. Usually the wrist is flexed and the fingers are hyperextended. Grimaces of the face may occur during the limb movements. This dyskinesia may be due to a lesion in the striatum, mainly in the putamen, following a birth injury. Such injury suggests that the striatum has an inhibitory role.

Torsion dystonia is a form of dyskinesia in which the athetoid movements are expressed largely by sustained contractions of the axial musculature. This results in an abnormal degree of fixity of postural configurations with severe torsion of the neck, shoulder girdle, and pelvic gridle. In contrast, athetosis is primarily expressed by spasticity of the musculature of the extremities.

Choreas (dances) are characterized by jerky, irregular, brisk, rapid, purposeless, continuous flow of different movements of the limbs accompanied by involuntary twitchings of the face. These movements are expressed primarily by the distal segments of the extremities. Muscles are hypotonic. In advanced cases, the patient is almost always in motion when awake. There is no reduction in muscle power. *Huntington's chorea* is a hereditary form which becomes progressively worse with age after its initial appearance, often in the late thirties. Damage to the striatum and the cerebral cortex are presumed to be causal. It is likely that some of the motor symptoms of Huntington's chorea are associated with reduction in the amount of the transmitter GABA in the striatonigral neurons.

Ballism ("throwing") is characterized by violent, abnormal, flail-like movements origi-nating mainly from the activity of the proximal appendicular muscles of the shoulder and pelvis. The movements cease during sleep. There is a marked reduction of muscle tone. These symptoms are exhibited unilaterally with a lesion in the contralateral subthalamic nucleus. The symptoms of ballism are an expression of a *release phenomenon* probably associated with the reduction or removal of the inhibitory action of glycine on the globus pallidus and substantia nigra.

Symptoms associated with the malfunctioning of the basal ganglia are usually observed bilaterally. However, symptoms on one side result from lesions in the contralateral basal ganglia; this is a consequence of the circuits by which the basal ganglia project to the ipsilateral cerebral cortex, which, in turn, relays its influences via the corticofugal pathways to the contralateral side (see the comments on ballism, above). The abnormal movements resulting from lesions in the basal ganglia circuitry are an expression of release phenomena in which the inhibitory influences on such structures as the globus pallidus or ventral lateral nucleus of the thalamus are lost or reduced. Surgical lesions of these "released structures" (globus pallidus and the VL nucleus) are known to ameliorate the symptoms in many patients. In this context, the loss of dopamine, noted in patients with Parkinsonism, is presumed to account for the reduction or loss of inhibitory influences upon the striatum.

It is not possible to state that any clinically observed "basal ganglia disease" is due to the damage of a certain nuclear structure or part of a structure. At autopsy, patients with these diseases are found to have extensive lesions of many regions, including many structures other than the basal ganglia. These observations contribute to the enigma concerning the precise role(s) of the basal ganglia. In addition, with the exception of ballism, none of the basal ganglia diseases has been reproduced by the experimental ablation of parts of the basal ganglia. Symptoms of ballism can be produced by an experimentally produced lesion in the subthalamic nucleus. It must be remembered that the symptoms observed in an organism with a lesion of a certain structure do not necessarily tell us what the normal functional role of the damaged structure is; rather the symptoms express the functional activity of the nervous system in the absence of the normal functioning of the damaged structure.

BIBLIOGRAPHY

Carpenter, M. B.: Anatomy of the basal ganglia and related nuclei: a review. Neurol, 14:7–48, 1976.

DeLong, M. R.: "Motor Functions of the Basal Ganglia: Single-Unit Activity During Movement," in F. O. Schmitt and F. G. Worden (eds.), *The Neurosciences—Third Study Program*, M.I.T. Press, Cambridge, Mass., 1974, chap. 28, pp. 319–325.

Denny-Brown, D.: *The Cerebral Control of Movement*, Charles C Thomas, Publisher, Springfield, Ill., 1966.

Evarts, E. V.: Brain mechanisms in movement. Sci Am, 241:164–179, 1979.

Fox, C., and J. A. Rafels: "The Striatal Efferents in the Globus Pallidus and in the substantia Nigra," in M. D. Yahr (ed.), *The Basal Ganglia*, Raven Press, New York, 1976, pp. 37–55.

Frigyesi, T. L., E. Rinvik, and M. D. Yahr (eds.): *Corticothalamic Projections and Sensorimotor Activities*, Raven Press, Hewlett, N.Y., 1972.

Goldman, P. S., and W. J. H. Nauta: An intricately patterned prefronto-caudate projection in the rhesus monkey. J Comp Neurol, 171:365–386, 1977.

Granit, R.: *The Basis of Motor Control*, Academic Press, Inc., New York, 1970.

———: *The Purposive Brain*, M.I.T. Press, Cambridge, Mass., 1977.

Haymaker, W.: *Bing's Local Diagnosis in Neurological Diseases*, 15th ed., The C. V. Mosby Company, St. Louis, 1968.

Kots, Y. M.: "The organization of voluntary movements," *Neurophysiological Mechanisms*, Plenum Press, New York, 1977.

Mettler, F. A.: Muscular tone and movement: their cerebral control in primates. Neurosci Res, 1:176–250, 1968.

Meyer-Lehmann, J., J. Hore, and V. B. Brooks: Cerebellar participation in generation of prompt arm movements. J Neurophysiol, 40:1038–1050, 1977.

Miles, F. A., and E. V. Evarts: Concepts of motor organization. Ann Rev Psychol, 30:327–262, 1979.

Nauta, H. J. W., and M. Cole: Efferent projections of the subthalamic nucleus. An autoradiographic study in monkey and cat. J Comp Neurol, 180:1–16, 1978.

Pearson, K.: The control of walking. Sci Am, 235:72–86, 1976.

Phillips, C. G., and R. Porter: *Corticospinal Neurons: Their Role in Movement*, Academic Press, London, 1977.

Purpura, D. P.: "Physiological Organization of the Basal Ganglia," in M. D. Yahr (ed.), *The Basal Ganglia*, Raven Press, New York, 1976, pp. 91–114.

Roberts, T. D. M.: *Neurophysiology of Postural Mechanisms*, Butterworth Scientific Publications, London, 1978.

Stein, P. S. G.: Motor systems with specific reference to the control of locomotion. Ann Rev Neurosci, 1:61–81, 1978.

Stelmach, G. E. (ed.): *Motor Control: Issues and Trends*, Academic Press, Inc. New York, 1976.

Szabo, J.: Projections from the body of the caudate nucleus in the rhesus monkey. Exp Neurol, 27:1–15, 1970.

Thach, W. T., Jr.: Timing of activity in cerebellar dentate nucleus and cerebral motor cortex during prompt volitional movement. Brain Res, 88:233–241, 1975.

Yahr, M. D., and D. P. Purpura (eds.): *Neurophysiological Basis of Normal and Abnormal Motor Activities*, Raven Press, Hewlett, N.Y., 1967.

CHAPTER FIFTEEN

THE OLFACTORY SYSTEM AND THE LIMBIC SYSTEM

THE OLFACTORY SYSTEM

Sense of smell

The sense of smell is a primordial modality with a long phylogenetic history. It remains as a dominant sensation in many modern vertebrates; many contemporary animals live largely in a world of odors. Olfaction is critical to the survival of many animals and species, e.g., in hunting for food, in finding a mate, in recognizing friends, and in warning against enemies. An animal often identifies another by the odor it generates. Vertebrates with a well-developed sense of smell are known as *macrosmatic*, and those with a poorly developed sense of smell are known as *microsmatic*. Even in microsmatic human beings, olfaction is a complex sense. Odors generate complex associations of ideas and images and personal interpretations modified by past experiences. The blind and deaf Helen Keller was able to describe a garden and other objects because of her acute sense of smell. Tea sniffers, wine tasters, and perfumers develop their sense of smell until it becomes finely discriminative.

The olfactory sensorium has a role in the emotional life, digestion, safety, and behavior of human beings. Odors can evoke such reflexes as salivation and hydrochloric acid secretion. Olfactory stimuli can act as reminders or recollections of past experiences. In the feeding infant, odors set in motion influences alerting the reticular activating system to aid in the maintenance of awareness or consciousness.

The olfactory system is more than just a perceiver of odors; it is an activator and a sensitizer of other neural systems—those which are substrates for emotional behavior patterns. The aromas emanating from many foods evoke salivation and lip smacking, the characteristic scent from a doe stirs responses in a buck deer in rut, and the olfactory sense can produce aggressive reactions in a dog. Even human reactions to many odors are instinctive.

Odors are describable only in subjective terms; there are no basic odors comparable to the primary colors or the notes of a scale. This explains the hazards inherent in predicting the smell of mixtures. The fragrance of flowers and the aroma of roast coffee are the product of complex interactions of literally scores of volatile chemicals.

The olfactory system can be activated by mere traces of excitants in the atmosphere. In humans, the sense of smell can be a more sensitive detector of certain chemicals than the most efficient chemical analytic techniques. Many odors are sensed immediately by smell in such minute concentrations that the most sophisticated chemical methods either cannot detect them or can identify them only after procedures requiring many days of analyses.

Odorous chemicals must be volatile, water-soluble, and lipid-soluble. These three qualities are essential, otherwise the odoriferous particles would not reach the nose, dissolve in the aqueous secretion coat of the olfactory region, and penetrate the final lipid barrier of the olfactory receptor cell. Although volatility is important for odor detection, the degree of volatility is not necessarily proportional to the intensity of smell. For example, highly volatile water has no odor, whereas poorly volatile musk is a powerful odorant used as a base in perfumes. The water solubility need be only infinitesimal. Nonvaporizing and lipid-insoluble chemicals do not produce odors. In addition, odoriferous chemicals are usually organic substances with molecular configurations that stimulate the olfactory receptor cells. These olfactory sensors will adapt rather quickly to a continuous stimulus. This explains why an unchanging odor may soon become unnoticed.

Sensitivity to odors may depend on obscure factors. For example, women can detect a certain steroid compound excreted in the urine by its odor. After an ovariectomy this ability is lost. However, this compound can be smelled by an ovariectomized woman given female sex hormones. The thresholds of smell detection can vary with phases in the menstrual cycle. Olfactory acuity is poorer during menstruation and is better in other phases of the cycle, especially around the time of ovulation.

The loss of the sense of smell does not have great significance in humans, as indicated by the fact there is no common expression for loss of smell (anosmia) as there is for the loss of sight (blindness) or for the loss of hearing (deafness). An impaired sense of smell, as experienced during a cold, is reflected in the bland taste of food; the aroma of food has an important role for the gourmet.

In addition to the commonly recognized sensory submodalities associated with the gustatory and olfactory systems, there is the so-called common chemical sense consisting of subjective responses to chemical stimulation of the nasal, oral, and pharyngeal cavities. Common chemical senses include sensations described as pungent, acrid, stinging, burning, and tickling. These are said to be mediated primarily by the trigeminal nerve with contributions from the glossopharyngeal and vagal nerves. The trigeminal fibers that terminate in the nucleus solitarius may be the nucleus to which some of these chemical senses may project (Chap. 8). The common chemical sense is thought to intrude on the "subtle world of olfaction." For example, the magnitude of perceived odors is consistently lower in the nostril with a lesion in the trigeminal nerve than in the normally innervated nostril. The olfactory sense is presumed to involve interaction

of an odor detector (olfactory system) and a common chemical stimulus.

Olfactory pathway

The olfactory receptor cells in humans are located in a small 2.5-cm² epithelial patch of the olfactory mucosa high up in each nostril; we sniff to help direct air to this olfactory mucosa. The olfactory epithelium is a tall, pseudostratified columnar epithelium consisting of three types of cells—receptor olfactory (bipolar) cells, sustentacular (supporting) cells, and small basal cells capable of undergoing mitosis. The more than 10 million receptor cells in humans are bipolar neurons, each of which is surrounded by sustentacular cells. The short dendrite of each olfactory cell (cell body within this layer) is directed peripherally. At its apical end is a bulbous olfactory knob which contains basal bodies out of which 6 to 8 long cilia (streamers or filaments) project in the form of a tuft. These long cilia are enmeshed with the cilia of other cells and with microvilli of the sustentacular cells in the odor-absorbing surface fluid coating the mucosa. The fluid is the secretion of the so-called glands of Bowman and of sustentacular cells; it furnishes the necessary solvent for the odoriferous substances which are much more soluble in lipids than in water.

The receptor sites where the *odorant-receptor interaction* takes place are probably located on the cilia and/or the microvilli on the free surfaces of these bipolar receptor neurons. The initial segment where the action potential (spike) is generated is located within the cell body. The axons project from the olfactory mucosa, forming the fascicles of the olfactory nerve which pass through the cribriform plate. These unmyelinated fibers are among the smallest and slowest-conducting fibers of the nervous system. They average about 0.2 μm in diameter. Groups of these unmyelinated axons are collectively enclosed in one sleeve of a neurolemma (Schwann) cell (see Fig. 2-15); hence axons are virtually in direct contact with one another (separated by 100-Å spaces). Cross-talk between these axons is theoretically possible. The receptor potentials are generated in the dendrites as a reaction to the odoriferous molecules acting at the olfactory

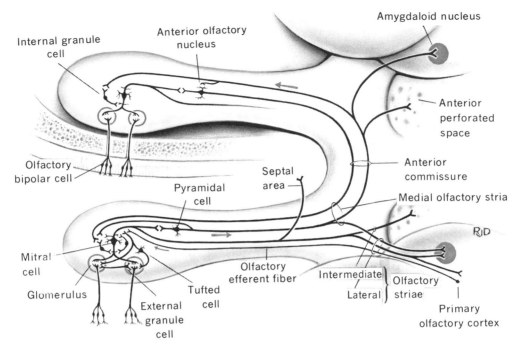

FIGURE 15-1 The olfactory pathways. The anterior olfactory nucleus is located in the posterior olfactory bulb and along the olfactory tract and striae.

hairs. The resulting action potentials are then transmitted via the axons to the olfactory bulb within the cranial cavity. Each bipolar cell acts in a dual role as an olfactory chemoreceptor cell and as the first-order olfactory neuron; each is a chemical detector, a transducer of a stimulus, and the transmitter of the nerve impulse. Each *sustentacular cell* has about 1000 microvilli on its free surface. These microvilli and the numerous organelles within these cells are indicative of the presumed secretory nature of these cells; the sustentacular cells are probably not just supporting cells.

The receptor neurons and sustentacular cells undergo constant regeneration. These new cells are apparently derived from small basal cells of the olfactory mucosal epithelium. When a degenerating receptor olfactory cell is replaced by a basal cell, the entire neuron, from receptor sites to axonal connections in the olfactory bulb, is replaced. Estimates indicate that throughout life there is an annual decrease of about 1 percent in the number of receptor neurons.

The concept of primary odors has not been verified. According to modern thought, each individual receptor cell in the olfactory mucosa reacts in a relatively broad response spectrum to molecules that evoke different odor sensations. The individual cells of the olfactory bulb are activated by more than a single odor; rather, they are both excited and inhibited by a range of odor compounds. In this respect, the quality of any one odor is probably encoded by a pattern of activity occurring in many cells simultaneously.

The *olfactory bulb* is the primary center in the central nervous system (see Fig. 15-1). The key structures of the bulb are the *glomeruli*. Each glomerulus is the complex synaptic "ball" where the terminal arborization of the axon of the receptor bipolar cell synapses with the dendritic arborization of the mitral cells (which resemble a bishop's miter in shape) and of the tufted cells of the olfactory bulb. The axon of a bipolar cell does not branch until it enters a glomerulus.

The *mitral cells* project axonal branches to the pyramidal cells in the anterior olfactory nucleus and project other branches through the olfactory tract and olfactory striae to the primary olfactory cortex, amygdaloid body, anterior perforated substance, and septal area. The anterior olfactory nucleus is composed of cells in the posterior part of the olfactory bulb, cells scattered along the olfactory tract and olfactory striae, and a few cells in the olfactory cortex and anterior perforated substance (Figs. 15-3 and 15-4).

The synaptic organization within the olfactory bulb may be summarized as follows (see Fig. 15-1).

1. The axons of all olfactory bipolar cells terminate within the glomeruli.
2. Within the glomeruli are tufts of dendrites of mitral cells; these are the main output cells from the bulb.
3. Each tuft arises from a mitral primary dendrite; other secondary dendrites ramify in the external plexiform layer.
4. Recurrent collaterals from the mitral cell axons also terminate in the external plexiform layer.
5. Within the external plexiform layer are cell bodies of tufted cells; these cells receive input from several glomeruli and from recurrent collateral branches of pyramidal cells of the anterior olfactory nucleus. In turn, they project axons to other glomeruli.
6. An external granule cell (periglomerular cell) has a dendrite tree in one glomerulus and an axon which terminates in a nearby glomerulus.
7. The axonless internal granule cells ramify within the external plexiform layer.
8. Rich dendrodendritic synapses (see Fig. 15-1) exist in the external plexiform layer between dendrites of mitral cells and internal granule cells and between tufted cells and internal granule cells, with most snyapses arranged as reciprocal pairs (see Fig. 2-9*D*).

The fact that the ratios of intrinsic neurons relative to principal neurons are high in the olfactory bulb supports the presumption that significant processing occurs within the intrinsic circuits of the bulb.

The axons of the mitral cells project via the olfactory tract and the olfactory striae to the primary olfactory cortex. The medial olfactory stria terminates largely in the cortex and nuclei of the septal region and in the contralateral olfactory bulb, while the lateral olfactory terminates mainly in the piriform cortex (uncus region-area 28) and in the amygdaloid body. These striae and the intermediate olfactory stria, when present, also end in the anterior perforated substance (olfactory tubercle). The olfactory tubercle is a small hillock in the rostral anterior perforated substance (see Fig. 15-4). Functionally the tubercle is related to the olfactory system and is connected with the limbic and hypothalamic structures.

The *primary olfactory cortex* comprises the cortex of the uncus and adjacent areas; this includes the rostral portions of the parahippocampal gyrus, periamygdaloid cortex (overlying the amygdaloid body), and the prepiriform cortex in the rostral uncus (see Figs. 15-3 and 15-4).

Little is known about the neural mechanisms by which odors are sensed and distinguished, and their intensities determined. The glomeruli have been implicated as being critical sites of this activity. The discharges from the olfactory epithelium and the feedback stimuli are integrated so that patterns of glomerular activity are expressed in the discharges of the mitral cells to the olfactory cortex. Each glomerulus sorts and integrates its input before relaying stimuli to the cortex.

Alone among the senses, *olfaction has no primary projection to the thalamus.* Because of this, the olfactory bulb has been considered to be an analogue of the thalamus. The primary olfactory cortex includes such cortical regions as the piriform area (rostral part of the uncus), the anterior perforated substance (sometimes called the "olfactory tubercle"), and the septal area. The olfactory bulb may project many fibers to the corticomedial nuclei of the amygdaloid body but none to the hippocampal formation or postuncal (area 36). This primary olfactory cortex has connections with such structures as the hypothalamus and reticular system (via the dorsal longitudinal fasciculus), amygdaloid body, and possibly through interconnections to the thalamus and to most of the limbic lobe. In addition, direct olfactory influences are conveyed to the hypothalamus via the stria terminalis and amygdalofugal fibers (see later on in chapter).

The term *rhinencephalon*, or "smell brain,"

is used in various ways. In its most restricted sense, the rhinencephalon is limited to the olfactory nerves, olfactory bulbs, and olfactory tracts, and to those neural structures receiving direct connections from the olfactory bulbs. The latter include the anterior perforated substance, prepiriform cortex, septal area, and corticomedial nuclei of the amygdaloid body. In the broadest definitions the rhinencephalon also includes the limbic cortex. The term *allocortex* is synonymous with *rhinencephalic cortex* (Chap. 16). The broad definition includes, at least in theory, all neural structures influenced by the sense of smell. Elimination of the term *rhinencephalon* has been suggested; after all, the terms "visual brain" and "auditory brain" are not used.

In theory, the *olfactory bulb is the crude indicator of smell* (as the thalamus produces crude awareness of pain), and the primary olfactory cortex and its associative cortex are the processors of finer odor discrimination. Electric recordings obtained from the olfactory bulbs of human subjects suggest that the quality of an odor is coded, at least in part, in the frequency patterns. The detection of an odor, following an adequate signal strength, is characterized by greater amplitude patterns. The complex neuronal interconnections operate to intensify,

enhance, and suppress the neural processing within the olfactory pathways. This includes the activities of the feedback circuits, reciprocal dendrodendritic synapses (Chap. 2), and the olfactory efferent (corticofugal) fibers from the olfactory cortex to the olfactory bulb (see Fig. 15-1).

One form of communication between individuals of the same species utilizes chemical messengers called *pheromones*. These substances are secreted externally by an organism and, in turn, elicit a specific influence upon the recipient—usually of a sexual behavioral nature. Pheromones are thought to be operant in human beings, in whom they are probably released by the skin, especially the axillary and pubic apocrine glands.

THE LIMBIC SYSTEM

Functional role

Many of the neuroanatomic substrates underlying the behavioral and emotional expressions of animals reside in the limbic system, otherwise known as the "visceral brain." This system is integral to those activities essential to the self-preservation of the organism, e.g., feeding,

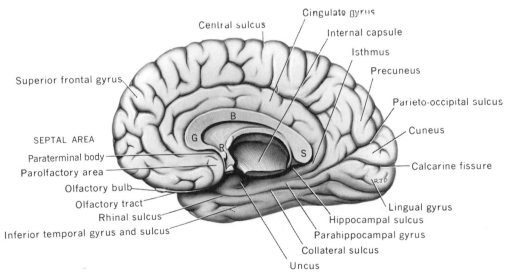

FIGURE 15-2 Median surface of the cerebral hemisphere. The internal capsule and the limbic lobe are exposed by the removal of the entire brainstem and cerebellum. The limbic lobe consists of the septal area, cingulate gyrus, isthmus, parahippocampal gyrus, and uncus. The corpus callosum is subdivided into a rostrum (R), genu (G), body (B), and splenium (S).

fight, and flight; and those essential to the preservation of the species, e.g., mating, procreation, and care of offspring. The limbic system is influenced by all sensory systems, including the olfactory, optic, auditory, and general exteroceptive and interoceptive systems. *The main outlet for its activity is via the pathways from the hypothalamus to the brainstem and spinal cord (largely via the autonomic nervous system), and the neural and vascular pathways to the hypophysis (endocrine gland).* The somatic motor system also serves as an outlet for the expression of the activities of the limbic system. Autonomic and somatic motor responses and feelings of a variety of sensations can be evoked by electrically stimulating structures belonging to the limbic system. Depending upon the structure stimulated and the nature of the stimulation, there are differences in the quality of the responses evoked.

1. *Somatic motor responses* evoked by limbic stimulation include (*a*) those associated with food acquisition and ingestion such as sniffing, licking, chewing, and swallowing movements; (*b*) those associated with behavioral patterns of activity such as grooming and goal-seeking searching movements; and (*c*) those associated with attack and defense such as snarling, clawing, and various posturing movements.
2. *Autonomic responses* include changes in the rate of the heartbeat, in blood pressure, in the motility and secretory activity of the gastrointestinal tract, and in the level of many hormones in the blood. Many hormonal effects of the autonomic nervous system are mediated via the hypothalamus and hypophysis (Chap. 11).
3. *Sensory modalities* evoked include the olfactory sensations (often sensed as an unpleasant quality), feelings of vertigo, and visceral sensations such as those felt within the abdomen. Other "sensory" responses evoked are emotional feelings noted later on in this chapter, under "'Pleasure Centers' and 'Punishing Centers.'"

Anatomy

The precise identification of all the structural elements associated with the limbic system is not possible at the present state of our knowl-

edge. This is so because it is difficult to establish morphologic correlates with the subtle physiologic and behavioral criteria by which the limbic system is characterized. The following are generally considered to be *core structures of the limbic system:*

The core structures
(Figs. 1-10 and 15-1 to 15-5)

1. The olfactory system and its pathways, comprising the olfactory nerve, olfactory bulb, olfactory tract and striae, and primary olfactory cortex (discussed at beginning of this chapter)
2. The septopreopticohypothalamoparamedian, midbrain, and upper pons complex including the septal area, preoptic area, hypothalamus, and paramedian tegmentum and periventricular gray of the midbrain and upper pons
3. The amygdaloid body and its major efferent pathways via the stria terminalis and ventral amygdalofugal fibers (pathway)
4. The hippocampal formation and its efferent pathways via the fornix system
5. The limbic lobe (Chap. 1)
6. The prefrontal cortex (lobe)

Septopreopticohypothalamoparamedian – midbrain – upper pons complex The neuronal complex extending from the septal region through the paramedian zone of the upper brainstem has a significant functional role in the limbic system. Anatomically it comprises the septal region, the preoptic (telecephalic) hypothalamus, the diencephalic hypothalamus, and the paramedian tegmentum and periaqueductal gray matter of the midbrain and upper pons. The septal and preoptic regions form a continuous unit. Of the several tracts associated with the hypothalamus, the medial forebrain bundle is most important (see Fig. 15-8). It extends as a multineuronal, multisynaptic pathway extending from the septal region through the lateral hypothalamus and paramedian upper pons. It transmits influences from the brainstem rostrally and from the septal and hypothalamic regions caudally. In a general sense, the lateral hypothalamus may be considered to be a specialization within the *bed nucleus of the median forebrain bundle* (see Fig. 15-8). Accompanying this bundle is an ascending pathway originating from aminergic cells in the

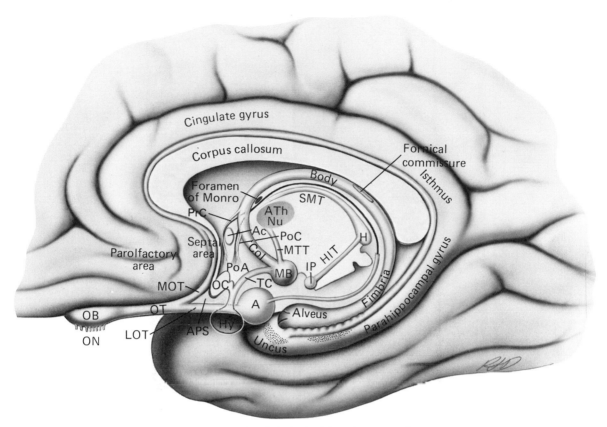

FIGURE 15-3 Some structures associated with the limbic lobe and system. Refer to Figs. 1-10, 15-2, and 16-4. The stippled areas represent the *entorhinal area* (area 28 of Brodmann) in the *uncus* and the *subiculum* in the *parahippocampal gyrus*. PrC and PoC are the pre- and postcommissural fibers of the fornix and stria terminalis (see Fig. 1-10). The fornix passes in front of and the bed nucleus and its stria terminalis pass behind the interventricular foramen (foramen of Monro). A, amygdala; Ac, anterior commissure; APS, anterior perforated substance; AThNu, anterior thalamic nuclear group; col, column of fornix; H, habenula; HIT, habenulointerpeduncular tract; Hy, hypophysis; IP, interpeduncular nucleus; LOT, lateral olfactory tract; MB, mamillary body; MOT, medial olfactory tract; MTT, mamillothalamic tract; OB, olfactory bulb; OC, optic chiasm; ON, olfactory nerve; OT, olfactory tract; PoC, postcommissural fibers; PrC, precommissural fibers; TC, tuber cinereum; SMT, stria medullaris thalami.

brainstem (raphe nuclei, locus coeruleus, and others (see Figs. 8-19 and 8-20, Chap. 8). Most of these fibers are passing through on their way to terminate in diencephalic and telencephalic nuclei including the cerebral cortex.

Functionally this septopreopticohypothalamoparamedian-midbrain complex contains the neural substrates through which the cerebral limbic system structures (cerebral cortex, amygdala, hippocampal formation, and others) are able to exert influences that are, in turn, expressed through the *endocrine system* and the *autonomic nervous system*. Broadly stated, this is accomplished (1) via the medial hypothalamus and its neural and vascular connections with the pituitary gland and (2) via the lateral hypothalamus and its caudal projections of the autonomic nervous system. Thus, the limbic system expresses itself largely through the endocrine system and the autonomic nervous system.

The *septal region* (*area*) or *septum* comprises those neural structures just anterior to the lamina terminalis and anterior commissure and extending dorsally. It includes the parolfactory and subcallosal gyri (called the *precommissural septum*) and the region surrounding and above the medial aspects of the anterior commissure (called the *postcommissural septum*). Ventral to

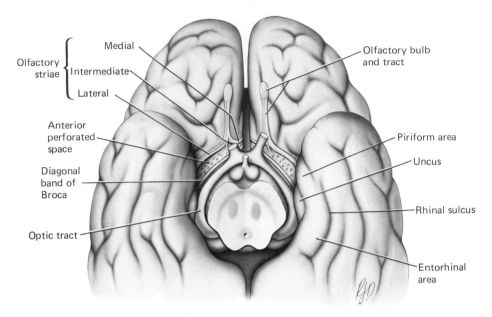

Olfactory striae
- Medial
- Intermediate
- Lateral

Olfactory bulb and tract

Anterior perforated space

Diagonal band of Broca

Optic tract

Piriform area

Uncus

Rhinal sulcus

Entorhinal area

FIGURE 15-4 Basal view of the cerebrum illustrating some of the structures associated with the olfactory and limbic systems. (*Modified from Nauta and Haymaker.*)

the septum is the anterior perforated space with its diagonal band of Broca (see Fig. 15-4). The septum pellucidum is a pair of thin, narrow plates composed of glial cells and a few fibers of the fornix; although technically a part of the postcommissural septum, it is generally considered to be a separate entity referred to as the *supracommissural septum.* The septal nuclei are located in the septum just above and rostral to the anterior commissure; they extend into the anterior parolfactory gyrus of the precommissural septum. There are two groups of septal nuclei, medial and lateral. The *medial septal nuclei* are found on either side of the midline; each is continuous with the nucleus of the diagonal band of Broca, which, in turn, blends into the amygdala (see Fig. 15-4). The *lateral septal nuclei* appear to be continuous with the neurons at the base of the septum pellucidum (see Fig. 15-6).

Intrinsic fibers of the septal nuclei and the septal–diagonal band complex interconnect the various septal nuclear subdivisions. Afferent input to the septal nuclei is derived primarily via the fornix from the hippocampal formation including the subiculum, via the median forebrain bundle from the hypothalamus and aminergic nuclei of the brainstem, and via the di-

agonal band from the amygdala. Olfactory influences are conveyed to the septal area through the medial olfactory stria (see Fig. 15-4). The efferent projections from the septal nuclei are directed primarily back via the fornix to the hippocampal formation, via the medial forebrain bundle to the hypothalamus and ventral midbrain tegmentum, via the stria medullaris thalami to the midline thalamic and habenular nuclei, and to the anterior thalamic nuclei, magnocellular dorsomedial thalamic nucleus, and periaqueductal gray (see Figs. 15-1 to 15-7). The septal nuclei are thought to be involved in motivational, emotional, and associative processes.

Amygdaloid body (amygdala, amygdaloid nuclear complex) The amygdaloid body is a large nuclear group located at the rostral end of the temporal lobe, so named because its shape resembles an almond (see Fig. 15-3; see also Figs. 1-8, 1-11, 1-20, and 1-26). Its large mass contributes to the bulge of the uncus. The fact that the amygdala is neither laminated in the cortical array nor located on the brain surface indicates that it is not a cortical structure. The amygdala is generally subdivided into three basic nuclear groups, namely (1) *corticomedial group* (*paleoa-*

mygdala), (2) *basolateral group (neoamygdala)*, and (3) *central amygdaloid nucleus*. The corticomedial group is located close to the putamen and the rostral tip of the caudate nucleus. Within the amygdala it is located dorsal and medial to the basolateral group.

The relatively small corticomedial group in humans is essentially continuous with the entorhinal cortex. It is usually subdivided into four nuclei: (1) *nucleus of olfactory tract*, (2) *medial amygdaloid nucleus*, (3) *anterior amygdaloid area*, and (4) *cortical amygdaloid nucleus*. The large basolateral group is usually subdivided into three nuclei: (1) *lateral amygdaloid nucleus*, (2) *basal amygdaloid nucleus*, and (3) *accessory basal nucleus*. The *central amygdaloid nucleus* is a separate entity.

The amygdala has numerous connections with many neural structures through a variety of afferent and efferent projections. A large proportion of these connections are made by axons which pass through two major pathways, namely, the *stria terminalis* (Fig. 1-10), and the ventral *amygdalofugal pathway* (see Fig. 15-6). Many details concerning the connections of the amygdala remain to be elucidated.

The *input to the amygdala* is panmodal in that the afferent influences are derived from olfactory, gustatory, and somatic sensory sources, from brainstem and diencephalic nuclei, and from the cerebral cortex. Intraamygdaloid fibers interconnect the corticomedial and basolateral nuclear groups. The olfactory input is both direct and indirect. Direct projections via the lateral olfactory stria terminate in the corticomedial group. Indirect projections are conveyed from the lateral olfactory stria to the piriform and entorhinal cortex (area 28) and from there to the basolateral group. The input from the gustatory and general visceral afferent systems is derived from the nucleus solitarius and its ascending pathway via the parabrachial (taste) nucleus in the midbrain (Fig. 8-18). Some fibers from this nucleus terminate in the basolateral and central amygdaloid nuclei. Visual, auditory, and tactile (extrasomatic) influences from the association cortical areas (Chap. 16) are conveyed to area 20 of the inferior temporal gyrus, from which they project to the basolateral amygdaloid groups. Area 20 is known to respond electrophysiologically to "meaningful" somatic stim-

uli; its ablation may result in visual agnosia (Chap. 16). Diencephalic regions such as the dorsomedial thalamic nucleus, rostral hypothalamus, and intralaminar thalamic nuclei send fibers to the amygdala via the stria terminalis and the ventral amygdalofugal pathway. The brainstem catecholamine nuclei have fibers projecting to the amygdala, especially to the basolateral and central nuclei. Dopaminergic input is derived from the medial substantia nigra and the adjacent ventral tegmental region. The substantia nigra may be a link associating the basal ganglia with the amygdala. The dopamine content of the central nucleus is high. The noradrenergic fibers to the amygdala originate largely in the locus coeruleus and to lesser degree from some cells in the lower brainstem reticular nuclei. The brainstem raphe nuclei give rise to serotoninergic fibers.

The diverse *output of the amygdala* (see Fig. 15-6) is primarily projected via two major pathways to subcortical loci: (1) the compact projection system or *stria terminalis* and (2) the *ventral amygdalofugal system (pathway)*.

In general, (1) the *corticomedial group* gives rise to fibers coursing via the stria terminalis and terminating primarily in the medial hypothalamus, whereas (2) the *basolateral group* projects via the amygdalofugal pathway to the lateral hypothalamus. The sequence of corticomedial group–stria terminalis–medial hypothalamus is conceived as being integrated in the hypothalamic–hypophyseal axis and expressing itself through the hormones of the pituitary gland (Chap. 11). In contrast, the sequence of basolateral group–amygdalofugal system–lateral hypothalamus is conceived as being integrated in the activity of the medial forebrain bundle and associated nuclei of the lateral hypothalamus and expressing primarily through the autonomic nervous system (Chap. 6).

Although the basolateral group may contribute a few fibers, the corticomedial group is the primary source of stria terminalis fibers (see Fig. 15-6; see also Fig. 15-3). The *stria terminalis* divides in the region above the anterior commissure into (1) the precommissural bundle of fibers passing in front of the commissure, (2) the postcommissural bundle passing behind the commissure, and (3) the fibers coursing with the anterior commissure to terminate in the contralateral corticomedial amygdala. The *precommissural fibers* terminate in the septal region including septal nuclei, medial preoptic region, and mesial hypothalamus. The *postcommissural fibers* terminate in the bed nucleus of the stria terminalis, anterior thalamic nuclei, and medial hypothalamus; some fibers continue via the stria medullaris thalami to the habenular nuclei. The *bed nucleus of the stria terminalis* is a scanty lamina of gray matter accompanying the stria from its origin in the amygdala to its enlarged termination in the preopticohypothalamic region. The term *bed nucleus* of the stria terminalis usually refers to the enlarged portion located in the caudal wall of the interventricular foramen around the anterior commissure lateral to the formix and in the preoptic area below the anterior commissure. The bed nucleus of the stria terminalis projects to all parts of the hypothalamus (via medial forebrain bundle), anterior nuclei of the thalamus, habenular nucleus, amygdala (via the stria terminalis, substantia inominata, Fig. A-26) and the nucleus accumbens septi. The latter is a nucleus located adjacent to the septum, inferiorly, at the junction of the caudate nucleus and the putamen (see Figs. A-23 and A-24). It may be striatal (ventral extension of caudate nucleus) or septal (ventral extension below anterior commissure). The bed nucleus also has connections via the median forebrain bundle with the midbrain tegmentum, brainstem raphe nuclei, and the locus coeruleus. The major input to the bed nucleus is via the stria terminalis from the amygdala and via the median forebrain bundle from the brainstem aminergic nuclei.

The amygdalofugal system spreads medially and rostrally below the lenticular nucleus to the septopreopticohypothalamus and its pathway system, the median forebrain bundle (Chap. 11). A major projection, largely reciprocal, is that with the magnocellular portion of the dorsomedian thalamic nucleus. This thalamic nucleus—through the parvocellular portion—is the gateway to the prefrontal lobe, which is the neocortical component of the limbic system (Nauta). It is through these indirect connections that the amygdala is in communication with the prefrontal lobe and may relate neocortical involvement of limbic system influences underlying emotional expression.

The amygdala has direct connections with the temporal lobe cortex, including the rostral portions of the superior, middle, and inferior temporal gyri and area 20 of the inferotemporal cortex. Direct connections are made with the caudal orbitofrontal cortex (area 13) of the frontal lobe (see Fig. 16-6).

The central amygdaloid nucleus is said to project fibers caudally to the brainstem as far as the level of the obex. These fibers terminate in the periaqueductal gray; reticular formation of the midbrain, pons, and medulla; and the dorsal vagal motor nucleus.

A nuclear group called the *substantia innominata of Reichert* extends caudally from the level of the amygdala and anterior perforated space beneath the lentiform nucleus (see Fig. A-26). It forms a plate of islands and small aggregates of cells. The *nucleus accumbens septi* is a mass of gray matter located medial to the junction of the caudate nucleus and the putamen near the septum (see Figs. A-23 and A-24). These structures are probably related either to the striatum or to limbic structures.

The hippocampal formation The *hippocampal formation* is generally described as composed of the dentate gyrus, hippocampus (hippocampus proper, ammon's horn, cornu ammonis, CA) and the subiculum (see Fig. 15-3; see also Fig. 1-10). The cortex of the formation is an archicortex (Chap. 16), with that of the subiculum being transitional with that of the adjacent entorhinal cortex of the neocortical parahippocampal gyrus. The hippocampus forms the floor of the temporal (inferior) horn of the lateral ventricle. The ventricular surface of the hippocampus is covered by a layer of white matter called the alveus, which consists of fibers of passage of the hippocampus and subiculum. (The *subiculum* is a cortical area in the parahippocampal gyrus.) These fibers converge to form (1) a flattened band called the fimbria of the fornix, which continues as the approximately 1.25 million fibers of the fornix and (2) the longitudinal stria of the supracallosal gyrus. The free border of the fimbria and fornix is continuous with the choroid plexus of the lateral ventricle (Figs. 1-22, 15-5). The hippocampal sulcus is located at the junction of the dentate gyrus and subiculum. In a cross section of the temporal lobe, note the sequence of V-shaped dentate gyrus, C-shaped hip-

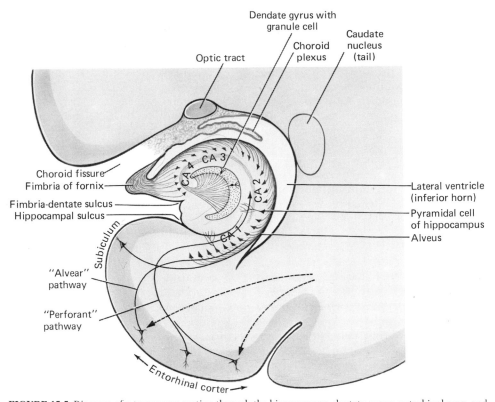

Optic tract

Dendate gyrus with
granule cell

Choroid
plexus

Caudate
nucleus
(tail)

Choroid fissure
Fimbria of fornix

Fimbria-dentate sulcus
Hippocampal sulcus

Subiculum

CA 4 CA 3

CA 2

CA 1

Lateral ventricle
(inferior horn)

Pyramidal cell
of hippocampus

Alveus

"Alvear"
pathway

"Perforant"
pathway

Entorhinal corter

FIGURE 15-5 Diagram of a transverse section through the hippocampus, dentate gyrus, entorhinal area, and subiculum. (1) Input to the entorhinal area and subiculum is derived from several areas of the temporal lobe cortex; (2) output from the entorhinal area and subiculum projects to the hippocampus, dentate gyrus via the alveus ("alvear" path) or via the perforant pathway passing through the "alvear" path; (3) connections of entorhinal area and subiculum with other cortical areas are often reciprocal; (4) axons of the pyramidal cells of the hippocampus pass through the alveus to the fimbria of the fornix; and (5) axons of the granule cells of the dentate gyrus terminate in the hippocampus. CA (cornus ammonis) refers to the four regions of the hippocampus.

pocampus, subiculum, and entorhinal cortex (area 28) of the parahippocampal gyrus (see Fig. 15-5; see also Fig. 1-28). On the basis of structural criteria the hippocampus is divided into fields CA1, CA2, CA3, and CA4. CA1 is continuous with the subiculum. CA4 is located in the hilus of the dentate gyrus. The cortex of the hippocampal formation is an archicortex (Chap. 16); it is composed of pyramidal cells and Golgi type II neurons. These cells are arranged in complex yet orderly arrangements, which have been described in exquisite detail by Lorente de Nó and others. Input fibers are the axons of pyramidal cells. The subiculum is often divided into subfields called the prosubiculum, subiculum, and presubiculum.

Afferent input to the hippocampal formation is largely derived from the neocortex of the temporal lobe (area 20) and the entorhinal area (area 28). Fibers from the medial part of area 28 pass along the subiculum to the alveus (take the "temporoalvear path") and terminate in the subiculum and CA1, synapsing with the basilar dendrites and cell bodies of the pyramidal cells (see Fig. 15-5). Fibers from the lateral part of area 28 take the direct temperoammonic (or perforant) path (perforant because its fibers pass through the alvear path) to terminate in CA1, CA2, and CA3 and synapse with the apical dendrites of pyramidal cells of the hippocampus (bypass CA4) and granule cells of the dentate gyrus. Fibers from the medial septal nucleus and lateral hypothalamus pass through the fornix and terminate topographically in CA3, CA4, and the dentate gyrus. Each hippocampus communicates with the contralateral hippocampus with fibers that pass through the fornix and the fornical (hippocampal) commissure and back through contralateral fornix. Aminergic fibers from the brainstem nuclei terminating in the hippocampus include noradrenergic fibers from the locus coeruleus and serotoninergic fibers from the brainstem raphe nuclei.

The *dentate gyrus* may be in the pivotal position in the sequential processing of information within the hippocampal formation as a whole (Swanson and Cowan). The input-output circuitry of the dentate gyrus is suggestive. The dentate gyrus is considered by some authorities not to be a cortical structure because its layer of nonpyramidal neurons (stellate cells) is not continuous with any other cortex. The major afferent input to the dentate gyrus is derived from the pan modal entorhinal cortex (see later on). Following the processing of this input, the dentate gyrus projects its output in a highly ordered manner solely to several regions of the hippocampus. Efferent fibers from the dentate gyrus and possibly CA4 do not terminate outside the hippocampus.

The *subiculum* of the parahippocampal gyrus is the neural link between the cortex of the temporal lobe and the hippocampus (see Fig. 15-3). It has direct connections with the temporal lobe cortex, hippocampus, dentate gyrus, diencephalon, and amygdala. Through these connections, the subiculum is presumed to act as pivotal center processing the output of the hippocampus and relaying it to widespread regions of the cerebrum. Many features of the subicular projections have only been recently recognized (Swanson and Cowan; VanHoesen, Rosene, and Mesulum; Siegel, Ohgami, and Edinger).

Although many of the connections noted below have been demonstrated in higher primates, some are based on evidence obtained from other mammals. In general, the subiculum receives its major input from large expanses of the temporal lobe both medial and lateral to the rhinal sulcus and from the hippocampus. The subicular output is conveyed (1) via direct connections to the temporal lobe cortex and (2)

via the fornix to the septal area and diencephalon. The cortical projections include the parahippocampal gyrus (enterhinal area 28 and perirhinal area 35), medial temporal gyrus and, in addition, the medial frontal cortex, caudal cingulate gyrus, isthmus, and fasciolar gyrus. Some direct connections terminate in the amygdala, mamillary bodies, and anterior thalamic nuclear group. Many subicular projections are reciprocal.

The fibers from the subiculum in the fornix pass (1) via the precommissural fornix to terminate in the septal area, medial frontal cortex (including gyrus rectus and subcallosal gyrus), and (2) via the postcommissural fornix to the anterior and lateral dorsal thalamic nuclei, bed nucleus of the stria terminalis, nucleus accumbens septi, ventral median hypothalamic nucleus, and mamillary body (see Figs. 15-3 and 15-7). The subiculum is probably the critical processing center associated with many of the behavioral expressions involving the hippocampal formation. It is well known that, in humans extensive injury to the hippocampal formation may result in severe memory defects, whereas localized lesions may be causally related with temporal lobe epilepsy (see "Amnestic Syndrome" later on).

The output from the hippocampus (CA1 to CA3) are not as extensive as previously claimed. Its efferent fibers project (1) via the precommissural fornix to the septal nuclei and (2) primarily to the subiculum. Some fibers also terminate in the entorhinal area 28, perirhinal area 35, and temporal pole cortex (see Fig. 16-8).

The neocortical *entorhinal area 28* of the parahippocampal gyrus is presumed to have a strategic functional role at the interface between the sensory systems and the limbic system (see Fig. 16-8). This cortical area receives inputs from many sources and projects fibers to both the amygdala and to the hippocampal formation. Of significance, this area has both indirect and direct access to the prefrontal lobe (Chap. 16)—the major neocortical representative of the limbic system (Nauta).

Areas 28 and 35 receive direct and indirect input from widespread areas of the cerebral cortex, especially those associated with sensory systems (see Fig. 16-8). Direct connections are derived from the hippocampal formation, amygdala, cingulate gyrus (via cingulum), and orbito-frontal cortex (via uncinate fasciculus, Chap. 16). The indirect sensory input comes (1) from the olfactory system from the primary olfactory cortex and the piriform lobe and (2) from the somatic sensory systems from area 20 of the inferior temporal gyrus. *Area 20* receives and processes sensory information from the visual, somatosensory, and auditory association cortical areas of the parietal, occipital, and temporal lobes before relaying it to area 28 (Chap. 16). Ablation of this area 20 has been implicated in agnosias (e.g., visual agnosia) of these sensory modalities. Thus, through its connections *area 28* is considered to be a neural station relaying processed information from several sensory systems to both the amygdala and the hippocampal formation.

The limbic lobe   The limbic lobe—*le grand lobe limbique de Broca*—comprises the cerebral convolutions on the medial surface forming the border around the diencephalon and corpus callosum. Limbic lobe literally means bordering lobe. It includes the parolfactory area, subcallosal gyrus, cingulate gyrus, isthmus, fasciolar gyrus, hippocampal formation (dentate gyrus, hippocampus, and subiculum), parahippocampal gyrus, and uncus (Figs. 15-2 and 15-3; also Figs. 1-10 and 16-4). Cytoarchitecturally the lobe consists of archicortex (hippocampal formation), paleocortex (pyriform cortex of uncus), and mesocortex or juxtallocortex (cingulate gyrus, isthmus, fasciolar gyrus, subcallosal gyrus, and parolfactory area) (see Chap. 16). The uncus is the hook-shaped formation just rostral to the parahippocampal gyrus. The uncal cortex covers the amygdala. The pyriform lobe consists of the uncus and the adjacent parahippocampal gyrus. It includes the piriform area (located adjacent to the lateral olfactory stria), the periamygdaloid area, and entorhinal area 28 (Fig. 15-4).

Prefrontal cortex (lobe)   (Figs. 16-7 and 16-8) The prefrontal cortex and orbitofrontal cortex (areas 9, 10, 11, 12, 24, 32, 46, and 47) have direct and indirect connections with the amygdala, hippocampal formation, and entorhinal cortex (area 20). The direct communication between the prefrontal and temporal cortices utilizes the association fibers of the uncinate fasciculus. The indirect communication is primarily via the dor-somedial (DM) nucleus of the thalamus (Chap. 13). This nucleus is the "gateway" to the prefrontal cortex. Because of the reciprocal interconnections between the prefrontal cortex and the DM nucleus, the cortex is also called the DM projection cortex. Inputs to the DM nucleus are derived from the septal area, preoptic area, hypothalamus, amygdala, hippocampal formation, periaqueductal gray, brainstem tegmentum (reticular formation), and several other thalamic nuclei. Polysensory influences are directed to DM via the amygdala and hippocampal formation (olfactory and somatic senses) and the periaqueductal gray and brainstem reticular formation.

General circuitry of the limbic system

The limbic structures of the telencephalon, just noted, are connected by pathways with the neocortex, diencephalon, and mesencephalon. The structures in the latter regions of the brain are considered to contain other morphologic substrates of the limbic system (Chap. 11). (1) The neocortex along the margin of the limbic lobe is interconnected with the limbic lobe; it particularly includes the neocortex of the orbitofrontal, medial temporal, and central lobe (insular) gyri. Even the prefrontal cortex may be considered to be a neocortical representation of the limbic system. (2) The major thalamic nuclei integrated into the limbic system include the dorsomedial nucleus (DM) and the anterior ventral nucleus of the anterior nuclear group. (3) Other important diencephalic structures comprise the fibers of the stria medullaris thalami and habenula of the epithalamus, and many nuclei of the hypothalamus. (4) The mesencephalic components of the limbic system are the interpeduncular nucleus, median midbrain reticular formation, dorsal and ventral tegmental nuclei of Gudden, superior central nucleus (brainstem raphe nucleus), and periaqueductal gray matter.

The complexities of the circuitry of the limbic system are schematized in this general account by outlining some interconnections associated with the amygdala (see Fig. 15-6), with the hippocampal formation (see Fig. 15-7), and with the paramedian cerebrum and upper brainstem (see Fig. 15-8). Reference to the input to these limbic structures from the central catechol-amine systems originating in the brainstem is omitted (Chap. 8).

Amygdala (Fig. 15-6) The corticomedial nuclear group of the amygdala receives input via the lateral olfactory tract from the olfactory system and via the stria terminalis from several diencephalic and limbic centers. The basolateral nuclear group receives input from extrasomatic sources (visual, auditory, and tactile), from cortical areas 28 and 20 of the temporal lobe, and via fibers of the ventral amygdalofugal pathway bundle from diencephalic and limbic centers. The corticomedial nuclear group projects its output primarily via the stria terminalis and its pre- and postcommissural bundles to the medial hypothalamus and other limbic centers. These fibers terminate in the hypothalamic centers which exert influences upon the activity of the pituitary gland. The basolateral nuclear group projects its output via the amygdalofugal fibers

to the lateral hypothalamus and other limbic centers; through these connections major influences are directed to the autonomic nervous system.

Hippocampal formation (Fig. 15-7) The input to the hippocampal formation (subiculum, hippocampus, and dentate gyrus) is derived largely from the entorhinal area (area 28) and via the fornix and longitudinal stria from several limbic centers. The output is conveyed from the subiculum and the hippocampus via the fornix (and its pre- and postcommissural bundles) and the longitudinal stria to many limbic centers including the septal nucleus and area, limbic cortex, some thalamic nuclei, the hypothalamus, and the paramedial midbrain. The hippocampus is interconnected with the subiculum and entorhinal area. The classic Papez circuit (1937) was postulated as consisting of the sequence of hippocampus via fornix to mamillary body via mamillothalamic tract to the anterior nuclear

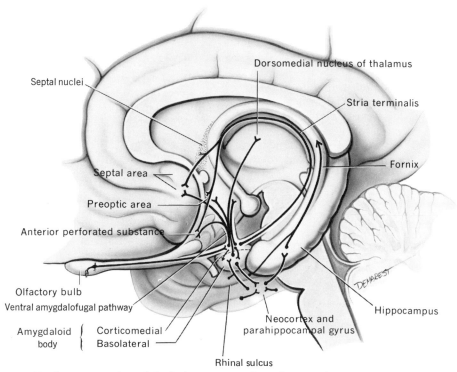

FIGURE 15-6 Some connections of the limbic system, with emphasis on the circuitry associated with the amygdaloid nucleus. Many are reciprocal.

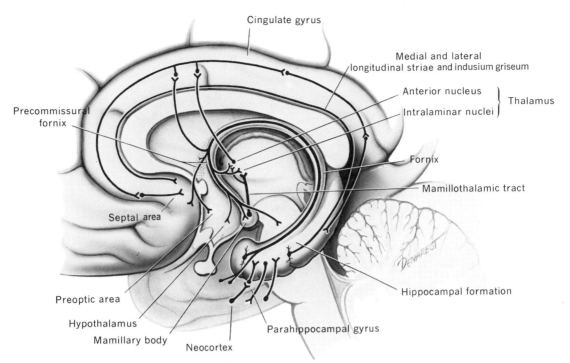

Cingulate gyrus

Medial and lateral
longitudinal striae and indusium griseum

Anterior nucleus

Intralaminar nuclei

Thalamus

Precommissural
fornix

Fornix

Mamillothalamic tract

Septal area

Preoptic area

Hippocampal formation

Hypothalamus

Mamillary body

Neocortex

Parahippocampal gyrus

FIGURE 15-7 Some connections of the limbic system, primarily those involving the subiculum and hippocampus. The "Papez circuit" includes the hippocampus via fornix → mamillary body via mamillothalamic tract → anterior thalamic nuclear group → cingulate gyrus hippocampus. Recent evidence demonstrates that the subiculum is a pivotal cortical area projecting to widespread regions of the cerebrum. Many connections are reciprocal.

group of the thalamus via thalamocingulate fibers to the cingulate gyrus via fibers of the cingulum to the hippocampus.

Paramedian cerebrum and upper brainstem (Fig. 15-8) The basic circuitry of this region is focused primarily on the centers associated with the medial forebrain bundle and the stria medullaris thalami. The medial forebrain bundle is the major pathway complex of fibers and centers conveying neural influences both rostrally and caudally to and from limbic centers. In a sense, this bundle is the key conduit for the limbic lobe (allocortex) and centers, as the internal capsule is for the neocortex and related subcortical centers (thalamus and corpus striatum). The medial forebrain bundle is a multineuron pathway extending throughout the septopreopticohypothalamoparamedian midbrain upper pons complex. Direct projections (not illustrated) pass through the bundle from the central catecholamine neuron system originating in

brainstem nuclei (Chap. 8). Paralleling the bundle is the dorsal longitudinal fasciculus, which extends from the hypothalamus caudally through the periventricular gray of the brainstem to the dorsal vagal nucleus and other centers. Another presumed pathway system comprises the sequence of septal and preoptic area via stria medullaris thalami to habenular nucleus via the fasciculus retroflexus (habenulopeduncular tract) to the interpeduncular nucleus of the midbrain and via fibers from this nucleus to the paramedian midbrain tegmentum.

Terminology An understanding of the terminology associated with emotion and behavior is basic to this discussion. Subjective terms should be distinguished from objective terms. *Feeling tone* and *affect* describe the subjective feeling state of an individual. When affect is prolonged in time, a mood sets in. *Emotion* generally refers to affect or a mood when it is accompanied by an active expression. The expression may be me-

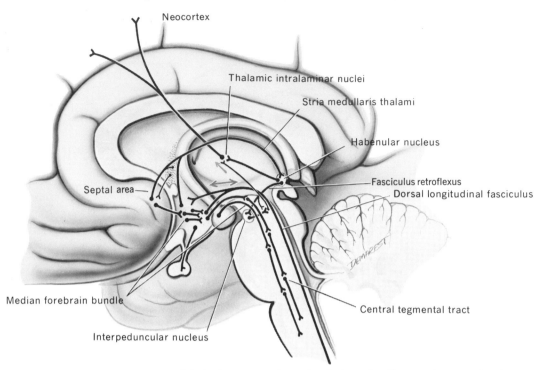

Neocortex

Thalamic intralaminar nuclei

Stria medullaris thalami

Habenular nucleus

Septal area

Fasciculus retroflexus
Dorsal longitudinal fasciculus

Median forebrain bundle

Central tegmental tract

Interpeduncular nucleus

FIGURE 15-8 Some connections of the limbic system. The median forebrain bundle is a multineuronal pathway extending from the septal area through the lateral hypothalamus to the brainstem tegmentum. Note the pathway system comprising the sequence of septal area and preoptic area → habenular nucleus → midbrain tegmentum and interpeduncular nucleus. The latter projects to the midbrain tegmentum.

diated through the autonomic nervous system (e.g., heart palpitations) or the somatic nervous system (e.g., fidgeting). In this context emotion combines subjective feelings (such as an empty feeling, pleasantness, unpleasantness, depression, elation, alertness, and contentment) with objective signs. *True rage* combines intense antagonistic subjective feelings (anger) with pronounced objective activity (the snarling or clawing of a cat). A *sham rage* (*pseudoaffective reflex*) is a rage without the subjective side but with the objective signs. An animal without a cortex may exhibit a sham rage because it presumably has no subjective feelings. *Behavior* is a constellation of expressions of an animal noted by an observer. Subjective signs are not observed, only inferred. Observed behavior includes the schooling of fish, the nesting of birds, and the stalking by lions. *Agonistic behavior* and *agonistic responses* refer to the behavior manifested by animals in an attack and defense contest during fight or flight. *Motivation* is the drive that urges

the animal to activity; it is reduced after the goal is reached, e.g., hunger is reduced following a meal. Several aspects of the relation of emotion and the limbic lobe and system will be outlined below.

Emotional behavior and putative neurotransmitters

The limbic system has an essential role in processing input which influences the activity of the autonomic and somatic motor systems. These influences act to suppress or to enhance those expressions of the organism which we interpret as emotional behavior. Some of the input to telencephalic limbic structures is conveyed via ascending pathways from the nuclei of the midbrain and the lower brainstem reticular formation. These include the adrenergic and serotoninergic pathways described in Chap. 8 (see Figs. 8-12 and 8-13). These pathways release norepinephrine, dopamine, and serotonin, which are putative neurotransmitters in many structures of the limbic system. These putative neurotransmitters are presumed to have a critical role in influencing emotional behavior. The tranquilizing and mood-elevating drugs probably exert their effects through action upon these pathway systems. Most of the mood-elevating drugs are known to be central antagonists of the catecholamines and serotonin.

A number of peptides, called *neuropeptides*, are presumed to be neurohormones, neurotransmitters, or neuromodulators found throughout the vertebrate nervous system. Until recently it was thought that these peptides (such as oxytocin and vasopressin) had specialized neuroendocrine roles limited to the hypothalamic-pituitary axis. Although it is established that many peptides, peptide receptors, and peptidergic neurons are ubiquitous in the nervous system, little is known about their specific roles in neuronal function. These peptides, among which are the endorphins, are said to be involved with many phases of behavior such as pain, euphoria, stress, thirst, learning, certain forms of mental illness, and aspects of pleasure and reward.

Klüver-Bucy syndrome Monkeys with the anterior temporal lobe ablated bilaterally (Klüver-Bucy syndrome) exhibit a constellation of emotional expressions. In the Klüver-Bucy syndrome the visual and other sensory systems are disconnected from the limbic lobe. This loss of the amygdaloid body, uncus, anterior pole of the temporal lobe, parts of the hippocampal formation, and the parahippocampus alters the animal's behavioral patterns. The animal is able to see and to locate objects visually, but it is unable to recognize objects by sight. (This visual agnosia in human beings with comparable damage is characterized by the loss of recognition of friends and places.) Animals in this condition probably have auditory and tactile agnosias, but these are difficult to determine. Such animals exhibit strong oral tendencies, expressed by a compulsiveness to examine objects with the mouth and lips. An object, once seen, is contacted, placed in the mouth, bitten, and often gently chewed. Unless edible, each object is immediately dropped. This overreacting animal is said to be stimulus-bound, as it has an irresistible impulse to touch every object in sight. Be-

havioral changes are profound and dramatic, for the animal is apparently released ("release phenomenon") from expressing fear. Wild or aggressive monkeys become tame and docile. The marked absence of emotional responses, such as anger or fear, is accompanied by the loss of the usually associated facial expressions and vocal protests. Monkeys that were formerly fearful of a mouse or a snake will pick up a live mouse or snake and handle it without fear. Dietary habits are altered; monkeys will eat fish and other food not usually eaten. Food is often consumed in excess. Hypersexual behavior is marked, with many manifestations of autosexual, homosexual, and heterosexual activities. Unilateral temporal lobe ablation does not produce such behavioral patterns, although it does make animals tamer.

Amygdaloid body Electrical stimulation of the amygdaloid body and the immediate region in the unanesthesized monkey produces a number of behavioral actions. Activities associated with nutrition are elicited, including sniffing, licking, biting, swallowing, and retching movements. A most common response is the "arrest reaction" in which all spontaneous ongoing activities cease and the animal assumes the attitude of aroused attention. This is similar to that obtained during activation of the brainstem reticular formation. This arrest reaction is assumed to be the initial phase of the fight and flight reactions associated with agonistic behavior. Monkeys exhibit agonistic behavior patterns. The peaceful monkey becomes a furious and aggressive animal that attacks and bullies. Once the stimulus is turned off, the peaceful monkey reappears. The stimulated cat is transformed into a ball of fury, with pupils dilated, claws extended, and back hair on end. Any approaching object is attacked. After the stimulus is turned off, the cat becomes a friendly, purring animal. Cats so stimulated can exhibit emotional behavior. If the amygdaloid body is stimulated in one of two cats, a fight ensues between the two animals. After this activity is repeated several times, the cats retain their newly acquired antagonism and will fight even without such stimulation. They are now emotionally driven.

An opposite response may be elicited. A stimulated cat may even express friendly behavioral patterns; it will sniff and lick, and nuzzle and rub other cats. In addition, such stimulation can inhibit a hungry and thirsty cat from eating and drinking and even prevent the hungry cat from sniffing food.

The increase in the secretion of digestive juices in the alimentary canal after repeated acute stimulations of the amygdaloid body may be followed by the appearance of erosions similar to peptic ulcers in the stomachs of monkeys and cats. The possibility of psychic excitation in the production of peptic ulcers in humans is implied.

Human beings with bilateral temporal lobe damage exhibit visual agnosia (associated with area 20), as seen in their lack of recognition of people and objects. They become docile and hypersexual. Nymphomania in the female and satyrism in the male are manifested. The behavior change may not be apparent to the casual observer, for the patient may be outwardly unchanged, with normal powers of reason and understanding. Stimulation of the amygdaloid body in humans produces the feeling tones of fear, anxiety, and rage.

Limbic lobe and neocortex Psychomotor epileptic seizures originating in the temporal lobe of humans illustrate the interplay and interaction that may occur between the limbic lobe and the neocortex. In a seizure, the patient may experience difficulty in speech (showing the influence of the neocortex) and may be in a confused state (showing the effect of the limbic lobe).

Limbic system and goal-directed behavior

The limbic system may act as a link between the sensorium and motivated activity. This linkage is probably an essential substrate in influencing the motor systems in goal-directed behavior. Some ingenious experimental studies with monkeys indicate that the amygdaloid body has a functional role in the motivational aspect of many motor responses. Monkeys whose amygdaloid body has been ablated can be demonstrated to have their mnemonic systems in normal working order. These animals react to visual stimuli; they are able to recognize objects and events in their environment. However, they do not respond behaviorally to these same visual

stimuli; they exhibit a loss in their emotional expression and in their ability to evaluate their environment. In summary, there is a definite loss in motivational behavior when mnemonic information is disconnected from the amygdaloid body; the latter may act as an intermediary between the neocortex and the parts of the limbic system. The hippocampus may contribute. For example, certain hippocampal cells may actively discharge when the animal is in a familiar locale, whereas other cells discharge when the animal senses a strange object or the absense of an anticipated one.

Memory The limbic lobe, especially the amygdaloid body and hippocampal formation, has been implicated in the memory for recent events. The neural mechanisms subserving the fleeting memory traces which are forgotten after a few minutes to several days are not known. The role of the hippocampus and the amygdaloid body in this phenomenon has been indicated by experimental work on animals and by human patients. Individuals with bilateral lesions of the amygdaloid body–hippocampal region of the temporal lobes retain memory of events prior to the surgical operation (long-term memory). Subsequent to the operation they may forget any information obtained ten or so minutes previously. These patients carry on normal conversations but cannot recall their content shortly thereafter. They are unable to commit anything to memory. If given a message to convey to another person, some patients can carry out this task only within a 5- or 10-min period after getting the instructions. After that, the message is forgotten. Lesions are found in the hippocampus in some cases of senile dementia. Patients with hippocampal lesions in the dominant hemisphere may have mild disturbances of memory. This may be related to the *amnestic (Korsakoff's) syndrome,* in which there is loss of recent memory and sense of time along with intellectual impairment. These patients have a tendency to fabricate and to become easily confused. For example, the subject forgets the question just asked and may reply with irrelevant answers (called *compensatory confabulation*).

The hippocampus is probably not the locale for the actual storage of the memory trace;

rather it may be thought of as being involved in the decision to tape and to store information for future recall. Information storage is thought to be a function of the entire brain or of many regions throughout the brain.

The neurons of the hippocampus are relatively more likely to be induced into convulsant activity, which can spread to other structures of the limbic system. In general, this activity tends to remain localized within limbic structures. This is an expression of the observation that hippocampal seizures generally do not become generalized epileptic seizures accompanied by loss of consciousness. It also accounts for the many bizarre changes in behavior observed in some patients during psychomotor attacks.

Stimulation of limbic lobe Stimulation of the hippocampus results in respiratory and cardiovascular changes and in a generalized arousal response. Such sexual activities as grooming and erection can be elicited. In this capacity, the hippocampus acts as a supplemental motor area by inducing such expressive somatic movements as facial grimaces, shoulder shrugging, and hand movements that are considered normal behavioral gestures. After the bilateral removal of the hippocampus, monkeys appear normal and feed themselves but are lethargic, apathetic, and slow to anger. They lack emotional tone.

Electric stimulation of the cingulate gyrus, the septal cortex, and other areas of the limbic lobe may evoke responses indicative of activity of the autonomic nervous system. Some responses include changes in the tone of the blood vascular system, in the activity of the digestive system, and in respiratory rhythms. These actions have even been observed in humans.

Aggressiveness can be inhibited or decreased in either monkeys or cats by electrical stimulation of the septal area or the caudate nucleus. The "boss" monkey in a colony of monkeys dominates the other members so that their behavior reflects their underdog position. The stimulation of the septal region of the boss monkey with implanted electrodes reduces the aggressive behavior of this dominant monkey. If this stimulation of the boss monkey is prolonged, the other monkeys sense this change. They lose their fear of the former bully and will take new liberties, such as securing a larger share of food or invading the boss monkey's territory. The former situation returns after the stimulation ceases. The aggressive monkey that attacks and bites becomes gentle when its caudate nucleus is electrically stimulated. This nonaggressive, easily handled, relaxed animal returns to its former self immediately after stimulation ceases.

The cortex of the cingulate gyrus is divisible into an *anterior* and a *posterior cingulate cortex*. The anterior cingulate cortex (area 24) receives its input primarily from the midline and intralaminar nuclei of the thalamus and the basolateral nuclear group of the amygdala (Vogt, Rosene, and Pandya). The posterior cingulate cortex (areas 23 and 29) receives its input mainly from the anterior and dorsolateral nuclei of the thalamus; the frontal, parietal, and temporal neocortices; and the subiculum of the hippocampal formation. The anterior cingulate cortex is involved with many complex visceral and somatic activities and in pain responses, whereas the posterior cingulate cortex is not. Stimulation of the anterior cingulate cortex can result in cardiac slowing, pupillary dilation, changes in the rate of respiration, and such integrated muscular responses as sucking and stretching. Surgical interruption of the fibers of the anterior cingulate gyrus in humans can eliminate the noxious aspects of pain without abolishing the perception of pain. This may be related to the input from the intralaminar nuclei which receive input from the spinothalamic pathways. Lesions of the intralaminar thalamic nuclei or the dorsomedial thalamic nucleus can also relieve the affective response to pain.

"Pleasure centers" and "punishing centers" The stimulation by implanted electrodes of certain regions of the limbic system of cats, dogs, dolphins, monkeys, apes, and human beings drives the subject to seek further stimulation. The animal will trip the lever over and over again and thus continually restimulate itself—*an expression of positive reinforcement on self-stimulation.* Such nodal sites have been named *pleasure centers* or *rewarding centers*. The stimulation of some regions excites the animal to avoid further stimulation—*an expression of neg-*

ative reinforcement on self-stimulation. Such sites have been named *punishing centers* or *aversion centers.* A "pleasure center" may be located a fraction of a millimeter from a "punishing center."

The general approach to locating these areas is to implant electrodes in the brain and to permit the animal to stimulate itself with small shocks by pressing a bar lever. Each press of the lever evokes a shock. With electrodes in the "pleasure centers" animals will press the lever thousands of times per hour (as many as 11,000 times per hour in some regions), hour after hour until physically exhausted. If an animal is permitted to indulge in this bar-pressing self-stimulating performance each day for an hour or so, the daily self-stimulation will be intensely performed for months on end with no indication of satiety. Such animals would rather press the lever than eat if hungry, or drink if thirsty. They will brave painful shocks to their feet to continue the self-stimulation ritual. This activity is in the nature of a positive feedback phenomenon. The several human beings whose septal areas were stimulated had feelings of pleasure or a "brightening of their attitude." They giggled, talked more, and expressed themselves more freely when the current was on. The stimulation changed their mood and made them "feel good." These so-called pleasure centers have been located within most of the limbic system, septal region, cingulate cortex, hippocampal formation, amygdaloid body, hypothalamic preoptic area, anterior nuclei of the thalamus, medial forebrain bundle, and midbrain tegmentum.

Shocks from electrodes within the "punishing centers" evoke behavioral patterns to which animals are averse. Monkeys grimace, quiver, and shake. They bite and tear objects with their mouths, their eyes dilate, and their hair stands on end. If stimulated for hours, the monkey becomes irritable, refuses to eat, and may become ill. These effects can be eliminated by stimulating a "pleasure center." If an animal is conditioned to expect a shock to a "punishing center" after a certain cue and it finds out that the shock can be avoided by some action such as pressing a lever, it becomes motivated to nullify the stimulus. Avoidance responses to the stimulation of these "aversion centers" are exhibited by rats and cats as well as by monkeys. The midbrain tegmentum and certain areas of the thalamus and hypothalamus are the sites of these "punishing centers." In human subjects, the response evoked is one of fear or terror.

Expressions of limbic system function The effects of electric stimulation or ablation of various regions of the limbic system are diverse and intricate. In effect, these regions are nodal sites that activate or inhibit many other functional complexes of the nervous system. Electric shocks to the area (or the ablation of a region) disturb, alter, and bias the dynamics of the preexisting physiologic and psychologic patterns. The effects are multifaceted—utilizing both the somatic nervous system and the autonomic nervous system. The responses can be expressed both subjectively and objectively, because the stimuli may modify the behavioral patterns, including moods and emotional states.

Uncinate fits are generally the consequence of involvement (by tumor or other disease process) of the uncus region and amygdaloid body. The immediate area is associated with the olfactory system and possibly with the gustatory system. A patient with a lesion in this area may have an olfactory aura; the hallucination usually consists of the smelling of a nonexistent disagreeable odor. Associated with this olfactory illusion is a difficult-to-describe fear of the unreality of the environment.

Prefrontal cortex as a limbic structure

The prefrontal cortex may be a major neocortical representative of the limbic system (Nauta). This interpretation is based on morphologic and behavioral criteria. The prefrontal cortex has multiple reciprocal connections with many core structures of the limbic system, including the cortex of the limbic lobe and the hypothalamus. The frontohypothalamic interconnection is the only known direct route from the neocortex to the hypothalamus. Functionally the prefrontal cortex may serve as a critical link between other regions of the cerebral cortex and the limbic system. This linkage is presumed to act as a channel through which the prefrontal cortex monitors and modulates limbic mechanisms and thereby influences the organism's affective and motivational states (Chap. 16).

BIBLIOGRAPHY

Beidler, L. M.: "Olfaction," in *Handbook of Sensory Physiology*, vol. IV, part 1, Springer-Verlag OHG, Berlin and New York, 1971, pp. 1–517.

Clemente, C. D., and M. H. Chase: Neurological substrates of aggressive behavior. Ann Rev Physiol, 35:329–356, 1973.

DeFrance, J. F. (ed): *The Septal Nuclei*, Plenum Press, New York, 1976.

Epple, G., and D. Moulton: "Structural Organization and Communicatory Functions of Olfaction in Nonhuman Primates," in C. R. Noback (ed.), *Sensory Systems of Primates*, Plenum Press, New York, 1978, chap. 1, pp. 1–22.

Grossman, S. P.: *Essentials of Physiological Psychology*, John Wiley & Sons, Inc., New York, 1973.

Haymaker, W. E., E. Anderson, and W. J. H. Nauta: *The Hypothalamus*, Charles C Thomas, Publisher, Springfield, Ill., 1969.

Hockman, C. H. (ed.): *Limbic System Mechanisms and Autonomic Function*, Charles C Thomas, Publisher, Springfield, Ill., 1972.

Klüver, H.: " 'The Temporal Lobe Syndrome' Produced by Bilateral Ablations," in E. E. Wolstenholm and C. M. O'Connor (eds.), *Neurological Basis of Behaviour*, Churchill, London, 1958, pp. 175–182.

Krettek, J. E., and J. L. Price: Amygdaloid projections to subcortical structures within the basal forebrain and brainstem. J Comp Neurol, 172:723–752, 1977.

Magoun, H. W.: *The Waking Brain*, 2d ed, Charles C Thomas, Publisher, Springfield, Ill., 1969.

Moulton, D. G., and L. M. Beidler: Structure and function in the peripheral olfactory system. Physiol Rev, 47:1–52, 1967.

Nauta, W. J. H.: "The Central Visceromotor System. A General Survey," in C. H. Hockman (ed.), *Limbic System Mechanisms and Autonomic Function*, Charles C Thomas, Publisher, Springfield, Ill., 1972, chap. 2, pp. 21–33.

Papez, J. W.: A proposed mechanism for emotion. Arch Neurol Psychiat, 38:725–743, 1937.

Rosene, D. L., and G. W. Van Hoesen: Hippocampal efferents to reach widespread areas of cerebral cortex and amygdala in the rhesus monkey. Science, 198:315–317, 1977.

Siegel, A., S. Ohgami, and H. Edinger: Projections of the hippocampus to the septum in the squirrel monkey. Brain Res, 99:247–260, 1975.

Swanson, L. W., and W. M. Cowan: An autoradiographic study of the organization of the efferent connections of the hippocampal formation in the rat. J Comp Neurol, 172:49–84, 1977.

———, and ———: The connections of the septal region in the rat. J Comp Neurol, 186:621–656, 1979.

Van Hoesen, G. W., D. L. Rosene, and M. M. Mesulum: Subicular input from temporal cortex in the rhesus monkey. Science, 205:608–610, 1979.

Vogt, B. A., D. L. Rosene, and D. N. Pandya: Thalamic afferents differentiate anterior and posterior cingulate cortex in the monkey. Science, 204:205–206, 1979.

Valenstein, E. S.: *Brain Stimulation and Motivation*, Scott, Foresman and Company, Chicago, 1973.

Valverde, F.: *Studies on the Piriform Lobe*, Harvard University Press, Cambridge, Mass., 1965.

CHAPTER SIXTEEN

THE CEREBRAL CORTEX

The cerebral cortex is the gray mantle of the cerebrum, composed of about 10 to 15 billion neurons and 50 billion glial cells (see Figs. 16-1 through 16-8). Its intricate networks are essential to our intellectual faculties and to the other higher neural expressions. This matrix has been likened to "an enchanted loom where millions of flashing shuttles weave a dissolving pattern" (Sherrington).

The cerebral cortex covers about $2\frac{1}{2}$ ft² of surface area. In thickness it varies from 4 mm in the precentral gyrus (motor cortex) to 1.5 mm in the primary visual cortex near the calcarine sulcus. Its total weight of 600 g—about 1 lb, or roughly 40 percent of the total brain weight—is estimated to be divisible into about 180 g of neurons, including their processes, and 420 g of glial cells and blood vessels.

The cortex of human beings achieves its maximal weight by the eighth year of life. No reliable data even suggest a relation between cortical weight (normal ranges) and intelligence.

ORGANIZATION OF THE CORTEX

Gross organization

The cerebral cortex has been parceled into a number of areas, depending on which structural and functional criteria are emphasized by an author.

On the basis of phylogenetic, ontogenetic, and functional criteria, the *cerebral cortex (palluim)* is subdivided into *archicortex (archipallium)*, *paleocortex (paleopallium)*, and *neocortex* (*neopallium*). The archicortex and paleocortex attain relatively large proportions early in mammalian evolution and during early development. The paleocortex has a significant role in olfaction (Chap. 15). The archicortex is integrated into the neural mechanisms associated with emotional and affective behavior.

The neocortex constitutes the bulk of the cortex (90 percent) in humans. Other names for it, besides *neopallium*, are *homogenetic cortex* and *isocortex*. This cortex has a six-layered laminated cytoarchitectural pattern (discussed below).

Allocortex (Figs. 1-10 and 15-3)

The paleocortex and archicortex are collectively known as the *heterogenetic cortex* or *allocortex* (Chap. 15). This ancient cortex either is nonlaminated or, if laminated, has fewer than six cytoarchitectural layers. Although the allocortex has a phylogenetically ancient history, many portions of it have become highly evolved in humans and the higher primates.

The archicortex is subdivided into hippocampus, dentate gyrus, and subiculum. The hippocampus forms the floor of the temporal horn of the lateral ventricle; the subiculum is a transitional area adjacent to the neocortex; and the dentate gyrus is wedged in between the hippocampus and the subiculum (see Fig. 15-3). The hippocampal formation consists of the hippocampus, dentate gyrus, and possibly the subiculum. The hippocampus is the ridge in the floor of the temporal horn of the lateral ventricle. It comprises (1) the pes hippocampi, which is the

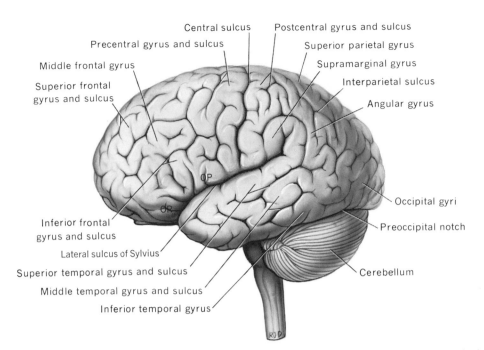

FIGURE 16-1 Lateral surface of the brain. The inferior frontal gyrus is subdivided into an opercular part (OP), triangular part (T), and orbital part (OR). The triangular and opercular parts are separated by the ascending ramus of the lateral sulcus, and the triangular and orbital parts by the horizontal ramus of the lateral sulcus.

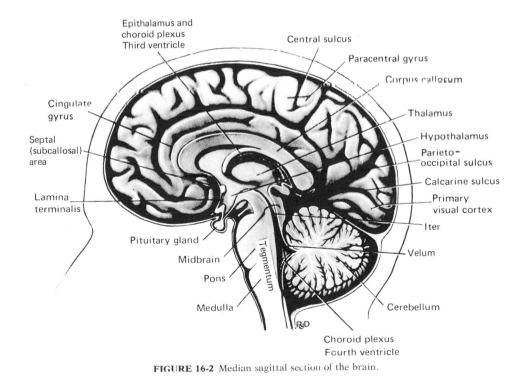

FIGURE 16-2 Median sagittal section of the brain.

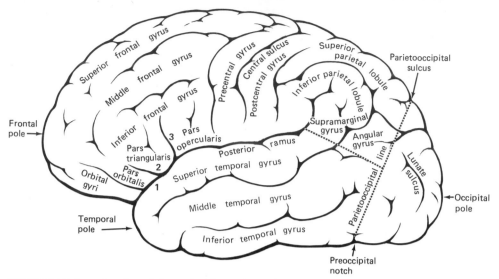

FIGURE 16-3. Lateral surface of the cerebral hemisphere. The lateral sulcus (fissure) is subdivided into (1) a stem, (2) a horizontal ramus, (3) an ascending ramus, and (4) a posterior ramus. The parietooccipital line is an arbitrary line separating the occipital lobe from the parietal and temporal lobes. The line from the posterior ramus of the lateral sulcus to the parietooccipital line is an arbitrary boundary between the parietal and temporal lobes. Refer to Fig. 1-2.

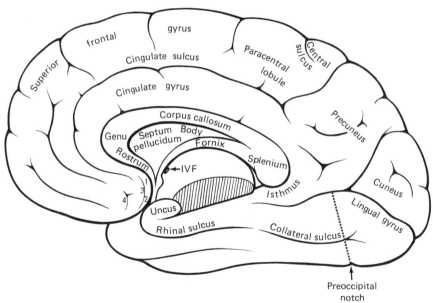

FIGURE 16-4 Median sagittal surface of the cerebral hemisphere. The numbered structures comprise (1) the subcallosal gyrus, (2) the anterior olfactory (paraterminal) gyrus or area, (3) the posterior olfactory sulcus, and (4) the anterior olfactory sulcus. The dotted line from the preoccipital notch is an arbitrary boundary between the occipital and temporal lobes. The corpus callosum is subdivided into the rostrum, genus, body, and splenium. Refer to Figs. 1-6, 1-7, and 1-8. IVF, interventricular foramen (foramen of Monro).

rostral extension; (2) the alveus hippocampi, which is a thin layer of white matter covering the ventricular surface of the hippocampus; and (3) the fimbria hippocampi (fimbria of the fornix), which is composed of many efferent and afferent fibers many of which project from and to the mamillary body (see Figs. 1-24, 15-3, and 15-4).

The *paleocortex* (essentially equivalent to the piriform area) is relatively and absolutely larger in humans than in other primates. It generally includes the uncus, parahippocampal gyrus medial to the rhinal sulcus, prepiriform cortex, anterior perforated substance, and some small adjacent areas of cortical tissue (see Figs. 1-8 and 15-2 to 15-4). The mesocortex (mesallocortex, juxtallocortex) includes the cortex of the cingulate gyrus (areas 23, 24, 29, and 33; see Fig. 16-5).

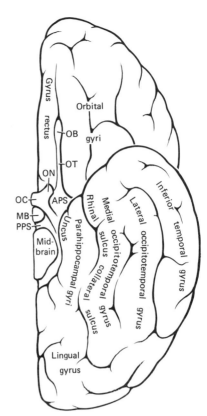

FIGURE 16-6 Basal view of the right cerebral hemisphere. APS, anterior perforated substance (space); MB, mamillary body; OB, olfactory bulb; OC, optic chiasm; ON, optic nerve; OT, olfactory tract; PPS, posterior perforated substance. Refer to Fig. 1-11.

NEOCORTEX

General organization

On the basis of cytoarchitectural criteria, the cortex has been parceled into 20 areas (Campbell), 47 areas (Brodmann), 109 areas (von Economo), and over 200 areas (Vogt). The numbered areas of Brodmann are commonly used (see Figs. 16-7 and 16-8). In a general way, the "motor" or "expressive cortex" is mainly located rostral to the central sulcus; the "sensory or receptive cortex" is mainly located occipital to the central sulcus.

The frontal lobe comprises the motor cortex (precentral gyrus, area 4), premotor cortex (area 6), prefrontal cortex, supplementary motor cor-

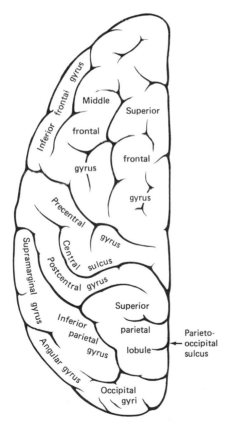

FIGURE 16-5 Surface view from above of the left cerebral hemisphere.

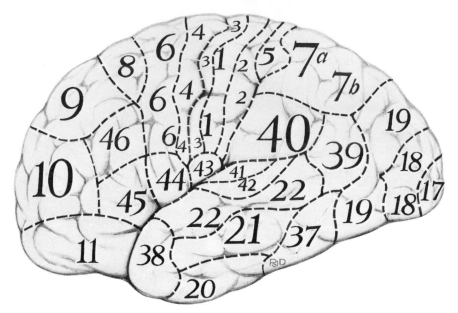

FIGURE 16-7 Cytoarchitectural map of the lateral surface of the human cerebral cortex. (Numbers represent the areas of Brodmann.)

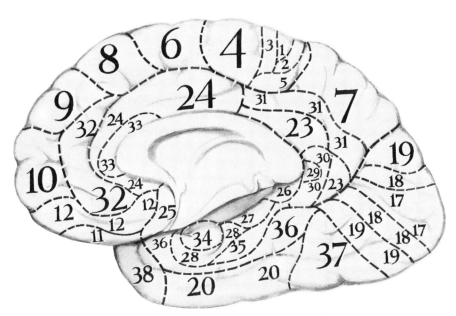

FIGURE 16-8 Cytoarchitectural map of the medial surface of the human cerebral cortex. (Numbers represent the areas of Brodmann.)

tex, and Broca's speech area (areas 44 and 45); the parietal lobe consists of a general somatic sensory cortex (postcentral gyrus, areas 1, 2, and 3), second sensory cortex (including part of area 4), and an association area; the occipital lobe consists of a primary visual cortex (area 17) and an association area (areas 18 and 19); and the temporal lobe consists of a primary auditory cortex (area 41) and an association area (areas 42 and 22). The association cortical areas of the parietal, temporal, and occipital lobes are concerned with the "higher integrative functions" of the general senses, vision, and audition. A wide area of the anterior temporal lobe association cortex has been called the "interpretive cortex." The association areas receive input from the adjacent primary and secondary sensory areas and are interconnected by reciprocal connections with several thalamic nuclei.

Horizontal organization The neocortex is laminated into six horizontal sheets. These conventionally recognized six laminae (see Figs. 16-9 to 16-12), beginning at the cortical surface, are lamina I, plexiform layer or molecular layer of nerve fibers oriented tangential to the cortical surface; lamina II, external granular layer, or layers of small pyramidal cells; lamina III, layer of medium-sized and large pyramidal cells, or external pyramidal layer; lamina IV, internal granular layer, or layer of small stellate and pyramidal cells; lamina V, inner or deep layer of large pyramidal cells; and lamina VI, spindle cell layer, layer of fusiform cells (modified pyramidal cells), or multiform layer.

The neocortex with each of the six laminae clearly evident is known as the *homotypic cortex* (generalized six-layered type), whereas the neocortex with the six laminae present but not clearly demarcated is known as the *heterotypic cortex*. The *heterotypic cortex* with a scant number of granule neurons (discussed below) is called the *agranular cortex*, while that with numerous granule (stellate) neurons is called the *granular cortex* (*koniocortex*). The primary visual cortex (area 17) is a heterotypic granular cortex; the primary auditory cortex (areas 41, 42) and the primary somesthetic cortex (areas 1, 2, and 3) are homotypic granular cortices; and the primary motor cortex (area 4) is a homotypic

agranular cortex. The heterotypic cortex is the more common neocortical pattern. Other cytoarchitectural schemas have been described.

Neocortical neurons Four basic neuronal types may be considered representative of the more than 60 cortical cell types that have been described (see Fig. 16-9). The pyramidal neurons and the stellate (granular) neurons are the most common. There are approximately 5.5 billion *pyramidal cells* and 4.5 billion *stellate cells*. The other basic neocortical cell types are the *horizontal cells of Cajal* and the *cells of Martinotti*. Each cortical cell is designated by convention as belonging to the lamina in which its cell body is located.

Each *pyramidal cell* has a pyramid-shaped cell body with its apex directed toward the cortical surface (see Figs. 16-9 and 16-13). The apex is continuous as the apical dendrite that terminates as several branches in the molecular layer. Short collateral branches extend horizontally from the apical dendrite. Several horizontally directed dendrites, known as basilar dentrites, extend laterally from the cell body. The branches of all dendrites have numerous spines, which increase the surface area of the neuron. The cell bodies (ranging from 10 to over 50 μm in diameter) of pyramidal cells are found in all cortical laminae except the molecular layer. The horizontal spread of the basilar dendrites and the distal branches of the apical dendrites generally range from 150 to 300 μm (see Fig. 16-13). The giant pyramidal cells, called Betz cells, are found in layer 5 of cortical area 4. The relative amount of synaptic activity on the dendrites as compared with that on the cell body of a pyramidal cell can be gauged from the estimate that 90 percent of the dendritic cell body surface area of each pyramidal cell is located on the dendrites.

Although a pyramidal cell is considered to be located in a particular lamina, its processes may extend into other laminae or even all laminae. Pyramidal cells of laminae V and VI have apical dendrites extending vertically up to lamina I and its basilar dendrites into laminae V and VI. In a sense the pyramidal cells "listen" through their dendrites to signals arriving in the layers superficial to and at the same level as its cell body.

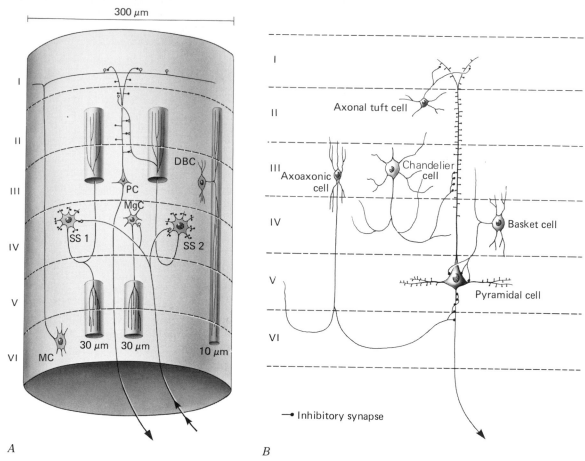

FIGURE 16-9 *A.* Schematic representation of the modular organization of the excitatory synaptic connections and of putative excitatory interneurons of the neocortex. The 300-μm-diameter cylinder represents spatial distribution of a corticocortical afferent fiber (both ipsilateral association and contralateral callosal fibers, Fig. 16-10A). This cylinder corresponds to the horizontal spread of the terminal branches of these corticocortical afferents in laminae II through VI. Stellate cells receive monosynaptic excitatory input from specific afferent fibers. The spiny stellate cell 1 (SS) has an axon which bifurcates into ascending and descending vertically directed branchings within a 30-μm-diameter cylinder. The spiny stellate cell 2 (SS 2) has a vertically directed axon with branchings outlining a 30-μm-diameter cylinder. Microgliaform cell (MgC) is a nonspiny stellate cell with a descending axon with branchings outlining a 30-μm-diameter cylinder. The double bouquet cell (DBC) is an interneuron with an axon having an ascending and a descending vertically directed axonal branching within a 10-μm-diameter cylinder. The Martinotti cell (MC) is a interneuron of lamina VI projecting excitatory input to lamina I. These cells have putative excitatory synaptic connections with pyramidal cells (PC); the neurons discharge from the cortex.

B. Schematic representation of the putative inhibitory interneurons of the neocortex. The axonal tuft cells have axonal branches which have inhibitory synaptic connections with the terminal branches of the apical dendrites of pyramidal cells. The chandelier cells have recurved axonal branches which make inhibitory synapses on the main shaft of the apical dendrite of the *pyramidal* cells. These chandelier cells may presumably act as an inhibitory "choke" on the apical dendrite within the territory of its dendritic aborization. The basket cells have axons which have inhibitory synaptic connections with the cell bodies of pyramidal cells. The axoaxonic cells have axons which terminate and synapse with the axon (axo-axonic synapses) just beyond the axon hillock of the pyramidal cells. These cells may act as the final central mechanism regulating the discharge of the pyramidal cells. (*After Szentágothai.*)

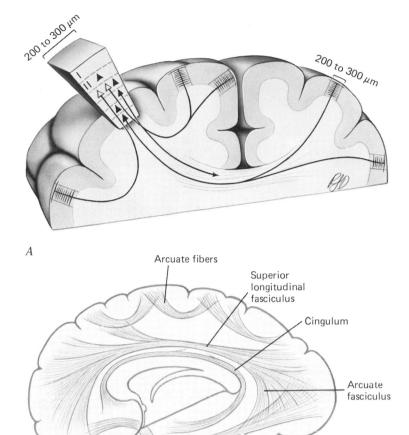

A

B

FIGURE 16-10 *A.* Diagrammatic representation illustrating the vertical columns (200 to 300 μm wide) as formed by the distribution of the association and commissural corticocortical projections. Neurons (open cells) from lamina III project to cortical columns in the ipsilateral hemisphere while other neurons (dark cells) of all laminae except lamina I project through the corpus callosum to cortical columns in the contralateral hemisphere. Each association fiber has terminal branches which spread laterally within each lamina (except lamina I) to the width of the cortical column. The spread in lamina I exceeds the width of the column. *B.* The principle associations (intrahemispheric) fibers of the cerebral hemispheres. (*A, after Szentágothai.*)

The axon of a pyramidal cell extends from the base of the cell body into the subcortical white matter. Before leaving the gray matter, all axons have one or more branches, called axon collateral branches, which project back (recurrent axon collaterals) or extend horizontally (horizontal axon collaterals) into the gray matter as intracortical association fibers (see Fig. 16-12). These collaterals synapse in the immediate vicinity with stellate neurons. The main axon

projects into the subcortical white matter. These axons project as (1) association fibers to other cortical areas in the same hemisphere; (2) commissural fibers to the same cortical areas in the opposite hemisphere; or (3) projection fibers to subcortical gray matter of the cerebral hemispheres (corpus striatum), diencephalon (thalamus), brainstem, and spinal cord (Fig. 16-10).

There are many varieties of pyramidal cells, including the fusiform cells of layer 6. Ontoge-

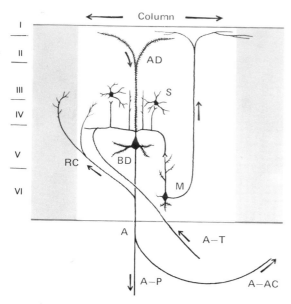

FIGURE 16-11 Schema of the vertical columnar organization of the cerebral cortex. The basic types of cortical neurons are indicated. A, axon of a pyramidal neuron; A-AC, axon of association or commissural fiber; AD, apical dendrite of a pyramidal neuron; A-P, axon of projection fiber; A-T, axon of neuron in a specific thalamic nucleus; BD, basilar dendrites of a pyramidal neuron; M, Martinotti cell; RC, recurrent collateral branch; S, stellate cell (granule, Golgi type II cell). Each pyramidal neuron may be an association neuron, commissural neuron, or projection neuron, but not all three. Arabic numerals indicate the six horizontal laminae of the neocortex.

netically, the pyramidal cells tend to mature in the following sequence: (1) the apical dendrites differentiate slightly before the basilar dendrites, and (2) the axodendritic synapses develop somewhat before the axosomatic synapses.

The *local circuit neurons (stellate cells, Golgi type II cells, interneurons)* are cells, each with a star-shaped soma, extensively branching dendrites, and an axon coursing, branching, and terminating wholly within the cortex (see Fig. 16-9). Most if not all of each local circuit neuron and its processes remains within a cortical column (see later on).

The local circuit neurons of the cortex have been divided in two functionally different groups, namely, excitatory neurons (group A) and inhibitory neurons (group B) (Szentágothai). The *putative excitatory cells* include spiny stellate cells of lamina IV, neurogliaform (microgliaform) stellate cells, and double bouquet cells

(cellule a double bouquette of Cajal). The *putative inhibitory cells* include axonal tuft cells, chandelier cells, basket cells, and axoaxonic cells. The excitatory neurons are so designated because they form type I synapses (see Fig. 2-11E, Chap. 2). Their putative excitatory synapses form asymmetric contacts between the pre- and postsynaptic neurons and have rounded vesicles in their presynaptic terminals. The putative inhibitory synapses are so designated because they form type II synapses (see Fig. 2-11F, Chap. 2). Their putative inhibitory synapses form symmetric contacts and have flattened vesicles in their presynaptic terminals. It is of importance to realize that, with the exception of some variations, the local circuit neurons of the cortex are, as far as is known, basically similar in the various species of mammals. The cells of Martinotti and the horizontal cells of Cajal are local circuit neurons which have not been classified as excitatory or inhibitory cells (Figs. 16-9 and 16-12).

EXCITATORY CELLS   The *spiny stellate cells* of lamina IV have extensively branched dendrites with numerous spines. Although most of these neurons are located in lamina IV, some are found in lamina III (see Fig. 16-9A). One type of stellate cell has an axon that bifurcates into an ascending and a descending branch. Another type has an axon that recurves and ascends. The ascending branch extends into lamina II and the descending branch into lamina VI. Each axonic branch has terminals that have a spatial arborization pattern outlining a vertically oriented cylinder about 30 μm in diameter (see Fig. 16-9A). These neurons receive direct monosynaptic excitatory input on their spines from axons of cells in the specific thalamic nuclei. The nonspinous portions of the dendrites also have synaptic contacts. Each axonic terminal of these stellate cells forms a climbing type repetitive synapse with many spines on the same apical dendrite of a pyramidal cell.

These repetitive synapses are incorporated into synaptic cartridges on pyramidal cell dendrites. A *synaptic cartridge* is a complex of excitatory and inhibitory synaptic endings on the spines and smooth surface between spines on a local segment of a dendrite; each cartridge is encapsulated by a glial sheath. These spiny stellate

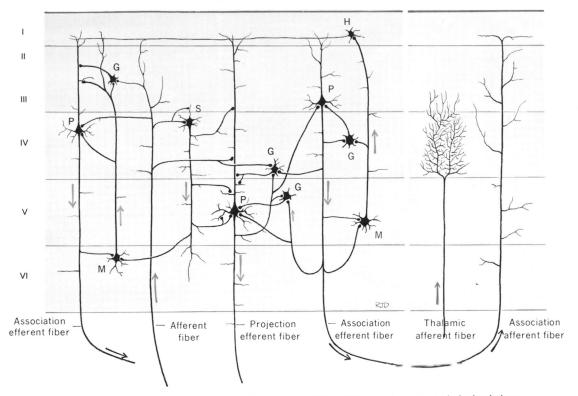

FIGURE 16-12 Some intracortical circuits of the neocortex. Afferent fibers to the cortex include the thalamo-cortical, commissural, and association fibers. Some stellate cells (S) have long axons which extend vertically to the deeper cortical layers. The Martinotti cells (M) have long axons which extend vertically to the superficial cortical layers. Other stellate cells (granule cells, G) have short axons which terminate in their immediate vicinity. Pyramidal cells (P) have long axons which, before emerging from the cortex, send recurrent and transverse collateral branches to terminate within the cortex. The horizontal cells of Cajal (H) are located in lamina I. (*Adapted from Lorento de Nó.*)

cells are the essential link between the excitatory input from the specific thalamic nuclei and other cells of the cerebral cortex.

The *neurogliaform cells* are cells located in laminae II through VI. They have a dense dendritic arbor with nonspinous dendrites. The descending axon has many branches and delicate beaded sub-branches that terminate in the deeper layers. The spatial arborization pattern of the axon terminals outlines a cylinder about 30 μm in diameter (see Fig. 16-9A).

The *double bouquet cells* are interneurons with fusiform cell bodies located in laminae II and III. Several dendrites emerge from the opposite poles of each cell body in the form of a vertically extending bouquet from each end (see Fig.

16-9A). The axon of each cell extends laterally a short distance where it bifurcates into an ascending and a descending branch extending from laminae II through VI. The axonal branches and their terminals have a spatial arborization pattern that outlines a vertically oriented cylinder roughly 10 μm in diameter.

INHIBITORY CELLS *Axonal tuft cells* are stellate neurons of lamina II (see Fig. 16-9). The axon of each cell arborizes and terminates (primarily in lamina I) on the spines of the distal segments of the apical dendrites of pyramidal cells. Each terminal branch may synapse on several distal segments of different pyramidal cells.

Chandelier cells are stellate interneurons (see

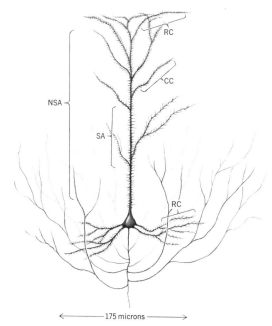

NSA

RC

CC

SA

RC

← 175 microns →

FIGURE 16-13 A pyramidal cell. Note the source of the input to the various regions of the dendritic arborization. The afferents from the specific afferent thalamic nuclei (SA) terminate on the central third of the apical shafts of cells with cell bodies in lamina V. The afferents of corpus callosal fibers (CC) are distributed to oblique branches of apical dendrites. The axon recurrent collaterals (RC) of other pyramidal cells are distributed on the tips of apical arches and basilar dendrites. The nonspecific afferents (NSA) terminate widely on the apical dendrites. (*Adapted from Scheibel and Scheibel.*)

Fig. 16-9). Each cell has an axon that descends and arborizes into several branches, each of which recurves and terminates in a serial synaptic arrangement on the smooth portions of the shaft of an apical dendrite. Each branch of the axon terminates on the apical dendrite of a different pyramidal cell.

Basket cells are local circuit neurons with short branching dendrites with a few spines located in laminae II through V (see Fig. 16-9). The axon of each basket cell divides into several branches, each of which has a terminal arborization synapsing with the cell body of a pyramidal cell. Each basket has such terminal contacts with many pyramidal cells. Small basket cells of lamina II have axons synapsing with pyramidal cells of lamina II and III. Large basket cells of laminae III, IV, and V have extensive axonal arborizations synapsing with pyramidal cells in laminae III, IV, and V.

Axoaxonic cells are neurons with vertically directed dendrites ascending and descending from each cell body (see Fig. 16-9). The descending axon of each cell divides into branches that extend laterally and terminate in ascending serial axoaxonic synapses on the pyramidal cell axon in the vicinity of the initial segment.

Cells of Martinotti are small, multipolar cells with short, branched dendrites with stubby spines (see Figs. 16-9*A* and 16-11). They are present in all but lamina I. Each cell has an axon that extends vertically and terminates in lamina I. Horizontal axonal branches terminate in the other laminae.

The *horizontal cells of Cajal* are small neurons of the molecular layer. These association cells have dendrites and axons that are parallel in direction to the cortical surface. These neurons, which are present in young but rarely in adult animals, are the only cortical neurons oriented entirely in the horizontal plane (see Fig. 16-12).

Input to the pyramidal neurons (Fig. 16-13) The afferent projections to the cortex terminate in organized patterns upon the pyramidal cells and other cortical neurons. These inputs are directed differentially to a number of sites of each pyramidal cell. The following is a general statement. The specific sensory afferent fibers synapse with the central third of the main shaft of the apical dendrites of pyramidal cells with cell bodies in the fifth cortical layer. Nonspecific afferent inputs from the thalamus and brainstem are exerted over the entire main shaft and some branches of the apical dendrites. The commissural fibers of the corpus callosum terminate upon oblique branches of the shaft of the apical dendrites. The recurrent collateral axonal branches of pyramidal cells are distributed to the outer segments of the basilar and apical dendrites of other pyramidal cells. Although much input to the pyramidal cells is through direct synaptic connections, most of it is conveyed to the cortical interneurons, e.g., stellate cells; they are intercalated between the association, projection, and commissural fibers and the pyramidal cells (see later on).

Nerve fibers which are oriented parallel to the cortical laminae form small bundles called *stripes*, *lines*, or *bands*. These horizontal stripes are more prominent in some layers than in others: the stripe of Kaes in lamina II, the inner stripe of Baillarger in lamina V, and the outer stripe of Baillarger in part of lamina IV. The two stripes of Baillarger form a common stripe called the *line of Gennari* in the primary visual cortex (17). These stripes are visible to the naked eye in some areas. The fibers that comprise these stripes include the basilar dendrites and myelinated horizontal axon collaterals of the pyramidal cells.

WHITE MATTER OF THE CEREBRUM

The white matter of the cerebrum is composed of association, commissural, and projection fibers.

Association, or intrahemispheric, fibers

The *association fibers* are the axons of pyramidal cells projecting to other cortical areas of the same hemisphere (see Fig. 16-10*A* and *B*). An innumerable number of short association fibers interconnect adjacent gyri or adjoining sectors within a gyrus. These short association fibers may remain wholly within the cortex (*intracortical*) or may pass through the white matter (*subcortical*). Long association fiber bundles reciprocally interconnect distant cortical areas within the same hemisphere.

The *intracortical association fibers* project their axonal branches (recurrent and transverse collateral branches) for short distances probably restricted to the confines of a cluster of vertical columns. The *subcortical association fibers* form bundles of fibers, called *arcuate* or *U association fiber bundles*, which pass from a cortical area of one gyrus to an area of an adjacent gyrus. These fibers course in an arc within the white matter deep and transverse to the sulcus between the gyri. Fibers do not pass lengthwise along the long axis of a gyrus. Some fascicles of arcuate fibers may extend deep to two or three sulci before terminating in the cortex.

The *long association fibers* form several named intrahemispheric bundles composed of both short and long fibers: superior longitudinal fasciculus, arcuate fasciculus, cingulum, superior occipitofrontal fasciculus, inferior occipitofrontal fasciculus, inferior longitudinal fasciculus, uncinate fasciculus, cingulum, and vertical occipital fasciculus. The fiber components of each fasciculus are organized precisely. The fibers originating from a limited area project and terminate in definite regions of the cortex. These regions of termination are usually located within cytoarchitecturally delimited zone(s) within a Brodmann area(s); this indicates that each Brodmann area projects fibers in an organized pattern to other Brodmann areas.

The *superior longitudinal fasciculus* interconnects most of the frontal lobe with the parietal and occipital lobes; the main mass of the fasciculus is located just above the insula and lateral to projection fibers of the internal capsule. The *arcuate fasciculus* is an extension of the superior longitudinal fasciculus which arcs around the insula and extends into the temporal lobe. The *cingulum* is a bundle of short and long fibers extending from the subcallosal and orbitofrontal areas, continuing through the cingulate gyrus, paralleling the corpus callosum and after curving around the splenium terminating in the parahippocampal gyrus, temporal pole, and basal occipital region. The superior occipitofrontal fasciculus is located roughly between the cingulum and the internal capsule; it interconnects the occipital and temporal cortical areas with the frontal and insular cortex. The *inferior occipitofrontal fasciculus* interconnects the inferior part of the frontal lobe with the temporal and occipital lobes; the main mass of the bundle passes beneath the lenticular nucleus and insula. The *uncinate fasciculus* is a compact arc of fibers which interconnects the cortex of the basal frontal lobe with the cortex of the temporal pole. The *inferior longitudinal fasciculus* is a fiber bundle extending from the temporal lobe to the occipital lobe. Posteriorly it is superficial to the optic radiations. Both the uncinate fasciculus and the inferior longitudinal fasciculus can be considered to be portions of the inferior occipitofrontal fasciculus. The *vertical occipital fasciculus* consists of fibers connecting the inferior parietal lobule and adjacent occipital lobe with the caudal portions of the temporal gyri and adjacent occipital cortex.

Commissural, or interhemispheric, fibers

The commissural fibers are pyramidal cell axons that generally interconnect an area of one hemisphere with its counterpart area of the contralateral hemisphere. They form the corpus callosum, anterior commissure, commissure of the fornix, and habenular commissure.

The corpus callosum is the massive commissure interconnecting most of the neocortical areas of one hemisphere with the other hemisphere (see Fig. 16-2; see also Fig. 1-25). The primary visual cortex (area 17), somatosensory cortex (areas 3, 1, and 2), part of the primary auditory cortex (area 41), and the regions of the motor cortex serving the upper and lower extremities (area 4) give rise to and receive few, if any, callosal fibers. The face, pectoral girdle, trunk, and pelvic girdle regions of the motor cortex (area 4) are the sites of the origin and termination of many callosal fibers. The fibers of the corpus callosum originate from pyramidal cells with cell bodies in laminae II to VI; they terminate in all laminae in a column in the contralateral cerebral cortex (see Fig. 16-10).

Callosal fibers may have many collateral branches in addition to those terminating in the several locales of the cortex (Fig. 16-10). This extensive collateralization may include projection fibers, which may terminate in the corpus striatum of either the same or the opposite side. Some projection fibers from the cortex may pass successively through the corpus callosum and internal capsule before terminating in the subcortical centers; these fibers do not have any collateral branches that terminate in the cortex.

The anterior commissure interconnects portions of the paleocortex and neocortex. The paleocortical regions connected by this commissure include the cerebral cortex medial to the rhinal sulcus. In humans there are, at the most, only sparse anterior commissural fiber connections between the amygdaloid bodies, olfactory bulbs, and anterior perforated substances of the two sides. A shift occurred during evolution so that in human beings, the anterior commissure is primarily a neocortical commissure. It interconnects neocortical areas which are not interconnected by the corpus callosum. Thus the anterior commissure is mainly a commissure for the neo-cortex of the anterior temporal cortex, which includes portions of the superior, middle, and inferior temporal gyri and the inferotemporal visual area of each side.

The *commissure of the fornix (of the hippocampus,* Chap. 15) consists of fibers that originate in the hippocampus, pass through the fimbria of the fornix, decussate across the midline (ventral to the splenium of the corpus callosum), pass through the fimbria, and terminate in the contralateral hippocampus. This is a commissure of the archicortex (see Fig. 15-3).

The habenular commissure consists of fibers of the stria medullaris thalami crossing to the contralateral habenular nucleus (see Fig. 15-8). Some fibers passing through the commissure are said to interconnect the habenular nuclei or the amygdaloid body or the hippocampal formation.

Projection fibers

The projection fibers include (1) the descending (corticofugal) pathways which originate in the cortex (axons of pyramidal cells) and project to the nuclei of the basal ganglia, diencephalon, brainstem, and spinal cord; and (2) the ascending (corticopetal) pathways which mainly originate from diencephalic nuclei, project to, and terminate in the cortex (see Fig. 16-14). These projection fibers are funneled through the fornix, external capsule, and internal capsule. The fornix conveys fibers to and from the hippocampus and subiculum (Chap. 15). The external capsule is partly made up of fibers projecting to the corpus striatum (corticostriate fibers) and to the brainstem tegmentum (corticotegmental, corticoreticular, or corticobulbar fibers). The internal capsule is the main "highway" for input to and output from the cerebral cortex.

The nonspecific fibers from the intralaminar thalamic nuclei and the monaminergic fibers from brainstem nuclei pass through all limbs of the internal capsule. Each nonspecific fiber terminates in all cortical laminae with spreads up to and possibly exceeding 3 mm. In contrast, specific thalamic fibers terminate within columns in laminae III and IV with spreads of only 200 to 500 μm. Fibers from the locus coeruleus ascend successively through the brainstem, tegmentum, external capsule, and subcortical white matter before arborizing in all laminae of the en-

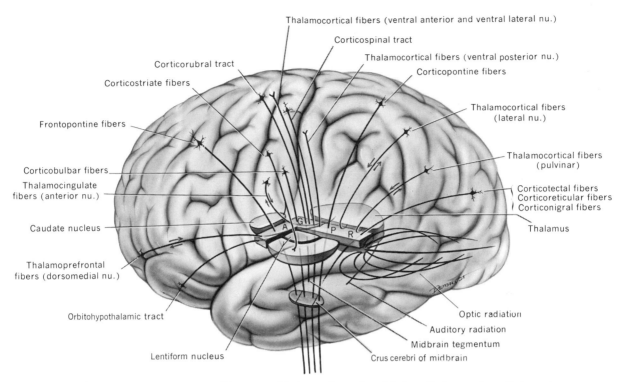

FIGURE 16-14 Some component fiber tracts of the internal capsule and their cortical connections. Reciprocal projections between a thalamic nucleus and a cortical area are indicated by arrows pointing in two directions. The nuclei refer to nuclei of the thalamus. A, anterior limb; G, genu; P, posterior limb; R, retrolenticular portion of the posterior limb.

Labels in figure:
- Thalamocortical fibers (ventral anterior and ventral lateral nu.)
- Corticospinal tract
- Corticorubral tract
- Thalamocortical fibers (ventral posterior nu.)
- Corticostriate fibers
- Corticopontine fibers
- Thalamocortical fibers (lateral nu.)
- Frontopontine fibers
- Thalamocortical fibers (pulvinar)
- Corticobulbar fibers
- Corticotectal fibers
- Thalamocingulate fibers (anterior nu.)
- Corticoreticular fibers
- Corticonigral fibers
- Caudate nucleus
- Thalamus
- Thalamoprefrontal fibers (dorsomedial nu.)
- Orbitohypothalamic tract
- Optic radiation
- Auditory radiation
- Lentiform nucleus
- Midbrain tegmentum
- Crus cerebri of midbrain

tire cerebral cortex. These coerulean fibers have collateral branches that innervate large portions of the diencephalon. After entering the cortex the fibers curve and then travel with a longitudinal trajectory from a more frontal location caudally. Thus, this coeruleocortical system parallels the horizontally continuous lamina of the cortex. In effect, the tangential noradrenergic fibers intersect the radially oriented array of cortical columns, thereby furnishing this projection with the capacity to modulate neuronal activity crossing cytoarchitectural and functional boundaries.

FUNCTIONAL CIRCUITRY OF THE CORTICAL NEURONS

The cortex has been classically conceived as being organized both in horizontal and vertical zones. An expression of the horizontal organization is subdivision into the laminae in the archicortex, paleocortex, and neocortex. The vertical organization is implied in the parcellation into cortical areas by Campbell (1906), Brodmann, von Economo, and the Vogts. These patterns of organization are primarily based on cyto- and myeloarchitectural criteria and only somewhat on functional correlates.

In recent years it has been demonstrated that the areas of parcellation of the neocortex are organized into neurophysiologically defined columns about 200 to 500 μm in diameter (width). These columns are known as ocular dominance and orientation columns in the primary visual cortex (area 17) (Chap. 12; Hubel and Wiesel) and the "tactile" and related columns of the somesthetic cortex (areas 3, 1, and 2) (Montcastle). These sensory columns are, in a way, a further refinement of the grosser parcellation of the cortical areas of Brodmann into smaller units.

Vertical or columnar organization Microelectrode studies of the primary somesthetic cortex (areas 3, 1, and 2) lead to the concept that the elementary organization of the cortex is a "column" of neurons (from one to several neurons thick) oriented vertically to the cortical surface (see Fig. 16-10 and 16-11). Many vertical cylinders of neurons constitute this cortical area. The primary visual cortex (area 17), the primary auditory cortex (areas 41, 42), and the primary motor cortex (area 4) are also organized as vertical columns of neurons. These vertical columns of neurons are connected with other areas of the cortex by association fibers and with subcortical nuclei by projection fibers. Each electrophysiologically defined column of neurons may be considered to be the ultimate in cortical parcellation.

The columns are not simple geometric arrangements but complexes of neurons and neuronal circuits. There is a morphologic basis for the cylindric columns of different sizes. The afferent fibers to the cortex terminate in cylindric spreads. Those from cells in the specific thalamic nuclei arborize in a plexus of about 200 to 500 μm in diameter, while the nonspecific thalamic afferent fibers terminate in spreads up to 3 mm in diameter. The pyramidal cells have dendrites which radiate from the central axis of the cell body and main shaft of the apical dendrite. The horizontal spread of the basilar dendrites and distal branches of the apical dendrites range from 150 to 300 μm (Figs. 16-9, 16-11, and 16-13), although spreads of 500 μm for the apical dendrites and 600 μm for the basilar dendrites have been reported. The axons of the stellate cells, Martinotti cells, and fusiform cells are generally oriented vertically within the cortex. They provide the essential circuitry for a vertical column.

The general organization of the fibers conveying input to and output from the cortex is consistent with the cortical columnar organization. Although the afferent fibers to the cortex form fasciculi which enter the cortical sheet at an angle (see Fig. 16-10), each afferent fiber, as noted above, terminates in a cylindric arborization. The efferent fibers emerge from the cortex as fasciculi oriented perpendicular to the neocortex (see Fig. 16-11).

Two-neuron and three-neuron loops

In theory the simplest loop that involves cortical neurons is a *two-neuron chain*. Such a loop, or circuit, would include a neuron with its cell body in the thalamus and a pyramidal neuron with its cell body in the cerebral cortex. The thalamic neuron from a specific thalamic nucleus synapses with a pyramidal cell that projects to a subcortical nucleus (see Fig. 16-12). In the analogy with the spinal arc, this thalamic neuron is comparable to a spinal ganglion neuron, and the pyramidal cell is the equivalent of the anterior horn motor cell of the spinal cord.

The pyramidal cell is integrated into another loop. The recurrent axon collateral (and the horizontal collateral) branch of each pyramidal cell feeds back and synapses with one (or more) of the stellate interneurons that, in turn, may synapse with the original pyramidal neuron. This circuit is similar to the spinal cord circuit, with the stellate interneuron playing a role similar to that of the Renshaw interneuron (Chap. 5). The essence of a *three-neuron chain* can be constructed from the sequence of thalamic afferent neuron to interneuron stellate cell to cortical pyramidal cell (see Fig. 16-12).

Column of the neocortex

The concept of the neocortex being parcelled into functional columns of from 200 to 500 μm in width is gaining acceptance. At present, two theories have been proposed regarding the basic definition of a column: (1) column based on thalamic input and (2) column based on association (corticocortical) fiber input.

Columns based on thalamic input are derived primarily from investigations of the primary visual cortex (Hubel and Wiesel) and the primary somesthetic cortex (Montcastle). The orientation columns and dominance columns of the visual cortex (Chap. 12) and of the sensory columns of the somesthetic cortex are delineated primarily by the afferent fiber projections from specific thalamic nuclei (lateral geniculate body and ventral posterior nucleus). In each thalamic-based cortical column, afferent fibers enter the cortex and terminate by arborizing in lamina IV and portions of lamina III (see Figs. 16-11 and 16-12). Microelectrode studies of the primary somesthetic cortex (areas 3, 1, and 2) are consistent with the concept that the elementary organization of the cortex is a column oriented vertically to the cortical surface (see Fig. 16-11). Many vertical columns constitute this cortical area. A specific column is activated by one and only one of the following stimuli: (1) movements of groups of hairs, (2) pressure on the skin, and (3) deformation of the tissues deep to the skin from a specific "spot" of the body. These columns are formed by the specific thalamic afferent fibers, each of which has an arborization spread within lamina IV of 200 to 500 μm—the width of a cortical column. In turn, the neuronal connections made by these afferent fibers with the local circuit neurons and the pyramidal cells form the core circuitry of these "sensory" columns. Whether the thalamic input is the primary basis has been questioned, in part, because the lower portions of the temporal lobe cortex—the "athalamic cortex"—receive no specific thalamic input (see Fig. 13-6).

Columns based on corticocortical input are derived primarily from recent studies of the nature of patterns of termination of corticocortical (association and commissural) fibers (see Fig. 16-10). This concept is applicable to all areas of the neocortex because all regions receive corticocortical input and all regions project to other cortical regions. This input terminates in all laminae in 200- to 300-μm wide columns (see next section for further details).

Organization of a corticocortical column (Szentágothai)

General statement Each corticocortical column is delineated primarily on the pattern of termination of the association and commissural fibers within the cortex. These fibers to each column originate from several cortical regions of both the ipsilateral and contralateral cerebral hemispheres (see Fig. 16-10). These columns are commonly of from 200 to 300 μm in diameter (range 120 to 500 μm). They are considered to be a cardinal feature of the mammalian cortex. Columnar organization reflects the pattern of intercortical fiber distribution that occurs in *all* types of cortices—namely, specific sensory, specific motor, association, and limbic cortex. It also ap-

plies to the short-U association fibers interconnecting neighboring gyri (Goldman and Nauta). These columns are present in such diverse mammals as rodents (rat), carnivores (cat), and primates (monkey). From either a small focal site or an extended area of cortex, corticocortical fibers project to many cortical targets; each of these targets constitutes a column (see Fig. 16-10).

These columns do not apparently overlap significantly, indicating that the cortex is *not* composed of a continuously shifting overlap of adjacent afferent fiber arborizations. A strong argument supporting the thesis that the corticocortical fibers are the substrates for the basic cortical circuitry and are the unifying morphologic construct of a column is the fact that roughly 99 percent of the afferent fibers entering the cortex are corticocortical axons. Only 1 percent of cortical afferents originate from cells in the thalamus or other subcortical regions.

The ipsilateral association fibers arise from pyramidal cells with cell bodies in laminae II and III, while commissural fibers arise from pyramidal cells in laminae II through VI. Each branch of a corticocortical fiber enters and passes vertically through a column with its side terminals extending laterally within each laminae. The spread in lamina I usually exceeds the width of the column (see Fig. 16-10).

The other input in the cortex is derived from the thalamus and the brainstem. With the possible exception of the "athalamic" lower temporal cortex, all neocortical areas receive input from specific thalamic nuclei via topographically organized thalamocortical fibers passing through the corona radiata. These fibers make monosynaptic excitatory contacts primarily with dendritic spines of spiny stellate and pyramidal cells within laminae IV and portions of III (Fig. 16-9A). The terminal arborization of a specific afferent fiber outlines a disk in laminae III and IV. Many cortical cells receive their main excitatory input from only one to possibly several specific fibers. Some synapses are made with nonspiny segments of the dendrites. The recurrent collaterals of pyramidal cells make excitatory synaptic contacts with local circuit neurons and with both apical and basilar dendrites of pyramidal cells. Most synapses within the cortex are "en passant" contacts.

Nonspecific fibers from the intralaminar thalamic nuclei terminate in laminae II through VI. The axons of cells in the locus coerleus ascend through the brainstem tegmentum, external capsule, and corona radiata to the cortex, where they branch and form collaterals located in all laminae in all cortical areas. These fibers have numerous regularly spaced varicosities. They terminate as T branches in lamina I.

The neurons within a column have been conceived as being organized into microcolumns (micromodules) by Szentágothai (Fig. 16-9A). Although many details of the synaptic connections within the circuitry of a column have not been resolved, the general outline of micromodules has a neuroanatomic and neurophysiologic basis. The excitatory corticocortical and thalamocortical inputs are integrated and processed through a columnar-oriented circuitry composed of excitatory and inhibitory neurons. The circuitry is directed to the pyramidal cells that are the discharge cells of the cortex whose axons convey excitatory influences to other cortical areas via association and commissural fibers and to other regions of the brain and spinal cord via projection fibers.

Excitatory modules within a column (Figs. 16-9 and 16-10) Each corticocortical fiber and its horizontal branches are distributed within the entire 200- to 300-μm width of the cylindrical column. Each afferent fiber from a specific thalamic nuclear cell has a terminal spatial pattern outlining a 300-μm diameter cylinder in laminae III and IV. This cylinder is located in two or more corticocortical columns. These excitatory fibers synapse with spiny stellate, microgliaform, and pyramidal cells. The *spiny stellate cells* are, according to their axonal distribution, of two types (Fig. 16-9). The first has an axon that bifurcates into an ascending and descending branch; each branch has a spatial arborization pattern outlining vertically oriented cylinders within laminae II and III (ascending branch) or within laminae V and VI (descending branch). The second has only an ascending axon with a spatial arborization pattern outlining a vertical cylinder in laminae II and III. Each *microgliaform cell* has a descending axon with a spatial arborization pattern outlining a vertical cylinder in laminae V and VI.

The cylinders formed by these axon terminals are roughly 30 μm in diameter. Each *double bouquet cell* has an axon that bifurcates into an ascending branch and a descending branch. The two branches have spatial arborization patterns outlining a vertical cylinder of about 10 μm in diameter and extending through laminae II through VI.

These putative excitatory local circuit neurons with their specialized distribution channels do form functional linkages that probably fractionate the input from widely dispersed afferents (each input fiber arborizes widely) to smaller microcolumns. In this way the circuitry selectively distributes neuron messages to subregions of the pyramidal cells and to the putative inhibitory cells of the inhibitory modules.

Inhibitory modules within a column (Fig. 16-9) The putative inhibitory neurons are so distributed as to exert inhibitory influences on selected segments of the pyramidal cells that are the excitatory output neurons of the cerebral cortex. According to Szentágothai's schema:

1. The main axon of an *axonal tufted cell* has a spatial arborization pattern outlining a flat cylinder in lamina I; its axon synapses with the branches of apical dendrites.
2. The main axon of a *chandelier cell* has a spatial arborization pattern outlining a flat cylinder; its axon terminals form serial synapses with the smooth portions of the shaft of an apical dendrite.
3. The main axon of an *axoaxonic cell* branches into a number of terminals, each of which forms serial axoaxonic synapses on different pyramidal cell axons in the region near the initial segment (trigger zone).
4. Each *basket cell* has an axon that branches into terminals, each of which forms several synapses in the form of a basket spray on the cell body of a pyramidal cell.

The outline of the spatial arborization patterns may be roughly a cube (100 μm on a side) in lamina II, a rectangular prism extending through laminae III, IV, and V (25 to 50 μm wide, 500 μm vertical side, and 500 to 1000 μm horizontal side) and a flat cylinder in lamina VI (50 μm in diameter). In this exquisite arrangement inhibitory influences are directed to different sectors of the apical and basilar dendrites and so differentially modulate and regulate the output of the pyramidal neurons (Fig. 16-9*B*).

Role of columnar organization

Two concepts for the role of the columnar organization connected by corticocortical fibers have been proposed. (1) Each column may be a unit in a system of columns with each column having closely related properties (e.g., orientation columns). Each entire system may be organized to process this specific information to a level for its utilization by one or more higher ordered macrosystems. (2) Each column may be a unit of a group or groups of columns organized to bring together several different types of information; these columns are presumed to have the role of integrating and elaborating a variety of functional properties. In this conceptualization, the interconnected columns are expressions of multichannel patterns of pathways that bring together various forms of content for further processing.

The linkage of cortical columns via corticocortical interconnections in the major visual cortical areas of the monkey gives an example of the probable role of the columnar organization (Wong-Riley). The corticocortical fibers entering the visual association areas terminate largely in laminae IV and in lesser degrees in the other laminae of cortical columns. This termination pattern resembles, in part, the thalamocortical (geniculostriate) projections that terminate primarily in lamina IV in a columnar pattern in the primary visual cortex. Apparently the vertical columns are the morphologic and functional units that process information and then can relate and communicate through corticocortical fibers with other columns in several functionally related areas of the cortex. The corticocortical fibers are the intercolumnar pathways linking the major visual cortical areas of both hemispheres with precise, topographical, and reciprocal connections. Again, this resembles, in part, the thalamocortical reciprocity where the primary visual cortex is precisely topographically and reciprocally connected with the lateral geniculate body. Following neuronal processing within each column the information is transferred to the pyramidal cells; these cells are the output units of the column through which the processed signals are conveyed from the column via projection, association, and commissure fibers.

NEUROPHYSIOLOGY OF CORTEX AND ELECTROENCEPHALOGRAM

The neurophysiologic activity of the brain induces variations in the electrical potentials that can be recorded with electrodes placed on the surface of the scalp. The record of these voltage shifts is known as an *electroencephalogram* (EEG). The fluctuating potential differences on the unshaven scalp surface usually range between such minute amounts as 50- to 100-millionth of a volt (microvolts). This is about one-tenth of the voltage induced by the heart on the body surface (electrocardiographic potentials of the ECG). From the EEG record of a patient lying quietly in bed in semidarkness, an encephalographer can tell if a patient is awake, asleep, or excited.

The brain waves recorded by the electroencephalogram are largely produced by the electrical activity at the axosomatic synapses, axodendritic synapses, and the all-or-none axon potentials in the cerebral cortex. These scalp surface recordings are the result of the algebraic summation of the excitatory postsynaptic potentials (deplorization), inhibitory postsynaptic potentials (hyperpolarization), and the axon spike (all-or none) potentials in the cerebral cortex. These activities are, in turn, influenced by the complex interactions derived from such subcortical stations as the specific thalamic nuclei and nonspecific thalamic nuclei, and from other cortical areas. The critical nature of the need of thalamic input for the maintenance of cortical rhythms, as recorded electrophysiologically, is demonstrated by the observation that rhythmicity of cortical neurons disappears following the deafferentation of the cortex. Such deafferentation denies the cortex of its thalamic influences.

The encephalogram is produced by the amplified electrical activity recorded as movement of a pen on a slowly moving sheet of paper. The EEG of an adult, like a fingerprint, is characteristic for the individual under standard conditions. However, it varies according to the state of the individual, i.e., alert, startled, drowsy, dreaming, or in deep sleep. The rhythms of children are less stable. The EEG pattern varies from one area to another area and from one person to another person.

The brain waves (rhythms) are described in terms of amplitude (in microvolts, one-millionth of a volt) and of frequency (number of oscillations or waves per second). When the subject is awake, frequencies of about 10 per second constitute a normal rhythm. This is the alpha rhythm of the EEG. This alpha rhythm is a high-voltage, slow-frequency rhythm (HVS) of 50 mV at a frequency of 8 to 14 per second. This rhythm is most prominent in the occipital region when the eyes are closed and is poorest in the frontal region. When an individual is alert, this resting alpha rhythm is replaced by an irregular, reduced-amplitude, rapid oscillation (desynchronization of alpha rhythm or alpha blocking) called the beta pattern. This rhythm is present during states of attention and problem solving. The beta rhythm is a low-voltage, fast-frequency rhythm (LVF) of 5 to 10 mV at a frequency of from 15 to 30 per second. This is most prominent in the frontal and parietal regions. The HVS activity is referred to as a "synchronized" EEG pattern, and the LVF activity is called a "desynchronized" EEG or "activation" pattern.

The desynchronization of the alpha rhythm to the beta rhythm results from activation. It can be induced by a set of stimuli that produces sudden arousal. This arousal reaction is probably produced by ascending reticular system activity. Visual stimuli and alerting stimuli desynchronize the alpha rhythm to the beta pattern. Mental concentration can abolish the alpha rhythm. Beta rhythms are present at birth; the alpha rhythms generally are not found until about 9 years of age. The typical adult EEG pattern is usually established at about 17 or 18 years of age.

The complexity of the EEG patterns is largely regulated by subcortical activity (Chap. 13). Although the details of the factors responsible for these cortical rhythms are not fully known, this rhythmicity is dependent on the integrity of the thalamus. As previously stated, the cortex deprived of thalamic connections exhibits no rhythmic patterns. Rhythms generated in thalamic reticular nuclei project their influences through the unspecific thalamocortical pathways utilizing recruiting activity (Chap. 3). Only after several (8 to 10) electrical stimuli are applied to thalamic reticular nuclei is the maximal effect recorded upon the cortex, apparently largely through axodendritic synapses of the stellate and pyramidal cells.

SLEEP

Normal consciousness is a state of psychologic awareness of the environment, sensations, and the self. Wakefulness, perception, and cognition are some of the qualities generally associated with consciousness. On the basis of subjective criteria, sleep seems to be quite different from the wakeful state. This is not so, for sleep is essentially an altered expression of consciousness. In one sense, sleep is a state of diminished consciousness in which, as compared to wakefulness, there is a change in the quality of the reactivity of the brain to events in the environment. During sleep mental activity does not cease and the capability to discriminate is retained. Actually the brain is not unaware. For example, even the muted cry of her baby will readily arouse the sleeping mother, whereas repetitive or insignificant, fairly loud sounds may not noticeably affect her sleep at all. Although sleep is essential for our well-being, the basic biologic significance of sleep is, as yet, unresolved.

The brain is often considered to be an organ that wants to sleep. This altered state of consciousness has been conceived as being induced (1) passively through the deprivation of sensory input (passive theory of sleep), or (2) actively through "sleep centers" (active theory of sleep). The two theories are not mutually exclusive.

Before 1950, sleep was thought to be primarily a passive phenomenon associated with a marked decrease in the amount of stimulation. According to this concept, the brain is said to fall asleep when it is not excited. The nature of the sensory influences conveyed from the periphery to the cerebrum via the ascending reticular pathways (Chap. 8) has profound effects on the sleep-wake cycle. When the cerebrum is deprived of this input by large lesions in the midbrain reticular formation, there is a drastic reduction in the sensory input to the cerebrum.

Patients and animals with such lesions are behaviorally and electrophysiologically (i.e., as seen in the EEG rhythm) in a permanent sleep state. In these preparations, the cerebrum, although lacking reticular input, presumably receives all the lemniscal input from the brainstem and spinal cord and sensory input from the olfactory and visual systems.

It is now known that sleep is the expression of active phenomena occurring within the brain. The activity of subcortical neuronal pools accounts for the rhythms expressed by the EEG during sleep (Chap. 13). Electrical stimulation of certain "hypnogenic regions" within the thalamus induces sleep; damage to such regions produces permanently awake, insomniac animals. Low-frequency stimulation of a "hypnogenic region" results in a sleeping animal, whereas high-frequency stimulation (about 100 Hz) in the same region arouses the sleeping animal to the awakened state. Low-frequency stimulation is comparable to the sleep induced following the rhythmic stimulation of vestibular receptors by the gentle to-and-fro motion of the rocking chair.

REM and NREM sleep

Sleep is not a unitary but rather a complex, multifaceted phenomenon. On the basis of electroencephalographic (EEG) behavior and psychologic criteria, two major types of sleep are recognized: rapid eye movement (REM) sleep and nonrapid eye movement (NREM or non-REM) sleep. The various types and stages of sleep can be differentiated from one another by differences (1) in the EEG wave patterns, (2) in behavior as expressed by somatic and autonomic activities and by the stimulus intensities required to awaken the sleeping subject, and (3) in psychologic manifestations of dreams and sensations related by an individual after arousal.

REM sleep is characterized by bursts of rapid conjugate eye movements accompanied by fluttering of the eyelids. It is called paradoxic sleep or behavioral sleep because the EEG exhibits a low-voltage fast EEG wave pattern (20 to 30 Hz), which is similar to that found in the aroused or awakened state. During REM sleep, vivid dreaming occurs, the heart rate and blood pressure are elevated, respiration is irregular and increased, and muscle tone is completely abolished. Cerebral blood flow is greater during dream sleep than during the waking state.

NREM or regular sleep is also called slow-wave sleep because the EEG potentials have a high-voltage, slow (1 to 10 Hz) wave pattern activity. During NREM sleep, the heart rate and blood pressure are somewhat reduced, respiratory rate is slow and regular, the pupil is constricted, and the motility and secretory activity of the gastrointestinal tract are normal. The somatic muscles are relaxed. Monosynaptic reflexes are slightly depressed. The antigravity muscles (e.g., neck, back, and extensors of the lower extremities) have less tone than those in the awake subject.

NREM sleep is divided into four stages. Stage 1 is characterized by slow rolling eye movements, regular respiration, drowsiness, decreased heart rate, and 7- to 10-Hz low-voltage EEG wave patterns. Stage 2 is characterized by light sleep from which the subject is readily aroused and by 3- to 7-Hz low-voltage EEG wave patterns with bursts of 12- to 14-Hz sleep spindles. (So-called K complexes occur; they are high-voltage bursts of waves before or after a sleep spindle.) Stage 3 is characterized by moderate-depth sleep, slow heartbeat, reduced blood pressure, constricted pupils, slightly depressed monosynaptic reflexes, and 1- to 2-Hz high-voltage EEG wave patterns with a few sleep spindles. Stage 4 is characterized by deep sleep, with 1- to 3-Hz high-voltage EEG wave patterns, which is similar to that occurring in a coma.

Sleep has rhythmicity. A normal night's sleep consists of from four to six sleep cycles. Each cycle lasts about $1\frac{1}{2}$ h and consists of an NREM period followed by a REM period. In an average sleep cycle an individual spends a few minutes in the "half-awake, half-asleep" lightest phase of sleep (stage 1) before reaching the "medium" kind of sleep (stage 2). Later the subject passes into the deep-sleep phases (stages 3 and 4) and then gradually eases into REM sleep. Stages 3 and 4 are thought to be the most restorative and recuperative sleep periods. The relative time spent by an average young adult in each of the stages of one cycle may be divided roughly as follows: 5 percent in stage 1 NREM, 50 percent in stage 2 NREM, 20 percent in stages 3 and 4 NREM, and 25 percent in the REM stage. The REM period of the first cycle is usually the shortest, lasting no more than 5 min (it may even be absent). The later REM periods may last from 30 to 60 min. Most NREM sleep occurs during the first third of a night's sleep, while most REM sleep takes place during the last third of sleep.

Ontogeny of sleep

The character of sleep changes with age. On the average, premature infants spend about 18 h per day in active sleep. This is reduced to about 12 to 16 h in the neonate, to about 8 h in the adolescent and young adult, and to less than 6 h in old age. The relative amount of NREM to REM sleep also shifts with age; neonates divide their sleep time equally between REM and NREM sleep, whereas old subjects spend only an hour in REM sleep. During REM sleep, babies grimace and smile in bursts; their rapid eye movements can be observed under the eyelids. The neonate and young child have a polyphasic sleep-wake pattern in which a sleep period alternates with an awake period. The newborn infant has about seven of these sleep-wake cycles, which alternate fairly regularly during a 24-h period. By the age of 4 this has been modified into a long night's sleep period supplemented by an afternoon nap. This grades into the monophasic sleep pattern of one sleep period per 24-h day. It is not certain whether this ontogenetic change from polyphasic to monophasic sleep is induced by learning or is a natural inborn maturation phenomenon.

Functional considerations of the sleep cycle

REM sleep is the dream stage. When awakened during this stage, four out of five individuals will describe a vivid, active dream colored by much imagery and some fantasies. Powerful inhibitory influences are exerted upon the lower motor neurons during REM sleep; this is a true paralysis, expressed by a marked decrease in the spontaneous and reflex somatic motor activity. The difficulty in making rapid movements (e.g., running) in a dream imagery is presumably the consequence of these inhibitory influences. REM sleep is the deepest state of sleep; it is more difficult to awaken a sleeping individual from REM sleep than from any of the NREM sleep stages.

Dreams with slight, if any, imagery may be experienced during NREM sleep. When awak-

ened from this type of sleep, the aroused individual may describe a dream related to thought processes or experiences associated with mental activity.

Normally, there is a reduction in gastric secretions during sleep. In contrast, patients with chronic duodenal ulcers experience an increase in gastric acid secretion during REM sleep. Individuals afflicted with nocturnal migrane headaches almost always experience these headaches upon waking during or just following REM sleep. Alcohol, tranquilizers, and sleeping pills inhibit the amount of REM sleep.

Somnambulism, enuresis (bedwetting), and frightening nightmare attacks (of the type associated with a suffocating feeling and terror) occur, surprisingly, during NREM sleep stage 4, not during REM sleep. These phenomena are not thought to be manifestations of dreams.

The serotoninergic neurons with cell bodies in the brainstem raphe nuclei (Chap. 8) may have a significant role in the sleep-wake cycle. The destruction of these serotoninergic neurons results in an animal that is almost continuously awake. Animals treated with drugs which elevate the serotonin levels of the brain experience an increase in the duration of the NREM stage and a reduction in the amount of the REM state. Serotonin may be involved with triggering REM sleep. Norepinephrine is believed to mediate REM sleep.

PRIMARY AND SECONDARY SENSORY AREAS

The areas of the cerebral cortex with the most direct afferent connections with the peripheral sensors are called the primary and secondary sensory areas (see Figs. 16-15 and 16-16). The primary somesthetic area is located in the postcentral gyrus (areas 1, 2, and 3); the primary visual area, in the cortex on both sides of the calcarine sulcus (area 17); the primary auditory area, in the transverse gyri of Heschl (areas 41, 42); the primary gustatory area, in the ventral part of the postcentral gyrus (area 43); the "primary vestibular area," probably in the temporal lobe near the primary auditory cortex; and the primary olfactory cortex, in the cortex in the region of the uncus.

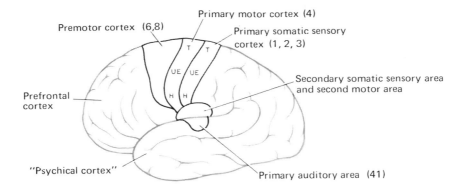

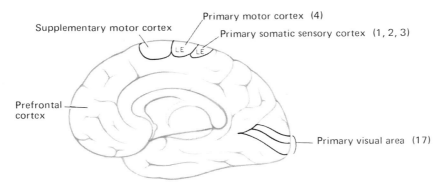

FIGURE 16-15 The location of several functional areas of the cerebral cortex. The representation of body parts on the primary motor and somatic sensory cortices includes the head (H), upper extremity (UE), trunk (T), and lower extremity (LE). Numbers represent areas of Brodmann.

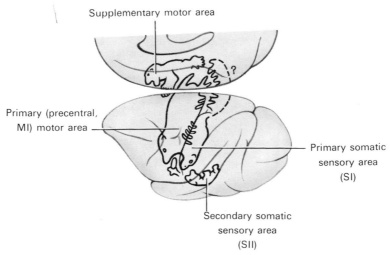

FIGURE 16-16 Some motor and sensory areas of the monkey cortex, with somatotopic representation. The upper portion represents the medial aspect. (*After Woolsey.*)

The secondary sensory areas are smaller than the primary sensory areas (see Fig. 16-16). Whereas ablation of the primary sensory areas results in dramatic deficits in sensory appreciation, the ablation of the secondary areas results in slight, if any, deficits. Information on the secondary sensory areas in humans is scant. A secondary somatic sensory area (somatic area II) is located in the cortex just above the lateral sulcus in the precentral and postcentral gyrus; a probable secondary auditory area (auditory area II) is located near the primary auditory area; and a probable secondary visual area (visual area II) is located on the lateral surface somewhere anterior to the primary visual cortex in areas 17 and 18.

Except for the olfactory cortex, the primary sensory area and the secondary sensory area receive their main input from the specific thalamic relay nuclei (ventral posterior nucleus, lateral geniculate body, and medial geniculate body). The primary olfactory cortex receives its input from the olfactory bulb.

PARIETAL LOBE

The parietal lobe has a major role in the higher-level processing of the general sensory modalities and in the integration of neural data from the auditory, visual, and somesthetic cortical areas; it has a lesser role in motor activities.

Primary somesthetic area (areas 1, 2, and 3)

The postcentral gyrus or the primary receptive somesthetic area (areas 1, 2, and 3, primary somatic sensory area, somatic area 1, Sl) receives its input from the ventral posterior nucleus of the thalamus. This primary projection area has a somatotopic localization pattern in the form of a sensory figurine (see Fig. 16-16). The amount of cortical area associated with a body area is proportional to the sensory innervation density of the body area rather than to the size of the area (e.g., lips, tongue, and thumb have a relatively large representation). Area 2 responds to stimuli from the deep tissues of the body, especially to movements of joints; this is significant for the appreciation of movement and position sense.

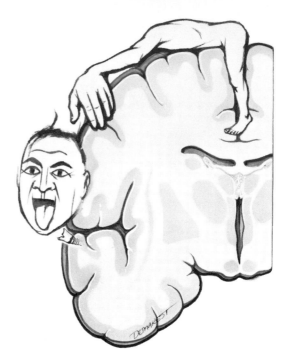

FIGURE 16-17 A motor homunculus on the precentral gyrus. It shows the somatotopic localization of motor activity (following focal cortical stimulation). The sensory homunculus has a similar configuration.

Area 3 responds to cutaneous stimuli. Most of the neurons of the ventral posterior thalamic nucleus project to area 3, and a lesser number to area 1. Most of the axons projecting to area 2 are apparently the collateral branches projecting to areas 3 and 1. The primary somesthetic area is often called a sensorimotor structure. This is so because 80 percent of the electric stimulations of its cortex in the awake human evoke sensations, while the remaining 20 percent evoke motor responses. Some fibers from this area project to such thalamic nuclei as the ventral posterior, ventral lateral, and reticular nuclei.

Some fibers originating in the postcentral gyrus descend via the pyramidal tract before terminating in the nuclei of the ascending pathways (refer to "Reflected Descending Fibers," later on in this chapter). These include the nuclei gracilis and cuneatus of the posterior column-medial lemniscal pathway. It is through these descending fibers that the somesthetic area influences this ascending pathway. This may explain why a monkey, following a lesion of the pyramidal tract, has a deficit in its ability to make certain kinesthetic discriminations.

Taste The primary area for taste is claimed to be located either at the base of the precentral gyrus and postcentral gyrus slightly rostral to the somesthetic area or in the immediate adjoining area of the insula (area 43). Stimulation of these areas may produce gustatory hallucinations.

Secondary somesthetic area

A secondary somesthetic area is apparently located at the base of the postcentral gyrus—occupying the same part of the cortex as the second motor area (Figs. 16-15 and 16-16). This area has been called the secondary somatic sensory area, somatic area II, SII, and supplementary sensory projection area. This area has been located in primates by electrophysiologic techniques and is presumed to be also present in human beings. The somatotypic patterns in this area are less precise than in the primary somesthetic area (somatic area I). The face, mouth, and throat are apparently not represented in the secondary sensory area.

Functional considerations Stimulation of the primary somesthetic area in human subjects evokes sensory effects on the contralateral side of the body. Numbness, absence of sensation, tingling, a feeling of electricity, or a sense of movement may result from focal stimulation. Patients do not inquire whether some object is in contact with the body region where sensation is felt. Actually the sensation is perceived as an unusual rather than a normal experience. Stimulation of somatic sensory area II may evoke sensations similar to those produced by stimulation of the primary somesthetic area except that the sensation may be felt bilaterally. This phenomenon may be explained by the fact that this sensory area receives input from the posterior thalamic region, which, in turn, receives input from both sides of the body.

Ablation of the postcentral gyrus is followed by loss of the finer and more subtle aspects of sensory awareness. When an object is handled (with the eyes closed) the patient can feel it but cannot appreciate its texture, estimate its weight, or gauge slight changes in its temperature. Difficulty is experienced in appreciating the position of one's body or its parts. The crude aspects of the general sensory modalities are apparently sensed in subcortical nuclei. The conscious recognition of pain, temperature, and gross contact sense are apparently functional correlates of the midbrain tectum and the thalamus in humans. Ablation of somatic sensory area II produces no known deficits. The primary receptive cortex integrates the information received from subcortical sources, and it is here that the more complex aspects of touch, deep sensibility, pain, and temperature are sensed. These perceptions include the appreciation of the location and position of a body part; the sensing of the movements of the body; the localization of the source of pain, temperature, and tactile stimuli; and comparison of these sensed modalities with those formerly experienced.

Somesthetic association area

Areas 5, 7, and 40 of the parietal lobe are known as the "somesthetic association area." These areas receive an extensive input from the postcentral gyrus. In addition they have well-developed reciprocal connections (thalamocortical and corticothalamic pathways) with the lateral nuclear group of the thalamus, including the pulvinar (Chap. 13). These areas also make a contribution to the descending pathways through some corticospinal, corticotegmental, and corticopontine fibers. The integration essential to the appreciation of the finer and more discriminative aspects of the somesthetic senses is a functional correlate of the somesthetic association cortex. The expression of this higher-level sensory station is the product of the processing of the information received from the receptive somesthetic cortex and the interaction with the lateral nuclear group of the thalamus.

The parietal associative cortex integrates and correlates impulses associated with the somesthetic modalities and those associated with the auditory, gustatory, and visual senses. The whole complex of associative patterns subserves the individual's knowledge and awareness of the environment. The conceptualization of qualities and quantities utilizes the basic somesthetic modalities. The qualities of shape, form, roughness, smoothness, size, and texture of an object (stereognosis) can be ascertained from a manual examination and can be ascertained from a manual examination and can even be imagined. Quantities that can be deduced include weight, temperature changes, and the degree of pressure sensations. Of great significance is the awareness of body image, of location of body parts, of postural relation of body parts, one to the other, and of one's self. The consciousness of one's physical being is a dimension of the general senses.

Supramarginal gyrus Lesions in area 40, called the supramarginal gyrus, especially on the dominant side, produce deficits in the sphere of higher general sensations—cortical astereognosis and the failure of the so-called *body scheme*. Cortical astereognosis (*tactile agnosia*) is the inability to recognize common objects through cues from the general sensory receptors; it is the failure to appreciate the significance of the sensory stimuli. The agnosia may be in the visual sphere (*visual agnosia*), in the tactile sphere (*tactile agnosia*), or in the auditory sphere (*auditory agnosia*). Agnosia refers to those disturbances in which there is a failure to recognize, to identify, or to discriminate somatic sensory, visual, auditory, smell, or taste information. It is presumed that patients with pure agnosia have no basic deficits within the afferent pathways and in the reception of the primary input at the cerebral cortical level.

When patients with lesions in the supramarginal gyrus feel a watch with the hand on the side opposite the lesions they do not recognize the object as a watch. The intact primary cortex is functional because such patients can tell that the watch is smooth, cold, and light in weight, and they may sense the vibrations of the watch movements. Recognition of position sense and fine discrinination are not impaired. However, in this tactile agnosia the patient is unable to integrate the bits of information into the concept of a watch. The recognition of an object through the general senses requires an intact parietal association cortex, whereas the awareness of the various sensory modalities can be brought into the conscious sphere through subcortical centers and the postcentral gyrus cortex.

A large lesion in the superior parietal cortex usually results in the failure to recognize the body scheme. The recognition of self is impaired. For example, patients with such a lesion may be unaware that the arm on the contralateral side of the lesion is their arm. In some patients the half of the face contralateral to the lesion is denied; that side may not be washed or shaved. Some mild motor effects such as hypotonia may be due to interruption of fibers originating from this area of the cortex and projecting to subcortical nuclei.

Angular gyrus (area 39) and Wernicke's area (area 22) (Fig. 16-15)

Areas 22 and 39 have rich connections with association fibers from the somesthetic (5 and 7), auditory (41 and 42), and visual (18 and 19) association cortex. These cortical areas subserve such complex expressions as the comprehension of the written word and the ability to conceive the symbols of language. The stimulation of these cortical areas in human subjects evokes no effects. A lesion of area 39 in the dominant hemisphere produces dysfunctions indicative of the significant role this part of the cortex has to communication in humans. Words are seen but not recognized (visual agnosia). The comprehension of the written word, whether in script or in type, is lost. This word blindness is expressed as the inability to read (*alexia*) or the inability to copy (*agraphia*). This is a form of *sensory* or *receptive aphasia*. In sensory aphasia, the patient is unable to comprehend the written or spoken language. This visual receptive aphasia is so severe that words written by patients themselves are not recognized as words. Note that area 39 is adjacent to visual association cortex 18.

Bilateral lesions of the angular gyrus may produce a disorientation of spatial discrimination. The location of objects and the relating of one to another in space are so misjudged that the patient gropes about and often runs into these "seen" objects.

Lesions in *Wernicke's area* of the dominant hemisphere produce defects of an even "higher" order of complexity (see Fig. 16-18). Patients lose the ability both to comprehend spoken words (auditory aphasia) and to express themselves through them. Auditory agnosia is more complete if the damage to area 22 is bilateral, probably because auditory input to the cortex is bilateral. The intelligent, thinking person with this injury is at a loss to communicate thoughts because words are unavailable. Such a patient has lost the tool of verbal expression and in effect is a mute, although technically all the motor facilities for speech are unimpaired. (See "Cerebral Dominance" and "'Twin-Brain' Human," below.)

OCCIPITAL LOBE

The occipital cortex is composed mainly of the visual cortex. It is subdivided into striate area 17, known as the primary visual cortex, parastriate area 18, and the peristriate area 19. Areas 18 and 19 are called the *visual association area*. A secondary visual area may be located in areas 17 and 18 in human beings.

The striate cortex receives its input from the lateral geniculate body via the optic radiation and in turn projects its output via associative fibers to the visual association area. The visual association area has massive reciprocal connections with the pulvinar of the thalamus.

Primary visual area (area 17)

The primary visual area (area 17, visual area 1) is the primary receptive area for visual stimuli. Its loss in humans results in complete blindness, indicating that our subcortical centers are not capable of elevating visual sensations to the conscious level. Patients can "see" with area 17 intact, even with massive lesions in the association visual area. They may even avoid walking into a table, but they are unable to identify or appreciate the significance of the table through visual cues. Stimulation of this area in the normal person evokes no elaborate hallucinations but rather flashes of lights, shadows, and colors with movements in the contralateral fields of vision.

Visual association area (areas 18 and 19)

Areas 18 and 19 subserve interpretive vision or the recognition of visual stimuli. Area 18 is often designated as visual area II (secondary visual area). Area 19 is often called visual area III. The objects "seen" by the striate cortex are processed

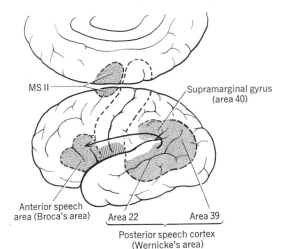

FIGURE 16-18 Location of some of the major functional association areas of the cerebral cortex. The line and arrow indicate the location of the arcuate association fibers interconnecting the association areas in the parietooccipitotemporal region with the frontal region. MSII, secondary somatic sensory and motor area. (*After Penfield and Roberts.*)

and made meaningful in the association area. With lesions of the visual association area, especially on the dominant side, *visual agnosia* or *psychic blindness* results. Such patients cannot recognize or name an object. They have difficulty in determining its function or appreciating its significance from visual cues.

Electrical stimulation of areas 18 and 19 evokes an imagery similar to that sensed from stimulation of area 17. Restimulation of the same cortical site may produce the same or a different visual sensation. Flashes, stars, streaks of light, whirling disks in color or in black and white are perceived. These visual sensations move about and vary in brightness. Similar images are visualized by patients with irritative lesions in these areas. Stimulation of the anterior temporal lobe produces complex images of scenes and people. (See "Temporal Lobe 'Psychical Cortex,'" further on.)

TEMPORAL LOBE

The temporal lobe cortex comprises the neocortex and the allocortex. The neocortex has a major role in the "higher" functions of audition. It is also concerned with the visual sense and the vestibular sense. The anterior temporal pole neocortex is involved in the sphere of behavior, emotion, and personality through its connections with the frontal and limbic lobes (Chaps. 13 and 15), and in the visual and auditory spheres through extensive interconnections with the visual and auditory association areas. The anterior pole of the temporal lobe has been called the *psychical cortex*.

The allocortex is integrated with the olfactory sense and with the limbic system (Chap. 15).

Primary auditory area (areas 41 and 42)

The transverse gyri of Heschl (areas 41 and 42) comprise the primary auditory cortex (auditory area I). A tonotopic pattern is present, with low tones localized laterally and high tones medially (see Fig. 10-7). A second auditory area (auditory area II) is probably located medial to the primary reception cortex. This auditory area II, identified in the monkey, has a reverse tonotopic representation and exhibits a higher threshold than the primary cortex. Area 22 of the superior temporal gyrus is the auditory association area.

The cortex of the superior temporal gyrus just rostral to the auditory cortex in humans may subserve a conscious phase of the vestibular activity. Stimulation of this cortical area can evoke dizziness and even make patients feel that they are rotating. This is considered to be the primary vestibular area.

Stimulation of the areas 41, 42, and 22 elicits sensations of sounds described as cricket chirping, bells, humming, buzzing, and whistling. The sounds may be heard as coming from the opposite ear. During stimulation, conversation picked up by the ears cannot be heard. At times, deafness may be subjectively sensed.

A patient can hear with areas 41 and 42 intact with a lesion in area 22 on the dominant side. Such patients have profound difficulty in the interpretation of sounds; the spoken language may be utterly meaningless or extremely difficult to comprehend. They are not deaf but cannot understand the conversation. This condition is known as *word deafness* and *auditory receptive aphasia*. The patient can speak but makes many mistakes without realizing it.

Lesion of areas 41 and 42, on one side, results in difficulty in locating the source of sound readily from auditory cues, but in only a slight loss of hearing. Subcortical centers and the redundancy in the central auditory pathways are functional and account for the high margin of physiologic safety (Chaps. 10 and 13).

Temporal lobe association cortex

The posterior cortex of the temporal lobe is an association cortex where integration of the input from auditory, visual, and somesthetic sources occurs. Large lesions of the association cortex on the dominant side result in visual and auditory aphasia. The patient loses the ability to comprehend the written and spoken word and the symbolism associated with language. Agnosia is a consequence. Deficits in the memory associated with these senses may occur (associated with hippocampus, Chap. 15). A deep lesion may interrupt the portion of the optic radiation which arcs into the temporal lobe (loop of Meyer); this results in a homonymous hemianopsia on the contralateral side (Chap. 12). The nonauditory cortex of the temporal lobe does not have such extensive connections with subcortical nuclei as does the association cortex of the occipital and parietal lobes.

Area 20 of the inferior temporal gyrus is a higher-ordered region receiving sensory of information from the visual, somatosensory, and auditory association areas of the occipital, parietal, and temporal lobes. Ablation of this area has been implicated in agnosias (such as visual agnosia) of the various sensory modalities. Area 20 sends input to the limbic system (Chap. 15).

Temporal lobe "psychical cortex"

The neocortex of the region in the vicinity of the temporal pole has been called the "psychical cortex," because responses obtained by stimulation of this area include associations relative to "experiences." Stimulation may elicit the recall of objects seen, or of music heard. Visual and auditory hallucinations may be produced, illusions which are similar to objects felt, seen, or heard in everyday experience. Feelings of fear may arise. The hallucination may be recall of an experience of the recent or distant past. It is a clear reenactment, unencumbered by confusion. A subsequent stimulation may evoke the same memory or a different memory. For example, the elicited experience may be a symphonic melody that is thought to be broadcast over a radio. Patients may, if requested, hum the tune at the tempo in which it is "heard." Later they will recall that they "heard" an orchestra playing the specific composition. The stimulation may evoke the recall of a conversation of a previous year. Patients with temporal lobe tumors may have auditory and visual hallucinations. They may see vivid scenery and friends not present and may hear songs not being sung. All these hallucinations can be consistent with experiences of reality because all could have been seen or heard in the past (*déjà vu*). The patient is cognizant of the hallucinations. Fearful feeling may ensue.

Motor activity and the temporal lobe

The temporal cortex may influence motor activity. Stimulation of this cortex, in humans, may elicit facial movements on the same and opposite sides. In primates, bilateral movements of each of the four extremities can be evoked by stimulation of the temporal lobe on one side.

INSULA

The cortex of the insula is somehow involved in both somatic and visceral functions. Its fiber connections are incompletely known. In the somatic sphere, the insula may have a supplementary motor area; stimulation of the insular cortex of a monkey may evoke somatic movements. The insula is apparently associated with visceral sensibility and visceral motor activity. Stimulation and irritation of this cortex (as in certain epileptic seizures) may produce some visceral sensations referable to many visceral organs. The insular cortex may have a role, probably minor, in such expressions as nausea, salivation, alteration in blood pressure and respiratory rhythms, piloerection, and desire to urinate, defecate, and belch.

CORTEX AND THE MOTOR PATHWAYS

Many areas of the cerebral cortex have roles in motor activity. These motor regions receive their main direct stimulation from the thalamus and from other cortical areas. The ventral lateral nucleus and the ventral anterior nucleus of the thalamus project powerful input to the cortex, mainly through axosomatic synapses with the pyramidal neurons, whereas the thalamic reticular nuclei exert their influences mainly through axodendritic synapses with the same cortical cells. The numerous association fibers from wide areas of the ipsilateral cortex and many callosal commissural fibers from the contralateral cortex are major sources of input to the motor cortex.

The motor areas project influences via a number of descending pathways to many subcortical nuclei and via association fibers and commissural (corpus callosum) fibers to many other areas of the cerebral cortex. The descending pathways include (1) the corticospinal tract, (2) corticobulbar fibers to cranial nerve motor nuclei, (3) corticoreticular fibers, (4) corticothalamic and corticostriate pathways, (5) corticonuclear fibers to nuclei of the ascending pathways, and (6) corticopontine tracts.

Corticospinal (pyramidal) tract

The corticospinal tract is composed of the axons of pyramidal cells located primarily in the frontal and parietal lobes (Chap. 5). These fibers collect to form the pathway that descends in order through the rostral part of the posterior limb of the internal capsule, crus cerebri of the midbrain, pons proper, pyramids of the medulla, and spinal cord (see Fig. 5-26). Approximately two-fifths of the fibers project from the motor and from the premotor cortex (areas 4 and 6), another one-fifth project from the postcentral gyrus (areas 1, 2, and 3), and the remaining two-fifths project from the association cortex of the parietal lobe and possibly from the temporal and occipital lobes. In the precentral gyrus are the 34,000 giant (Betz) pyramidal cells which probably give rise to the small percentage of fast-conduction fibers of the pyramidal cells tract. Many collateral branches terminate in subcortical nuclei of the brainstem (Chap. 14). Roughly 90 percent of the 1 million fibers of the pyramidal tract cross over in the pyramidal decussation and terminate mainly on spinal cord interneurons, which, in turn, synapse with both alpha and gamma motor neurons (Chap. 5).

Corticobulbar fibers to cranial nerve motor nuclei

The corticobulbar fibers consist of the axons of pyramidal cells located in several neocortical areas. For example, the frontal cortex (area 8), lower aspect of the precentral gyrus (area 4), and occipital association area can influence eye movements. Most of these axons descend through the genu of the internal capsule and terminate mainly on brainstem reticular formation interneurons, which, in turn, synapse with the lower motor neurons of the cranial nerves (see Fig. 8-22, Chap. 8). The course of the fiber groups of this pathway in the brainstem varies in different individuals. Bundles of corticobulbar fibers are found in both the basilar and tegmental portions of the brainstem. Because the fibers of this pathway synapse with interneurons in the reticular formation, they may be included with the corticoreticular fibers.

Corticoreticular fibers

The corticoreticular fibers arise from pyramidal cells of wide areas of the neocortex, many from areas 4 to 6. These fibers pass through the internal capsule and terminate in the brainstem tegmentum. Many fibers terminate in the red nucleus (corticorubral tract), the tectum (corticotectal tract), and other tegmental nuclei. This system exerts influences on the reticular nuclei of the pons and medulla, especially on those nuclei projecting to the spinal cord via the reticulospinal tracts (Chap. 5). Other descending fibers exert influences on the ascending reticular activating system (Chap. 8).

Corticothalamic pathways and corticostriate pathways

The cortex has connections with many of the subcortical nuclei, especially with certain thalamic nuclei, the corpus striatum, nucleus centrum medianum, subthalamus, substantia nigra, and some nuclei in the brainstem (Chaps. 13 and 14). The primary somesthetic cortex projects fibers to the ventral posterior thalamic nucleus, the primary visual cortex to the lateral geniculate body, the primary auditory cortex to the medial geniculate body, and the primary motor cor-

tex (area 4) to the ventral lateral thalamic nucleus. The reciprocal interconnections of the neocortex with the other thalamic nuclei are discussed in Chap. 13 (see Figs. 13-4 and 13-6). The cortex has many reciprocal connections with the thalamic nuclei. They do not form reverberating circuits.

The corticostriate fibers from widespread cortical areas have connections with the caudate nucleus and putamen. These pathways are integrated in the complex feedback circuitry that includes the globus pallidus and ventral anterior thalamic nucleus (Chap. 14).

Reflected descending fibers (descending fibers from cortex to nuclei of ascending pathways) (Chap. 5)

Many corticofugal fibers synapse, either directly or through interneurons, with the nuclei of the ascending pathways. These pathways transmit information that influences the processing occurring within these nuclei (Chaps. 3, 8, and 13). Included are the neocortical projections from the primary sensory areas to the ventral posterior thalamic nucleus (general senses), to the lateral geniculate body (vision), and to the medial geniculate body (audition). These descending pathways from the cortex also terminate in (1) the nucleus gracilis, nucleus cuneatus, and ventral posterior thalamic nucleus of the posterior column-medial lemniscus system; (2) the nucleus of the inferior colliculus, medial geniculate body, and other nuclei of the auditory pathways; (3) such brainstem nuclei as the cranial nerve nuclei of the trigeminal nerve; and (4) such spinal cord nuclei as the thoracic (Clarke's) nucleus and the gray matter of the posterior horn (Chaps. 5, 8, and 10). Because these fibers project from the cortex to subcortical nuclei, they are called reflected descending pathways.

Corticopontine tracts

The corticopontine tracts are pathways which arise from the neocortex of all cerebral lobes, descend in order through the internal capsule, corona radiata, and crus cerebri before terminating within the ipsilateral pontine nuclei. These tracts are integrated into the feedback circuitry of the cerebellum with cerebral cortex (Chap. 9).

MOTOR AREAS AND SPINAL CORD

The pathways from the motor areas of the cortex to the spinal cord may be divided functionally into three groups.

1. The corticoreticulospinal pathways relaying via the pontine and medullary nuclei of the brainstem reticular formation are a component of the anteromedial system within the spinal cord (see Fig. 8-21). The fibers of these tracts terminate on interneurons of the spinal gray matter. This system is primarily concerned with axial movements, maintenance of posture, integrated movements of body with limbs and total limb movements.
2. The corticorubrospinal pathway relaying via the magnocellular portion of the red nucleus constitutes a lateral pathway system (lateral in spinal cord; see Fig. 8-21). This system adds another motor dimension by fractionating movements of the extremities such as the independent use of the extremities and especially of the hands. (Because the corticorubrospinal and corticoreticulospinal pathways parallel the pyramidal tract, they are also called *parapyramidal pathways*.)
3. The corticospinal (pyramidal) tract (Fig. 5-26) increases and amplifies control of delicate hand movements. The high degree of fractionation of movements as expressed by the independent finger movements is, in part, accomplished through the direct synaptic connections of corticospinal fibers with the alpha motor neurons innervating the distal segments of the extremities. The corticobulbar components of this pathway are likewise crucial to the independent movements of the facial and tongue muscles.

FRONTAL LOBE

The cortex of the frontal lobe is subdivided into several areas; each subserves one or more roles.

1. The motor areas comprise the cortex of the precentral gyrus and the adjacent cortical areas of the superior, middle, and inferior frontal gyri (cortical areas 4, 6, and 8). They are associated with certain somatic motor activities.
2. The prefrontal cortex includes the cortex rostral to areas 6 and 8. It is somehow functionally integrated in circuits basic to many expressions of emotion and behavior (Chap. 15).
3. The orbitofrontal cortex on the inferior surface of the frontal lobe (areas 11 and 12) is apparently the site of the linkage between the ascending reticular pathways and the neocortex (Chap. 15).
4. Broca's speech area is the cortical area of the opercular and triangular parts of the inferior frontal gyrus (areas 44 and 45). It is involved with the formulation of speech (Fig. 16-18).

Primarily on the basis of observations of movements evoked by electrical stimulation of the cerebral cortex, several so-called motor areas have been designated. Ablation of these regions may result in changes in the qualities of the movements. These motor areas include (1) the primary motor area (area 4, MI, "the motor cortex"), which is the cortex of the precentral gyrus; (2) the premotor cortex (areas 6 and 8), located just rostral to the precentral gyrus; (3) the secondary motor area (second motor area, MII), located at the base of the precentral and postcentral gyri adjacent to the lateral sulcus, and coextensive with somatic sensory area II; and (4) the supplementary motor area, which is the portion of area 6 on the medial surface of the superior frontal gyrus rostral to area 4 (see Figs. 16-15, 16-16, and 16-18). The supplementary motor area is designated as MII by some authors.

The primary, secondary, and supplementary motor areas are somatotopically organized in caricature figurines. Each figurine is called a *homunculus* (see Fig. 16-17). The head and body image represented by the MI homunculus is large as compared with images represented by the MII and supplementary motor homunculi. The MI figurine is oriented "upside down" on area 4, with the head located near the lateral sulcus and the lower extremity in the paracentral lobule (see Fig. 16-16). In a general way, motor area MI faces sensory area SI as mirror images, with the line of the central sulcus acting as an interface. The body image of MII in humans is presumed to be oriented with the upper body located rostrally and the lower extremity caudally. The homunculus of the supplementary motor cortex is sequentially organized with the head located rostrally and the lower extremity caudally. Although electrical stimulation of each of these areas normally evokes a motor response, such stimulation does, at times, evoke a sensation; hence these motor areas are often called sensorimotor areas.

Association fibers interconnect some of the motor areas with one another and with somesthetic sensory areas. The primary motor area projects topographically to MII, supplementary motor area, premotor area, and somesthetic sensory areas SI and SII. The premotor cortex has connections with MI, MII, and adjacent prefrontal cortex. The supplementary motor area has topographic connections with MI and the premotor cortex. The corticofugal projections from these motor areas to the subcortical nuclei, brainstem, and spinal cord are conveyed via several descending fiber pathways.

Primary motor area (MI)

The primary motor area, often called the "motor cortex," is located in area 4 of the precentral gyrus. Direct topical electrical stimulation of this region evokes movements of the voluntary muscles. A map of this electrically excitable motor cortex produces the configuration of a homunculus indicative of the somatotopical representation of different parts of the body (see Fig. 16-17). In addition to its major projection via the pyramidal tract to the spinal cord, cortical area 4 projects to many subcortical nuclei, including the ventral lateral thalamic nucleus, nucleus centrum medianum, subthalamic nucleus, red nucleus, substantia nigra, and many brainstem reticular nuclei. Many of these connections are via collateral branches of the corticospinal fibers. MI receives subcortical input from the ventral lateral thalamic nucleus.

In a general way this homunculus is upside down, with the head region near the lateral sulcus and with the lower extremity on the medial surface in the paracentral lobule. The homunculus reveals that larger proportions of motor cortex are associated with those cortical regions evoking movements of the face, larynx, tongue, and hand as compared with the smaller regions associated with the trunk and lower extremities. The detailed representation of the thumb and fingers is consistent with the para-

mount importance of manual dexterity in the primacy of the human species. The amount of the motor cortex devoted to specific regions is roughly proportional to the delicacy of control that is possible in each body region.

Small foci of neurons in the motor cortex, called *discrete efferent zones*, are known through physiologic stimulation to control the contraction of individual muscles. This indicates the preciseness of the connectivity of a few cortical neurons with the motor neurons innervating a specific muscle—such as a lumbricle or an interosseous hand muscle. This efferent zone is also precisely connected with the periphery; it receives afferent input from the particular muscle which the efferent zone controls. In addition, the efferent zone receives feedback from the joint following the movement.

The pyramidal neurons of the corticospinal tract are driven by central motor programs generated prior to their discharge that evokes a volitional movement. These central programs invoke the basal ganglia, cerebellum, and other subcortical structures. The activity of the pyramidal tract neurons coactivates the alpha and the gamma motor neurons. The alpha motor neuron discharge results in a contraction of the extrafusal muscles accompanied by a decrease in the discharge of the muscle spindles (length receptor). The gamma motor neuron discharge results in a contraction of the intrafusal muscle fibers accompanied by an increase in the discharge of the muscle spindles. Neuromuscular spindle discharge via group Ia afferent fibers excites the alpha motor neurons. In essence, the activity of the neuromuscular spindles within a gamma loop is basically a negative feedback circuit (Chap. 5). An analogous negative feedback circuit is also relayed to the cortical pyramidal cells giving rise to the corticospinal tract. Some physiologic evidence suggests that some degree of independent control of the alpha motor neurons and gamma motor neurons may be projected by different pyramidal motor neurons.

Stimulation of the motor cortex generally elicits phasic activity in groups of muscles, rather than from individual muscles per se. Experimentally induced movements include changes in facial expression, swallowing, torsion of the body, rotation of an extremity, and flexion of limbs. Focal stimulation may occasionally produce the contraction of individual muscles, such as an adductor muscle of the thumb. Flexor responses occur more frequently than extensor responses. The specific localized movements are usually expressed on the side of the body opposite the cortical stimulation, although some ipsilateral activity may be elicited. Stimulation of the postcentral gyrus (areas 1, 2, and 3) in humans may evoke motor responses when area 4 is intact. The responses are similar to those obtained from stimulating area 4, but weaker.

The ablation of the precentral gyrus in a monkey produces an initial paralysis; a monkey with an ablated precentral gyrus exhibits an immediate severe impairment of voluntary movements, hypotonia, and diminished reflexes on the contralateral side. With the passage of time, the monkey has a good return of function, but with a persistent flaccidity and some impairment of skilled actions. The paresis is accompanied by an almost normal tonus, no major increase in the deep tendon reflexes, and no clonus. The main loss is of the fine voluntary movement, particularly of the fingers and feet. However, the monkey has sufficient manual dexterity to be able to pick up objects by the apposition of the thumb with the index finger. Effects are more pronounced in the distal muscles than in the proximal muscles of a limb.

The abnormal stimulation of the motor cortex may produce patterned convulsions. The *Jacksonian seizure* (*epilepsy*) offers a vivid example of such responses. In a focal seizure, the convulsive movement of a group of muscles may be manifested. The repeated contractions may be restricted to the muscles of the face, an arm, or a leg, taking the form of tonic and clonic movements, such as a twitch of the cheek, finger, or ankle. In the Jacksonian march, the seizure, which may commence with a finger twitch, spreads in an orderly progression from the distal to the proximal muscles of the limb, down the same side of the body, down the lower extremity, across to and up the other lower extremity, up the body to the upper extremity and face, following the order of representation of the homunculus of one side and then the homunculus of the opposite side. Consciousness is lost, unless the seizure is confined to one side. During a seizure, the patient can see and hear but cannot communicate.

Premotor cortex (premotor area)

The premotor cortex comprises areas 6 and 8 on the lateral surface of the hemisphere. Area 6 on the medial surface of the frontal lobe is the supplementary motor area. The major subcortical input to area 6 is derived from the ventral anterior nucleus of the thalamus. Electrical stimulation of part of area 6 in humans may produce motor responses which are similar to those evoked by stimulating the primary motor cortex. These responses may be elicited through relays via association fibers to the primary motor area and then via the corticospinal, corticobulbar, and corticoreticular pathways to the brainstem and spinal cord.

Stimulation of area 6 on the lateral cerebral surface often produces adversive movements which are different from the precise movements obtained from stimulation of area 4. *Adversive movements* or *orientation movements* are generalized actions, such as turning the head and eyes, twisting movements of the trunk, and general flexion or extension of the limbs. These movements are thought of as directional—the motor reaction to attention. Stimulation of area 8 (just rostral to area 6) results in conjugate movements of the eye to the opposite side. This frontal eye field influences the volitional eye movements. Adversive movements may be elicited by stimulating other regions of the cortex. Stimulation of areas 9 and 10, which project fibers to the caudate nucleus, inhibits the deep tendon reflexes and movements in progress. Ablation limited to area 6 on the lateral hemispheric surface (avoiding the primary motor and supplementary motor areas) does not produce a monkey with paresis, motor impairment, hypotonia, hypertonia, or grasp reflexes. The ablation of premotor area and primary motor area results in a flaccid paralysis.

Secondary motor area (second motor area, MII)

The secondary motor area is the small cortical region at the base of the pre- and postcentral gyri (see Fig 16-15); its precise function in motor activity is unknown. Electrical stimulation of this area generally produces sensations rather than motor responses. This greater prominence of sensory phenomena following its stimulation suggests that the role of the MII area in motor activity is minimal. When motor responses are evoked, they are usually elicited on the contralateral side, especially of the more distal segments of the extremities. At times ipsilateral and bilateral responses can also be evoked. The electrical stimulation of this area may elicit in humans the desire to make a specific movement. No obvious sensory or motor deficits have been observed in experimental animals with this cortical area ablated. This is probably so because the secondary motor area is functionally overpowered by the primary motor area.

Supplementary motor area

The supplementary motor area is found on the medial surface of the superior frontal gyrus (area) rostral to the paracentral lobule (see Fig. 16-15). Stimulation of this area outlines a small homunculus with its head located rostrally. The motor responses in humans evoked by electrical stimulation are largely bilateral movements of a tonic or postural nature, resulting from the activity of the axial, pectoral girdle, and pelvic girdle musculature. These generalized responses are slow and outlast the stimulation for a short time. They include such posturing movements as turning the head contralaterally and raising the contralateral upper extremity. The stimulation can also evoke vocalization as well as fine movements of the thumb, fingers, and hand.

These bilateral responses elicited by the stimulation of each supplementary motor area are probably evoked through influences conveyed by the corticospinal and corticoreticulospinal pathways from both sides. These pathways can be activated directly or indirectly by some of the following known connections from each supplementary motor area: (1) direct corticoreticular fibers projecting to the brainstem, (2) association fibers projecting to the brainstem, motor area and premotor cortex of the same side, (3) corpus callosal fibers projecting to the contralateral supplementary motor area, and (4) corticofugal fibers projecting bilaterally to the ventral lateral and intralaminar nuclei of the thalamus (the decussating fibers cross through

the anterior commissure). There are no direct projections from the supplementary motor area to the spinal cord.

The bilateral removal of both supplementary motor areas produces an animal exhibiting hypertonus, hyperactive deep tendon reflexes, spasticity, and increased resistance to passive movements of the extremities; there is no paralysis. The ablation of only one supplementary motor area results in a monkey with only minimal symptoms, such as weak but transient grasp reflexes, lasting slowness of movement of the contralateral extremities, and moderate hypotonia of the shoulder musculature. The removal of the contralateral supplementary motor area six or more months later produces an animal exhibiting minimal effects, with no spasticity. Reasons for these phenomena are unknown. However, the simultaneous ablation of the supplementary motor cortex and the motor cortex on the same side produces a monkey that exhibits symptoms of upper motor neuron paralysis accompanied by marked spasticity, without paresis. The ablation of the entire cortex on both frontal lobes in the monkey results in an animal with spastic paralysis symptoms, including clonus and hyperactive deep tendon reflexes. These animals are unable to stand up, walk, or feed themselves.

These observations are similar to those obtained in monkeys and chimpanzees with bilaterally transected pyramids in the medulla (Chap. 8). When all corticospinal tract fibers are interrupted at this site, the animals are characterized by a marked impairment of their motor activities. They can move about and feed themselves. They exhibit slow, stereotyped movements accompanied by hypotonus and no clonus.

The motor areas are not absolutely essential to movement. After bilateral ablation of the primary, supplementary, and premotor areas (areas 4 and 6), adult monkeys can walk and right themselves.

The following statements based on experimental evidence in the monkey are of relevance to motor symptoms in patients with lesions in the central nervous system. (1) The phenomenon of spasticity (Chap. 5) is probably not a manifestation of pure pyramidal disease or of complete lesions of the pyramids in the medulla. A lesion limited to the medullary pyramids in the monkey produces a hypotonic paralysis. In time, the animal gains control of most voluntary movements accompanied by a persistent slowness of all movements and a loss of control of the individual movements of the fingers. These observations are consistent with the concept that voluntary movements depend, in part, upon parapyramidal pathways such as the corticorubrospinal and corticoreticulospinal systems. (2) In human patients spasticity, paresis, and paralysis occur together following lesions in the internal capsule (stroke). However, evidence suggests that spasticity can be dissociated from paresis and paralysis. Following a bilateral ablation of the supplementary motor cortices, hypertonus, hyperactive deep tendon reflexes, and clonus develop after 2 to 4 weeks, but paresis does not occur. On the other hand, a unilateral ablation of precentral (motor) and supplementary motor cortex results in time in hypertonus with exaggerated myotatic reflexes. As yet, the precise influence of the subdivisions of the cortical motor areas on motor symptoms associated with lesions in the central nervous system are not fully understood.

Prefrontal cortex

The prefrontal cortex (areas 9 through 13, 24, 32, 46, and 47) is well developed in higher primates. This cortex has rich reciprocal connections with the parvocellular part of the dorsomedial (DM) nucleus of the thalamus (Chap. 13). Hence, the prefrontal cortex has been referred to as the DM-projection cortex. Many complex reciprocal projections are made with other neocortical and limbic areas, both of the same and opposite side. Brodmann's areas 32 and 24 have corticocortical connections with the entorhinal cortex and presubiculum. Efferent fibers project to such subcortical regions as the midline thalamic nuclei, hypothalamus, and paramedian midbrain tegmentum.

The bilateral ablation of areas of the prefrontal cortex or the interruption of white matter deep to the cortex in both prefrontal lobes (*prefrontal lobotomy, leukotomy*) may produce permanent changes in an individual. The patient may become less excitable and less creative. The relief from anxiety is accompanied by a change in the patient's outlook and disposition. Less altruism toward others and a release from many inhibitions make patients free to express themselves frankly, often without the restraint demanded by society. A neat, precise individual may become indifferent and sloppy in appearance. Surprisingly, this change in personality, including a reduction in the awareness of self, is generally accompanied by no real change in mental processes. Drive, not intelligence, is altered.

Alleviation of suffering from pain may follow a lobotomy. Relief from intractable pain and other effects of a phantom limb is also obtained. The pain remains, but the patient is unconcerned about it; it can be ignored, for the psychic feeling associated with the intensity of the pain is lost.

The prefrontal lobe may be thought of as a regulator of the depth of feeling of an individual. Basically it is involved not in the perception of sensations, but rather in the "affect" associated with the sensation. The special quality of "feeling tone" or state of mind is apparently the result of the processing of the input from the numerous subcortical and cortical sources. This may form the basis for many of the emotional aspects associated with behavioral responses. The relative pitch of one's being is influenced in this region. The complex responses of an individual from calmness to ecstasy, from gloom to elation, from friendliness to disagreeableness—have their roots in areas 9 to 12. One concept suggests that the prefrontal cortex is the neocortical representation of the limbic system; this view is based on (1) the rich direct and indirect interconnections between this lobe and limbic structures, and (2) the similarities of the functional expressions of the prefrontal cortex and the limbic system. The autonomic responses associated with various emotional states are probably mediated through the frontopreoptic tract, frontohypothalamic tract, and frontodorsomedian thalamic nuclear hypothalamic pathways (Chap. 13). The hypothalamus exerts its effects on the blood pressure, respiratory rate, and gastrointestinal activity through the autonomic nervous system (Chap. 11).

FUNCTIONAL CONSIDERATIONS OF THE NEOCORTEX

The functional role of an ablated area of the cortex should not and cannot be objectively inferred from observations of the residual activity of the organism. The expressions remaining following the ablation of an area may be taken to indicate, in effect, the performance of the nervous system without the influences of this missing region. Additionally it may reveal the prior expression of the rest of the nervous system plus the degree to which the nervous system compensates.

The activity evoked from focal stimulation does not necessarily tell the real function of the area stimulated. The stimulation acts as a nodal site which sets off a complex of other integrated systems with its multiplicity of inhibitory, excitatory, and feedback effects. Each cortical area actually functions in conjunction with many other cortical and subcortical regions. The specific part stimulated is a segment integrated into the complex circuitry of the brain. The cortical influences are exerted not directly on the end organs (muscle cells and glands) but actually through intermediaries of from one to many intercalated nuclear complexes.

Autonomic nervous system and the neocortex

Cortical activity is also expressed through the autonomic nervous system, e.g., those behavior patterns colored by emotion. Intellectual decisions, all cortically derived, are set in an emotional environment. All lobes of the cerebrum contribute primarily through connections with the hypothalamus, limbic system, and midbrain tegmentum (Chap. 15). The autonomic expressions elicited during emotional states can be evoked by the electrical stimulation of the neocortex. Among these responses are cardiovascular effects (vasodilatation, vasoconstriction, and blood pressure changes), digestive influences (salivation, peristalsis, and gastric discomfort), temperature changes, and alterations of pupillary size. These actions have their emotional counterpart in heart palpitations, cold sweat, paleness, and blushing.

Role of the cortex in "highest-order" activities

The cortex is essential in the neural processing underlying the loftiest activities of the nervous system. Among these activities are the fullest comprehension of the afferent input, expression through the symbolisms of communication of the unique nuances of each personality, and abstract creativity. Only a few indications of the role of the cortex in these spheres will be made.

The cortex of the parietal lobe, occipital lobe, and temporal lobe is necessary for the comprehension of the afferent input. Defects in these lobes produce individuals with receptive aphasias. These patients receive input from visual, auditory, and somesthetic pathways—can see, hear, and feel. The receptive aphasia is indicated when they are unable to process this information in order to comprehend the written word, the spoken word, or the felt object. Visual aphasia, auditory aphasia (word deafness), and somesthetic aphasia are expressions of malfunction in the highest levels of neural integration in the neocortex.

The ultimate of afferent processing in the cerebrum of humans is seen in the neural activities expressed as abstract and creative thought. These highest expressions may not necessarily be accompanied by any overt motor activity.

The motor aspect of expression through the symbolism of language is in part a function of the frontal lobe. The motor aphasias (motor apraxias) are indications that these regions are essential to the performance of these activities. Broca's speech area (areas 44 and 45 of the inferior frontal gyrus) is a nodal site concerned with ability to produce the spoken word. Lesions of Broca's area, especially of the left dominant hemisphere, may result in motor or expressive aphasia. More often these lesions lead to a transient speech defect. This loss of articulate speech occurs even though there is no demonstrable paralysis of any muscles associated with speech. Complete loss of articulate speech—the ability to say only several words, mispronunciation of common everyday words, or repetition of the same word over and over again—may be a consequence of the total destruction of Broca's speech area. At times these patients may express themselves with better facility when under emotional stress.

The "sensory" association cortex has a role in subtle motor activity. Injury to the somesthetic association cortex (supramarginal gyrus) may result in a sensory apraxia. Such patients are capable of performing the various separate movements of a sequence but may not be able to carry out volitionally all the movements of the sequence in their intended or proper order. They know what and how to execute the sequence but are unable to do it volitionally or on command. They are unable to handle a screwdriver although they can explain its use. They may be able to brush their teeth, comb their hair, and tie their shoes automatically but are unable to perform these tasks when instructed to do so.

Blood flow in the cortex

The mean blood flow in the brain of normal individuals is 50 mL per 100 g of brain tissue per minute (Chap. 1). However, at any given moment, the blood flow through a specific region may either be greater, the same as, or less than the mean blood flow through the region. To state it otherwise, the brain is similar to other body tissues in that the flow of blood varies with the level of metabolism and functional activity within the tissue. The pattern of blood flow through the various regions of the neocortex is not uniform in a normal individual who is at rest and awake with eyes closed in a quiet room and is not touched or spoken to (Larsen, Ingvar, and Skinhøz). In such a condition, the flow in the prefrontal and premotor areas (called hyperfrontal region) of the dominant hemisphere may exceed the mean flow by 20 to 30 percent. In turn, a corresponding reduction in flow is taking place in the parietal lobe and adjoining areas of the occipital and temporal lobes. This means that in the so-called resting brain, the flow rate in the hyperfrontal cortex can be as much as 50 percent higher than in the posterior cortex. When this relaxed subject opens the eyes and gazes at an object, a 20 percent increase in blood flow occurs in the frontal eye fields (area 8) and in the visual association cortex (areas 18 and 19). An increase in blood flow takes place in the primary and association auditory cortex (areas 41 and 42) of tem-

poral lobes when loud and meaningless sounds are heard. A simple, understandable spoken work is associated with a further increase in blood flow in the auditory cortex in both hemispheres and in Wernicke's area (areas 39 and 40) in the left hemisphere. During a verbal conversation blood flow in Brocas (areas 44 and 45) increases.

Stimulated tactile receptors can affect blood flow. An object in the palm of a motionless hand is accompanied by an increase in blood flow in the hand area of the contralateral postcentral gyrus and adjacent association cortex of parietal lobe.

Dynamic movements of the hand evoke blood flow increases in several cortical areas involved with hand movements and with sensory signals from sensors in the skin, joints, and muscles associated with the movements. Blood flow increases occur in the contralateral "hand" region of the motor cortex (area 4) and postcentral gyrus (somesthetic cortex) and of both ipsilateral and contralateral premotor and supplementary motor (areas 6 and 8) cortex.

The motor and sensory activities involved with the acts of reading aloud and listening result in an increase in blood flow in both the ipsilateral and contralateral auditory cortex, motor and somatosensory cortex (face and mouth areas), premotor and supplementary motor cortex, Borca's speech area, frontal eye fields (area 8), and visual association cortex.

Cerebral dominance

Cerebral dominance refers to the fact that the control of certain forms of learned behavior in humans is exerted predominantly by one of the two cerebral hemispheres. Handedness, perception of language, performance of speech, and appreciation of spatial relations are, in all but a few individuals, primarily expressions of one or the other hemisphere.

By convention, speech is used as a measure of hemispheric dominance, with the left hemisphere being dominant for speech in most individuals. Although it is often assumed that speech, handedness, and hemispheric dominance are causally related, such is probably not the case. The left hemisphere is speech dominant

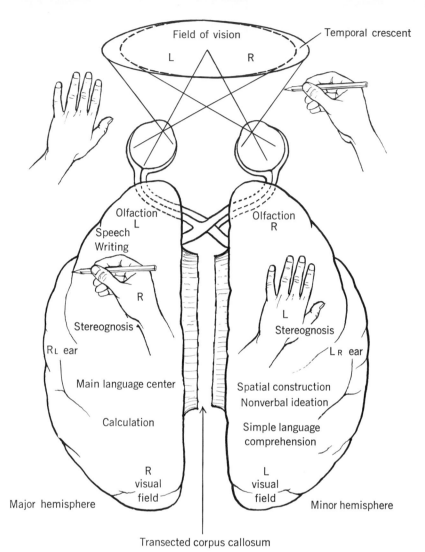

Field of vision

Temporal crescent

L   R

Olfaction
L

Olfaction
R

Speech
Writing

R

Stereognosis

L

Stereognosis

R L ear

L R ear

Main language center

Spatial construction
Nonverbal ideation

Calculation

Simple language
comprehension

R
visual
field

L
visual
field

Major hemisphere

Minor hemisphere

Transected corpus callosum

FIGURE 16-19 Some of the roles of the major and minor cerebral hemispheres as established in "twin-brain" humans. General senses from one hand and from half of the visual field are projected to the contralateral hemisphere. The olfactory sense is conveyed to the ipsilateral hemisphere. Hearing is largely projected to the contralateral hemisphere. (*Adapted from Sperry.*)

in about 90 percent of right-handed, 65 percent of left-handed, and 60 percent of ambidextrous individuals. The right hemisphere is speech dominant in about 20 percent of left-handed, 10 percent of right-handed, and 10 percent of ambidextrous individuals. Both hemispheres are dominant in about 30 percent of ambidextrous, 15 percent of left-handed, and no right-handed individuals. These figures were obtained in awake subjects who received a unilateral carotid

artery injection of the short-acting anesthetic agent sodium amytal (amobarbital).

Roughly 90 percent of the adult population is right-handed. Except for a few ambidextrous individuals, the remainder is left-handed. In the right-handed population the left hemisphere is dominant because the motor centers on this side control the right hand. In the left-handed population, the right hemisphere is considered to be dominant for handedness. In about 98 percent of the adult population, comprehension of the spoken and written word as well as motor control of language are expressions of the left cerebral hemisphere. Only in about 2 percent of the population are the "speech centers" located in the right hemisphere.

The differences in the functional roles expressed by the two hemispheres have been ascertained from studies on a variety of human subjects (see Fig. 16-19).

1. Patients with cerebral lesions: Over 96 percent of adult aphasics with language disorders have brain damage in the left hemisphere.
2. Twin-brain individuals: Studies on these human subjects indicate that the left hemisphere is adapted for linguistic expression through speech and writing whereas the right hemisphere is specialized to sense and appreciate spatial relations.
3. Subjects treated with the short-acting anesthetic agent sodium amytal (amobarbital): When amobarbitol is injected into the left carotid artery, the left hemisphere is temporarily anesthetized, whereas the right hemisphere is not affected. On the basis of responses from patients so exposed to sodium amytal, it can be demonstrated that, in right-handed individuals, the left hemisphere controls handedness, perception of language, and performance of speech. In some left-handed people (less than half the total), language is controlled by the right hemisphere, while in the remainder language functions reside in the left hemisphere.

Evidence indicates that the lateralization of the so-called speech centers (e.g., Broca's area, see Fig. 16-18) in the left hemisphere is not causally related to handedness. Most left-handed individuals have their "speech centers" located in the left hemisphere. Stated otherwise, speech functions are lateralized in the left hemisphere in most adults, regardless of hand preference. Some right-handed individuals are said to have their speech centers in both hemispheres.

On the basis of observations of these subjects, *the left hemisphere has been called the dominant or major hemisphere* and *the right hemisphere has been called the nondominant or minor hemisphere*. The major hemisphere has essential roles in the verbal and analytic abilities of humans; the minor hemisphere has crucial roles in nonverbal and artistic expressions (see "Twin-Brain Human," further on in this chapter).

The major hemisphere has the substrates and memory traces relevant to thoughts and knowledge expressed and symbolized through language and our highest analytic powers. Through its influence on handedness, the hemisphere is involved in the control of the opposite hand and fingers for precise and delicate grips and movements. By means of this role the human race has evolved manipulative manual skills, which are often enhanced through the use of tools. There is no known microscopic (ultramicroscopic), neuroanatomic, or neurophysiologic basis for the dominance of this hemisphere in handedness and speech.

Several gross anatomic differences between the hemispheres have been reported; the functional significance of them has been inferred but not demonstrated. The asymmetry between the hemispheres has been demonstrated in the temporal lobes and in the posterior part of the inferior frontal gyrus of a number of brains. The superior surface of the temporal lobe just behind the transverse temporal gyrus of Heschl is larger on the left side in about 65 percent of brains; it is larger on the right side in about 11 percent of brains. This region—called the *planum temporale*—is adjacent to the temporal speech area of Wernicke (see Fig. 1-4).

The triangular and opercular portions of the inferior frontal gyrus, which are called Broca's speech area, are apparently larger in about 80 percent of the left cerebral hemispheres. Note that these enlargements do not occur in 98 percent of the brains, as expected from the lateralization of speech in the left hemisphere. The gross asymmetry of these regions is also present in the newborn infant; this occurs before language learning and unimanual preference are expressed behaviorly. According to some investigators, this suggests that the newborn infant may be programmed with the capacity to process speech sounds.

Ontogeny of cerebral dominance The young infant is, to a degree, presumed to be a split-brain individual. This is so because the interhemispheric communication through the fibers of the anterior commissure and corpus callosum is, at the most, slight in the newborn infant. The interhemispheric communication through these commissures increases with age; it is apparently fairly well developed by the second and third year of age. The two hemispheres of the neonate have essentially equipotential capabilities. Cerebral dominance probably develops gradually during childhood and does not become relatively well fixed until the end of the first decade of life. On the basis of the use of hands in manipulatory play it seems that, after the age of 2, the duplication of learning by both hands becomes less frequent and the lateralization of handedness becomes more pronounced. Apparently the language and speech capabilities in young children reside in both sides of the brain, expressing the tendency for each hemisphere to evolve independently as a duplicate of the other. The natural twin-brain of the growing child explains, in part, why a left-handed child can be readily taught to write with the right hand, and why some athletes who have been trained in childhood are ambidextrous. This also explains why a child with a damaged dominant hemisphere can be trained to become left-handed and proficient in language and speech, whereas the older patient with a cerebral infarction of the major hemisphere finds it difficult or impossible to become left-handed and to relearn lost language and speech abilities.

Studies on twin-brain subjects suggest that language learned in early childhood by the minor hemisphere will, during later development, be suppressed and even lost completely. Some skills controlled predominantly by one hemisphere tend to suppress the same skill by the other hemisphere; "excellence in one tends to interfere with top level performance in the other" (Sperry). According to one concept, those individuals who mature into "major hemisphere types" are equipped to function more effectively in a verbal and analytic way, while those who evolve into "minor hemisphere types" will be able to express themselves more effectively nonverbally in many of the creative arts.

Speech may be relearned in some human subjects following injury to the cortical areas involved with speech (e.g., Broca's area). Damage to the left hemisphere accompanied by a definite

impairment of speech in children below the age of 10 can be followed by the assumption of essentially normal speech. However, the degree of recovery from cortical damage decreases rapidly with age. From none to a minimal amount of recovery occurs from such injury in later ages. The complete recovery in the young is presumed to occur because the other hemisphere assumes the functional role in speech. It is thought that linguistic centers mature bilaterally during early life and later consolidate in the left hemisphere. In a sense, the child has a split brain. This is another example of a critical developmental period prior to which the brain is malleable and language centers can be established in either hemisphere. Following the critical period, the verbal centers become fixed and rigid. Injury to these centers at this postcritical period results in subjects who cannot reestablish language.

FUNCTIONAL ROLE OF ASSOCIATION FIBERS AND COMMISSURAL FIBERS ("SPLIT-BRAIN ANIMALS")

The interactions of the billions of association and commissural cortical neurons have a significant role in the higher integration of the cerebral cortex. These multitudes of connections suggest that the cortex may function in overall patterns of mass action. This could be a consequence of the continuous spread of impulses through the white matter to other cortical areas. However, experimental evidence indicates that the interruption of large bundles of association fibers by surgical incisions, especially in the association areas in many regions of the same brain, produces few objective symptoms. Monkeys, dogs, and rats with many association fibers interrupted show slight defects or none in the learning and retention of maze-trained habits. Multiple transections of the cortex and underlying association fibers coming from "motor" areas in a monkey do not essentially alter motor coordination. Any functional depression following such lesions is usually temporary and transient.

The presence of several commissures in the cerebrum—one of them, the massive corpus callosum, with its more than 300 million fibers in humans, is the largest fiber tract of the brain—

suggests that interhemispheric fiber pathways are of crucial significance to the functioning of the brain. Yet, when the corpus callosum is completely transected surgically, even in humans, no functional alterations can be detected, even after careful neurologic and psychologic examinations. Behavior patterns are not noticeably disturbed. Complex activities, such as playing musical instruments (piano, violin, and others), typing, and writing, are performed with the same dexterity as prior to sectioning of the corpus callosum.

An experimental animal with a transected corpus callosum and other commissures (anterior commissure and commissure of the fornix) is, in a way, an animal with two brains; such animals are called "twin-brain" animals or "split-brain" animals. Such cats and monkeys behave normally. These animals are alert and curious and exhibit good muscular coordination. They perceive, learn, and retain learned activities as do ordinary animals. Normal expressions are still observed because the input of complex information from the periphery is apparently projected to both hemispheres and therefore each hemisphere receives sufficient input to operate efficiently by itself.

Experimental animals may be trained in such a way that information may be relayed to only one hemisphere. In this way it is possible to train one of the divided hemispheres with one set of data and the other hemisphere with other data; or one hemisphere with certain information and the other hemisphere without this information. For example, this can be accomplished by sectioning the optic chiasma in cats and in monkeys so that all decussating fibers from the eye are cut and the nondecussating fibers from the eye are intact. In such animals each eye projects only to its ipsilateral hemisphere. By blindfolding one eye, and training the animal with visual stimuli directed to only one eye, visual information is conveyed to only the ipsilateral hemisphere. This experiment has many variations.

Studies of such split-brain monkeys have been conducted so that the input from the periphery has been projected to only one hemisphere. The memory for the perceptual and motor learning in these animals is confined to the hemisphere to which the sensory information was relayed, and from which the motor output was projected. However, if the corpus callosum was intact this memory is found to be utilized for motor expression by both hemispheres. Apparently the engram, or memory trace, laid down in the directly trained hemisphere is transferred via the callosal fibers to the opposite hemisphere and a second engram is laid down in the contralateral hemisphere. The inference is that the function of the corpus callosum is to transfer information from one hemisphere to the other and to equate the newly acquired engrams of the neocortex of each hemisphere. The corpus callosum may be utilized by the uneducated hemisphere to tap the engram of the trained hemisphere. A double set of engrams is not necessarily always laid down equally in both hemispheres. The lateralization of language functions in the human brain to one hemisphere indicates that some functional expressions are largely confined to one hemisphere. This is in line with the concept of cerebral dominance of one hemisphere.

With training, the split-brain animal can use its two "half-brains" independently or simultaneously to perform different tasks. Each half-brain performs its own perceptual, learning, and memory processes. The animal may have one half-brain trained to respond one way to a specific visual cue from the one half-brain and to respond in the opposite way to the same visual cue from the other half-brain. If this cue is visualized simultaneously by both half-brains, hesitancy is displayed by the animal, but marked conflict does not occur. One hemisphere will express itself, and later a shift will occur and the other hemisphere will express itself. A split-brain animal may utilize both half-brains together or in alternation. The behavioral responses of a split-brain animal with an ablated amygdaloid body are informative. The bilateral removal of the amygdaloid body converts an excitable, temperamental, and wild monkey into a placid and docile animal, whereas the unilateral removal of the amygdaloid body produces little, if any, observable change in a primate (Chap. 15). A split-brain monkey (one with midline transection of the corpus callosum, anterior commissure, and habenular commissure) with a unilateral ablation of the amygdaloid body exhibits interesting behavioral responses. When an aggravating visual stimulus is presented to the eye on the side with the intact amygdaloid body (with the opposite eye blindfolded), the monkey responds in an emotional, aggressive, and belligerent manner. When the same visual stimulus is presented to the eye on the side with the ablated amygdaloid body, the monkey shown no emotional or aggressive responses but remains docile and tame. This is in line with the concept that the commissures act to transfer information from one hemisphere to the other.

"Twin-brain" humans

Commissurotomy of the corpus callosum and commissure of the fornix (hippocampal commissure) has been performed in a number of patients in order to prevent the interhemispheric spread of severe epileptic seizures. The normal behavior of these patients is unaffected by the surgical section. These subjects with "two minds in one head" are alert and curious. They perceive, learn, and retain learned experiences as well as normal people. Careful testing reveals that the two hemispheres are almost completely independent with respect to learning, memory, perception, and ideation. *Language, speech, and handedness are almost exclusively lateralized in these subjects to the major hemisphere.*

The minor hemisphere can perceive tactile, auditory, and visual information. Although it does think, this mute hemisphere is unable to communicate through verbal language. However, it can respond and communicate by gestures (e.g., pointing) or emotional activity (e.g., fidgeting or blushing). *The minor hemisphere is specialized to appreciate spatial dimensions, to grasp the totality of a scene, and to recognize the faces of people better than the major hemisphere. This mute hemisphere is presumed to have an essential role in creative acts associated with musical, poetic, and imaginative expressions.*

Hemispheric specialization has interesting consequences. The twin-brain subject cannot describe orally an unseen object felt by the left hand because the minor hemisphere, which receives this information, is unable to relay the knowledge to the speech areas of the major hemisphere. On the other hand, such people cannot draw accurately with their right hands because the motor centers of the major hemisphere do not receive the critical guidance of spatial knowledge from the minor hemisphere.

When a visual image is presented to the monocular crescent of the retina of one eye, visual information is projected only to the visual cortex of the ipsilateral hemisphere. This is done by permitting the crescent of the eye to view an object several times tachistoscopically for only from 0.01 to 0.1 s. Such a quick view prevents other portions of the eye from viewing the object if the eye moves. If a word (e.g., "cat") or an object (e.g., an apple) is so presented to the monocular crescent of the right eye, this information is conveyed to the minor hemisphere. Under appropriate testing conditions, twin-brain subjects will be able to write "cat" with their left hands or identify the apple by selecting the correct object from a variety of fruits viewed by both eyes.

The cerebral commissures—anterior commissure and corpus callosum—are thought to have a critical role in conveying information between the hemispheres that has a role in providing a unity to the thought processes. In the split-brain subject, two independent thought processes can occur simultaneously in the one individual. Thus the "mute" hemisphere communicates. The words and objects cannot be named verbally because the minor hemisphere is unable to communicate with the "talking" major hemisphere.

Several basic conclusions concerning the roles of the cerebral hemispheres obtained from studies of "twin-brain" subjects (see Fig. 16-19) are (1) perception and memory can be performed independently in both hemispheres; (2) language and speech are almost exclusively the roles of the major hemisphere; (3) the minor hemisphere is superior to the major hemisphere in the recognition and appreciation of spatial dimensions; (4) the primary role of the cerebral commissures is in the bilateral integration of the two hemispheres for linguistic functions; (5) it is through the major hemisphere that humans can have thoughts and knowledge expressed through language, and (6) the commissures are essential for maintaining the unity of the higher sensory and motor functions of the cerebrum. The following is a rather simplistic summary of roles of the two hemispheres. The left (major) hemisphere may be considered to be the analytical, rational, and verbal half of the cerebrum. It is analytic as used in language recognition. The right (minor) hemisphere is the synthetic, intuitive, and nonverbal half. It is nonanalytic as used in perceptual recognition.

An interesting illustration of visual perception by a split-brain subject (commissurotomy of the corpus callosum) is expressed in the response to the observation of a chimeric figure in which the right half is a male face and the left half is a female face. Upon fixating on the center of the figure, the assumption is that the male half is projected to the left hemisphere and the female half to the right hemisphere. When queried, subjects usually say they see a male face but point to the female face with the left hand.

Recent studies of twin-brain humans support the concept that the two cerebral hemispheres are (1) essentially equal and holistic in their perceptual capabilities but (2) unequal in their expressive (motor) capabilities. For example, when the left hemisphere "sees" an object, this hemisphere can respond to a question concerning the object by giving the appropriate answer by talking or by writing with the right hand. In contrast, when the right (mute) hemisphere sees an object, this hemisphere cannot respond with an appropriate answer to the same question by talking but can by drawing, gesturing, or pointing to one out of many answers on a panel with the left hand. When asked a question about an object seen by the right hemisphere, these patients respond with an inappropriate verbal answer because the talking hemisphere does not have access to the information locked in the mute hemisphere. In essence, the patient employs the strategy of using lateralized responses with the motor resources available to the hemisphere. Thus the two hemispheres are said to exhibit perceptual equality but motor response inequality. Both hemispheres are capable of expressing emotional responses through the limbic system.

Language

The organizational complexities of the neuroanatomic, neurophysiologic, and psychologic substrates associated with language and speech are, as yet, only slightly known. Much of the current understanding is derived from studies of patients with disturbances of language function re-sulting from damage to the brain; these disturbances are called aphasias. They are commonly classified as (1) *receptive (posterior or Wernicke's) aphasias* and (2) *expressive (anterior or Broca's) aphasia.* This simple classification is not accepted by many neurologists because aphasias are known to result also from brain injuries located outside Wernicke's and Broca's areas. *Wernicke's area* is located in the posterior part of the superior temporal gyrus (area 22) adjacent to the auditory cortex (see Fig. 16-18). This area is involved in the recognition of the patterns of the spoken language. *Broca's area* is located in the inferior frontal gyrus (orbital and opercular parts) just rostral to that region of the motor cortex with representation for the musculature associated with speech muscles of the face, tongue, lips, palate, and vocal chords. Speech can be arrested when Broca's area is electrically stimulated in the conscious person.

A patient with a lesion involving Wernicke's area of the dominant hemisphere usually has a *receptive aphasia*, expressed as a failure in understanding both the spoken and the written word. In such subjects the inputs to the cortex from the auditory and visual systems are apparently unimpaired. They speak rapidly, maintain natural speech rhythms, and have normal nuances of articulation. The conversational output sounds normal, but it is actually devoid of meaningful content. Key words are omitted; they are substituted by empty meaningless words, or replaced by related words ("knife" for "fork"), or unrelated words ("hammer" for "book").

In contrast, patients with a lesion presumably in Broca's area have an *expressive aphasia,* which is primarily a failure in the formulation of speech. They have a normal comprehension of language. Speech is labored and crudely articulated. The omission of small words and of the endings of nouns and verbs results in a telegraphic style or delivery. The muscles involved in speech are not paralyzed; this is demonstrated by the fact that many of these patients can often sing a formerly known song rapidly, correctly, and even with feeling.

To explain these aphasias, it is presumed that several areas of the cortex are associated and linked with one another in the following ways. Meaningful sounds are conveyed from the inner ears via auditory pathways to the auditory cortex in the temporal lobe. This processed information is relayed to Wernicke's area, which has a significant role in the conscious recognition of the spoken language. In a sense, spoken words are "understood" in Wernicke's area. The words to be spoken are then projected via association fibers of the arcuate fasciculus to Broca's area, where the articulatory phrases of speech are formulated. This information is relayed to the motor cortex of area 4, which is involved with the control and regulation of the musculature associated with speech. In order to spell a word orally, it must be visualized. This is accomplished by transferring the processed information of a word that is heard and understood in Wernicke's area to the angular gyrus, where the patterns of words are visualized. From the angular gyrus, the information is conveyed successively to Wernicke's area, Broca's area, and the "speech centers" of the primary motor cortex. On the other hand, the processed information obtained from reading written and spoken words is conveyed via the visual pathways to the primary, association, and inferotemporal areas and then to the angular gyrus. The visualized form within the angular gyrus is projected to Wernicke's area for conversion to the auditory form. This is consistent with the concept that *the comprehension of the written word involves the activation of the auditory form within Wernicke's area*, where it is understood.

Following a lesion of the angular gyrus, patients lose the ability to read (*alexia*) and write (*agraphia*). They can comprehend the spoken language and speak, but to them the written word is meaningless. Patients with alexia and agraphia are unable to recognize words spelled orally to them, nor can they spell aloud and write the spoken word.

In human beings, speech and language symbolisms of the written and spoken word are lateralized, even though the cortical areas associated with these activities have extensive connections through the corpus callosum. Both the dominant (or "talking") hemisphere and the nondominant ("mute") hemisphere can comprehend, but normally only the dominant hemisphere "talks."

Within the numerous variations of the basic neuronal types in the various regions of the neo-

cortex, there "is a basic constancy in the general organization of the cortical afferents, intracortical neurons and intracortical distribution of the axons. What remains constant is the arrangement of the plexuses of dendritic and axonal branches; i.e., of the synaptic articulations through which nerve impulses are transmitted" (Lorente de Nó).

BIBLIOGRAPHY

Brazier, M. A. B., and H. Petsche (eds.): *Architectonics of the Cerebral Cortex*, International Brain Research Organization (IBRO) Monograph Series, 3:1–486, Raven Press, New York, 1978.

Brodmann, K.: "Feinere Anatomie des Grosshirns," *Lewandowsky's Handbuch der Neurologie*, 1910, vol. 5, pp. 206–307.

Campbell, A. W.: *Histological Studies on the Localization of Cerebral Function*, Cambridge University Press, Cambridge, 1905.

Ebner, F. F., and R. Myers: Corpus callosum and the interhemispheric transfer of tactual learning. J Neurophysiol, 25:380–391, 1962.

Eccles, J. C.: *The Understanding of the Brain*, McGraw-Hill Book Company, New York, 1977.

Gazzaniga, M. S.: *The Bisected Brain*, Appleton-Century-Crofts, Inc., New York, 1970.

———, and J. E. LeDoux: *The Integrated Mind*, Plenum Press, New York, 1978.

Geschwind, N.: Specializations of the human brain. Sci Am, 241:180–201, 1979.

Goldman, P. S., and W. J. H. Nauta: Columnar distribution of cortice-cortical fibers in the frontal association, limbic and motor cortex of the developing rhesus monkey. Brain Res, 122:393–413, 1977.

Hartmann, E. I.: *The Functions of Sleep*, Yale University Press, New Haven, 1973.

Hubel, D. H., and T. N. Wiesel: Brain mechanisms of vision. Sci Am 241:150–162, 1979.

Lassen, N. A., D. H. Ingvar, and E. Skinhøj: Brain function and blood flow. Sci Am, 239:62–71, 1978.

Lorente de Nó, R.: "Cerebral Cortex: Architecture, Intracortical Connections, Motor Projections," in J. F. Fulton (ed.), *Physiology of the Nervous System*, Oxford University Press, New York, 1949, chap. 15, pp. 288–330.

Mountcastle, V. B.: "An Organizing Principle for Cerebral Function: The Unit Module and the Distribution System," in G. E. Edelman and V. B. Montcastle (eds.), *The Mindful Brain*, The M.I.T. Press, Cambridge, Mass., 1978, pp. 7–50.

Nauta, W. J. H.: The problem of the frontal lobe: a reinterpretation. J Psychiat Res 8:167–187, 1971.

Pandya, D., P. Dye, and N. Butters: Efferent cortico-cortical projections of the prefrontal cortex in the rhesus monkey. Brain Res, 31:35–44, 1971.

Penfield, W., and L. Roberts: *Speech and Brain Mechanisms*, Princeton University Press, Princeton, N. J., 1959.

Schaltenbrand, G., and C. N. Woolsey: *Principles of Cerebral Localization and Organization*, University of Wisconsin Press, Madison, 1964.

Scheibel, M. E., and A. B. Scheibel: "Elementary Processes in Selected Thalamic and Cortical Subsystems: The Structural Substrates," in F. O. Schmitt et al. (eds.), *The Neurosciences—Second Study Program*. Rockefeller University Press, New York, 1970.

Sperry, R. W.: *Mental Unity Following Surgical Disconnection of the Cerebral Hemispheres*, Harvey Lectures, Academic Press, Inc., New York, 1966–1967.

Szentágothai, J.: The neuron network of the cerebral cortex: a functional interpretation. Proc Roy Soc Lond, series B, 201:219–248, 1978.

Towe, A. L.: "Motor ortex and the pyramidal system," in J. D. Maser (ed.), *Efferent Organization and Integration of Behavior*, Academic Press, Inc., New York, 1973, pp. 67–97.

Valenstein, E. S.: *Brain Control: A Critical Examination of Stimulation and Psychosurgery*, John Wiley and Sons, Inc., New York, 1973.

Vogt, C., and O. Vogt: Allgemeine Ergebnisse unserer Hirnforschung. J Psychol Neurol, 25:279–461, 1919.

von Economo, C.: *The Cytoarchitectonics of the Human Cerebral Cortex*, Oxford University Press, London, 1929.

Woolsey, C. N.: "Organization of Somatic Sensory and Motor Areas of the Cerebral Cortex," in H. F. Harlow and C. N. Woolsey (eds.), *Biological and Biochemical Bases of Behavior*, The University of Wisconsin Press, Madison, 1958, pp. 63–81.

Wong-Riley, M.: Columnar cortico-cortical interconnections within the visual system of the squirrel and macaque monkeys. Brain Res, 162:201–217, 1979.

Zaidel, D., and R. W. Sperry: Memory impairment after commissurotomy in man. Brain, 97:263–272, 1974.

ATLAS 1

TRANSVERSE SECTIONS THROUGH THE BRAINSTEM

Drawing of the lateral view of the brainstem indicating the level and plane of the transverse sections in Figs. 8-4 through 8-13 and A-1 through A-22. (*Figures A-1 through A-11 after E. Villiger: Atlas of Cross Section Anatomy of the Brain, Blakiston Co., New York, 1951; Figs. A-11 to A-22 through courtesy of Dr. Joyce E. Shriver, Department of Anatomy, Mount Sinai School of Medicine, New York.*)

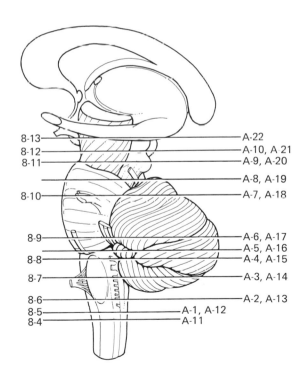

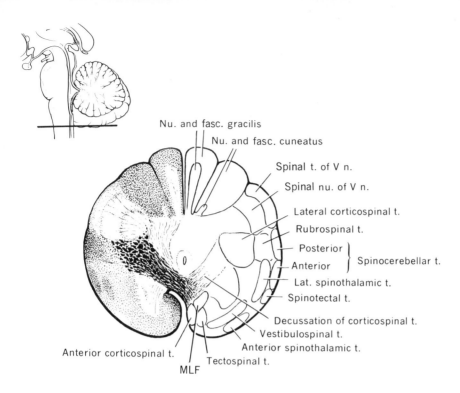

Nu. and fasc. gracilis

Nu. and fasc. cuneatus

Spinal t. of V n.

Spinal nu. of V n.

Lateral corticospinal t.

Rubrospinal t.

Posterior ⎫
Anterior ⎭ Spinocerebellar t.

Lat. spinothalamic t.

Spinotectal t.

Decussation of corticospinal t.

Vestibulospinal t.

Anterior spinothalamic t.

Anterior corticospinal t.

Tectospinal t.

MLF

FIGURE A-1 Transverse section of the lower medulla at the middle of the corticospinal (pyramidal) decussation. MLF, medial longitudinal fasciculus; n., nerve; nu., nucleus; t., tract. Refer to Figs. 8-3 and A-12. (*After Villiger.*)

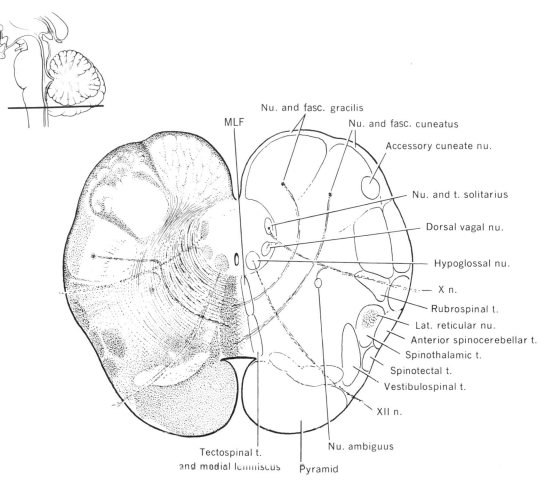

Nu. and fasc. gracilis

MLF

Nu. and fasc. cuneatus

Accessory cuneate nu.

Nu. and t. solitarius

Dorsal vagal nu.

Hypoglossal nu.

X n.

Rubrospinal t.

Lat. reticular nu.

Anterior spinocerebellar t.

Spinothalamic t.

Spinotectal t.

Vestibulospinal t.

XII n.

Nu. ambiguus

Tectospinal t.
and medial lemniscus

Pyramid

FIGURE A-2 Transverse section of the lower medulla at the level of the decussation of the medial lemniscus. Refer to Figs. 8-6 and A-13. (*After Villiger.*)

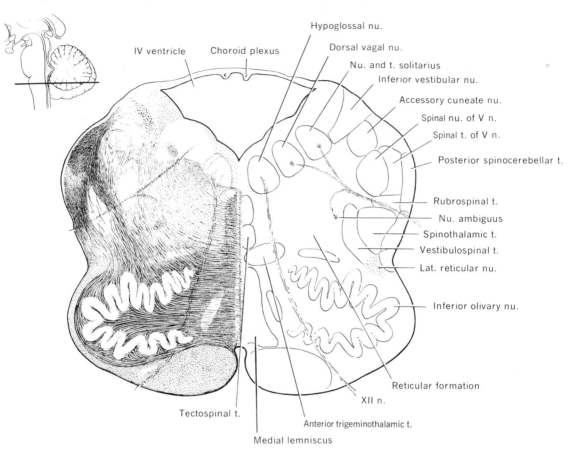

IV ventricle Choroid plexus

Hypoglossal nu.

Dorsal vagal nu.

Nu. and t. solitarius

Inferior vestibular nu.

Accessory cuneate nu.

Spinal nu. of V n.

Spinal t. of V n.

Posterior spinocerebellar t.

Rubrospinal t.

Nu. ambiguus

Spinothalamic t.

Vestibulospinal t.

Lat. reticular nu.

Inferior olivary nu.

Reticular formation

XII n.

Tectospinal t.

Anterior trigeminothalamic t.

Medial lemniscus

FIGURE A-3 Transverse section of the medulla at the level of the middle of the olive. Refer to Figs. 8-7 and A-14. (*After Villiger.*)

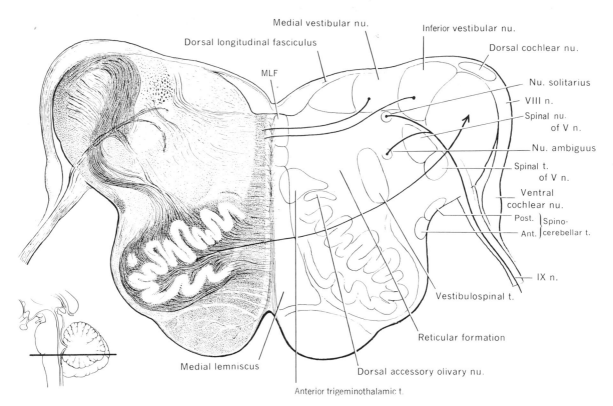

Dorsal longitudinal fasciculus

Medial vestibular nu.

Inferior vestibular nu.

Dorsal cochlear nu.

MLF

Nu. solitarius

VIII n.

Spinal nu. of V n.

Nu. ambiguus

Spinal t. of V n.

Ventral cochlear nu.

Post. } Spino-
Ant. } cerebellar t.

IX n.

Vestibulospinal t.

Reticular formation

Dorsal accessory olivary nu.

Medial lemniscus

Anterior trigeminothalamic t.

FIGURE A-4 Transverse section of the upper medulla at the level of the entrance of the cochlear nerve and the glossopharyngeal nerve. The nerve fibers from the medial and inferior vestibular nuclei join the medial longitudinal fasciculus (MLF). The fiber from the inferior olivary nucleus represents the olivocerebellar fibers which join the contralateral inferior cerebellar peduncle located deep to cranial nerve VIII. Refer to Figs. 8-8 and A-15. (*After Villiger.*)

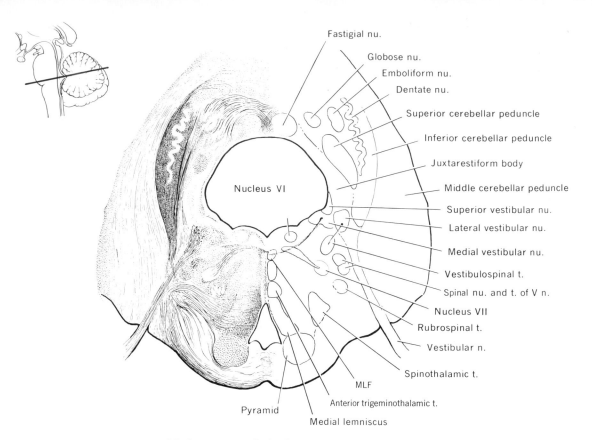

Fastigial nu.
Globose nu.
Emboliform nu.
Dentate nu.
Superior cerebellar peduncle
Inferior cerebellar peduncle
Juxtarestiform body
Middle cerebellar peduncle
Superior vestibular nu.
Lateral vestibular nu.
Medial vestibular nu.
Vestibulospinal t.
Spinal nu. and t. of V n.
Nucleus VII
Rubrospinal t.
Vestibular n.
Spinothalamic t.
Nucleus VI
MLF
Anterior trigeminothalamic t.
Pyramid
Medial lemniscus

FIGURE A-5 Transverse section of the lower pons at the level of the entrance of the vestibular nerve and of the cerebellum through the deep cerebellar nuclei. Refer to Fig. A-16. (*After Villiger.*)

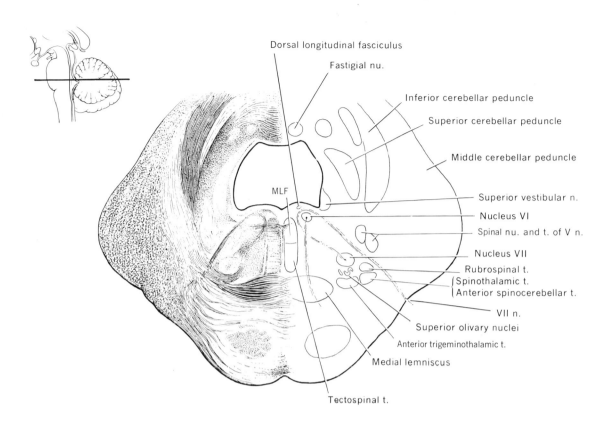

Dorsal longitudinal fasciculus

Fastigial nu.

Inferior cerebellar peduncle

Superior cerebellar peduncle

Middle cerebellar peduncle

MLF

Superior vestibular n.

Nucleus VI

Spinal nu. and t. of V n.

Nucleus VII

Rubrospinal t.
Spinothalamic t.
Anterior spinocerebellar t.

VII n.

Superior olivary nuclei

Anterior trigeminothalamic t.

Medial lemniscus

Tectospinal t.

FIGURE A-6 Transverse section of the pons at the level of the facial colliculus, abducent (VI) nucleus, and the superior olivary nuclei. Refer to Figs., 8-9 and A-17. (*After Villiger.*)

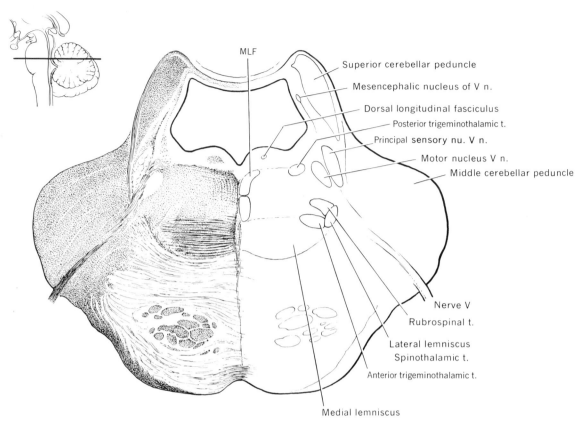

MLF

Superior cerebellar peduncle

Mesencephalic nucleus of V n.

Dorsal longitudinal fasciculus

Posterior trigeminothalamic t.

Principal sensory nu. V n.

Motor nucleus V n.

Middle cerebellar peduncle

Nerve V

Rubrospinal t.

Lateral lemniscus

Spinothalamic t.

Anterior trigeminothalamic t.

Medial lemniscus

FIGURE A-7 Transverse section of the pons at the level of the entrance of the fifth cranial nerve. Refer to Figs. 8-10 and A-18. (*After Villiger.*)

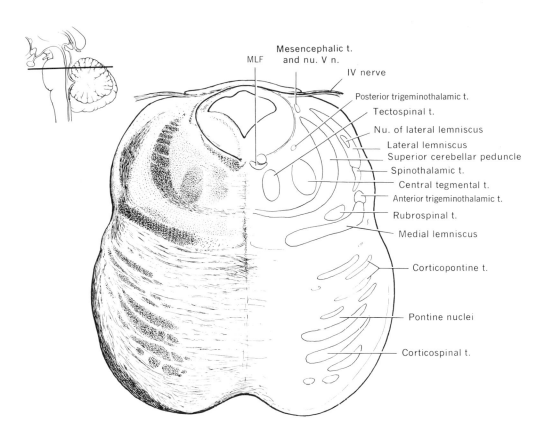

MLF

Mesencephalic t.
and nu. V n.

IV nerve

Posterior trigeminothalamic t.

Tectospinal t.

Nu. of lateral lemniscus

Lateral lemniscus

Superior cerebellar peduncle

Spinothalamic t.

Central tegmental t.

Anterior trigeminothalamic t.

Rubrospinal t.

Medial lemniscus

Corticopontine t.

Pontine nuclei

Corticospinal t.

FIGURE A-8 Transverse section of the isthmus region at the level of the decussation and emergence of the trochlear (IV) nerve and of the upper pons. Refer to Fig. A-19. *(After Villiger.)*

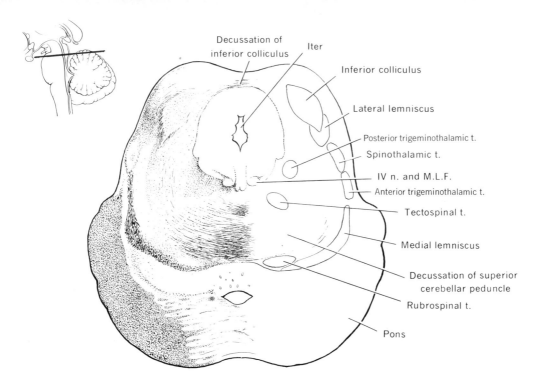

FIGURE A-9 Transverse section of the lower midbrain at the level of the inferior colliculus and decussation of the superior cerebellar peduncle. Refer to Figs. 8-11 and A-20. (*After Villiger.*)

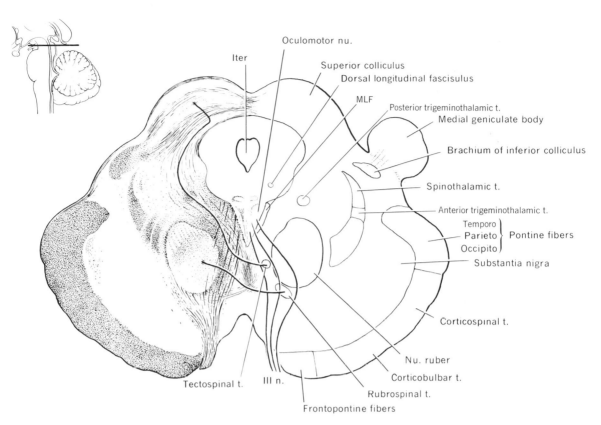

Oculomotor nu.

Iter

Superior colliculus

Dorsal longitudinal fascisulus

MLF

Posterior trigeminothalamic t.

Medial geniculate body

Brachium of inferior colliculus

Spinothalamic t.

Anterior trigeminothalamic t.

Temporo
Parieto } Pontine fibers
Occipito

Substantia nigra

Corticospinal t.

Nu. ruber

Corticobulbar t.

Tectospinal t.   III n.

Rubrospinal t.

Frontopontine fibers

FIGURE A-10 Transverse section of the upper midbrain at the level of the superior colliculus and the oculomotor (III) nerve. Refer to Figs. 8-12 and A-21. (*After Villiger.*)

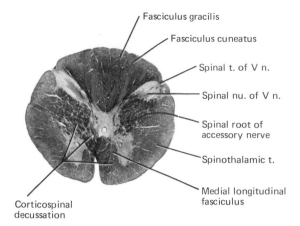

Fasciculus gracilis

Fasciculus cuneatus

Spinal t. of V n.

Spinal nu. of V n.

Spinal root of accessory nerve

Spinothalamic t.

Medial longitudinal fasciculus

Corticospinal decussation

FIGURE A-11 Transverse section in the region of the spinal cord–medulla junction at the caudal level of the corticospinal (pyramidal) decussation. Weigert myelin stain. Refer to Fig. 8-4.

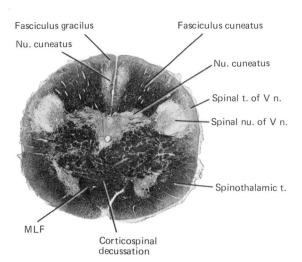

Fasciculus gracilus

Nu. cuneatus

Fasciculus cuneatus

Nu. cuneatus

Spinal t. of V n.

Spinal nu. of V n.

Spinothalamic t.

MLF

Corticospinal decussation

FIGURE A-12 Transverse section of the lower medulla at the middle of the corticospinal (pyramidal) decussation. Weigert myelin stain. Refer to Figs. 8-5 and A-1.

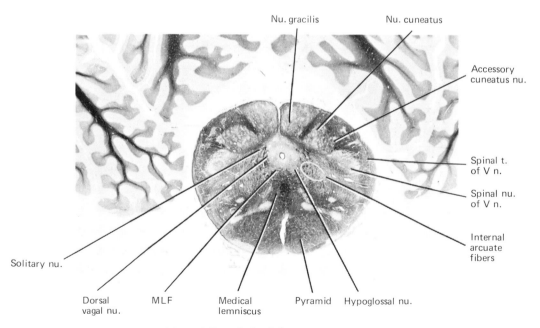

Nu. gracilis

Nu. cuneatus

Accessory cuneatus nu.

Spinal t. of V n.

Spinal nu. of V n.

Internal arcuate fibers

Solitary nu.

Dorsal vagal nu.

MLF

Medical lemniscus

Pyramid

Hypoglossal nu.

FIGURE A-13 Transverse section of the medulla at the level of the decussation of the medial lemniscus (internal arcuate fibers). Weigert myelin stain. Refer to Figs. 8-6 and A-2.

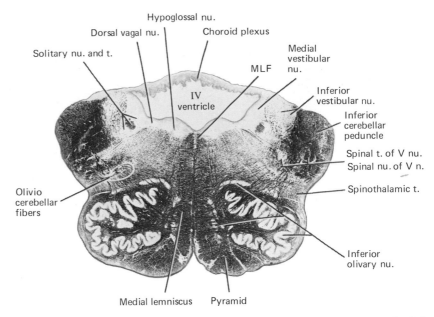

FIGURE A-14 Transverse section of the medulla at the level of the middle of the olive. Weigert myelin stain. Refer to Figs. 8-2 and A-3.

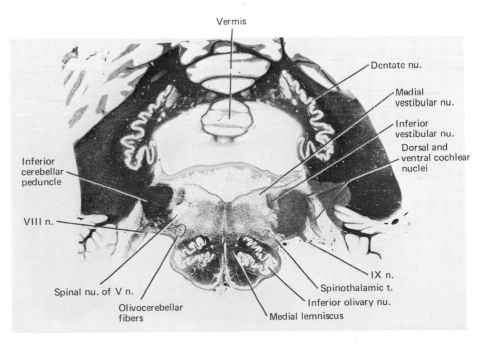

FIGURE A-15 Transverse section of the upper medulla at the level of the entrance of the cochlear nerve and the glossopharyngeal (IX) nerve. Weigert myelin stain. Refer to Figs. 8-8 and A-4.

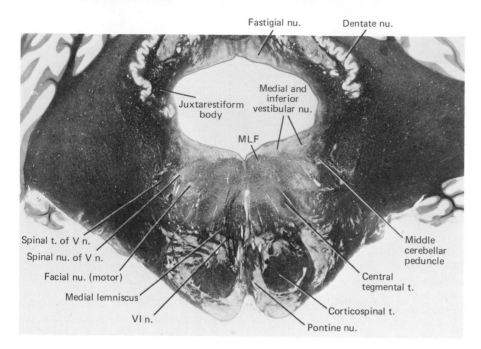

FIGURE A-16 Transverse section of the lower pons at the level of the facial motor nucleus and portions of the abducent nerve. Weigert myelin stain. Refer to Fig. A-5.

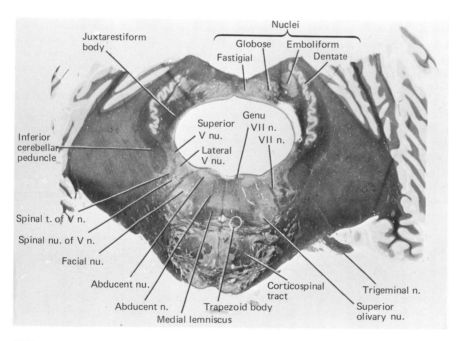

FIGURE A-17 Transverse section of the lower pons at the level of the facial (abducent) colliculus. Weigert myelin stain. Refer to Figs. 8-9 and A-6.

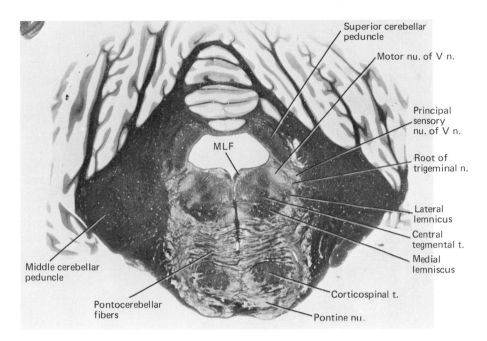

FIGURE A-18 Transverse section of the pons at the level of the motor and principal sensory nucleus of the trigeminal nerve. Weigert myelin stain. Refer to Figs. 8-10 and A-7.

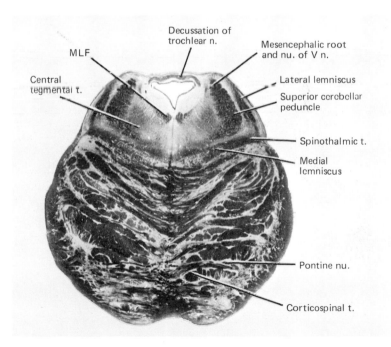

FIGURE A-19 Transverse section of the isthmus region at the level of the trochlear (IV) nerve and upper pons. Weigert myelin stain. Refer to Fig. A-8.

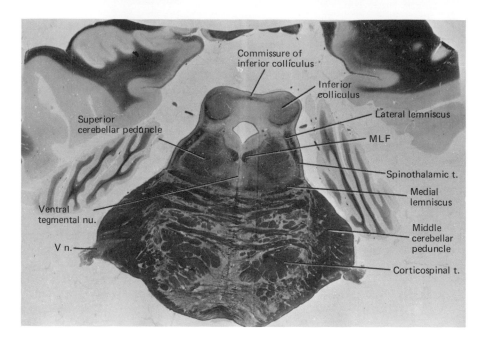

FIGURE A-20 Transverse section of the lower midbrain at the level of the inferior colliculus. Weigert myelin stain. Refer to Figs. 8-11 and A-9.

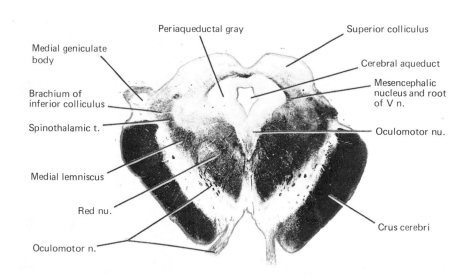

FIGURE A-21 Transverse section of the upper midbrain at the level of the superior colliculus and the oculomotor (III) nerve. Weigert myelin stain. Refer to Figs. 8-12 and A-10.

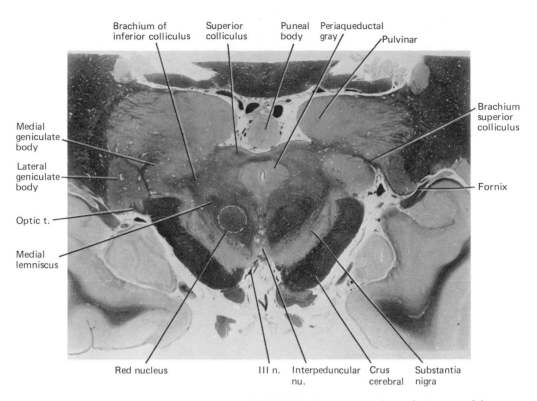

Brachium of inferior colliculus

Superior colliculus

Puneal body

Periaqueductal gray

Pulvinar

Medial geniculate body

Lateral geniculate body

Optic t.

Medial lemniscus

Brachium superior colliculus

Fornix

Red nucleus   III n.   Interpeduncular nu.   Crus cerebral   Substantia nigra

FIGURE A-22 Transverse section at the junction of the upper midbrain and the diencephalon. Weigert myelin stain. Refer to Fig. 8-13.

ATLAS 2

CORONAL (FRONTAL) SECTIONS THROUGH THE CEREBRUM

Drawing of the median sagittal section of the brain indicating the level and plane of coronal sections in Figs. A-23 through A-32.

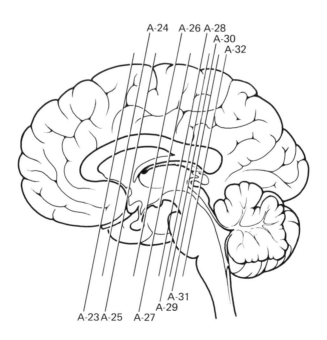

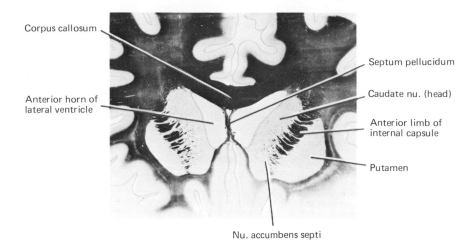

Corpus callosum

Anterior horn of
lateral ventricle

Septum pellucidum

Caudate nu. (head)

Anterior limb of
internal capsule

Putamen

Nu. accumbens septi

FIGURE A-23 Coronal section of cerebrum through head of
caudate nucleus and putamen. Weigert stain.

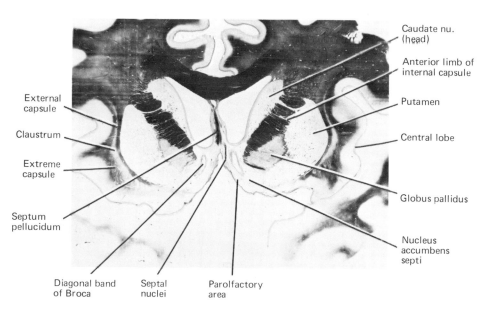

External
capsule

Claustrum

Extreme
capsule

Septum
pellucidum

Caudate nu.
(head)

Anterior limb of
internal capsule

Putamen

Central lobe

Globus pallidus

Nucleus
accumbens
septi

Diagonal band
of Broca

Septal
nuclei

Parolfactory
area

FIGURE A-24 Coronal section of cerebrum through head of
caudate nucleus, putamen, and globus pallidus. Weigert stain.

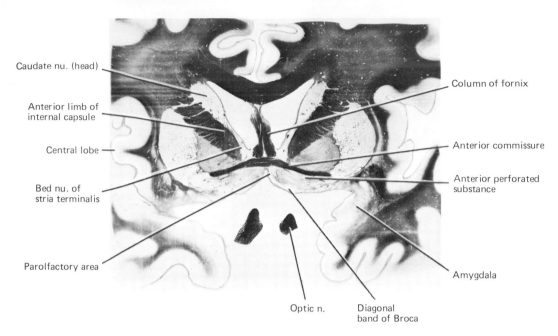

Caudate nu. (head)

Anterior limb of
internal capsule

Central lobe

Bed nu. of
stria terminalis

Parolfactory area

Column of fornix

Anterior commissure

Anterior perforated
substance

Amygdala

Optic n.

Diagonal
band of Broca

FIGURE A-25 Coronal section of cerebrum through anterior
commissure and parolfactory area. Weigert stain.

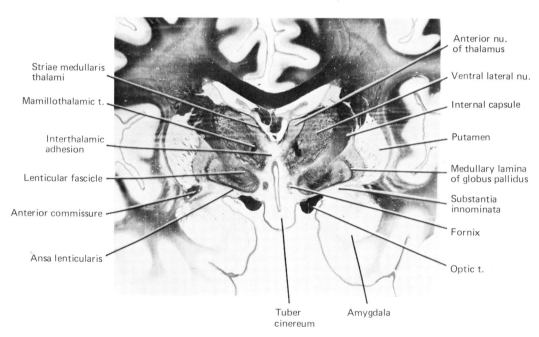

Striae medullaris
thalami

Mamillothalamic t.

Interthalamic
adhesion

Lenticular fascicle

Anterior commissure

Ansa lenticularis

Anterior nu.
of thalamus

Ventral lateral nu.

Internal capsule

Putamen

Medullary lamina
of globus pallidus

Substantia
innominata

Fornix

Optic t.

Tuber
cinereum

Amygdala

FIGURE A-26 Coronal section of cerebrum through rostral
thalamus and tuber cinereum of hypothalamus. Weigert stain.

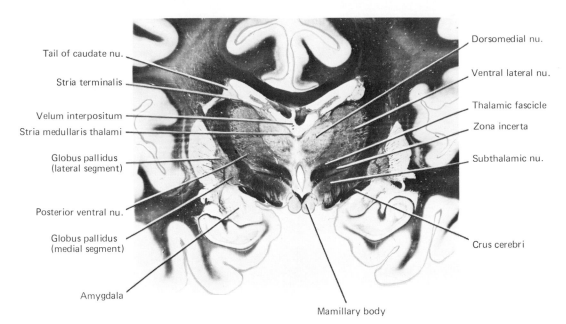

Tail of caudate nu.

Stria terminalis

Velum interpositum

Stria medullaris thalami

Globus pallidus
(lateral segment)

Posterior ventral nu.

Globus pallidus
(medial segment)

Amygdala

Dorsomedial nu.

Ventral lateral nu.

Thalamic fascicle

Zona incerta

Subthalamic nu.

Crus cerebri

Mamillary body

FIGURE A-27 Coronal section of cerebrum through thalamus and mamillary body. Weigert stain.

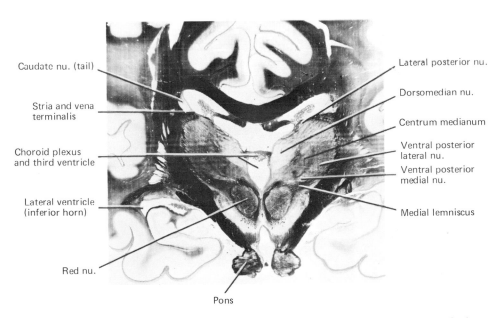

Caudate nu. (tail)

Stria and vena
terminalis

Choroid plexus
and third ventricle

Lateral ventricle
(inferior horn)

Red nu.

Pons

Lateral posterior nu.

Dorsomedian nu.

Centrum medianum

Ventral posterior
lateral nu.

Ventral posterior
medial nu.

Medial lemniscus

FIGURE A-28 Coronal section through thalamus, cerebral peduncle, and rostral basilar pons. Weigert stain.

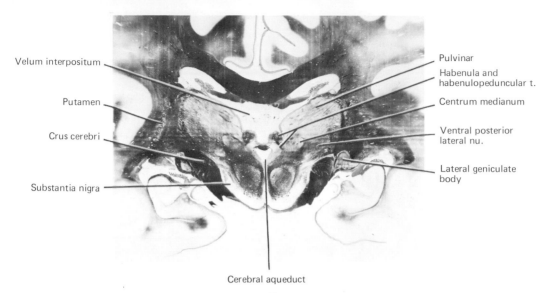

Velum interpositum

Putamen

Crus cerebri

Substantia nigra

Pulvinar

Habenula and
habenulopeduncular t.

Centrum medianum

Ventral posterior
lateral nu.

Lateral geniculate
body

Cerebral aqueduct

FIGURE A-29 Coronal section through pulvinar, centrum medianum, and cerebral peduncle. Portions of the basal midbrain and pons are missing from the section. Weigert stain.

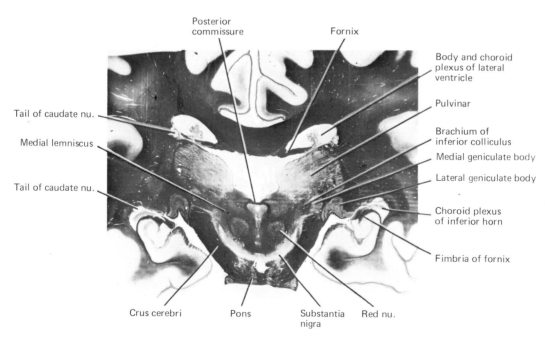

Posterior
commissure

Fornix

Tail of caudate nu.

Medial lemniscus

Tail of caudate nu.

Body and choroid
plexus of lateral
ventricle

Pulvinar

Brachium of
inferior colliculus

Medial geniculate body

Lateral geniculate body

Choroid plexus
of inferior horn

Fimbria of fornix

Crus cerebri   Pons   Substantia   Red nu.
                              nigra

FIGURE A-30 Coronal section through pulvinar, posterior commissure, and cerebral peduncle. Weigert stain.

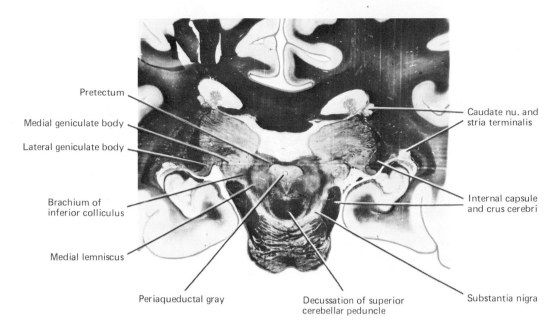

Pretectum

Medial geniculate body

Lateral geniculate body

Brachium of
inferior colliculus

Medial lemniscus

Periaqueductal gray

Caudate nu. and
stria terminalis

Internal capsule
and crus cerebri

Decussation of superior
cerebellar peduncle

Substantia nigra

FIGURE A-31 Coronal section through pulvinar, geniculate bodies, and decussation of superior cerebellar peduncle. Weigert stain.

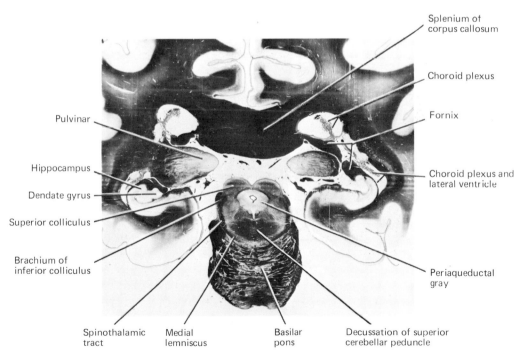

Pulvinar

Hippocampus

Dendate gyrus

Superior colliculus

Brachium of
inferior colliculus

Splenium of
corpus callosum

Choroid plexus

Fornix

Choroid plexus and
lateral ventricle

Periaqueductal
gray

Spinothalamic
tract

Medial
lemniscus

Basilar
pons

Decussation of superior
cerebellar peduncle

FIGURE A-32 Coronal section through splenium of corpus callosum, superior colliculus, and basilar pons. Weigert stain.

ATLAS 3

HORIZONTAL SECTIONS THROUGH THE BRAIN

Drawing of the median sagittal section of the brain indicating the level and plane of horizontal sections in Figs. A-33 through A-39.

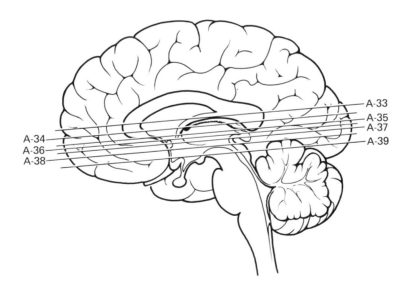

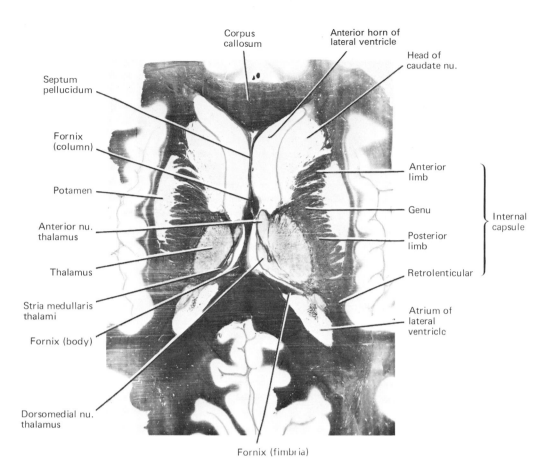

Septum
pellucidum

Fornix
(column)

Potamen

Anterior nu.
thalamus

Thalamus

Stria medullaris
thalami

Fornix (body)

Dorsomedial nu.
thalamus

Corpus
callosum

Anterior horn of
lateral ventricle

Head of
caudate nu.

Anterior
limb

Genu

Posterior
limb

Internal
capsule

Retrolenticular

Atrium of
lateral
ventricle

Fornix (fimbria)

FIGURE A-33 Horizontal section of the brain passing through the head of caudate nucleus, internal capsule, putamen, body of fornix, and thalamus.

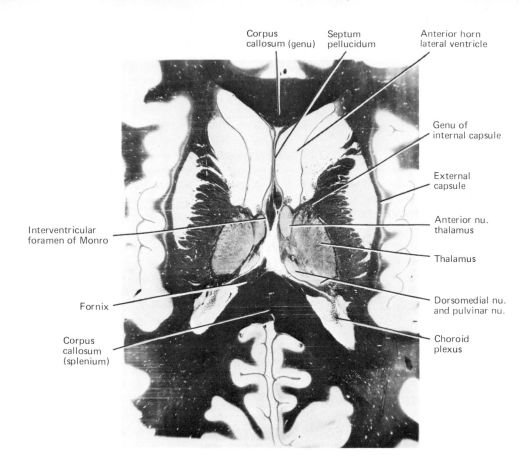

Corpus callosum (genu)

Septum pellucidum

Anterior horn lateral ventricle

Genu of internal capsule

External capsule

Anterior nu. thalamus

Thalamus

Interventricular foramen of Monro

Dorsomedial nu. and pulvinar nu.

Fornix

Choroid plexus

Corpus callosum (splenium)

FIGURE A-34 Horizontal section of the brain passing through the head of caudate nucleus, putamen, internal capsule, interventricular foramen of Monro, and thalamus.

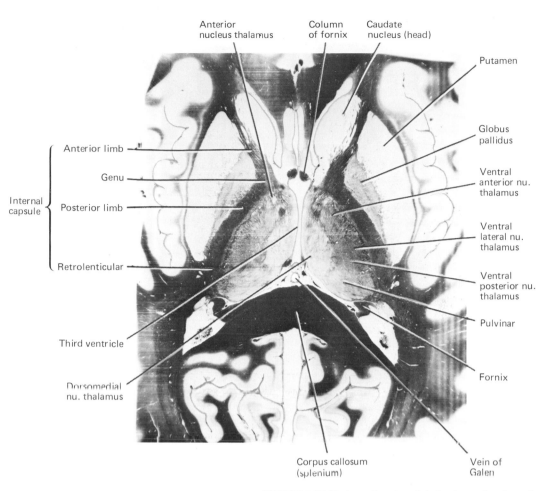

Anterior nucleus thalamus

Column of fornix

Caudate nucleus (head)

Putamen

Globus pallidus

Ventral anterior nu. thalamus

Ventral lateral nu. thalamus

Ventral posterior nu. thalamus

Pulvinar

Fornix

Vein of Galen

Anterior limb

Genu

Posterior limb

Internal capsule

Retrolenticular

Third ventricle

Dorsomedial nu. thalamus

Corpus callosum (splenium)

FIGURE A-35 Horizontal section of the brain passing through the head of caudate nucleus, internal capsule, third ventricle, putamen, globus pallidus, and thalamus.

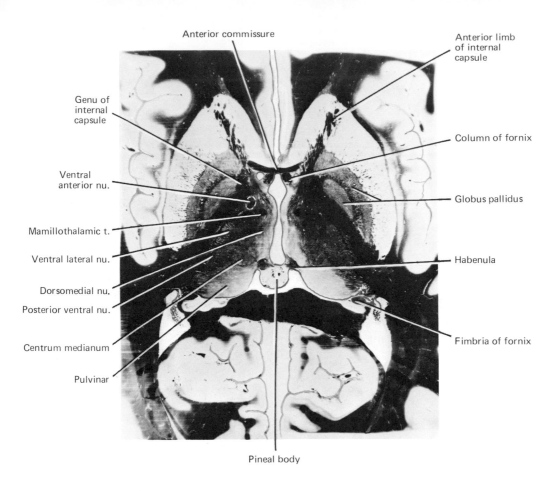

Anterior commissure

Anterior limb
of internal
capsule

Genu of
internal
capsule

Column of fornix

Ventral
anterior nu.

Globus pallidus

Mamillothalamic t.

Ventral lateral nu.

Dorsomedial nu.

Habenula

Posterior ventral nu.

Centrum medianum

Pulvinar

Fimbria of fornix

Pineal body

FIGURE A-36 Horizontal section of the brain passing through the head of caudate nucleus, anterior commissure, third ventricle, centrum medianum of thalamus, and pineal body.

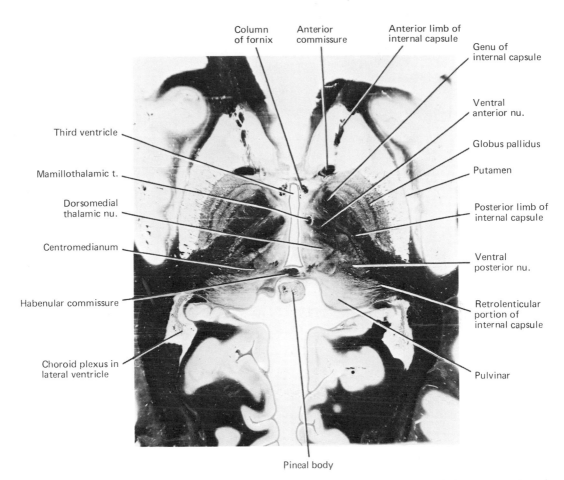

Column
of fornix

Anterior
commissure

Anterior limb of
internal capsule

Genu of
internal capsule

Ventral
anterior nu.

Globus pallidus

Putamen

Posterior limb of
internal capsule

Ventral
posterior nu.

Retrolenticular
portion of
internal capsule

Pulvinar

Third ventricle

Mamillothalamic t.

Dorsomedial
thalamic nu.

Centromedianum

Habenular commissure

Choroid plexus in
lateral ventricle

Pineal body

FIGURE A-37 Horizontal section of the brain passing through the head of caudate nucleus, anterior commissure, internal capsule, third ventricle, globus palllidus, thalamus, and pineal body.

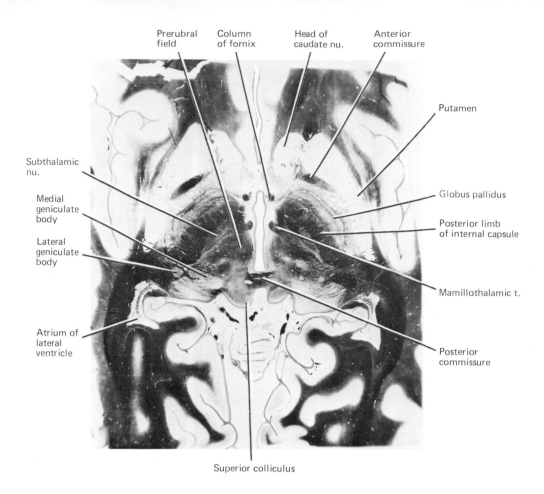

Prerubral field · Column of fornix · Head of caudate nu. · Anterior commissure · Putamen · Subthalamic nu. · Globus pallidus · Medial geniculate body · Posterior limb of internal capsule · Lateral geniculate body · Mamillothalamic t. · Atrium of lateral ventricle · Posterior commissure · Superior colliculus

FIGURE A-38 Horizontal section of the brain passing through the anterior commissure, putamen, globus pallidus, red nucleus, third ventricle, and superior colliculus.

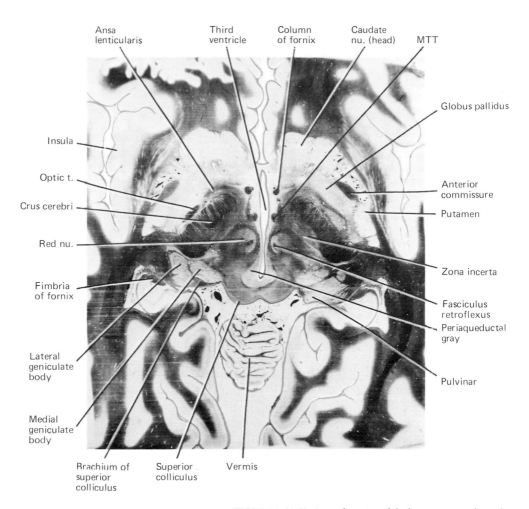

Ansa lenticularis

Third ventricle

Column of fornix

Caudate nu. (head)

MTT

Globus pallidus

Insula

Anterior commissure

Optic t.

Putamen

Crus cerebri

Red nu.

Zona incerta

Fimbria of fornix

Fasciculus retroflexus

Periaqueductal gray

Lateral geniculate body

Pulvinar

Medial geniculate body

Brachium of superior colliculus

Superior colliculus

Vermis

FIGURE A-39 Horizontal section of the brain passing through the caudate nucleus, putamen, globus pallidus, third ventricle, red nucleus, and superior colliculus. MTT, mamillothalamic tract.

SAGITTAL SECTIONS
THROUGH THE BRAIN

Drawing of median sagittal section through the brain indicating the level and plane of sagittal sections in Figs. A-40 through A-45.

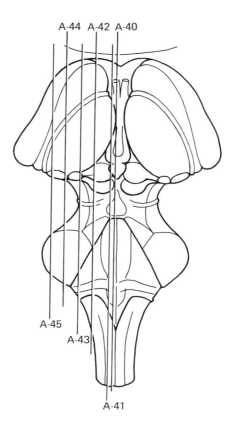

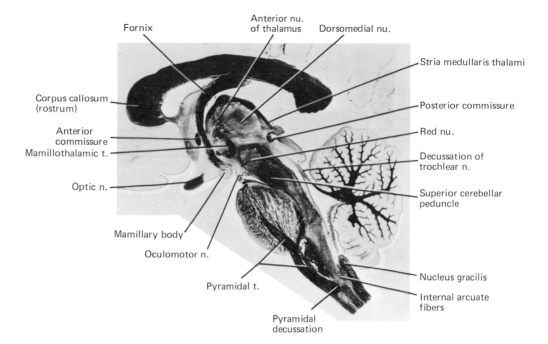

Fornix

Anterior nu.
of thalamus

Dorsomedial nu.

Stria medullaris thalami

Corpus callosum
(rostrum)

Posterior commissure

Anterior
commissure
Mamillothalamic t.

Red nu.

Optic n.

Decussation of
trochlear n.

Superior cerebellar
peduncle

Mamillary body

Oculomotor n.

Nucleus gracilis

Internal arcuate
fibers

Pyramidal t.

Pyramidal
decussation

FIGURE A-40 Parasaggital section of brainstem through column of fornix, oculomotor nerve, and pyramidal decussation.

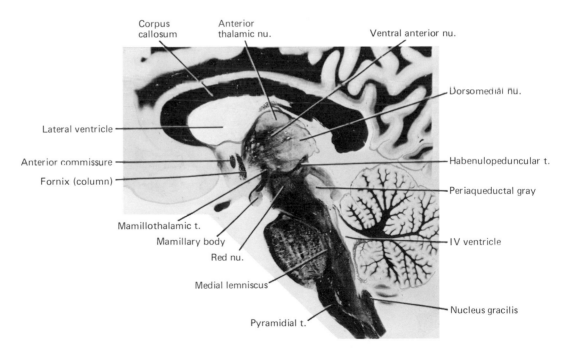

Corpus
callosum

Anterior
thalamic nu.

Ventral anterior nu.

Dorsomedial nu.

Lateral ventricle

Anterior commissure

Habenulopeduncular t.

Fornix (column)

Periaqueductal gray

Mamillothalamic t.

Mamillary body

Red nu.

IV ventricle

Medial lemniscus

Pyramidial t.

Nucleus gracilis

FIGURE A-41 Parasagittal section of brainstem through anterior nucleus of thalamus, medial lemniscus, and nucleus gracilis.

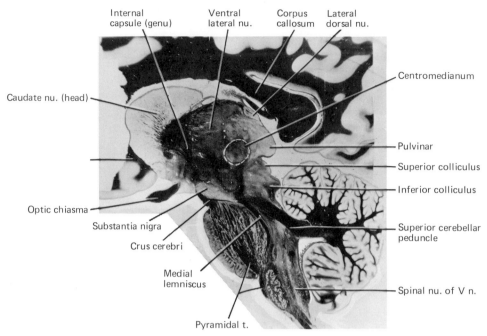

Internal
capsule (genu)

Ventral
lateral nu.

Corpus
callosum

Lateral
dorsal nu.

Centromedianum

Caudate nu. (head)

Pulvinar

Superior colliculus

Inferior colliculus

Optic chiasma

Substantia nigra

Crus cerebri

Superior cerebellar
peduncle

Medial
lemniscus

Spinal nu. of V n.

Pyramidal t.

FIGURE A-42 Parasagittal section of brainstem through optic chiasm, centromedianum, and spinal nucleus of trigeminal nerve.

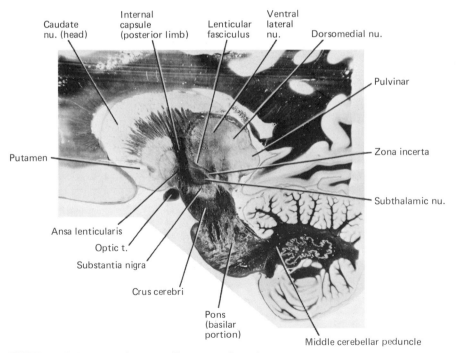

Caudate
nu. (head)

Internal
capsule
(posterior limb)

Lenticular
fasciculus

Ventral
lateral
nu.

Dorsomedial nu.

Pulvinar

Putamen

Zona incerta

Subthalamic nu.

Ansa lenticularis

Optic t.

Substantia nigra

Crus cerebri

Pons
(basilar
portion)

Middle cerebellar peduncle

FIGURE A-43 Parasagittal section of brainstem through medial globus pallidus, subthalamic nucleus, and crus cerebri.

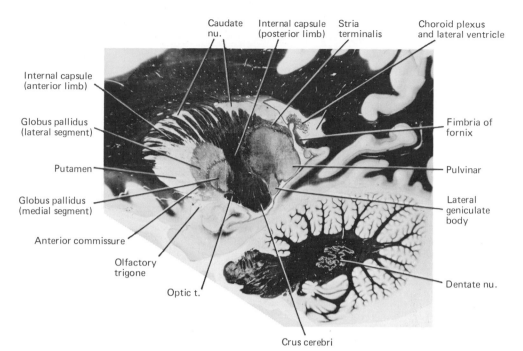

FIGURE A-44 Parasagittal section of brainstem through putamen, lateral geniculate body, and dentate nucleus of cerebellum.

Labels for Figure A-44:
- Caudate nu.
- Internal capsule (posterior limb)
- Stria terminalis
- Choroid plexus and lateral ventricle
- Internal capsule (anterior limb)
- Globus pallidus (lateral segment)
- Putamen
- Globus pallidus (medial segment)
- Anterior commissure
- Olfactory trigone
- Optic t.
- Crus cerebri
- Fimbria of fornix
- Pulvinar
- Lateral geniculate body
- Dentate nu.

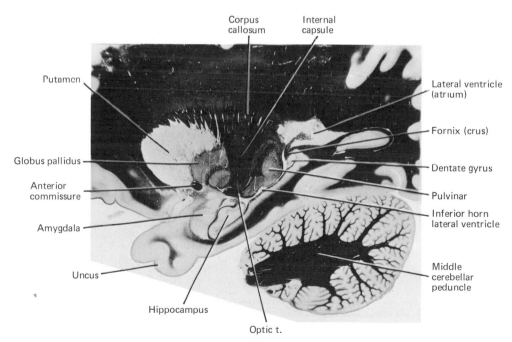

FIGURE A-45 Parasagittal section of brainstem through amygdaloid nucleus, lateral globus pallidus, dentate gyrus, and lateral cerebellum.

Labels for Figure A-45:
- Corpus callosum
- Internal capsule
- Putamen
- Globus pallidus
- Anterior commissure
- Amygdala
- Uncus
- Hippocampus
- Optic t.
- Lateral ventricle (atrium)
- Fornix (crus)
- Dentate gyrus
- Pulvinar
- Inferior horn lateral ventricle
- Middle cerebellar peduncle

INDEX

INDEX

Page numbers in *italic* refer to illustrations.

Autonomic nervous system:
sympathetic, 220–229, *221*
anatomy of, 220–225
compared to parasympathetic
system, 224–225
efferent segmental distribution of outflow, 225
interneurons in ganglia of,
225
physiology of, 226–227
reflex arc in, 225, *226*
trophic effects of, 241–242
and visceral learning, 242
Aversion centers, 480
Axes:
of brain, 22–23
optical, 390
visual, 390
Axolemma, 51
Axons, 50, 57, 58, 60
collateral sprouting of, *86*, 87–
88, 131, 137, 489
development and growth of, 131
blueprint hypothesis of, 131
hillock of, *52, 53*, 58, 60
potential at, *92*
initial segment of, 58, 60
long, *50*, 60
myelinated, *52*, 60, *94*
reaction after transection, 85
regeneration of, 86–87
synapses of (*see* Synapse)
terminal of, 60
unmyelinated, 60, *94*
Axoplasm transport and flow,
61–62

Ballism, 457, 459
Band, diagonal, of Broca, 11, 468,
468
Barr body, 55
Barrier:
blood-brain, 45, 75–78
meningeal, 78
Basal ganglia, 26–27, *291, 446,*
447–452
ablation of, 457
archistriatum, 448
connections and circuits for,
452–455
functional and clinical considerations, 452, 458–460
globus pallidus, 448–451
neurotransmitters associated
with, 455–456

Basal ganglia:
stimulation of, 457
striatum (neostriatum), 448–
449
substantia nigra, 451
subthalamic nucleus, 451
Basket cells (*see* Cells, basket)
Behavior and emotions, 476
agonistic, 476
basal ganglia ablation affecting,
457
goal-directed, limbic system affecting, 478–480
hormones affecting, 138–140
hypothalamus affecting, 238,
383–384
limbic lobe role in, 13
prefrontal lobe role in, 12
and putative neurotransmitters,
476–477
in split-brain animals, 521–522
terminology for, 475–476
Bell's palsy, 259–260, 320
Benedikt syndrome, 319
Biceps brachii muscle, innervation of, 157
Biofeedback, 242
Bladder:
automatic, 236
reflex, 214, 236
Blindness:
congenital, 140
monocular, 421
psychic, 507
Blocking agents:
competitive, 238
depolarizing, 238
Blood:
hyperosmotic, 382
hypotonic, 382
Blood-brain barrier, 45, 75–78
Blood flow in brain, 517
Blood supply:
of brain, 28–40
of brainstem, 316
of hypophysis, 375
of spinal cord, 205–207
Blood vessels, innervation of, 234
Body:
amygdaloid (*see* Amygdala)
Barr, 55
basal, of hair cells of organ of
Corti, 346, *346*
carotid, 220, *261*, 262
chemoreceptors in, 29
ciliary, 389, *389, 390*, 392

Body:
of corpus callosum, 11, *484*
of fornix, 9, *24, 427*
geniculate: lateral, *16*, 18, *18,
24, 31, 285, 287, 351*, 353,
354, 408, 409, 410, *411*, 412,
431, 432, 434, 435, *438*
medial, *18*, 269, *287, 431, 432,
434*, 435, *438*
Herring, 377
juxtarestiform, 280, *281, 332,
333, 334, 365*
of lateral ventricle, 21, *21*, 26,
32, 427
mammillary, 7, *8, 12, 24*, 245,
369, *370, 373, 467, 475, 485*
Nissl, 55
Pacchionian, 46
paraterminal, 10–11
pineal, 7, *18, 34*, 269, *287*, 385,
386, *438*
restiform, 19
trapezoid, *351*, 352
vitreous, 389, *390*
Body scheme, failure of, 506
Botulinus toxin and acetylcholine
release, 103
Boutons, synaptic, 60
Brachialis muscle, innervation of, 157
Brachium:
conjunctivum (*see* Peduncle,
cerebellar, superior)
of inferior colliculus, *18*, 18–19,
19, 269, *284, 285*
pontis (*see* Peduncle, cerebellar,
middle)
of superior colliculus, 18, *18,
19, 409*
Bradycardia, 233
Brain, 1–47
anatomy of: gross, 1–47
microscopic, 49–88
arterial supply of, 30–38
ascending pathways from spinal
cord, 169–173
axes of, 22–23
barriers in, 75
basal aspects of, *13*, 15–17
blood supply of, 28–40
CAT scan of, 47
core structures and arc structures of, 23–25
development of, 142–146
postnatal, *145*, 145–146
prenatal, *142, 143, 144*, 142–
145

Position sense, pathways for, 180
Posture, 337 – 338, 443 – 445
Potassium:
    diffusion across plasma membrane, 91 – 95
    sodium-potassium pump, 54, *54*, 93, 95, 111
Potential:
    action, 90 – 91, 93 – 98
    all-or-none, 57, 90, *92*, 117
    baby, 96
    and cable property, 94, 97
    and decremental conduction, 94, 97 – 98
    dendritic, 106
        postsynaptic, 91
    graded, 91, *92*
        excitatory, 101
        inhibitory, 101
    input, 91
    integrated, 90, 93, 94
    and local or graded response, 94, 97, *102*
    miniature end plate (MEPP), 102
    nonpropagating, 91, *92*
    and obligatory response, 101, 107
    optional, 107
    postsynaptic, 97
        dendritic, 91
        excitatory (EPSP), *92*, 101, *103*, 106, 120
        inhibitory (IPSP), *92*, 101, *103*, 106, 120
    presynaptic, 97
    propagated, 91
    receptor (generator), 91, 98 – 99, 108 – 109, 119
    and refractory periods, 96
    regenerative, 93
    resting, 90, *91*, 91 – 93
    and saltatory conduction, 95 – 96
    transducer, 91
Precuneus, *465*, *484*
Presbyacusis, 355
Pressoreceptors, 29, 108, 167, 262, 310
Pretectum, *269*, 271
Process, spinous, *153*
Processing in nervous system, 119 – 123
Prolactin-inhibiting factor (PIF), 376
Prolactin-releasing factor (PRF), 376

Prosencephalon (forebrain), 1, 127
    prenatal development of, *142*
Protein:
    deficiency of, 138
    ionic channels composed of, 91, 93, 111
    in plasma membrane, 54, 110 – 111
    receptor, 100, 111
    turnover in brain, 131
Psalterium, 10
Ptosis of eyelids, 254
Pulvinar, 18, *18*, *24*, *287*, *408*, *434*, *436*, *495*
Pump, sodium-potassium, 54, *54*, 93, 95, 111
Puncture, spinal, 42, 46, 154
Punishing centers, 479 – 480
Pupil:
    Argyll-Robertson, 421
    constriction of, 417 – 418
    dilatation of, 418 – 419
    paradoxical reaction of, 240
Purkinje cells (*see* Cells, Purkinje)
Purkinje effct, 407
Pursuit movements, smooth, 420
Putamen, 27, *28*, *31*, *34*, *306*, *427*, *438*, *446*, *448*, *449*, *450*, *453*, *454*
    ablation of, 457
Pyramid, *6*, *7*, *12*, *16*, 17, *17*, *26*, *198*, *245*, *271*, *272*, *274*, *276*, *324*, *437*

Quadriceps femoris muscle, innervation of, 157
Quadriplegia, 213

Radiation:
    auditory, *438*, *495*
    optic, *26*, *30*, *32*, *33*, *34*, 412 – 413, *422*, *437*, *438*, *495*
    thalamic, 438
Rage:
    sham, 383 – 384, 376
    true, 476
Ramus:
    gray, 223
    of spinal nerves, 154 – 155
        dorsal, 154, *155*
        ventral, 154 – 155, *155*
    white, *155*, 223
Reaction, arrest, 477
Rebound phenomenon, 339

Receptors:
    acetylcholine, 238 – 239
    adrenergic, 239 – 240
        alpha, 240
        beta, 240
    central, 310
    chemoreceptors, 29, 108, 167, 262, 310
    cold, 79
    exteroceptive, 167
    hypothalamic, 377 – 379, 382
    interoceptive, 167
    muscarinic, 239
    nicotinic, 238 – 239
    nociceptors, 173
    olfactory, 462
        interaction with odorant, 462
    opiate, 175, 296 – 297
    osmoreceptor cells, hypothalamic, 382
    peripheral, physiology of, 107 – 110
    photoreceptors, 388, 397 – 398
    potential, 98 – 99, 108 – 109, 119
    pressoreceptors, 29, 108, 167, 262, 310
    proprioceptive, 167
    sensory (afferent), 108, 118, 167, 168
    sites in postsynaptic membranes, 100 – 101
    vestibular, 357 – 358
    visual, 388, 397 – 398
Recess:
    of fourth ventricle, lateral, *19*, 20, *21*
    infundibular, *7*, *21*
    pineal, *21*
    supraoptic, *7*, *21*
Recruitment, 114 – 115, 429, 431, 441
Rectal function disorders, 236
Reflex:
    acoustic, 344
    areflexia, 209, 210
    Babinski, 211
    bladder, 214, 236
    carotid, 262
    cerebral ischemic, 30
    clasp-knife, 211
    corneal, 257
    cough, 233
    crossed extensor, 193, *194*, 195
    disynaptic, 158
    extensor, monosynaptic, 188 – 190

Striae:
  semicircularis (*see* terminalis, *below*)
  terminalis, 10, *10*, *18*, *25*, *31*, *269*, *287*, *427*, *469*, *474*
  vascularis, *343*
Striatum (neostriatum), 27, 448–449
  stimulation of, 457
Striola of maculae of saccule and utricle, *357*, 359
Stripe, Hensen's, 346, *347*
Subiculum, 8, *8*, 470, 472, 482
Subnucleus caudalis, 294
Substance:
  Nissl, 52, *53*, 55
  perforated: anterior, 15, 16, *245*, *368*, *368*, *463*, *467*, *474*, *485*
    posterior, 16, *245*, *485*
Substance P, 175, 297
Substantia:
  alba (*see* White matter)
  gelatinosa, 162, *163*, 174–175, *247*
  grisea (*see* Gray matter)
  innominata, of Reichert, 470
  nigra, 15, *31*, 272, 285, *285*, *287*, *306*, *446*, 448, 450, 451, *454*
    and globus pallidus, 451–452
    pars compacta, *285*, 451, 454
    pars reticularis, *285*, 451, 454
Subthalamus, 14, *31*, *427*, 448
Sulcus (sulci), 3
  anterolateral, of spinal cord, 154, *162*
  calcarine, 7, *8*, *30*, *33*, *409*, *483*
  central, of Rolando, *2*, *4*, *4*, *5*, *6*, *6*, *8*, *465*, *483*, *484*
    prenatal development of, *143*
  cingulate, *8*, *484*
  collateral, *10*, 12, 15, *245*, 465, *484*, 485
  of corpus callosum, *8*
  dorsal: intermediate, *19*
    lateral, *19*
    median, *19*
  fimbria-dentate, *471*
  frontal: inferior, 5, *483*
    superior, 4–5, *483*
  hippocampal, *465*, *471*
  hypothalamic, *6*, *370*
  interparietal, 5, *483*
  intraparietal, 5
  lateral, *2*, 4, *483*
  limitans, *19*, *126*, 133, *278*
  lunate, 6

Sulcus (sulci):
  olfactory, anterior, 10
  orbital, 11
  parietooccipital, 7, *465*, *483*, *484*, *485*
  postcentral, 5, *483*
  posterior: intermediate, 154, *162*
    median, 153–154
  posterolateral, of spinal cord, 154, *162*
  precentral, *2*, *483*
  preolivary, 16
  rhinal, *10*, 12, 15, *465*, *468*, *474*, *484*, *485*
  temporal: inferior, *245*, *465*
    middle, *483*
Summation:
  spatial, 97, 114
  temporal, 97, 114
Sweat glands, innervation of, *218*, 232, 234
Sweating:
  of palms, adrenergic, 234
  spinal reflex, 214
Sympathetic nervous system (*see* Autonomic nervous system, sympathetic)
Synapse, *52*, 62–67, *76*, *488*
  adrenergic, 66, *230*
  asymmetrical, 67
  axoaxonic, *61*, *63*, *64*
  axodendritic, *51*, *53*, *61*, *63*, *64*, *66*, 98
  axosomatic, *50*, *51*, *63*, *64*, 66, 98
    en passant, 60, *61*
  chemical, 62, 64–66
    asymmetric, *62*
    physiology of, 98
    serial, *62*
  cholinergic, 65, *230*
  cross-over, 327, 328
  dendrodendritic, 66
    reciprocal, *61*, *62*, 66
  developmental formation of, 130–131
  electrical, *56*, 62, 66
    symmetric, *62*
  en passant, 60, *61*, 83
  excitatory, 102
  inhibitory, 102
  interneuronal, 63, 66–67
  neuroglandular, 63
  neuromuscular, 63, 101–105
    and contraction activation, 104
    involuntary muscles, 104–105
    and motor end plate, *51*

Synapse:
  neuromuscular: and relaxation, 104
    voluntary muscle, 101–104
  in pyramidal cells, 66–67
  retinal, 398–399
  ribbon, of rods and cones, 399, 401
  somatoaxonic, *61*, 66
  somatodendritic, 66
  somatosomatic, *61*
  symmetrical, *62*, 67
  as transformation function, 119
Syncytium, electrical, 232
Syringomyelia, 213
System:
  auditory, 342–355
  autonomic (*see* Autonomic nervous system)
  central nervous, 71–78
  cholinergic, ascending, 305–307
  craniosacral, 229
  dopaminergic, 305
  endocrine, 90
  enteric nervous, 220
  exteroceptive, head ganglion of, 322
  extrapyramidal, 447
  hypophyseal portal, *373*, 375
  hypothalamohypophyseal portal, 381
  hypothalamoneurohypophyseal, 381
  lemniscal, of brainstem, 286–287
  limbic, 465–480
  motor, somatic, 443–460
  noradrenergic: ascending, 303
    descending, 303
  oculomotor, 361–364, 419–420
  olfactory, 372, 461–465
  optic, 388–423
  peripheral nervous (*see* Nervous system, peripheral)
  photoneuroendocrine, 379
  proprioceptive, head ganglion of, 322
  pyramidal, 446–447
  reticular, 272, 286–293, 305
  serotoninergic: ascending, 305
    descending, 303
  sympathoadrenal, 235
  thalamocortical projection, 429
  thoracolumbar, 220
  ventricular, 1, 21
  vergence, 420
  vestibular, 355–361, 420
  visual, 388–423